# OSTEOARTHRITIS

Other companion titles in the *Rheumatology* series:

*Ankylosing Spondylitis and the Spondyloarthropathies*

*Osteoporosis and the Osteoporosis of Rheumatic Diseases*

*Psoriatic and Reactive Arthritis*

*Systemic Lupus Erythematosus*

# OSTEOARTHRITIS

## A Companion to *Rheumatology*
*First Edition*

**Leena Sharma, MD**
Professor of Medicine
Feinberg School of Medicine
Northwestern University
Chicago, llinois

**Francis Berenbaum, MD, PhD**
Faculty of Medicine Pierre & Marie Curie—Paris VI
Head of the Department of Rheumatology
Saint-Antoine Hospital
Paris, France

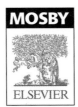

MOSBY

ELSEVIER

1600 John F. Kennedy Blvd.
Ste 1800
Philadelphia, PA 19103-2899

OSTEOARTHRITIS: A COMPANION TO RHEUMATOLOGY      ISBN 13: 978-0-323-03929-1
**Copyright © 2007 by Mosby, Inc., an affiliate of Elsevier Inc.**

---

**Notice**

Knowledge and best practice in this field are constantly changing. As new research and experience broaden our knowledge, changes in practice, treatment and drug therapy may become necessary or appropriate. Readers are advised to check the most current information provided (i) on procedures featured or (ii) by the manufacturer of each product to be administered, to verify the recommended dose or formula, the method and duration of administration, and contraindications. It is the responsibility of the practitioner, relying on their own experience and knowledge of the patient, to make diagnoses, to determine dosages and the best treatment for each individual patient, and to take all appropriate safety precautions. To the fullest extent of the law, neither the Publisher nor the Authors assumes any liability for any injury and/or damage to persons or property arising out or related to any use of the material contained in this book.

The Publisher

---

**Library of Congress Cataloging-in-Publication Data**
Osteoarthritis : a companion to Rheumatology / [edited by] Leena Sharma, Francis Berenbaum. -- 1st ed.
p. ; cm.
Companion v. to: Rheumatology / edited by Marc C. Hochberg . . . [et al.]. 3rd ed. 2003.
Includes bibliographical references and index.
ISBN 978-0-323-03929-1
1. Osteoarthritis. 2. Rheumatology. I. Sharma, Leena. II. Berenbaum, Francis. III. Rheumatology .
[DNLM: 1. Osteoarthritis. WE 348 O8465 2007]
RC931.O6708843 2007
616.7'223--dc22

2006037786

*Publishing Director:* Kim Murphy
*Developmental Editor:* Denise LeMelledo
*Project Manager:* Bryan Hayward

# Contributors

**Kim Bennell, BAppSci, PhD**
Professor
Centre for Health, Exercise, and Sports
   Medicine
School of Physiotherapy
University of Melbourne
Melbourne, Victoria, Australia

**Francis Berenbaum, MD, PhD**
Faculty of Medicine Pierre & Marie
   Curie—Paris VI
Head of the Department of
   Rheumatology
Saint-Antoine Hospital
Paris, France

**Lan X. Chen, MD**
Clinical Assistant Professor
Department of Medicine
University of Pennsylvania;
Attending Physician, Penn Presbyterian Medical
   Center
Philadelphia, Pennsylvania

**Maxime Dougados, MD**
Faculty of Medicine
University Paris-Descartes;
Attending Physician, Hospital Cochin
Paris, France

**Patrick Garnero, PhD, DSc**
Senior Scientist
INSERM Research Unit 664;
Vice President and Scientific Director
Molecular Markers
Synarc
Lyon, France

**Mary B. Goldring, PhD**
Associate Professor of Medicine
Harvard Medical School;
Associate Professor of Medicine,
Beth Israel Deaconess Medical Center;
Senior Scientist
New England Baptist Bone and Joint Institute
New England Baptist Hospital
Boston, Massachusetts

**Nicola J. Goodson, MB, ChB, PhD**
Senior Lecturer in Rheumatology
University of Liverpool;
Honorary Consultant Rheumatologist
University Hospital Aintree
Liverpool, Merseyside, United Kingdom

**Rana S. Hinman, BPhysio, PhD**
Lecturer
Center for Health Exercise and Sports Medicine
The University of Melbourne
Melbourne, Victoria, Australia

**Daniel Lajeunesse, PhD**
Professor
Department of Medicine
University of Montreal;
Senior Researcher
Department of Rheumatology
Hospital Norte-Dame
Montreal, Quebec, Canada

**Marie-Pierre Hellio Le Graverand, MD, DSc, PhD**
Senior Director
Clinical Research and Development, Inflammation
Pfizer Global Research and Development
Ann Arbor, Michigan

**Grace H. Lo, MD, MSc**
Assistant Professor
Department of Medicine
Division of Rheumatology
Tufts University;
Assistant Professor
Department of Medicine
Division of Rheumatology
New England Medical Center
Boston, Massachusetts

**Richard F. Loeser, Jr., MD**
Professor
Department of Internal Medicine
Division of Molecular Medicine
Wake Forest University School of
 Medicine
Winston-Salem, North Carolina

**L. Stefan Lohmander, MD, PhD**
Department of Orthopaedics
Lund University Hospital
Lund, Sweden

**Didier Mainard, MD, PhD**
Professor
Laboratory of Pharmacology
Faculty of Medicine;
Head of Department of Orthopaedic and
 Trauma Surgery
Centre Hospitalo-Universitaire
Nancy, France

**Lisa A. Mandl, MD, MPH**
Assistant Professor of Medicine
Department of Public Health
Weill Medical College of Cornell
 University;
Assistant Attending Physician
Division of Rheumatology
Hospital for Special Surgery
New York, New York

**Jean-Pierre Martel-Pelletier, MD**
Professor
Department of Medicine
University of Montreal;
Director, Osteoarthritis Research Unit
Research Centre, University of Montreal
 Hospital Centre
Notre-Dame Hospital
Montreal, Quebec, Canada

**Johanne Martel-Pelletier, PhD**
Professor
Department of Medicine
University of Montreal;
Director, Osteoarthritis Research Unit
Research Centre, University of Montreal Hospital
 Centre
Notre-Dame Hospital
Montreal, Quebec, Canada

**Timothy E. McAlindon, MD, MPH**
Associate Professor of Medicine
Division of Rheumatology
Tufts University;
Chief, Division of Rheumatology
New England Medical Center
Boston, Massachusetts

**Timothy J. Mosher, MD**
Associate Professor of Radiology
Penn State University College of Medicine;
Chief, Musculoskeletal Imaging, and Magnetic
 Resonance Imaging
Department of Radiology
Penn State Milton S. Hershey Medical Center
Hershey, Pennsylvania

**Patrick Netter, MD, PhD**
Professor
Laboratory of Pharmacology, Faculty of Medicine
University of Nancy
Vandoeuvre les Nancy, France

**George Nuki, MB, FRCP**
Emeritus Professor of Rheumatology
The Queen's Medical Research Institute
University of Edinburgh;
Honorary Consultant Rheumatologist
Western General Hospital
Edinburgh, Scotland, United Kingdom

**Pascale Pottie, PhD**
Professor
Laboratory of Pharmacology, Faculty of Medicine
University of Nancy
Vandoeuvre les Nancy, France

**Nathalie Presle, PhD**
Professor
Laboratory of Pharmacology, Faculty of Medicine
University of Nancy
Vandoeuvre les Nancy, France

**Pascale Reboul, PhD**
Assistant Professor of Medicine
University of Montreal
Montreal, Quebec, Canada

**Donald M. Salter, BSc, MD, FRCPath, FRCPE**
Professor of Osteoarticular Pathology
University of Edinburgh;
Consultant Pathologist
Edinburgh Royal Infirmary
Edinburgh, Scotland, United Kingdom

**Leena Sharma, MD**
Professor of Medicine
Feinberg School of Medicine
Northwestern University
Chicago, llinois

**Daniel H. Solomon, MD, MPH**
Associate Professor of Medicine
Division of Rheumatology
Division of Pharmacoepidemiology
Harvard Medical School;
Associate Physician
Brigham and Women's Hospital
Boston, Massachusetts

**Bernard Terlain, PharmaD**
Professor
Laboratory of Pharmacology, Faculty of Medicine
University of Nancy
Vandoeuvre les Nancy, France

**Amanda M. Tiffany, MD, MPhil**
Johns Hopkins University
House Staff
Johns Hopkins Bayview Medical Center
Baltimore, Maryland

**Eric Vignon, MD**
Professor
Department of Rheumatology
Claude Bernard University;
Head of Rheumatology
Centre Hospitalier Lyon Sud
Lyon, France

**Frank A. Wollheim, MD, PhD, FRCP**
Department of Rheumatology
Lund University Hospital
Lund, Sweden

**Tim V. Wrigley, BSc, MSc**
Director, Movement Research Laboratories
Centre for Health, Exercise and Sports Medicine
School of Physiotherapy
University of Melbourne
Melbourne, Victoria, Australia

# Preface

The most common type of arthritis that humans acquire is osteoarthritis (OA). The World Health Organization estimates that OA is a cause of disability in at least 10% of the world population over age 60 years. In 2006, we have at best a rudimentary understanding of how to modify its course or how to prevent function loss and disability in those who have it. There are at least three major reasons for our current level of understanding.

First, OA is a difficult disease to study and is heterogeneous in its presentation, style and rate of progression, and manifestations. Second, the field of investigators dedicated to the study of osteoarthritis has been small. Third, although there is much discussion in the literature about the need for multidisciplinary teams to study osteoarthritis most studies reflect a perspective dominated by one discipline.

This book consists of chapters written by authors who are leaders in their fields, who are innovative thinkers, and who come from several disciplines relevant to OA. Their words speak for themselves.

This is an important time—a time ripe for a substantial increase in knowledge concerning OA. In presenting this book, we have several goals and hopes: that this book serve as a source of information and ideas for those already involved in OA investigation and patient care (as well as for a new generation of clinicians and researchers), that it stimulate patient care approaches and research that arise from equal engagement of the key disciplines, and that it and others like it synergize with the landmark public data release known as the Osteoarthritis Initiative to accelerate the pace of travel toward more meaningful and effective prevention and treatment strategies for OA.

# Acknowledgements

We would like to acknowledge the wonderful work and contributions of the authors and the masterful editorial assistance of Faith Brody.

# Contents

**I.   EPIDEMIOLOGY**

1.   Epidemiology of Osteoarthritis, 1
     *Lisa A. Mandl*

**II.  PATHOGENESIS**

2.   The Role of Subchondral Bone in Osteoarthritis, 15
     *Johanne Martel-Pelletier, Daniel Lajeunesse, Pascal Reboul, and Jean-Pierre Pelletier*

3.   The Impact of Mechanical Stress on the Pathophysiology of Osteoarthritis, 33
     *George Nuki and Donald Salter*

4.   Update on the Chondrocyte Lineage and Implications for Cell Therapy in Osteoarthritis, 53
     *Mary B. Goldring*

5.   Aging Cartilage and Osteoarthritis Cartilage: Differences and Shared Mechanisms, 77
     *Richard F. Loeser*

6.   Adipokines in Osteoarthritis, 85
     *Nathalie Presle, Pascale Pottie, Didier Mainard, Patrick Netter, and Bernard Terlain*

7.   Pathology and Animal Models of Osteoarthritis, 104
     *Frank A. Wollheim and L. Stefan Lohmander*

**III. CLINICAL ASPECTS**

8.   Biochemical Markers of Osteoarthritis, 113
     *Patrick Garnero*

9.   Radiographic Imaging in Osteoarthritis of the Hip and Knee, 131
     *Eric Vignon and Marie-Pierre Hellio Le Graverand*

10.  Magnetic Resonance Imaging in Osteoarthritis, 143
     *Timothy Mosher*

**IV.  TREATMENT**

11.  Nonsteroidal Anti-inflammatory Drugs for Osteoarthritis, 178
     *Daniel H. Solomon and Nicola J. Goodson*

12.  Complementary and Alternative Medicine in Osteoarthritis, 202
     *Amanda Tiffany and Lan X. Chen*

13.  Future Directions in Physical Therapy for Knee Osteoarthritis, 217
     *Kim Bennell, Rana Hinman, and Tim Wrigley*

14.  Management of Limb Osteoarthritis, 232
     *Maxime Dougados*

15.  Nutritional and Nutritional Supplement Interventions for Osteoarthritis, 247
     *Timothy E. McAlindon and Grace H. Lo*

Index, 267

# Color Plates

# PLATE 1

### NORMAL

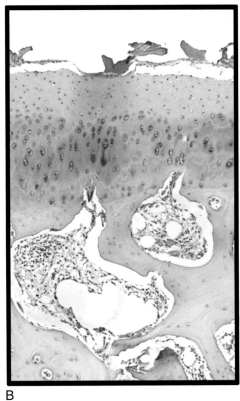

Cartilage

Subchondral bone

A

### EARLY OSTEOARTHRITIS

B

### LATE OSTEOARTHRITIS

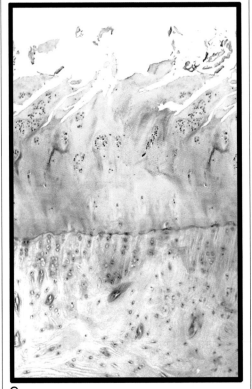

C

**Fig. 2.1** Representative sections of subchondral bone and cartilage from normal, early osteoarthritis and late osteoarthritis specimens. (A) shows a normal specimen with uniform thick cartilage and a subchondral bone section composed of large trabeculae. (B) shows a similar section in early stages of osteoarthritis with thinning of articular cartilage, expansion of the subchondral bone plate, and invasion of blood vessels into the subchondral region. (C) depicts late-stage osteoarthritis with severe cartilage lesions and thinning of the subchondral bone plate (H & E stain; original magnification × 60). (See Pages 18-19.)

**PLATE 2**

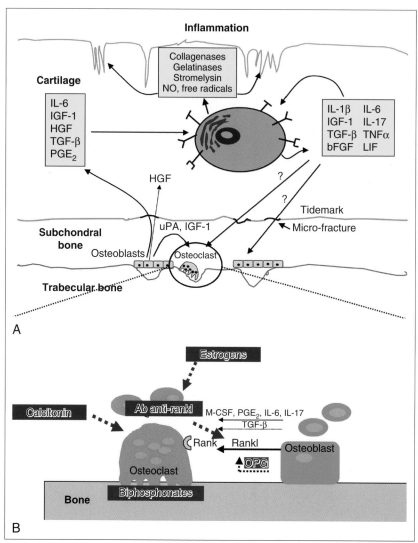

**Fig. 2.2** Illustration of the major pathophysiological pathways involved in osteoarthritis: (A) at the cartilage and subchondral bone interface and (B) in subchondral bone tissue remodelling. In B, potential therapeutic interventions that could modulate these pathways are identified in blue rectangles. Definitions: bFGF (basic fibroblast growth factor), LIF (leukemia inhibitory factor), IGF-1 (insulin-like growth factor 1), IL-1/IL-6/IL-17 (interleukin-1, -6, -17), M-CSF (macrophage colony stimulating factor), NO (nitric oxide), OPG (osteoprotegerin), PGE$_2$ (prostaglandin E$_2$), RANK (receptor activator of NF-κB), RANKL (receptor activator of NF-κB ligand), TGF-β (transforming growth factor β), TNF-α (tumor necrosis factor α), uPA (urokinase plasminogen activator). (See Page 23.)

PLATE 3

**Fig. 4.2** Cellular organization of the growth plate of mouse femur at embryonic day 17 of endochondral development. Distinct morphologies are observed in the different zones by histologic staining with hematoxylin and eosin. The periarticular proliferating chondrocytes are also called reserve chondrocytes. (See page 55.)

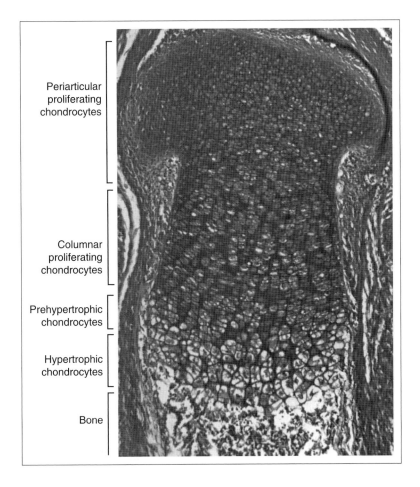

Periarticular proliferating chondrocytes

Columnar proliferating chondrocytes

Prehypertrophic chondrocytes

Hypertrophic chondrocytes

Bone

PLATE 4

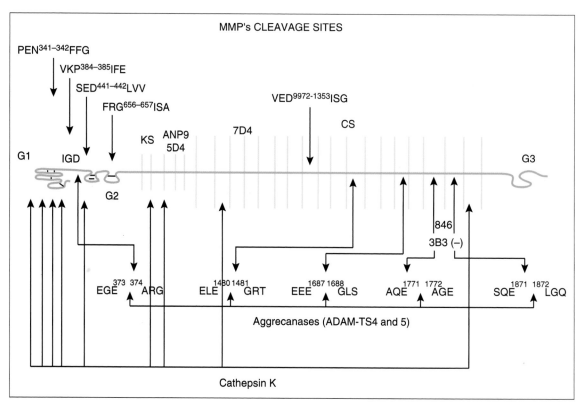

**Fig. 8.2** Schematic illustration of the aggrecan molecule, localization of the epitopes of antibodies used to assess its turnover, and proteolytic cleavage sites. A central core protein is substituted with about 100 glycosaminoglycan chains of chondroitin sulfate (CS) and keratan sulfate (KS). Specific domains include an N-terminal hyaluronate binding domain (G1), a homologous domain (G2), an interglobular domain (IGD), a KS-rich region, a CS-rich region, and a C-terminal domain (G3). This latter may be absent as a result of proteolytic cleavage. Several proteolytic cleavage sites have been identified for matrix-metalloproteases (MMPs), aggrecanases (including members of ADAMTS), and cysteine proteases such as cathepsin K. Antibodies against these various cleavage sites and other motifs (ANP9, 5D4, 7D4, 846, and 3B3 [-]) have been developed and used to investigate aggrecan turnover. (See page 115.)

PLATE 5

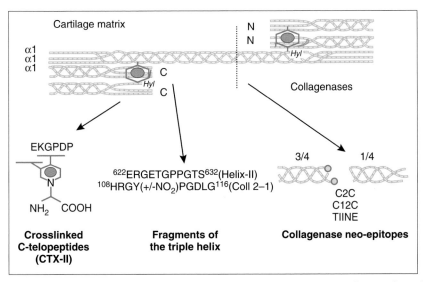

**Fig. 8.3** Type II collagen fragments as specific biologic markers of cartilage degradation. Type II collagen is formed by the association of three identical α1 chains in triple helix except at the ends (telopeptides). In the extracellular matrix of cartilage, collagen molecules are cross-linked by pyridinoline (PYD) involving the telopeptide regions. During cartilage degradation, different molecules are released in synovial fluid, serum, and urine. These include neoepitopes generated by the collagenases (e.g., C2C, C12C, and TIINE), fragments of the triple helix (Helix-II and Col 2-1), and C-terminal cross-linking telopeptides (CTX-II). See text for details. (See page 119.)

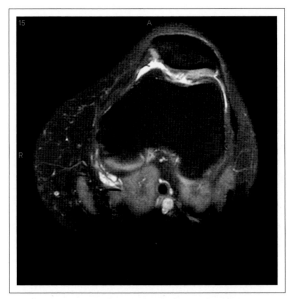

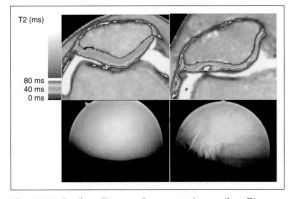

**Fig. 10.12** Cartilage T2 maps. Representative cartilage T2 maps and corresponding arthroscopy images are presented for a 29-year-old female with normal cartilage (left) and a 67-year-old female with grade III ulceration of the lateral patellar facet (right) confirmed at arthroscopy. Normal cartilage demonstrates spatial variation in cartilage T2, with short T2 values observed near bone (blue: 30 to 40 ms). Because of lower anisotropy of collagen fibers in the transitional zone of cartilage, T2 values increase near the articular surface (yellow: 50 to 60 ms). Focal degeneration of the collagen matrix elevates cartilage T2—in this example to values greater than 80 ms. (See page 166.)

**Fig. 10.10** Grade III lesion. 3.0-T axial fat-suppressed proton density image of the patella demonstrates a large area of cartilage erosion and fibrillation involving the medial patellar facet and median ridge. Although cartilage thickness of the more peripheral lateral facet is preserved, the diffusely increased signal intensity is consistent with degenerative change in the collagen matrix. (See page 157.)

PLATE 6

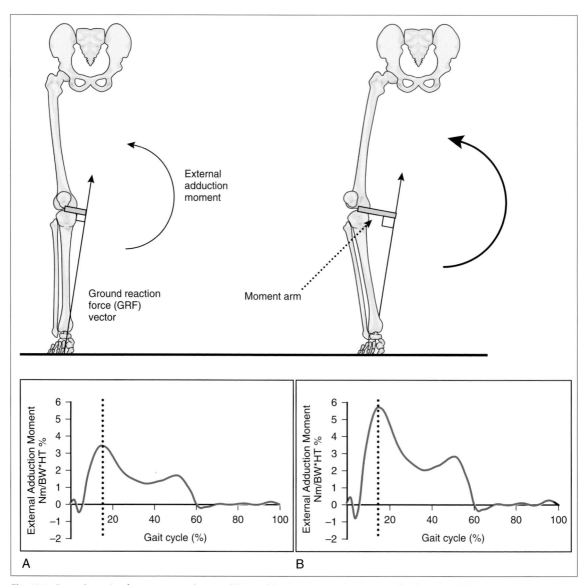

**Fig. 13.1** Ground reaction force vector and external knee adduction moment in (a) normally aligned and (b) varus mal-aligned knees. The external knee adduction moment is greater in the varus mal-aligned knee because the moment arm between the ground reaction force vector and the knee joint center is longer. (See page 219.)

# 1 Epidemiology of Osteoarthritis

Lisa A. Mandl

## BACKGROUND

Osteoarthritis (OA) is the most common joint disease in the world, with an age-associated increase in both incidence and prevalence.[1] In the United States, "arthritis and rheumatism" (largely OA) is the single largest reason for disability among those over 18. This is more than double the number of people disabled by cardiac disease.[2] OA affects predominantly older adults, and by the year 2020 the population 65 and over in developed countries is projected to increase by 71%.[3]

Already a major public health and economic problem costing the United States at least $15.5 billion per year,[4] this demographic shift will cause the prevalence of OA to skyrocket over the next decade. It is estimated that the population burden of disease due to OA will be greater than either human immunodeficiency virus (HIV) or chronic obstructive pulmonary disease (COPD).[3] It will, therefore, become increasingly important to define and study OA to better understand risk factors for disease, find the best treatment for symptoms, and discover new therapies to slow down or even prevent disease progression.

## DEFINITIONS OF OSTEOARTHRITIS

### Anatomic/Etiologic Definition

OA can be broadly divided into primary, or idiopathic disease, and OA secondary to another condition. Primary OA may be localized to one joint, or in a generalized form to several joints. Definitions of generalized OA vary in the literature and commonly include small joint involvement of the hands coupled to involvement of one or more large joints (Table 1.1).

### Radiographic/Functional Definitions

Determining population rates of OA is not a straightforward endeavor, because the incidence and prevalence of OA vary dramatically depending on how one defines disease. The inconsistent relationship between clinical symptoms and X-ray findings can make identifying cases difficult. For example, it is estimated that

people aged 63 to 93 years have a 33% prevalence of radiographic knee OA, but only 9.5% are symptomatic.[5] The converse is also true: patients can have debilitating OA pain with minimal or no radiographic findings.

The most commonly used method for evaluating and defining radiographic OA is the Kellgren and Lawrence system (Table 1.2).[6] This grading system is applied to specific joints by comparing a patient's radiograph with that of a standard radiographic atlas. A Kellgren–Lawrence grade of 2 or greater is the most commonly used definition of radiographic OA.[7] However, using radiographs alone to define OA will capture many individuals who have minimal or no symptoms of disability. Therefore, most functional definitions rely on a combination of clinical and radiographic findings. The most common epidemiologic definition is radiographic evidence of OA and pain on most days of a month within the past year.

The American College of Rheumatology (ACR) has developed consensus criteria to define clinically relevant OA of the hand, knee, and hip (Table 1.3). These widely used criteria allow the identification of similar groups of patients for randomized controlled trials and other studies. The ACR criteria were derived from actual OA patients, and are the most suitable criteria for identifying OA patients in clinical practice.

The uncoupling of symptomatology and imaging (at least early in the disease process) may be partially a function of technology.[8] Radiographs, which cannot image soft tissues, are unable to identify early pathologic changes in the joint and thus provide only a gross estimate of joint disease. Although joint space narrowing, an important measure of OA progression, can be reliably measured by X-rays,[9] it is important to realize that this technique depends not just on cartilage volume but on the integrity of associated ligaments, tendons, synovial tissue, and menisci.[10] In contrast, magnetic resonance imaging (MRI) not only images bone but can provide important information on cartilage and other soft tissues. Specifically, MRI can identify very subtle changes in soft tissues that occur early

| TABLE 1.1  DEFINITIONS OF OSTEOARTHRITIS |
|---|
| **Primary OA** |
| Idiopathic: |
| • Localized |
| • Generalized (three or more joints) |
| **Secondary OA** |
| Examples include: |
| 1. Developmental |
| • Congenital hip dislocation |
| • Legg-Calves-Perthes disease |
| • Congenital hip dislocation |
| • Epiphyseal dysplasias |
| 2. Mechanical |
| • Hypermobility syndromes (Ehlers-Danlos, hyperlaxity syndromes) |
| • Leg length discrepancy |
| • Mal-alignment |
| 3. Trauma (acute or chronic) |
| • Accidental |
| • Sports injury |
| • Occupational |
| • Iatrogenic (post-surgical) |
| 4. Metabolic |
| • Hemachromatosis |
| • Wilson's disease |
| • Mucopolysaccharidoses |
| • Amyloidosis |
| • Ochronosis |
| • Gout |
| • Pseudogout |
| • Calcium crystal deposition |
| 5. Endocrine |
| • Acromegaly |
| • Hyperparathyroidism |
| • Hypothyroidism |
| 6. Inflammatory |
| • Any systemic rheumatic disease |
| • Septic arthritis |
| 7. Miscellaneous |
| • Hemophilias |
| • Paget's disease |
| • Osteonecrosis |
| • Neuropathic arthropathy |

| TABLE 1.2  KELLGREN–LAWRENCE RADIOGRAPHIC GRADING SYSTEM FOR OSTEOARTHRITIS | |
|---|---|
| Grade | Radiographic Description |
| 0 | Normal |
| 1 | Possible osteophyte |
| 2 | Definite osteophytes, possible joint space narrowing |
| 3 | Moderate osteophytes, definite narrowing, some sclerosis, possible attrition |
| 4 | Large osteophytes, marked narrowing, severe sclerosis, definite attrition |

correlation between loss of cartilage volume, as measured by MRI, and joint space narrowing.[15] As more work is done using MRI to study the development and evolution of OA, it is likely that future definitions of OA will incorporate MRI features.

## INCIDENCE AND PREVALENCE OF OSTEOARTHRITIS

### Prevalence of Pathologic Osteoarthritis

Some damage to joint cartilage is probably unavoidable in later life. A 1926 series of 1,000 autopsies found evidence of OA in almost all people over 65.[16] Autopsy studies show that knee OA is almost universally present after age 60, and is associated with increasing age.[17] Postmortem studies show that up to 50% of postmenopausal Caucasian women have almost complete obliteration of the carpometacarpal (CMC) joint, and an additional 25% have severe damage to the cartilage.[18] However, the link between such pathology and clinical symptoms is still poorly understood.

Another autopsy study found that although 48% of knees had moderate to severe histologic OA medical record review revealed that only 10% of these patients had any clinical manifestation of knee OA.[19] Future studies should evaluate the relationship between specific anatomic areas of cartilage destruction, the integrity of joint-associated soft tissues, the anatomic alignment of joint components, and clinical symptoms.

### Prevalence of Radiographic Osteoarthritis

Population-based studies consistently show high prevalence rates of radiographic OA in older adults. However, there may be significant geographic and ethnic differences in rates of radiographic OA, although it is difficult to make absolute comparisons due to differences in case ascertainment and radiographic assessment. To identify real differences among populations, future studies will need to be able to control for important potential

in the disease process and which radiographs alone are not sensitive enough to discern.[11]

These two techniques can provide very different information. Cross-sectional data show that MRI identifies cartilage changes that are unable to be seen on plain radiographs.[12] MRI has also been shown to be a more sensitive method of measuring cartilage changes over time compared with radiographs.[13,14] In one study that followed OA patients for two years there was no

| TABLE 1.3 AMERICAN COLLEGE OF RHEUMATOLOGY DEFINITIONS OF OSTEOARTHRITIS |
| --- |

**ACR Classification Criteria for Osteoarthritis of the Hand[a]**

Hand, pain, aching, or stiffness and three or four of the following features.

- Hard tissue enlargement of two or more of ten selected joints*
- Hard tissue enlargement of two or more DIP joints
- Fewer than three swollen MCP joints
- Deformity of at least one of ten selected joints*

*Second and third DIPs, PIPs, and first CMC joints bilaterally

94% sensitive

87% specific

**ACR Combined Clinical and Radiographic Classification for Criteria for Osteoarthritis of the Hip[b]**

Hip pain and at least two of the following three features.

- ESR <20 mm/hr
- Radiographic femoral or acetabular osteophytes
- Radiographic joint space narrowing (superior, axial, and/or medial)

89% sensitive

91% specific

**ACR Criteria for Classification of Idiopathic Osteoarthritis of the Knee[c]**

| Clinical and Laboratory | Clinical and Radiographic | Clinical[d] |
| --- | --- | --- |
| Knee pain | Knee pain | Knee pain |
| + at least 5 of 9: | + at least 1 of 3: | + at least 3 of 6: |
| • Age >50 years | • Age >50 years | • Age >50 years |
| • Stiffness <30 minutes | • Stiffness <30 minutes | • Stiffness <30 minutes |
| • Crepitus | • Crepitus | • Crepitus |
| • Bony tenderness | • Osteophytes | • Bony tenderness |
| • Bony enlargement | | • Bony enlargement |
| • No palpable warmth | | • No palpable warmth |
| • ESR <40 mm/hr | | |
| • RF <1:40 | | |
| • SF OA | | |
| 92% sensitive | 91% sensitive | 95% sensitive |
| 75% specific | 86% specific | 69% specific |

[a]Altman R, Alcaron G, Appelrouth D, Bloch D, Borenstein D, Brandt K, et al. The American College of Rheumatology criteria for the classification and reporting of osteoarthritis of the hand. Arthritis Rheum 1990;33:1601–10.
[b]Altman R, Appelrouth D, Bloch D, Borenstein D, Brandt K, et al. The American College of Rheumatology criteria for the classification and reporting of osteoarthritis of the hip. Arthritis Rheum 1991;34:505–14.
[c]Altman R, Asch E, Bloch D, Borenstein D, Brandt K, et al. The American College of Rheumatology criteria for the classification and reporting of osteoarthritis of the knee. Arthritis Rheum 1986;29:1039–49.
[d]Alternative for the clinical category would be 4 of 6, which is 84% sensitive and 89% specific.

confounders such as body weight, physical activities, and genetic background.

Radiographic evidence of hand OA is common. A Dutch survey found that 75% of women 60 to 70 years old had distal interphalangeal joint OA.[20] The U.S. National Health Examination Survey (1960 to 1962) revealed that in the population aged 25 to 74 years 29.5% had radiographic evidence of hand OA.[21] Interestingly, hand arthritis has been shown to be much lower in the elderly Beijing Chinese population than in Caucasians of the same age in the United States (the reasons for this are unclear).[22]

Radiographic knee OA is also common in older adults. The Framingham cohort (based on the U.S. study of 1983 to 1985) found that 31% of men and 34% of women between the ages of 63 and 93 had signs of radiographic knee OA.[5] A Swedish study revealed similar rates of radiographic knee OA among those over 75 years: 33% in men and 45% in women.[23] In contrast to hand OA, radiographic evidence of lateral knee OA is more than twice as prevalent among Beijing Chinese subjects as a similar U.S. population.[24]

Radiographic hip OA is less prevalent than knee OA. In a large Swedish cohort, the prevalence of hip OA was between 4.4 and 5.3% in individuals 60 years and older.[25] In the United States, the crude prevalence rate of radiographic hip OA is estimated at 3.1%, with no difference found in rates between Caucasian and African Americans.[26] The prevalence of radiographic hip OA has been reported to be much lower in some non-Western populations, including Nigerians, Liberians, black South Africans, and Hong Kong Chinese.[27] Recent studies have also shown that residents of Beijing aged 60 to 89 years have very low prevalence of radiographic hip OA (0.9% in women and 1.1% in men).[28] Studies of Turkish patients show similar rates of moderate or severe radiographic hip OA (1.1% overall in a random sample of Turkish patients 40 years or older).[29] By contrast, Icelandic patients have up to five times increased prevalence of radiographic hip OA compared to a similar Swedish population.[30,31]

## Incidence of Symptomatic Osteoarthritis

A study of hand, hip, and knee OA among members of a community health plan found that for both men and women the incidence of symptomatic OA increased dramatically with age, especially after 50. This increase continued until age 80, after which there was a leveling off or decline (Fig. 1.1).[1] The annual incidence of knee OA was <1%/year for women aged 70 to 89. The overall female/male ratio for OA at all sites was 2:1. Similar rates are seen in other cohorts.[5,20] There are a number of theories for the sex-based differences in OA rates.

Women may have a larger center-edge angle, a measure of acetabular depth that predisposes them to hip OA.[32] Female distribution of fat tissue may lead to disadvantageous distribution of mechanical forces across weight-bearing joints. Leptin, a small cytokine-like protein associated with obesity, is up-regulated in OA and may contribute to osteophyte formation.[33] Because women have proportionally more adipose tissue than men, and therefore have higher relative leptin levels, leptin may mediate the OA gender differential.[34] Female hormones may be chondroprotective, leading to a rapid increase in incident OA at menopause.[35]

## Prevalence of Symptomatic Osteoarthritis

The prevalence of symptomatic OA has important implications for population health. In the United States, an estimated 9.5% of people between age 63 and 93 years have symptomatic knee OA,[5] and symptomatic knee OA is associated with long-term disability.[36] Symptomatic hip OA affects 4.4% of people over age 55 (hip pain predicts locomotor disability).[37,38] Estimates of symptomatic hand OA vary widely, from 2.4% of people aged 25 to 75 years[37] to 80% of women over 80.[39] Hand arthritis can lead to loss of hand function, and diminished

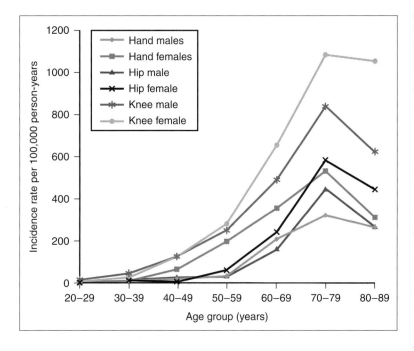

**Fig. 1.1** Incidence of osteoarthritis of the hand, hip, and knee in members of the Fallon Community Health Plan (1991 to 1992) by age and sex. (Redrawn from a figure in Oliveria et al. Incidence of OA in an HMO population. Arthritis & Rheumatism 1995;38(8): 1134–1141.)

hand function predicts future functional limitation and dependency.[40] Therefore, OA at a variety of common anatomic locations has both present and well-defined future costs. As the developed world's population ages, OA-related disability and impairment will place significant strains on nations' health care infrastructures.

## KEY OUTCOMES IN OA EPIDEMIOLOGY

To fully appreciate the impact of OA on both the individual and the community, investigators must be able to evaluate all dimensions of this disease. This requires measures of all relevant outcomes in OA, using accurate and reliable measurement tools. As discussed previously, the incidence and prevalence of OA are usually measured with a combination of imaging studies and symptom scales. Rates will vary depending on the method of case ascertainment, which is one reason for the widely varying estimates over time and between centers.

Once present, the progression of OA is extremely important, and the predictors of disease progression may be different from the risk factors for incident disease. Although functional impairment can be a direct result of structural joint disease, it does not have a linear relationship with disease stage and is particularly influenced by an individual's co-morbidities. Finally, disability (or how well a patient can function given the impairments he or she has) reflects not simply structural disease but access to medical and surgical care, coping skills, personality, and an individual's social support network.

## RISK FACTORS FOR OSTEOARTHRITIS

### Constitutional Risk Factors
#### Hereditary and Genetic Factors
Genetic factors appear to influence risk of developing primary OA. Population-based studies have found that Heberden's nodes are two to three times more frequent among mothers and sisters of individuals with hand OA than would be predicted by chance.[41] Twin studies suggest that generalized OA in women has a heritability rate of 39 to 65%, with a concordance rate in monozygotic twins of 0.64.[42] Others have estimated that siblings of patients undergoing total knee or hip replacements have an increased relative risk of primary OA of 2.3, with a heritability rate of severe OA of 27%.[43] Genetic factors may influence disease differently in men and women. A Finnish twin study showed an OA concordance rate among monozygotic twin pairs of 0.44 in women but only 0.34 in men.[44]

It is difficult to separate the influence of environment from that of genetics when performing family and twin studies. However, studying immigrant populations is one means of circumventing this problem. For example, not only do Chinese individuals in China have a lower rate of radiographic hip OA than the U.S. population but persons with Chinese surnames living in San Francisco have dramatically lower rates of hip replacements compared with other people utilizing the same hospital system.[45]

Although the lack of clear genetic linkage for most families points to a multifactorial etiology for primary OA, there are some rare cases for which there is evidence of direct linkage. Primary OA at multiple sites in a Dutch family appears to have been transmitted in an autosomal dominant fashion, and has been linked to microsatellite markers on chromosome 2q.[46] Severe hip OA in a Dutch South African family also traveled in an autosomal dominant fashion, and has been mapped to chromosome 4q35.[47] Severe hip OA in an Icelandic family may also be chromosomally linked.[46] Although there are no suspected candidate genes in the mapped regions, it is possible that these families actually have an as yet undescribed genetic chondrodysplasia, and in fact have secondary OA.

Some case-control studies have looked at defects in genes coding for components of collagen synthesis, or genes that might be involved with the regulation of subchondral bone density. Genes coding for or regulating types I, II, and IX collagen; bone morphogenic protein; the vitamin D receptor; estrogen receptors; and insulin-like growth factor 1 have all been found by some investigators to be associated with an increased risk of primary OA.[48-52] Recently, functional variants within the gene coding for secreted frizzled-related protein 3 have been associated with primary hip OA in women.[53]

Secreted frizzled-related protein 3 is an antagonist of wingless (wnt) signaling (which regulates the expression of target genes by activating a conserved signal transduction pathway), and likely contributes to the production of abnormal articular cartilage via decreasing osteoblast proliferation.[54,55] Studies of potential candidate genes are difficult, as gene frequencies are likely to vary among different populations, case findings differ between studies, and genes likely have significant interactions with environmental triggers. However, the identification of genes associated with primary OA could significantly improve our understanding of the pathogenesis of this disease and provide evidence for targeted interventions.

How genes specifically influence incidence, progression, and disability associated with OA is difficult to ascertain with the present data. Genetic studies of OA use different definitions of OA (including radiographic changes, self-reported OA, and joint replacement) as evidence of disease. More specific outcome measures of OA are needed to help us better understand the effect of genetics on different stages of joint destruction.

### Congenital and Developmental Disorders

Any disorder that prevents the development of normal joint anatomy can lead to joint incongruity and/or deformity and secondary OA. Childhood disorders of the hip joint (such as congenital hip dysplasia, Legg-Calve-Perthes disease, and slipped capital femoral epiphyses) are relatively common and important because they are modifiable risk factors if identified early. If untreated, these disorders result in anatomic irregularities of the femoral head and acetabulum, which lead to the premature development of hip OA.[56]

Mild versions of these disorders may account for a portion of "idiopathic" hip OA.[57] In adults, evidence of hip dysplasia on X-rays is strongly associated with prevalent hip OA.[58] Acetabular dysplasia is a strong independent predictor of incident hip OA in patients with and without baseline pain. Rare genetic disorders that affect the growth plate, such as multiple epiphyseal dysplasia and achondroplasia, result in abnormal bone growth and often severe OA.

## Activity-related Risk Factors

### Occupational/Repetitive Activities

Jobs associated with repetitive movements coupled with excessive joint loading have long been associated with OA. Miners, dock workers, farmers, firefighters, mail carriers, and female housekeepers all have been reported to have high rates of knee and sometimes hip OA.[59-64] However, the inherent difficulties in retrospectively studying occupational risk factors resulted in some flawed research. For example, it is likely that early studies used less specific definitions of disease.

A critical review of the literature through 1994 found serious problems with many studies evaluating the relationship between occupational activities and OA. However, a review of the most reliable studies did show an overall positive relationship between work involving knee bending and knee OA in men (range of odds ratio of 1.4 to 6). The data were not strong enough to conclude a similar relationship among women.[63] In addition, this review found that work-related exposures, such as farming, were only weakly associated with hip OA. By 2000, however, larger and more rigorous studies still identified agricultural workers and housekeepers as having significant excess prevalence of OA.[64] This study, which examined the prevalence of symptomatic OA in any joint, showed a latency of 10 to 20 years between occupational exposure and the onset of symptoms (with agricultural workers having earlier onset of symptoms than any other occupational category).[64]

The most specific data are from studies of the Framingham cohort, which found that severe knee OA (defined as needing knee surgery) was associated with lifting at least 10 kg more than 10 times per week, kneeling for >1 hour a day, and squatting for >1 hour a day regardless of type of employment (even after adjusting for multiple confounders such as body mass index, previous knee injury, and the presence of Heberden's nodes).[65,66] A recent systematic review also determined that hip OA is also associated with heavy occupational workload, and found a clear dose-response gradient in 10 of 16 studies reviewed.[67]

The effect of occupation on hand OA is less clear. Mill workers who perform frequent repetitive motions have been found to have patterns of hand arthritis consistent with their assigned job.[68] Some studies have found increased prevalence of OA in the dominant hand, whereas others have not.[69-72] Routine use of chopsticks has been associated with increased prevalence of finger OA, especially the interphalangeal (IP) joint of the thumb.[73] Among a Finnish cohort, physical stress at work (including measures of continuously repeated series of movements) was associated with OA in any finger in women (but not in men).[74]

A study comparing rates of hand OA between female dentists and teachers found overall lower rates of hand OA among dentists, despite their greater use of repetitive hand movements. However, the dentists were more likely to develop severe OA in joints of the thumb and index and middle fingers, which are used to grip dental instruments.[72] Further investigations need to be done to better elucidate the true effect of physical stress on the development of hand OA. To date, there are no data on the effect of vocational activities and the progression of established OA.

### Sports and Recreational Activity

There has been a great deal of interest in how physical activity and sports influence the development of OA. This information is particularly important for physicians because physical activity is often recommended to patients for its cardiovascular fitness and weight loss benefits. Animal data show that there are differences among moderate increases in the use of normal joints, extreme increases in the use of normal joints, and increased abnormal impact loading across a normal joint. Having beagles run 3 km/hr for 75 minutes 5 days a week for 527 weeks with weighted jackets did not lead to any increased joint damage compared with caged control dogs.[75] Running dogs moderately, without added weight, increased cartilage thickness and proteoglycan content.[108] Intense running led to decreased cartilage proteoglycan content and remodeling of subchondral bone, but the cartilage surfaces of the joints remained intact (without evidence of early OA).[76-78] However, repeat non-physiologic impact loading of animal joints (given so that the animals cannot provide any compensatory protection to the joint) rapidly leads to signs of early OA.[79]

Most observational human studies corroborate these animal data: regular physical activity does not appear to increase the risk or progression of hip or knee OA. Recreational runners show no increased risk in incident radiographic hip OA compared with non-runners over a nine-year period.[80] Students who participated in organized running in college report no higher rates of hip pain than students who were college swimmers, after a mean follow-up of 25 years.[81] A small case-control study also found that serious recreational runners who run 12 to 24 miles a week for a median of 40 years have no higher rates of radiographic or symptomatic hip OA than controls.[82] The data are similar for knee OA.[80-82] One study suggests that among women increased physical activity when young increases the risk of both symptomatic and radiographic hip OA.[83] However, such retrospective case-control studies are at high risk of recall bias in that activity questions are asked decades after the fact.

By contrast, elite runners may be at higher risk. Women who are ex–elite runners have higher rates of lower extremity OA compared to age-matched controls.[86] One study suggests that only men less than 50 years old running at least 20 miles per week increase their risk of future OA.[84] Another retrospective case-control study took two radiographs 15 years apart on long-distance runners (averaging 60 miles per week at the time of first X-ray), bobsledders, and healthy controls and found higher rates of hip OA in runners.[85] The number of miles run at baseline was the only modifiable risk factor that predicted incident hip OA. However, data on running are conflicting. For example, male runners who competed at national and international levels were not shown to have higher rates of knee OA when compared with other elite athletes.[86,87]

There have also been studies evaluating the risk of OA among professional athletes, and elite athletes who compete at world-class levels in other sports. Male athletes who represented Finland in wrestling or soccer between 1920 and 1965 had higher rates of hospital admissions for ankle, knee, or hip OA than matched healthy male controls.[88] The same study also found high rates of OA among elite hockey players and weight lifters, although these athletes were compared to an unmatched control group.[88] Swedish soccer players had higher rates of hip OA than an age-matched control groups, with the highest rates in elite players.[89] Between 32 and 49% of retired English soccer players had a (self-reported) diagnosis of OA.[90,91] Up to 80% of professional gridiron football players had signs of OA 10 to 30 years after retiring.[92]

Baseball players may be at increased risk of shoulder and elbow OA.[93] Elite javelin throwers and high jumpers were found to have high rates of radiographic hip OA.[94] One retrospective study of female athletes included fourteen ex–elite tennis players (two of whom were Wimbledon singles champions). These players had a non-significant increase in osteophytes at the tibiofemoral and hip joints compared with ex–elite runners, whereas the runners had more osteophytes and narrowing at the patellofemoral joints.[84] Weightlifters have also been shown to have an increased prevalence of tibiofemoral (and particularly patellofemoral) OA, although this may be confounded by high body mass index (BMI).[86,87]

An important confounder of sports and OA is joint injury. Professional or elite athletes may have a higher incidence of significant joint injuries, and are more likely to continue playing despite pain. The result of rupturing an anterior cruciate ligament (ACL), an easily identifiable clinical event, has been particularly studied. Soccer players with a ruptured ACL are much more likely to develop knee OA than those players whose ACL is intact.[95]

Interestingly, an observational study of soccer players with ACL-deficient knees found that the risk of subsequent OA is significantly increased regardless of whether the ACL is surgically repaired.[96] (However, ACL repair may be more effective in non-elite athletes. Early ACL reconstruction appears to decrease rates of subsequent meniscal and cartilage injuries in young healthy adults,[97] and other studies suggest early ACL repair does minimize the risk of knee OA.[98]) These observational findings should be confirmed in randomized controlled trials, although growing secular beliefs in the benefit of ACL repair may make such studies impossible. However, previous damage is clearly not the entire story because an association between some sports (such as soccer) and future risk of OA exists independently of injury.[99]

### Non Sports-related Trauma

Joint injuries significantly increase future risk of OA in non-athletes as well. This association has been seen in many cross-sectional and retrospective studies, and a few prospective studies show similar results.[100-102] For example, one prospective trial showed that having a self-reported knee injury dramatically increased subsequent risk of OA in that joint. There was a similar but not statistically significant trend for hip injuries leading to later hip OA.[103]

The same study also showed that retrospectively reporting a knee injury as a child or young adult indicated a significantly increased risk of having knee OA by age 65. A second prospective study documented that incident knee OA but not OA progression is significantly associated with previous knee injury.[104] Iatrogenic injury can also increase the risk of OA. Patients who had a partial meniscectomy for an isolated meniscal tear were found to have a significantly increased risk of OA 21 years later compared with matched controls.[105]

## Local Mechanical Factors

### Body Mass Index

Having a high weight or BMI (defined as weight in kilograms/height per meters[2]) strongly increases the rate of developing symptomatic and radiographic incident knee OA.[106,107] Cross-sectionally, obesity is associated with both radiographic and symptomatic knee OA in a stepwise dose-dependent manner. Obesity is a stronger risk factor in woman than in men, and is more strongly related to bilateral than to unilateral knee OA.[108,109] Fifty percent of women 65 to 74 years of age who are obese have radiographic evidence of OA, compared with <6% of non-obese women the same age.[108,109]

The risk of knee OA increases approximately 15% for each additional kg/m[2] over 27.[109] Increasing BMI, even within a normal range, is associated with increased rates of knee OA. Men with a BMI of 23 to 25 have a fourfold increased risk of OA compared with men with a BMI of <23.[110] Recent longitudinal studies suggest that higher BMI also increases the risk of progression of radiographic knee OA.[106] Interestingly, the effect of BMI on knee OA progression may depend on alignment, as recent data suggest high BMI causes progression only in mal-aligned but not neutrally aligned knees.[111]

A disease-modifying effect of weight loss on knee OA, although intuitive, is not as definitively proven. Weight loss does decrease loading across the knee joint,[112] appears to decrease the risk of developing symptomatic knee OA,[108] and may modestly decrease the risk of radiographic progression.[113] Interestingly, it may be that body mass composition rather than absolute weight or BMI is an important determinant of disease progression. In the knee of subjects without OA, muscle mass appears to protect against loss of tibial cartilage (after controlling for BMI).[114] These data suggest that maintaining muscle, despite being denser than adipose tissue, may decrease the risk of incident knee OA. All weight may not be created equal, at least in terms of knee OA.

Obesity not only increases the risk of radiographic hip OA (especially the incidence of bilateral hip OA) but significantly increases the risk of symptomatic hip OA.[26,111,115] Moderate to severe obesity at least doubles the risk of clinical symptoms of hip OA.[116] In addition, studies using total hip arthroplasty as a proxy for symptomatic primary hip OA show a strong association between BMI at time of surgery or BMI in early adulthood and having a hip replacement.[117,118] This has important public health implications, as these data suggest that the present epidemic of childhood obesity could result in an exponential increase in the need for total joint arthroplasty as this population ages. However, one recent prospective trial found that BMI was not associated with either incident or progression of hip OA.[106] These results may have been due to the fact that this trial had very few patients in the highest BMI categories. The bulk of evidence suggests that obesity is likely a stronger risk factor for knee than hip OA.

The relationship between obesity and hand OA has been the subject of debate. Some studies have shown no association or association only in men.[119-122] However, the preponderance of evidence, including prospective studies, suggests that obesity is a significant risk factor for symptomatic hand OA.[123,124] This is an important observation, as it implies a metabolic rather than exclusively mechanical component in OA pathogenesis.

### Muscle Weakness

A painful joint results in joint disuse, muscle atrophy, and secondary muscle weakness, and it is well known that painful knee OA is associated with weak quadriceps.[125] However, some data suggest that muscle weakness may actually contribute to the development of OA. One prospective study showed that, after adjusting for body weight, quadricep weakness preceded radiographic knee OA in women, although the number of incident cases was small.[126] Cross-sectional studies also support this hypothesis by showing that quadricep weakness is present in pain-free knees with radiographic OA, in addition to being associated with symptomatic knee OA.[127]

A larger cross-sectional study of Chinese subjects showed that quadricep weakness was significantly associated with radiographic OA in both the patellofemoral and tibiofemoral compartments in men and women, although the strength of association was attenuated when symptomatic subjects were excluded.[128] This evidence suggests that pain is an important effect modifier of quadricep weakness. Conversely, one prospective study found that greater quadricep strength at baseline was associated with increased likelihood of tibiofemoral OA progression in mal-aligned knees and lax knees.[129]

Others have found that quadricep strength does not appear to predict radiographic progression of knee OA in women.[130] The true role of muscle activity in terms of risk of incident or progressive knee OA remains to be seen, and may differ in normal and mal-aligned knees. This work is a high priority, given the modifiability of muscle parameters.

### Alignment

Local mechanical factors play a major role in the progression of knee OA. Valgus and varus alignment result in a significant threefold increased risk of tibiofemoral OA progression, after controlling for potential confounders such as age, sex, and BMI.[131] Knee alignment also predicts functional decline in patients with knee OA. Patients with bilaterally mal-aligned knees are two times more likely to have deterioration in their physical function over 18 months compared to those without mal-alignment.[131] Knee alignment is also associated with progression of patellofemoral OA, with increased odds ratios about half that seen in tibiofemoral disease.[132] The effect of alignment on incident knee OA, or on OA incidence or progression in other joints, has not been reported.

## Behavioral and Hormonal Factors

### Smoking

The association of smoking and OA remains ambiguous. Studies in the prospective Framingham cohort have found that previous smoking is associated with a lower prevalence of knee OA and that smoking also protects against the development of incident knee OA.[133,134] Other cross-sectional and cohort studies have also suggested that smoking may be protective against knee OA,[135] DIP OA in men, and symptomatic but not radiographic DIP OA in women.[74] However, still other prospective cohort studies have found no association between smoking and developing OA of either the knee or hand.[136,137] Smoking is not associated with an increased risk of needing a knee replacement.[138] It also has no association with radiographic joint space width in the hip of an asymptomatic population without hip OA.[139] Further prospective cohort studies, with well-validated cases of symptomatic and radiographic OA, are needed to resolve this issue.

### Estrogen

The prevalence of OA in women increases dramatically after menopause. This temporal observation has contributed to the theory that decreased estrogen levels play a role in OA pathogenesis, and there is some pathophysiologic data to support this hypothesis. Human articular chondrocytes express estrogen receptors,[140] and treating cultured chondrocytes in vitro with estrogen increases the synthesis of proteoglycans.[141] Estrogen may also influence the balance of matrix metalloproteinases and tissue inhibitors of metalloproteinases in chondrocytes, providing some chondroprotection.[142]

However, epidemiologic studies have not shown a consistently protective relationship between estrogen and OA, or estrogen replacement therapy (ERT) and OA. Some well-done cross-sectional studies found that current use of ERT was associated with lower rates of hip OA[143] or knee OA,[144] and that users of ERT appeared to have more knee cartilage than nonusers.[145] Conversely, other studies have shown that women using ERT had a higher prevalence of hip, hand, and knee OA.[135,146]

One prospective cohort, which used *self-reported* physician-diagnosed OA as the primary outcome, found increased rates of incident OA in users of ERT, and that the risk was proportional to the amount of time on ERT.[147] However, still other cross-sectional studies found no association between the use of estrogens and the prevalence of hip OA, the prevalence of "generalized OA" (severe symptomatic knee or hip OA plus radiologic hand OA),[148,149] or the severity of hand OA.[150] The prospective Framingham study found no association between estrogen replacement and the prevalence of radiographic knee OA,[151] and a protective but non-significant trend between ERT and both incidence and progression of radiographic knee OA.[152]

Unfortunately, there are no randomized controlled trials that look at the relationship between OA and estrogen. A sub-analysis of the Heart and Estrogen/Progestin Replacement study (a randomized double-blind placebo-controlled trial of estrogen and progestin in women with heart disease) evaluated the relationship between knee pain and disability and the use of estrogen replacement therapy. No significant association was found.[153]

Despite the prevailing wisdom that estrogen use is protective against OA, most studies supporting this view are cross-sectional (with results that do not achieve significance). The most rigorous prospective epidemiologic data to date do not support any convincing association between estrogens and OA. However, this is an area in which prospective randomized controlled trials would be extremely useful, especially given the modifiability of this risk factor. There is a clear biologic mechanism to support the hypothesis that estrogen protects against OA, as estrogen can affect cartilage via binding to estrogen receptors in a dose-dependent fashion.[154] It is possible that existing studies were underpowered and thus unable to show significance. However, given the potential cardiovascular risks associated with ERT a trial to definitively answer this question may not be feasible.

## Local Osseous Factors

### Bone Marrow Lesions

A well-known but little understood disconnect exists between radiographic evidence of OA and clinical symptoms. Severe OA on plain films can be relatively asymptomatic. Conversely, very mild radiographic disease can be disabling. Bone marrow lesions are characterized by discrete areas of hyperintense-T2-weighted fat-suppressed MRI images adjacent to subcortical bone. The presence of bone marrow lesions results in a 3.3-fold increase in the odds that a patient with mild to moderate radiographic knee OA will have pain, after controlling for other radiographic features, effusion, sex, and age.[155] Large lesions increase the odds of pain almost sixfold.[155]

Importantly, the presence of these bone marrow lesions in a specific compartment of the knee predicts progression of joint space narrowing in that compartment.[156] BML also appear to correlate with levels of C-terminal cross-linking telopeptide of type II collagen (CTX-2, a potential marker of OA progression).[157] In a recent prospective study of patients with painful knee OA, higher baseline levels of CXT-2 predicted worse BML at 3 months (and there was a significant positive correlation between changes in CXT-2 and changes in BML at 3 months).[158] Bone marrow lesions in the knee also correlate with higher levels of bone density in the adjacent tibia, supporting the hypothesis that local loading factors are an important mechanism in the development of OA.[159]

### Bone Mineral Density

Many studies have suggested that OA is inversely related to osteoporosis or low bone mineral density (BMD).[160,161] A recent prospective study supports this relationship. These investigators found that high BMD in the femoral neck or lumbar spine increases the risk of incident knee OA, and high lumbar spine BMD also increased the risk of progression of knee OA.[162] Having a prevalent isolated vertebral fracture was highly associated with lower risk of both the incidence and progression of knee OA.[162] A prospective study has also shown that higher bone density at the lumbar spine and hip predict the development of knee osteophytes.[163]

However, the relationship of OA and bone mineral density is likely more complex. The presence of OA does not preclude osteoporosis, and women with OA are not protected from osteoporotic fractures.[164] One study of postmenopausal Caucasian women undergoing elective hip replacement for severe OA found that 25% had unsuspected osteoporosis.[165] Another prospective cohort study found that although high bone density is associated with a higher risk of incident knee OA it may be protective against disease progression.[166] However, the protective effect was largely due to reduced joint space loss.

These conflicting data may be a function of OA disease definition. Radiographs are traditionally used to evaluate OA, and although they are excellent for evaluating osteophytes they are a poor measure of cartilage volume. Using MRI to evaluate knees of subjects without OA, tibial knee cartilage volume (which reflects joint space narrowing) has actually been found to positively correlate with bone mineral density.[167] The opposite relationship of tibial cartilage volume and osteophytes to bone mineral density points out the importance of evaluating these components separately, and suggests that different biologic mechanisms coexist in OA pathogenesis.

## SUMMARY

OA is a common disorder with significant functional and economic sequelae.[168] Because OA does not affect all older adults uniformly, it can no longer be regarded simply as an inevitable consequence of aging. A better understanding of OA epidemiology will direct investigators toward promising areas of potential therapeutic intervention and provide individuals with evidence-based lifestyle recommendations, such as avoiding obesity and exercising regularly (which will target modifiable risk factors).

## REFERENCES

1. Oliveria SA, Felson DT, Reed JI, Cirillo PA, Walker AM. Incidence of symptomatic hand, hip, and knee osteoarthritis among patients in a health maintenance organization. Arthritis Rheum 1995; 38(8):1134–41.
2. CDC. Prevalence of disabilities and associated health conditions among adults: United States, 1999. MMWR 2001;50:120–25.
3. Murray CJ, Lopez AD. Alternative projections of mortality and disability by cause 1990–2020: Global Burden of Disease Study. Lancet 1997;349(9064):1498–1504.
4. Yelin E. The economics of osteoarthritis. In Brandt KD, Doherty M, Lohmander LS (ed.), Osteoarthritis. New York: Oxford University Press 1998:23–30.
5. Felson DT, Naimark A, Anderson J, Kazis L, Castelli W, Meenan RF. The prevalence of knee osteoarthritis in the elderly: The Framingham Osteoarthritis Study. Arthritis Rheum 1987;30(8): 914–18.
6. Kellgren JH, Lawrence JS. Radiological assessment of osteoarthrosis. Ann Rheum Dis 1957;16(4):494–502.
7. Felson DT. An update on the pathogenesis and epidemiology of osteoarthritis. Radiol Clin North Am 2004;42(1):1–9, v.
8. Altman RD. Measurement of structure (disease) modification in osteoarthritis. Osteoarthritis Cartilage 2004;12(A):S69–76.
9. Altman RD, Fries JF, Bloch DA, Carstens J, Cooke TD, Genant H, Groth H, McShane DJ, Murphy WA, et al. Radiographic assessment of progression in osteoarthritis. Arthritis Rheum 1987;30(11):1214–25.
10. Adams JG, McAlindon T, Dimasi M, Carey J, Eustace S. Contribution of meniscal extrusion and cartilage loss to joint space narrowing in osteoarthritis. Clin Radiol 1999;54(8): 502–06.
11. Jones G, Ding C, Scott F, Glisson M, Cicuttini F. Early radiographic osteoarthritis is associated with substantial changes in cartilage

volume and tibial bone surface area in both males and females. Osteoarthritis Cartilage 2004;12(2):169–74.

12. Beattie KA, Boulos P, Pui M, O'Neill J, Inglis D, Webber CE, Adachi JD. Abnormalities identified in the knees of asymptomatic volunteers using peripheral magnetic resonance imaging. Osteoarthritis Cartilage 2005;13(3):181–86.

13. Pessis E, Drape JL, Ravaud P, Chevrot A, Dougados M, Ayral X. Assessment of progression in knee osteoarthritis: Results of a 1 year study comparing arthroscopy and MRI. Osteoarthritis Cartilage 2003;11(5):361–69.

14. Cicuttini F, Hankin J, Jones G, Wluka A. Comparison of conventional standing knee radiographs and magnetic resonance imaging in assessing progression of tibiofemoral joint osteoarthritis. Osteoarthritis Cartilage 2005;13(8):722–27.

15. Raynauld JP, Martel-Pelletier J, Berthiaume MJ, Labonte F, Beaudoin G, De Guise JA, Choquette D, et al. Quantitative magnetic resonance imaging evaluation of knee osteoarthritis progression over two years and correlation with clinical symptoms and radiologic changes. Arthritis Rheum 2004;50(2): 476–87.

16. Cooper C. Osteoarthritis and related disorders: Epidemiology. In Klippel JH, Dieppe PA, Arnett FC, et al. (ed.), Rheumatology, Second Edition. London: Mosby International 1998:8.2.6.

17. Gupta RC, Gupta SC, Misra US, Singhal AK, Khanduri OP. An etiology and morbid anatomical changes in osteoarthrosis of the knee joint in Indians: An autopsy study. Indian J Med Res 1979;69:301–07.

18. Pellegrini VD Jr. Osteoarthritis of the trapeziometacarpal joint: The pathophysiology of articular cartilage degeneration. I. Anatomy and pathology of the aging joint. J Hand Surg [Am] 1991;16(6):967–74.

19. Gordon GV, Villanueva T, Schumacher HR, Gohel V. Autopsy study correlating degree of osteoarthritis, synovitis and evidence of articular calcification. J Rheumatol 1984;11(5):681–86.

20. van Saase JL, van Romunde LK, Cats A, Vandenbroucke JP, Valkenburg HA. Epidemiology of osteoarthritis: Zoetermeer survey. Comparison of radiological osteoarthritis in a Dutch population with that in 10 other populations. Ann Rheum Dis 1989;48(4):271–80.

21. Engle A. Osteoarthritis in adults by selected demographic characteristics, United States, 1960–1962. Vital Health Statistics 1966;11:20.

22. Zhang Y, Xu L, Nevitt MC, Niu J, Goggins JP, Aliabadi P, Yu W, Lui LY, Felson DT. Lower prevalence of hand osteoarthritis among Chinese subjects in Beijing compared with white subjects in the United States: The Beijing Osteoarthritis Study. Arthritis Rheum 2003;48(4):1034–40.

23. Bergstrom G, Bjelle A, Sundh V, Svanborg A. Joint disorders at ages 70, 75 and 79 years: A cross-sectional comparison. Br J Rheumatol 1986;25(4):333–41.

24. Felson DT, Nevitt MC, Zhang Y, Aliabadi P, Baumer B, Gale D, Li W, Yu W, Xu L. High prevalence of lateral knee osteoarthritis in Beijing Chinese compared with Framingham Caucasian subjects. Arthritis Rheum 2002;46(5):1217–22.

25. Jacobsen S, Sonne-Holm S, Soballe K, Gebuhr P, Lund B. Radiographic case definitions and prevalence of osteoarthrosis of the hip: A survey of 4 151 subjects in the Osteoarthritis Substudy of the Copenhagen City Heart Study. Acta Orthop Scand 2004;75(6):713–20.

26. Tepper S, Hochberg MC. Factors associated with hip osteoarthritis: Data from the First National Health and Nutrition Examination Survey (NHANES-I). Am J Epidemiol 1993;137(10): 1081–88.

27. Lawrence JS Sebo M. The Geography of Osteoarthritis. In G Nuki (ed.), The Aetiopathogenesis of Osteoarthrosis. Baltimore: University Park Press 1980:155–83.

28. Nevitt MC, Xu L, Zhang Y, Lui LY, Yu W, Land NE, Qin M, Hochberg MC, Cummings SR, Felson DT. Very low prevalence of hip osteoarthritis among Chinese elderly in Beijing, China, compared with whites in the United States: The Beijing osteoarthritis study. Arthritis Rheum 2002;46(7):1773–79.

29. Goker B. Radiographic osteoarthritis of the hip joint in Turkey. Rheumatol Int 2001;21(3):94–6.

30. Ingvarsson T, Hagglund G, Lohmander LS. Prevalence of hip osteoarthritis in Iceland. Ann Rheum Dis 1999;58(4): 201–07.

31. Lau EM, Symmons DP, Croft P. The epidemiology of hip osteoarthritis and rheumatoid arthritis in the Orient. Clin Orthop Relat Res 1996;(323):81–90.

32. Ledingham J, Dawson S, Preston B, Milligan G, Doherty M. Radiographic progression of hospital referred osteoarthritis of the hip. Ann Rheum Dis 1993;52(4):263–67.

33. Dumond H, Presle N, Terlain B, Mainard D, Loeuille D, Netter P, Pottie P. Evidence for a key role of leptin in osteoarthritis. Arthritis Rheum 2003;48(11):3118–29.

34. Teichtahl AJ, Wluka AE, Proietto J, Cicuttini FM. Obesity and the female sex, risk factors for knee osteoarthritis that may be attributable to systemic or local leptin biosynthesis and its cellular effects. Med Hypotheses 2005;65(2):312–15.

35. Spector TD, Campion GD. Generalised osteoarthritis: A hormonally mediated disease. Ann Rheum Dis 1989;48(6):523–27.

36. Ettinger WH, Davis MA, Neuhaus JM, Mallon KP. Long-term physical functioning in persons with knee osteoarthritis from NHANES. I: Effects of comorbid medical conditions. J Clin Epidemiol 1994;47(7):809–15.

37. Lawrence JS, Bremner JM, Bier F. Osteo-arthrosis. Prevalence in the population and relationship between symptoms and X-ray changes. Ann Rheum Dis 1966;25(1):1–24.

38. Odding E, Valkenburg HA, Algra D, Vandenouweland FA, Grobbee DE, Hofman A. Associations of radiological osteoarthritis of the hip and knee with locomotor disability in the Rotterdam Study. Ann Rheum Dis 1998;57(4):203–08.

39. Kelsey JL. Upper Extremity Disorders: A Survey of Their Frequency and Cost in the United States. St. Louis: Mosby 1980.

40. Hughes S, Gibbs J, Dunlop D, Edelman P, Singer R, Chang RW. Predictors of decline in manual performance in older adults. J Am Geriatr Soc 1997;45(8):905–10.

41. Stecher R. Heberden's nodes: Heredity in hypertrophic arthritis of the finger joints. Am J Med Sci 1941;210:801–09.

42. Spector TD, Cicuttini F, Baker J, Loughlin J, Hart D. Genetic influences on osteoarthritis in women: A twin study. BMJ 1996;312(7036):940–43.

43. Chitnavis J, Sinsheimer JS, Clipsham K, Loughlin J, Sykes B, Burge PD, Carr AJ. Genetic influences in end-stage osteoarthritis: Sibling risks of hip and knee replacement for idiopathic osteoarthritis. J Bone Joint Surg Br 1997;79(4):660–64.

44. Kaprio J, Kujala UM, Peltonen L, Koskenvuo M. Genetic liability to osteoarthritis may be greater in women than men. BMJ 1996;313(7051):232.

45. Hoaglund FT, Oishi CS, Gialamas GG. Extreme variations in racial rates of total hip arthroplasty for primary coxarthrosis: A population-based study in San Francisco. Ann Rheum Dis 1995;54(2):107–10.

46. Loughlin J. Genetic epidemiology of primary osteoarthritis. Curr Opin Rheumatol 2001;13(2):111–16.

47. Roby P, Eyre S, Worthington J, Ramesar R, Cilliers H, Beighton P, Grant M, Wallis G. Autosomal dominant (Beukes) premature degenerative osteoarthropathy of the hip joint maps to an 11-cM region on chromosome 4q35. Am J Hum Genet 1999;64(3):904–08.

48. Loughlin J, Sinsheimer JS, Mustafa Z, Carr AJ, Clipsham K, Bloomfield VA, Chitnavis J, Bailey A, Sykes B, Chapman K. Association analysis of the vitamin D receptor gene, the type I collagen gene COL1A1, and the estrogen receptor gene in idiopathic osteoarthritis. J Rheumatol 2000;27(3):779–84.

49. Southam L, Dowling B, Ferreira A, Marcelline L, Mustafa Z, Chapman K, Bentham G, Carr A, Loughlin J. Microsatellite association mapping of a primary osteoarthritis susceptibility locus on chromosome 6p12.3–q13. Arthritis Rheum 2004;50(12):3910–14.

50. Uitterlinden AG, Burger H, Huang Q, Yue F, McGuigan FE, Grant SF, Hofman A, et al. Vitamin D receptor genotype is associated with radiographic osteoarthritis at the knee. J Clin Invest 1997;100(2):259–63.

51. Ushiyama T, Ueyama H, Inoue K, Nishioka J, Ohkubo I, Hukuda S. Estrogen receptor gene polymorphism and generalized osteoarthritis. J Rheumatol 1998;25(1):134–37.

52. Zhai G, Rivadeneira F, Houwing-Duistermaat JJ, Meulenbelt I, Bijkerk C, Hofman A, van Meurs JB, Uitterlinden AG, Pols HA, Slagboom PE, van Duijn CM. Insulin-like growth factor I gene promoter polymorphism, collagen type II alpha1 (COL2A1) gene, and the prevalence of radiographic osteoarthritis: The Rotterdam Study. Ann Rheum Dis 2004;63(5):544–48.

53. Loughlin J, Dowling B, Chapman K, Marcelline L, Mustafa Z, Southam L, Ferreira A, Ciesielski C, Carson DA, Corr M. Functional variants within the secreted frizzled-related protein 3 gene are associated with hip osteoarthritis in females. Proc Natl Acad Sci USA 2004;101(26):9757–62.

54. Chung YS, Baylink DJ, Srivastava AK, Amaar Y, Tapia B, Kasukawa Y, Mohan S. Effects of secreted frizzled-related protein 3 on osteoblasts in vitro. J Bone Miner Res 2004;19(9):1395–1402.

55. Loughlin J. Polymorphism in signal transduction is a major route through which osteoarthritis susceptibility is acting. Curr Opin Rheumatol 2005;17(5):629–33.

56. Weinstein SL. Natural history and treatment outcomes of childhood hip disorders. Clin Orthop Relat Res 1997;(344):227–42.

57. Wedge JH, Wasylenko MJ, Houston CS. Minor anatomic abnormalities of the hip joint persisting from childhood and their possible relationship to idiopathic osteoarthrosis. Clin Orthop Relat Res 1991;(264):122–28.

58. Jacobsen S, Sonne-Holm S. Hip dysplasia: A significant risk factor for the development of hip osteoarthritis: A cross-sectional survey. Rheumatology (Oxford) 2005;44(2):211–18.

59. Kellgren JH, Lawrence JS. Rheumatism in miners. II. X-ray study. Br J Ind Med 1952;9(3):197–207.

60. Partridge RE, Duthie JJ. Rheumatism in dockers and civil servants: A comparison of heavy manual and sedentary workers. Ann Rheum Dis 1968;27(6):559–68.

61. Vingard E, Alfredsson L, Goldie I, Hogstedt C. Occupation and osteoarthrosis of the hip and knee: A register-based cohort study. Int J Epidemiol 1991;20(4):1025–31.

62. Croft P, Coggon D, Cruddas M, Cooper C. Osteoarthritis of the hip: an occupational disease in farmers. BMJ 1992;304(6837): 1269–72.

63. Maetzel A, Makela M, Hawker G, Bombardier C. Osteoarthritis of the hip and knee and mechanical occupational exposure: A systematic overview of the evidence. J Rheumatol 1997;24(8):1599–1607.

64. Rossignol M, Leclerc A, Hilliquin P, Allaert FA, Rozenberg S, Valat JP, Avouac B, Coste P, Savarieau B, Fautrel B. Primary osteoarthritis and occupations: A national cross sectional survey of 10 412 symptomatic patients. Occup Environ Med 2003;60(11):882–86.

65. Coggon D, Croft P, Kellingray S, Barrett D, McLaren M, Cooper C. Occupational physical activities and osteoarthritis of the knee. Arthritis Rheum 2000;43(7):1443–49.

66. McAlindon TE, Wilson PW, Aliabadi P, Weissman B, Felson DT. Level of physical activity and the risk of radiographic and symptomatic knee osteoarthritis in the elderly: The Framingham study. Am J Med 1999;106(2):151–57.

67. Lievense A, Bierma-Zeinstra S, Verhagen A, Verhaar J, Koes B. Influence of work on the development of osteoarthritis of the hip: A systematic review. J Rheumatol 2001;28(11):2520–28.

68. Hadler NM, Gillings DB, Imbus HR, Levitin PM, Makuc D, Utsinger PD, Yount WJ, Slusser D, Moskovitz N. Hand structure and function in an industrial setting. Arthritis Rheum 1978;21(2):210–20.

69. Neame R, Zhang W, Deighton C, Doherty M, Doherty S, Lanyon P, Wright G. Distribution of radiographic osteoarthritis between the right and left hands, hips, and knees. Arthritis Rheum 2004;50(5):1487–94.

70. Lane NE, Bloch DA, Jones HH, Simpson U, Fries JF. Osteoarthritis in the hand: A comparison of handedness and hand use. J Rheumatol 1989;16(5):637–42.

71. Acheson RM, Chan YK, Clemett AR. New Haven survey of joint diseases. XII. Distribution and symptoms of osteoarthrosis in the hands with reference to handedness. Ann Rheum Dis 1970;29(3):275–86.

72. Solovieva S, Vehmas T, Riihimaki H, Luoma K, Leino-Arjas P. Hand use and patterns of joint involvement in osteoarthritis: A comparison of female dentists and teachers. Rheumatology (Oxford) 2005;44(4):521–28.

73. Hunter DJ, Zhang Y, Nevitt MC, Xu L, Niu J, Lui LY, Yu W, Aliabadi P, Felson DT. Chopstick arthropathy: The Beijing Osteoarthritis Study. Arthritis Rheum 2004;50(5):1495–500.

74. Haara MM, Manninen P, Kroger H, Arokoski JP, Karkkainen A, Knekt P, Aromaa A, Heliovaara M. Osteoarthritis of finger joints in Finns aged 30 or over: Prevalence, determinants, and association with mortality. Ann Rheum Dis 2003;62(2):151–58.

75. Newton PM, Mow VC, Gardner TR, Buckwalter JA, Albright JP. The effect of lifelong exercise on canine articular cartilage. Am J Sports Med 1997;25(3):282–87.

76. Kiviranta I, Tammi M, Jurvelin J, Saamanen AM, Helminen HJ. Moderate running exercise augments glycosaminoglycans and thickness of articular cartilage in the knee joint of young beagle dogs. J Orthop Res 1988;6(2):188–95.

77. Kiviranta I, Tammi M, Jurvelin J, Arokoski J, Saamanen AM, Helminen HJ. Articular cartilage thickness and glycosaminoglycan distribution in the canine knee joint after strenuous running exercise. Clin Orthop Relat Res 1992;(283):302–08.

78. Arokoski J, Kiviranta I, Jurvelin J, Tammi M, Helminen HJ. Long-distance running causes site-dependent decrease of cartilage glycosaminoglycan content in the knee joints of beagle dogs. Arthritis Rheum 1993;36(10):1451–59.

79. Radin EL, Martin RB, Burr DB, Caterson B, Boyd RD, Goodwin C. Effects of mechanical loading on the tissues of the rabbit knee. J Orthop Res 1984;2(3):221–34.

80. Lane NE, Oehlert JW, Bloch DA, Fries JF. The relationship of running to osteoarthritis of the knee and hip and bone mineral density of the lumbar spine: A 9 year longitudinal study. J Rheumatol 1998;25(2):334–41.

81. Sohn RS, Micheli LJ. The effect of running on the pathogenesis of osteoarthritis of the hips and knees. Clin Orthop Relat Res 1985;(198):106–09.

82. Konradsen L, Hansen EM, Sondergaard L. Long distance running and osteoarthrosis. Am J Sports Med 1990;18(4):379–81.

83. Lane NE, Hochberg MC, Pressman A, Scott JC, Nevitt MC. Recreational physical activity and the risk of osteoarthritis of the hip in elderly women. J Rheumatol 1999;26(4):849–54.

84. Cheng Y, Macera CA, Davis DR, Ainsworth BE, Troped PJ, Blair SN. Physical activity and self-reported, physician-diagnosed osteoarthritis: Is physical activity a risk factor? J Clin Epidemiol 2000;53(3):315–22.

85. Marti B, Knobloch M, Tschopp A, Jucker A, Howald H. Is excessive running predictive of degenerative hip disease? Controlled study of former elite athletes. BMJ 1989;299(6691):91–3.

86. Spector TD, Harris PA, Hart DJ, Cicuttini FM, Nandra D, Etherington J, Wolman RL, Doyle DV. Risk of osteoarthritis associated with long-term weight-bearing sports: A radiologic survey of the hips and knees in female ex-athletes and population controls. Arthritis Rheum 1996;39(6):988–95.

87. Kujala UM, Kettunen J, Paananen H, Aalto T, Battie MC, Impivaara O, Videman T, Sarna S. Knee osteoarthritis in former runners, soccer players, weight lifters, and shooters. Arthritis Rheum 1995; 38(4):539–46.

88. Kujala UM, Kaprio J, Sarna S. Osteoarthritis of weight bearing joints of lower limbs in former elite male athletes. BMJ 1994; 308(6923):231–34.

89. Lindberg H, Roos H, Gardsell P. Prevalence of coxarthrosis in former soccer players: 286 players compared with matched controls. Acta Orthop Scand 1993;64(2):165–67.

90. Drawer S, Fuller CW. Propensity for osteoarthritis and lower limb joint pain in retired professional soccer players. Br J Sports Med 2001;35(6):402–08.

91. Turner AP, Barlow JH, Heathcote-Elliott C. Long term health impact of playing professional football in the United Kingdom. Br J Sports Med 2000;34(5):332–36.

92. Buckwalter JA, Martin JA. Sports and osteoarthritis. Curr Opin Rheumatol 2004;16(5):634–39.

93. Adams JE. Injury to the throwing arm: A study of traumatic changes in the elbow joints of boy baseball players. Calif Med 1965;102:127–32.

94. Schmitt H, Brocai DR, Lukoschek M. High prevalence of hip arthrosis in former elite javelin throwers and high jumpers: 41 athletes examined more than 10 years after retirement from competitive sports. Acta Orthop Scand 2004;75(1):34–9.

95. Neyret P, Donell ST, DeJour D, DeJour H. Partial meniscectomy and anterior cruciate ligament rupture in soccer players: A study with a minimum 20-year follow-up. Am J Sports Med 1993;21(3):455–60.

96. von Porat A, Roos EM, Roos H. High prevalence of osteoarthritis 14 years after an anterior cruciate ligament tear in male soccer players: A study of radiographic and patient relevant outcomes. Ann Rheum Dis 2004;63(3):269–73.

97. Dunn WR, Lyman S, Lincoln AE, Amoroso PJ, Wickiewicz T, Marx RG. The effect of anterior cruciate ligament reconstruction on the risk of knee reinjury. Am J Sports Med 2004;32(8): 1906–14.

98. Jomha NM, Borton DC, Clingeleffer AJ, Pinczewski LA. Long-term osteoarthritic changes in anterior cruciate ligament reconstructed knees. Clin Orthop Relat Res 1999(358):188–93.

99. Roos H, Lindberg H, Gardsell P, Lohmander LS, Wingstrand H. The prevalence of gonarthrosis and its relation to meniscectomy in former soccer players. Am J Sports Med 1994;22(2):219–22.

100. Lundberg M, Messner K. Ten-year prognosis of isolated and combined medial collateral ligament ruptures: A matched comparison in 40 patients using clinical and radiographic evaluations. Am J Sports Med 1997;25(1):2–6.

101. Honkonen SE. Degenerative arthritis after tibial plateau fractures. J Orthop Trauma 1995;9(4):273–77.

102. Sahin V, Karakas ES, Aksu S, Atlihan D, Turk CY, Halici M. Traumatic dislocation and fracture-dislocation of the hip: A long-term follow-up study. J Trauma 2003;54(3):520–29.

103. Gelber AC, Hochberg MC, Mead LA, Wang NY, Wigley FM, Klag MJ. Joint injury in young adults and risk for subsequent knee and hip osteoarthritis. Ann Intern Med 2000;133(5): 321–28.

104. Cooper C, Snow S, McAlindon TE, Kellingray S, Stuart B, Coggon D, Dieppe PA. Risk factors for the incidence and progression of radiographic knee osteoarthritis. Arthritis Rheum 2000;43(5): 995–1000.

105. Roos H, Lauren M, Adalberth T, Roos EM, Jonsson K, Lohmander LS. Knee osteoarthritis after meniscectomy: Prevalence of radiographic changes after twenty-one years, compared with matched controls. Arthritis Rheum 1998;41(4):687–93.

106. Reijman M, Belo JN, Lievense AM, Hazes JM, Pols HA, Bierma-Zeinstra SM. Is BMI associated with the onset and progression of osteoarthritis of the knee and hip?: The Rotterdam Study. Osteoarthritis Cartilage 2007;15(A):S28.

107. Oliveria SA, Felson DT, Cirillo PA, Reed JI, Walker AM. Body weight, body mass index, and incident symptomatic osteoarthritis of the hand, hip, and knee. Epidemiology 1999;10(2):161–66.

108. Felson DT, Anderson JJ, Naimark A, Walker AM, Meenan RF. Obesity and knee osteoarthritis: The Framingham Study. Ann Intern Med 1988;109(1):18–24.

109. Anderson JJ, Felson DT. Factors associated with osteoarthritis of the knee in the first national Health and Nutrition Examination Survey (HANES I): Evidence for an association with overweight, race, and physical demands of work. Am J Epidemiol 1988;128(1):179–89.

110. Holmberg S, Thelin A, Thelin N. Knee osteoarthritis and body mass index: A population-based case-control study. Scand J Rheumatol 2005;34(1):59–64.

111. Felson DT, Goggins J, Niu J, Zhang Y, Hunter DJ. The effect of body weight on progression of knee osteoarthritis is dependent on alignment. Arthritis Rheum 2004;50(12):3904–09.

112. Messier SP, Gutekunst DJ, Davis C, DeVita P. Weight loss reduces knee-joint loads in overweight and obese older adults with knee osteoarthritis. Arthritis Rheum 2005;52(7): 2026–32.

113. Dougados M, Gueguen A, Nguyen M, Thiesce A, Listrat V, Jacob L, Nakache JP, Gabriel KR, Lequesne M, Amor B. Longitudinal radiologic evaluation of osteoarthritis of the knee. J Rheumatol 1992;19(3):378–84.

114. Cicuttini FM, Teichtahl AJ, Wluka AE, Davis S, Strauss BJ, Ebeling PR. The relationship between body composition and knee cartilage volume in healthy, middle-aged subjects. Arthritis Rheum 2005;52(2):461–67.

115. Saville PD, Dickson J. Age and weight in osteoarthritis of the hip. Arthritis Rheum 1968;11(5):635–44.

116. Felson DT. Obesity and vocational and avocational overload of the joint as risk factors for osteoarthritis. J Rheumatol Suppl 2004;70:2–5.

117. Karlson EW, Mandl LA, Aweh GN, Sangha O, Liang MH, Grodstein F. Total hip replacement due to osteoarthritis: The importance of age, obesity, and other modifiable risk factors. Am J Med 2003;114(2):93–8.

118. Jacobsen S, Sonne-Holm S. Increased body mass index is a predisposition for treatment by total hip replacement. Int Orthop 2005;29(4):229–34.

119. Hochberg MC, Lethbridge-Cejku M, Plato CC, Wigley FM, Tobin JD. Factors associated with osteoarthritis of the hand in males: Data from the Baltimore Longitudinal Study of Aging. Am J Epidemiol 1991;134(10):1121–27.

120. Hochberg MC, Lethbridge-Cejku M, Scott WW Jr., Plato CC, Tobin JD. Obesity and osteoarthritis of the hands in women. Osteoarthritis Cartilage 1993;1(2):129–35.

121. Sturmer T, Gunther KP, Brenner H. Obesity, overweight and patterns of osteoarthritis: The Ulm Osteoarthritis Study. J Clin Epidemiol 2000;53(3):307–13.

122. Sayer AA, Poole J, Cox V, Kuh D, Hardy R, Wadsworth M, Cooper C. Weight from birth to 53 years: A longitudinal study of the influence on clinical hand osteoarthritis. Arthritis Rheum 2003; 48(4):1030–33.

123. Carman WJ, Sowers M, Hawthorne VM, Weissfeld LA. Obesity as a risk factor for osteoarthritis of the hand and wrist: A prospective study. Am J Epidemiol 1994;139(2):119–29.

124. Sowers M, Zobel D, Weissfeld L, Hawthorne VM, Carman W. Progression of osteoarthritis of the hand and metacarpal bone loss: A twenty-year followup of incident cases. Arthritis Rheum 1991;34(1):36–42.

125. O'Reilly SC, Jones A, Muir KR, Doherty M. Quadriceps weakness in knee osteoarthritis: The effect on pain and disability. Ann Rheum Dis 1998;57(10):588–94.

126. Slemenda C, Heilman DK, Brandt KD, Katz BP, Mazzuca SA, Braunstein EM, Byrd D. Reduced quadriceps strength relative to body weight: A risk factor for knee osteoarthritis in women? Arthritis Rheum 1998;41(11):1951–59.

127. Slemenda C, Brandt KD, Heilman DK, Mazzuca S, Braunstein EM, Katz BP, Wolinsky FD. Quadriceps weakness and osteoarthritis of the knee. Ann Intern Med 1997;127(2):97–104.

128. Baker KR, Xu L, Zhang Y, Nevitt M, Niu J, Aliabad P, Yu W, Felson D. Quadriceps weakness and its relationship to tibiofemoral and patellofemoral knee osteoarthritis in Chinese: The Beijing osteoarthritis study. Arthritis Rheum 2004;50(6):1815–21.

129. Sharma L, Dunlop DD, Cahue S, Song J, Hayes KW. Quadriceps strength and osteoarthritis progression in malaligned and lax knees. Ann Intern Med 2003;138(8):613–19.

130. Brandt KD, Heilman DK, Slemenda C, Katz BP, Mazzuca SA, Braunstein EM, Byrd D. Quadriceps strength in women with radiographically progressive osteoarthritis of the knee and those with stable radiographic changes. J Rheumatol 1999; 26(11):2431–37.

131. Sharma L, Song J, Felson DT, Cahue S, Shamiyeh E, Dunlop DD. The role of knee alignment in disease progression and functional decline in knee osteoarthritis. JAMA 2001;286(2): 188–95.

132. Cahue S, Dunlop D, Hayes K, Song J, Torres L, Sharma L. Varus-valgus alignment in the progression of patellofemoral osteoarthritis. Arthritis Rheum 2004;50(7):2184–90.

133. Felson DT, Anderson JJ, Naimark A, Hannan MT, Kannel WB, Meenan RF. Does smoking protect against osteoarthritis? Arthritis Rheum 1989;32(2):166–72.

134. Felson DT, Zhang Y, Hannan MT, Naimark A, Wissman B, Aliabadi P, Levy D. Risk factors for incident radiographic knee osteoarthritis in the elderly: The Framingham Study. Arthritis Rheum 1997;40(4):728–33.

135. Sandmark H, Hogstedt C, Lewold S, Vingard E. Osteoarthrosis of the knee in men and women in association with overweight, smoking, and hormone therapy. Ann Rheum Dis 1999;58(3): 151–55.

136. Wilder FV, Hall BJ, Barrett JP. Smoking and osteoarthritis: Is there an association? The Clearwater Osteoarthritis Study. Osteoarthritis Cartilage 2003;11(1):29–35.

137. Hart DJ, Doyle DV, Spector TD. Incidence and risk factors for radiographic knee osteoarthritis in middle-aged women: The Chingford Study. Arthritis Rheum 1999;42(1):17–24.

138. Dawson J, Juszczak E, Thorogood M, Marks SA, Dodd C, Fitzpatrick R. An investigation of risk factors for symptomatic osteoarthritis of the knee in women using a life course approach. J Epidemiol Community Health 2003;57(10):823–30.

139. Jacobsen S, Sonne-Holm S, Soballe K, Gebuhr P, Lund B. The relationship of hip joint space to self reported hip pain: A survey of 4.151 subjects of the Copenhagen City Heart Study. The Osteoarthritis Substudy. Osteoarthritis Cartilage 2004;12(9):692–97.

140. Ushiyama T, Mori K, Inoue K, Huang J, Nishioka J, Hukuda S. Association of oestrogen receptor gene polymorphisms with age at onset of rheumatoid arthritis. Ann Rheum Dis 1999;58(1):7–10.

**13**

141. Richmond RS, Carlson CS, Register TC, Shanker G, Loeser RF. Functional estrogen receptors in adult articular cartilage: Estrogen replacement therapy increases chondrocyte synthesis of proteoglycans and insulin-like growth factor binding protein 2. Arthritis Rheum 2000;43(9):2081–90.

142. Lee YJ, Lee EB, Kwon YE, Lee JJ, Cho WS, Kim HA, Song YW. Effect of estrogen on the expression of matrix metalloproteinase (MMP)-1, MMP-3, and MMP-13 and tissue inhibitor of metalloproteinase-1 in osteoarthritis chondrocytes. Rheumatol Int 2003;23(6):282–88.

143. Nevitt MC, Cummings SR, Lane NE, Hochberg MC, Scott JC, Pressman AR, Genant HK, Cualey JA. Association of estrogen replacement therapy with the risk of osteoarthritis of the hip in elderly white women: Study of Osteoporotic Fractures Research Group. Arch Intern Med 1996;156(18):2073–80.

144. Spector TD, Nandra D, Hart DJ, Doyle DV. Is hormone replacement therapy protective for hand and knee osteoarthritis in women?: The Chingford Study. Ann Rheum Dis 1997;56(7):432–34.

145. Wluka AE, Davis SR, Bailey M, Stuckey SL, Cicuttini FM. Users of oestrogen replacement therapy have more knee cartilage than non-users. Ann Rheum Dis 2001;60(4):332–36.

146. Von Muhlen D, Morton D, Von Muhlen CA, Barrett-Connor E. Postmenopausal estrogen and increased risk of clinical osteoarthritis at the hip, hand, and knee in older women. J Womens Health Gend Based Med 2002;11(6):511–18.

147. Sahyoun NR, Brett KM, Hochberg MC, Pamuk ER. Estrogen replacement therapy and incidence of self-reported physician-diagnosed arthritis. Prev Med 1999;28(5):458–64.

148. Dennison EM, Arden NK, Kellingray S, Croft P, Coggon D, Cooper C. Hormone replacement therapy, other reproductive variables and symptomatic hip osteoarthritis in elderly white women: A case-control study. Br J Rheumatol 1998;37(11):1198–1202.

149. Erb A, Brenner H, Gunther KP, Sturmer T. Hormone replacement therapy and patterns of osteoarthritis: Baseline data from the Ulm Osteoarthritis Study. Ann Rheum Dis 2000;59(2):105–09.

150. Cauley JA, Kwoh CK, Egeland G, Nevitt MC, Cooperstein L, Rohay J, Towers A, Gutai JP. Serum sex hormones and severity of osteoarthritis of the hand. J Rheumatol 1993;20(7):1170–75.

151. Hannan MT, Felson DT, Anderson JJ, Naimark A, Kannel WB. Estrogen use and radiographic osteoarthritis of the knee in women: The Framingham Osteoarthritis Study. Arthritis Rheum 1990;33(4):525–32.

152. Zhang Y, McAlindon TE, Hannan MT, Chaisson CE, Klein R, Wilson PW, Felson DT. Estrogen replacement therapy and worsening of radiographic knee osteoarthritis: The Framingham Study. Arthritis Rheum 1998;41(10):1867–73.

153. Nevitt MC, Felson DT, Williams EN, Grady D. The effect of estrogen plus progestin on knee symptoms and related disability in postmenopausal women: The Heart and Estrogen/Progestin Replacement Study, a randomized, double-blind, placebo-controlled trial. Arthritis Rheum 2001;44(4):811–18.

154. Gokhale JA, Frenkel SR, Dicesare PE. Estrogen and osteoarthritis. Am J Orthop 2004;33(2):71–80.

155. Felson DT, Chaisson CE, Hill CL, Totterman SM, Gale ME, Skinner KM, Kazis L, Gale DR. The association of bone marrow lesions with pain in knee osteoarthritis. Ann Intern Med 2001;134(7):541–49.

156. Felson DT, McLaughlin S, Goggins J, LaValley MP, Gale ME, Totterman S, Li W, Hill C, Gale D. Bone marrow edema and its relation to progression of knee osteoarthritis. Ann Intern Med 2003;139(5 Pt 1):330–36.

157. Reijman M, Hazes JM, Bierma-Zeinstra SM, Koes BW, Christgau S, Christiansen C, Uitterlinden AG, Pols HA. A new marker for osteoarthritis: Cross-sectional and longitudinal approach. Arthritis Rheum 2004;50(8):2471–78.

158. Garnero P, Peterfy C, Zaim S, Schoenharting M. Bone marrow abnormalities on magnetic resonance imaging are associated with type II collagen degradation in knee osteoarthritis: A three-month longitudinal study. Arthritis Rheum 2005;52(9):2822–29.

159. Lo GH, Hunter DJ, Zhang Y, McLennan CE, Lavalley MP, Kiel DP, McLean RR, Genant HK, Guermazi A, Felson DT. Bone marrow lesions in the knee are associated with increased local bone density. Arthritis Rheum 2005;52(9):2814–21.

160. Nevitt MC, Lane NE, Scott JC, Hochberg MC, Pressman AR, Genant HK, Cummings SR. Radiographic osteoarthritis of the hip and bone mineral density: The Study of Osteoporotic Fractures Research Group. Arthritis Rheum 1995;38(7):907–16.

161. Dequeker J, Boonen S, Aerssens J, Westhovens R. Inverse relationship osteoarthritis-osteoporosis: What is the evidence? What are the consequences? Br J Rheumatol 1996;35(9):813–18.

162. Bergink AP, Uitterlinden AG, Van Leeuwen JP, Hofman A, Verhaar JA, Pols HA. Bone mineral density and vertebral fracture history are associated with incident and progressive radiographic knee osteoarthritis in elderly men and women: The Rotterdam Study. Bone 2005;37(4):446–56.

163. Hart DJ, Cronin C, Daniels M, Worthy T, Doyle DV, Spector TD. The relationship of bone density and fracture to incident and progressive radiographic osteoarthritis of the knee: The Chingford Study. Arthritis Rheum 2002;46(1):92–9.

164. Arden NK, Nevitt MC, Lane NE, Gore LR, Hochberg MC, Scott JC, Pressman AR, Cummings SR. Osteoarthritis and risk of falls, rates of bone loss, and osteoporotic fractures: Study of Osteoporotic Fractures Research Group. Arthritis Rheum 1999;42(7):1378–85.

165. Glowacki J, Hurwitz S, Thornhill TS, Kelly M, LeBoff MS. Osteoporosis and vitamin-D deficiency among postmenopausal women with osteoarthritis undergoing total hip arthroplasty. J Bone Joint Surg Am 2003;85-A(12):2371–77.

166. Zhang Y, Hannan MT, Chaisson CE, McAlindon TE, Evans SR, Aliabadi P, Levy D, Felson DT. Bone mineral density and risk of incident and progressive radiographic knee osteoarthritis in women: The Framingham Study. J Rheumatol 2000;27(4):1032–37.

167. Cicuttini F, Wluka A, Davis S, Strauss BJ, Yeung S, Ebeling PR. Association between knee cartilage volume and bone mineral density in older adults without osteoarthritis. Rheumatology (Oxford) 2004;43(6):765–69.

168. McKenna MT, Michaud CM, Murray CJ, Marks JS. Assessing the burden of disease in the United States using disability-adjusted life years. Am J Prev Med 2005;28(5):415–23.

# 2

# The Role of Subchondral Bone in Osteoarthritis

Johanne Martel-Pelletier, Daniel Lajeunesse, Pascal Reboul, and Jean-Pierre Pelletier

## INTRODUCTION

Arthritis is the most frequently diagnosed chronic medical condition worldwide. Osteoarthritis accounts for 40 to 60% of degenerative illnesses of the musculoskeletal system. On the whole, approximately 15% of the population suffers from osteoarthritis. Of this number approximately 65% are 60 years of age and over. The high incidence of this illness is rather disturbing at this time because its frequency increases gradually with the aging of the population. As a result, it is a major medical problem at present and for the foreseeable future. Although it is the most common joint disease, osteoarthritis is often difficult to define. The disease develops and changes slowly, and clinically it is a heterogeneous group of disorders often referred to as osteoarthritic diseases. The absence of objective and definitive biochemical markers has also been a major barrier to clinical and therapeutic research.

Research remains the most efficient means of tackling this illness and reducing its impact. At present, no disease-modifying treatment exists for osteoarthritis. Current treatments are palliative and only provide symptomatic relief without preventing the progression of the disease. Investigating its pathophysiologic mechanisms and specific treatments is an obvious priority in medical research. Over the last few decades, significant progress has been made with respect to new concepts about the pathogenesis of osteoarthritis. Findings with regard to the physiologic and pathologic mechanisms have made it possible to better target therapeutic approaches that could lead to the development of treatments to reduce or stop the progression of the disease.

At this point in time, one may question the rationale of such a chapter on the role of subchondral bone in osteoarthritis. We believe it represents a logical approach to the understanding of the pathophysiology and future treatment of the disease. For a long time, the belief was that the focal characteristic pathologic feature of osteoarthritis was the destruction of articular cartilage. Consequently, it is not surprising that investigations have concentrated for a few decades on the mechanisms involved in the destruction of the cartilage. More than 30 years ago, Radin et al.[1] suggested that changes in the bone might be a cause for osteoarthritis. Since that time, there has been substantial evidence provided from preclinical and clinical studies that changes in the metabolism of the bony skeleton, and in particular at the subchondral bone area, are an integral part of the disease process.

Recent advances in this field of research have clearly shown the global involvement in osteoarthritis of all of the major tissues of the joints; namely, cartilage, synovial membrane, and subchondral bone. In addition to cartilage loss, which is mainly related to matrix degradation, the participation and the role of synovial inflammation in the progression of the structural changes of this disease are now widely accepted. Although synovitis is considered secondary to the changes in other tissues such as cartilage, some data indicate that synovial inflammation could be a component of the early events leading to the clinical stage of osteoarthritis.[2]

However, the question remains as to whether subchondral bone alterations are the cause or a consequence of cartilage degeneration. Some studies have reported that subchondral bone changes preceded cartilage lesions and could be responsible for the evolution of these tissue lesions.[3-5] Others reported that subchondral bone changes occur simultaneously or even follow cartilage changes and therefore could only be a phenomenon secondary to cartilage degradation.[6-8] However, evidence from human and animal models is accumulating and suggests that alterations at the subchondral bone level precede cartilage damage.

15

Radin and Rose[5] speculated that the increase in bone mass and thickness could have modified the biomechanical properties of the tissue and favored the appearance/progression of articular cartilage structural changes. Many studies have demonstrated that the subchondral bone is the site of a number of active morphologic changes that may vary during the evolution of the disease and appear to be part of the disease process.[3,4,7,9,10] These changes are allied with many local abnormal biochemical pathways that are likely involved in bone changes and may contribute (in association with anatomic and biomechanical changes) to cartilage degradation.[11-18]

Determining whether cartilage or bone is the primary tissue altered in the pathogenesis of osteoarthritis in humans is not trivial because at the clinical stage of the disease, cartilage degeneration is generally well advanced, by which time it is too late to determine the early events. Studies done in spontaneous osteoarthritic animal models (including those with STR/ORT mice[19] and guinea pigs[20-22]) clearly demonstrated that increased bone remodeling preceded cartilage degradation. This concept is supported by studies with the cynomolgus macaque, in which thickening of the subchondral bone occurs before fibrillation of the articular cartilage (and the extent of thickening can be related to the onset of cartilage fibrillation).[3,23] Additional evidence has been found in a rabbit model of progressive osteoarthritis in which sub-fracture insults applied to the patellofemoral joint showed that the progressive increase in subchondral plate thickness was evident much earlier (months) than any significant cartilage changes.[24]

One could argue that the morphologic changes seen early in osteoarthritis are only age related. However, changes associated with osteoarthritis and those associated only with aging are distinctly different: in the latter condition there is a decrease in bone density and the number of trabeculae (with a reduction in trabecular separation without a change in trabecular thickness), whereas well-established osteoarthritis demonstrated increased apparent bone density and fewer but thicker trabeculae without a change in trabecular separation. These differences, in addition to the data from animal models, lend credence to the notion that subchondral bone changes in osteoarthritis are a component of the cause. Moreover, and in support of the role of subchondral bone in the pathology of osteoarthritis, cross-talk between this tissue and cartilage has revealed intricate molecular networks between these two tissues which adds a new dimension to the complexity of the mechanism of cartilage/bone degradation/repair.

To better understand the mechanisms responsible for the pathologic subchondral bone changes in osteoarthritis, this chapter first reviews the bone structure and the cellular, biochemical, and molecular mechanisms involved in the physiologic remodeling of this tissue. This chapter also reviews the pathologic mechanisms occurring in the subchondral bone during osteoarthritis, the importance of these tissue changes in this disease, and the possibility of a cross-talk between bone and cartilage. Studies on the therapeutic influence of specific drugs on bone metabolism in animals and humans are also reviewed.

## NORMAL BONE PHYSIOLOGY

### Normal Bone Structure

Bone tissue serves three functions: (1) mechanical support and site of muscle attachment for locomotion, (2) protector of vital organs and bone marrow, and (3) metabolic reservoir (especially for calcium and phosphate) that helps maintain serum homeostasis. As in all connective tissue, bone consists of cells and an abundant extracellular matrix. The extracellular matrix is composed of collagen fibers and noncollagenous proteins that have the unique ability to calcify. Two types of bones are distinguished in the skeleton: flat bones and long bones. Flat bones are derived through intramembranous development, whereas the growth and development of long bones involve both intramembranous and endochondral processes. Long bones are composed of two wider extremities (the epiphyses), a mid section composed of a more or less cylindrical tube (the diaphysis), and the metaphysis or developmental zone between the first two sections. A layer of epiphyseal cartilage (also called the growth plate) separates the epiphysis and the metaphysis, originating from two independent ossification centers in growing bone. This is responsible for the longitudinal growth of the long bones. The epiphyseal cartilage is progressively calcified and remodeled and finally replaced by bone by the end of the growth period.

The cortex or compact bone forms the thick and dense outer layer of bone that encloses the hematopoietic bone marrow in the diaphysis. In the metaphysis and the epiphysis, the cortex becomes progressively thinner and the inner space is filled with a network of calcified trabeculae (the cancellous or trabecular bone). Hematopoietic bone marrow also fills the spaces between the trabeculae and is in continuity with the medullary cavity of the diaphysis. The epiphysis is covered with a layer of articular cartilage that does not calcify. The articular cartilage is separated from the end of the epiphysis by a very thin cortical-like bone structure. In adults, this calcified growth plate or subchondral bone plate separates the cancellous bone and the articular cartilage.

### Bone Formation/Osteogenesis

Bone formation occurs via two distinct developmental processes: intramembranous ossification and endochondral ossification.[25] Intramembranous ossification takes place in several craniofacial bones and in the lateral part of clavicles, whereas endochondral ossification occurs in the long bones of the limbs, basal parts of the skull, vertebrae, ribs, and medial part of the clavicles. Osteoblasts differentiate directly from mesenchymal condensations in intramembranous ossification. In endochondral ossification, an intermediate step is crucial, involving cartilaginous templates that give rise to the future skeletal elements and play a major role in regulating the developing skeletal elements. In both processes, osteoblasts play a central role in the production of a characteristic extracellular matrix.

Osteoblasts also regulate the differentiation of osteoclasts, the bone resorbing cells. Therefore, osteoblasts play a pivotal role in $Ca^{2+}$ homeostasis. Early histological, cell biological, and biochemical studies performed mainly using cells in culture indicated that the osteoblast-differentiation pathway involved several transitional stages. Such studies indicated that collagen type I and alkaline phosphatase are molecular markers of early-stage differentiation, whereas osteocalcin and mineralization are markers of late-stage differentiation. However, a tight control of collagenous to noncollagenous proteins must take place for normal mineralization to occur. The control of skeletal development also involves a number of signaling molecules that play a role in patterning many embryonic structures such as members of the bone morphogenetic protein (BMP), members of the transforming growth factor-beta (TGF-β) superfamily, fibroblast growth factors, and members of the hedgehog family.[26-28]

BMPs are able to promote osteogenesis, chondrogenesis, and adipogenesis, whereas they inhibit myogenesis from mesenchymal cells.[29] Among the dozens of BMPs known, BMP-2 applied to a matrix carrier protein subcutaneously implanted drives mesenchymal cells recruited from the tissues to degrade the matrix and develop into trabecular bone and cartilage.[30] This BMP-2-dependent bone formation is self-limited, suggesting the presence of endogenous inhibitors of bone formation.[31] TGF-β is present in bone in three isoforms (TGF-β1, -2, and -3) of similar bioactivity.[32] TGF-β has both positive and negative effects on bone. It can induce bone formation when injected in rodents,[33,34] whereas transgenic mice overexpressing TGF-β2 in bone exhibit an osteoporotic phenotype characterized by impaired mineralization.[35] TGF-β modulates the expression and transcriptional activity of Runx2[36] to promote osteoblast differentiation.

## Role of the Subchondral Bone

Articular cartilage is bordered at its base by the subchondral bone plate (or the cortical end plate or the articular bone plate), which is a very thin cortical bone structure. The subchondral bone plate possesses an irregular surface to which the articular cartilage is keyed in. The trabecular subchondral bone is situated under this thin end-plate zone. It contains fatty bone marrow and trabecular bone. Many arterial terminal branches, probably end arteries, are present in the subchondral bone plate and end in sinusoids of uneven caliber and an irregular distribution. These sinusoids terminate in venous radicles forming a transverse sinus, perpendicular to the tiny venous branches.

This venous plexus is very vulnerable to compressive or shearing forces. Tiny vessels penetrate the cortical end plate and can invade the calcified cartilage zone up to the tidemark. In humans, vascular perfusion slowly declines until about the age of 70.[37] However, this perfusion declines not only due to age but individually within joints and in load-bearing areas. As the blood flow in the subchondral bone is 3 to 10 times higher than in trabecular bone,[38] this normal perfusion allows for approximately 50% of the glucose, oxygen, and water requirements of articular cartilage.[39,40] Hence, as this perfusion drops with age it is possibly leading to a decreased nutrition of the deep layers of articular cartilage.

The thickness of the subchondral bone end plate varies also as the vascular supply with age, body weight, location, function, and genetics. However, it is generally much thicker in the central weight-bearing area. Although bone is a harder tissue than articular cartilage it is actually a better shock absorber and hence the normal subchondral bone tissue protects articular cartilage against damage caused by excessive loads. Indeed, articular cartilage deforms less over a stiff and dense bone structure (whereas inhomogeneities in stiffness or in density will deform it more).

## Normal Bone Matrix and Mineral

Bone is formed of an abundant extracellular matrix largely composed of collagen type I (representing 90% of the total protein) and of noncollagenous proteins. Crystals of hydroxyapatite $[3Ca_3(PO_4)_2(OH)_2]$ form the mineral matrix network bound on collagen fibers and in the ground substance. Collagen type I is usually oriented in a preferential direction and hydroxyapatite crystals also tend to be in the same orientation. The ground substance is composed of complexes of glycoproteins and proteoglycans. These anionic complexes are thought to play an important role in the calcification process and the fixation of hydroxyapatite crystals to the collagen fibers via their high ion-binding capacity. The role played by noncollagenous proteins is still not fully characterized, although their presence is essential for the mineralization process. These proteins are for the most part synthesized de novo by bone-forming cells except for a number of plasma proteins preferentially absorbed by the bone matrix (such as α2-HS-glycoprotein synthesized in the liver).

Alternate layers of collagen fibers give adult bone a typical lamellar structure, allowing the highest density of collagen per unit volume of tissue. Two different structures of lamellar bone are known: when lamellae are parallel to each other on a flat surface or when lamellae are concentric around a channel centered on a blood vessel (harvesian canal). During rapid remodeling, fracture healing, or development, collagen fibers do not have a preferential organization. Oriented in bundles and not tightly packed, this type of bone is called woven bone as opposed to lamellar bone.

## OSTEOARTHRITIC BONE AND SUBCHONDRAL BONE

### Bone/Subchondral Bone Structure and Function in Osteoarthritis

In normal joint articular tissue, the subchondral bone is composed of large trabecules with small trabecular space (see Fig. 2.1). Contrasting, in early osteoarthritis there is a thinning of the subchondral bone plate, excessive resorption with reduction of trabecular bone thickness, and increased trabecular space. There is invasion of blood vessels in the cartilage. The late stage of osteoarthritis involves a thinning of the subchondral bone plate and trabecular spaces.

Using macroscopic and histologic methods, the first observation of human osteoarthritic bone tissue is that it is sclerotic and shows increased bone density. However, the apparent density of bone is the bone mass per total volume of tissue. It is suggested that as the volume of tissue increases in osteoarthritis the apparent density follows. Histomorphometric data show that bone volume and total volume increase in osteoarthritis.

This increase in trabecular bone tissue can reach 10 to 15%. This is mainly related to an increase of the thickening of the trabeculae but also may stem from an actual increase in trabecular number. Indeed, the diameter of osteoarthritic long bones and trabeculae

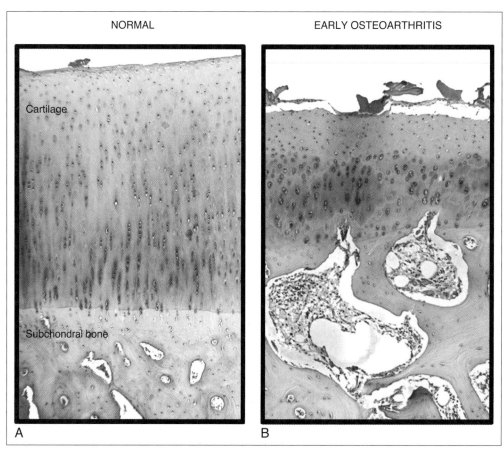

| NORMAL | EARLY OSTEOARTHRITIS |

Cartilage

Subchondral bone

A                                    B

**Fig. 2.1** Representative sections of subchondral bone and cartilage from normal, early osteoarthritis and late osteoarthritis specimens. (A) shows a normal specimen with uniform thick cartilage and a subchondral bone section composed of large trabeculae. (B) shows a similar section in early stages of osteoarthritis with thinning of articular cartilage, expansion of the subchondral bone plate, and invasion of blood vessels into the subchondral region. (C) depicts late-stage osteoarthritis with severe cartilage lesions and thinning of the subchondral bone plate (H & E stain; original magnification × 60). (See Color Plate 1.)

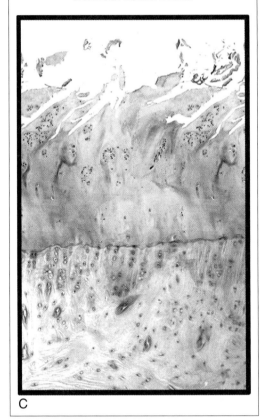

LATE OSTEOARTHRITIS

C

**Fig. 2.1,** cont'd. (See Color Plate 1.)

is wider than normal and would contribute to better strength and fewer fragility fractures. This should then lead to an increase in the apparent bone density and real bone density, as proposed by Dequeker et al.[38] However, density fractionation profiles[4,41] and biochemical studies[15] have demonstrated that subchondral cortical bone and trabecular bone of osteoarthritic patients are less mineralized than age-matched or younger control subjects. Hence, bone density in osteoarthritis would actually decrease, not increase.

One possible explanation for this decrease could be that bone remodeling is increased in osteoarthritis such that bone does not have the opportunity to fully mineralize. A number of studies also indicated that stiffness and bone density are not uniform in osteoarthritic bone tissue and that actually only the bone closest to the articular cartilage influences the integrity of cartilage. Indeed, increased stiffness and bone density only affect stresses in the overlying cartilage if within 3 mm of the osteochondral junction.[42] Moreover, the trabecular bone underlying the subchondral bone plate shows decreased trabecular number and increased intertrabecular spacing in osteoarthritic femoral heads. Trabeculae further away than 3 mm are thicker. Hence, variable stiffness and density of the bone tissue in osteoarthritis may be causing more damage to cartilage integrity than any of these parameters under normal conditions.[43,44]

When considering the contribution of bone in osteoarthritis, we cannot underestimate the role of the subchondral cortical bone plate and the subchondral trabecular bone as key players in the pathophysiology of the disease. Indeed, a large number of studies have explored the structural changes taking place in the subchondral bone during the evolution of osteoarthritis. Correlation has been established between the progression of the disease and patients' symptoms. Most of the clinical correlations are derived from technologies such as X-rays, CT scans, magnetic resonance imaging (MRI), scintigraphy, and biomarkers. Buckland-Wright et al. reported from quantitative microfocal radiography that the earliest anatomic change in osteoarthritic joints is the thickening of the subchondral cortical plate, which precedes changes in the thickness of the articular cartilage measured radiographically as joint space narrowing.[45]

Using labeled bisphosphonate in a scintigraphic study, Dieppe et al.[46] demonstrated an elevated bone cell activity that progressed to severe osteoarthritis. They also showed that an increased bone scintigraphic signal in the affected knee was predictive of the progression of osteoarthritis in the following 5 years.[46] The same authors reported similar results for osteoarthritis of the hand.[47] More recently, these investigators showed that in knee osteoarthritis the scintigraphic abnormalities correlated with synovial fluid levels of osteocalcin (a marker of bone formation).[48]

To test the hypothesis that increased subchondral bone turnover is a determinant of the progression of osteoarthritis, Bettica et al.[9] conducted a study in which the level of urinary N-terminal type I collagen telopeptides (NTX) and C-terminal type I collagen telopeptides (CTX-1)—which are validated markers of bone resorption—were measured at three different time points in patients with knee osteoarthritis. The results from this study demonstrate that over time bone resorption is increased in patients with progressive knee osteoarthritis and is not in those with nonprogressive knee osteoarthritis. The increase in bone resorption biomarkers seen in patients with progressive knee osteoarthritis had a similar profile as the one observed in patients with osteoporosis.

MRI is ideal in assessing global structural changes in osteoarthritis, particularly in longitudinal studies of cartilage and bone and early changes that have been overlooked by less sensitive imaging technologies. It is now possible to quantify the trabecular architecture and generate information such as the trabecular number and width in the trabecular bone volume fraction and trabecular separation.[49,50] The main findings from these studies have been that the increased bone turnover, subchondral bone marrow edema-like lesions, and bone attrition are very strong predictors of structural worsening of knee osteoarthritis.[51-53]

A number of studies have focused on the exploration of the subchondral trabecular bone structural changes in knee osteoarthritic patients. In a cross-sectional study, Beuf et al.[54] found that in osteoarthritis the loss of femoral trabecular bone was correlated to the severity of the disease. Blumenkrantz et al.[55] in a 2-year longitudinal study in knee osteoarthritic patients using high-definition MRI found that the loss of cartilage volume/thickness and the deterioration of the subchondral bone structure were interdependent. In these patients, a positive correlation was established between the loss of cartilage and the subchondral bone sclerosis and osteopenia of the underlying trabecular bone.

The observation that alterations of the bony bed preceded cartilage changes in the *Macaca fascicularis* primate model of osteoarthritis[3,23] and in the Dunkin–Hartley guinea pig model also strongly support the concept that osteoarthritis is a more generalized bone metabolic disease. Moreover, an increase in both bone formation and resorption indices in osteoarthritis patients has been obtained[15,56-61] and could explain abnormal remodeling and low mineralization.

The exact roles of subchondral bone remodeling and osteophyte formation, which are well-recognized manifestations of human osteoarthritis, remain largely unknown. It is suggested that osteophyte formation may play a compensatory role in the redistribution of biomechanical forces to provide articular cartilage protection. The mechanisms responsible for osteophyte formation in osteoarthritis have not yet been elucidated. However, in the murine knee joint it was shown that TGF-β and interleukin-1β (among other factors) might be implicated.[62] It is also of note that TGF-β levels are elevated in osteoarthritic subchondral bone compared to normal and that in vitro osteoarthritic osteoblasts release more TGF-β1 than normal osteoblasts.[12]

Although it is currently suggested that subchondral bone alterations may be more intimately related to the osteoarthritis process rather than merely a consequence of the disease,[63] the question that still remains to be answered is whether changes in subchondral bone induce or participate in disease progression. Healing of trabecular microfractures in osteoarthritic subchondral bone could generate a stiffer bone that no longer functions as an effective shock absorber.[5,64] Indeed, studies in knee osteoarthritis have shown that subchondral stiffening can increase trabecular bone strain in the proximal tibial plateau[65,66] and distal tibia.[67]

However, no direct experimental evidence of cartilage lesions due to bone strain has been provided.

Despite this limitation, bone strain could lead to subsequent cartilage lesions, especially in individuals with already compromised articular cartilage. Hence, a steep stiffness gradient in the underlying subchondral bone may be an initiating mechanism of osteoarthritis, as the integrity of the overlying articular cartilage depends on the mechanical properties of its bony bed. Indeed, inhomogeneities in density or stiffness of the subchondral bone are key factors that could modulate cartilage loss. The articular cartilage that is above a less dense and more compliant bone will deform more than that above a denser and stiffer bone. Such a deformation can then stretch the articular cartilage at the edge of the joint contact area, generating tensile and shear stresses.[7]

Reports indicate that the subchondral bone remodeling occurring in osteoarthritis involves both bone resorption and bone formation. Several studies have demonstrated that in the more advanced stage of the disease bone formation was predominant in the different layers of the tissues.[68,69] In contrast in the early phase, studies identified a remodeling process that primarily favors bone resorption.[6,8-10,14,21,70] Most of the later findings came from experimental models allowing for a chronologic evaluation of events. In the early phase of experimental osteoarthritis, the subchondral plate and the underlying trabecular bone become thinner (indicating excess bone resorption).[6,8-10,21] These changes are associated with an increase in the number and size of the remodeling units.[8] Moreover, in experimental dog osteoarthritis osteoblasts isolated from subchondral bone were shown to produce an excess of many biochemical factors[11,71] previously demonstrated to favor either the maturation and activation of osteoclasts and/or the resorption of bone matrix.[72]

Bone remodeling is a tightly controlled mechanism that involves coupling between a mineralized collagen type I bone matrix laid down by osteoblasts and osteoclasts resorbing this matrix. Although late-stage osteoarthritis is associated with a thickening of subchondral bone, explants of the femoral head of osteoarthritic patients at autopsy showed a low mineralization pattern compared to normal.[4] However, the trabecular thickening observed in osteoarthritic subchondral bone could reflect osteoid volume increases and not an increase in bone mineralization.[4,15,73,74]

Of note, the distribution of cancellous bone microdamage in the proximal femur of osteoarthritic patients is higher than normal individuals at autopsy,[75] consistent with the reported material property differences for osteoarthritis.[41] Such a situation would then retard normal remodeling by uncoupling bone formation and resorption. Indicators of bone remodeling are also increased in osteoarthritic patients. Therefore, the increase in indices of both bone formation and resorption in osteoarthritic patients could explain abnormal remodeling and low mineralization. An increase in material density but not in mineral density would retard normal remodeling by uncoupling bone formation and resorption. Abnormal mineralization in osteoarthritis may then be viewed as an osteoblast problem.

## Osteoarthritic Subchondral Osteoblasts

### Phenotypic Features and Metabolic Activity

The morphologic alteration in osteoarthritic subchondral osteoblasts does not appear to be the consequence of a change in serum levels of humoral factors or hormones[76] but of an alteration in local signals. Several studies have provided strong evidence that even in the early stage of osteoarthritis phenotypic differences in subchondral osteoblasts are present and these cells are metabolically more active. Indeed, a large number of factors (including inflammatory and growth factors and proteases) are produced in excessive amounts in this disease tissue. In addition, the collagen synthesized differs from the one synthesized by normal osteoblasts.[73] The latter may likely have a deleterious effect on the mechanical properties and the mineralization of the subchondral bone due to the loose packing of the fibers.

Determination of synovial fluid osteocalcin (a marker of bone formation) and serum osteopontin (a bone-specific matrix protein) suggests that new bone synthesis exceeds degradation in osteoarthritis.[48] In that osteopontin increases shortly following trauma, these findings imply that alterations in bone cell activity may occur quite early in the disease. Gevers and Dequeker[77] showed elevated serum osteocalcin levels in cortical bone explants in women with hand osteoarthritis. This group also reported that insulin-like growth factors (IGF) 1 and 2 and TGF-β levels are higher in samples of iliac crest bone of patients with osteoarthritis,[18] and hence at a site distant from weight-bearing joints (suggesting a generalized bone metabolic dysfunction).

An imbalance between collagen and non-collagen protein synthesis (such as osteocalcin by osteoarthritic osteoblasts) can lead to an increase in bone volume without a concomitant increase in the bone mineralization pattern. Abnormal collagen content may also lead to abnormal mineralization because only native collagen type I fibrils can mineralize. Although Mansel et al.[15] reported that the collagen type I content was elevated in trabecular bone of femoral heads of osteoarthritic patients, further data showed that these collagen properties were abnormal. Collagen type I is composed of a heterotrimer of α1 and α2 chains at an average ratio of 2.4:1 in normal bone, yet this was found to vary from 4:1 to 17:1 (α1 versus α2) in osteoarthritic bone tissue.[73]

A reduction in α2 chains may lead to a tighter packing of collagen fibers, and coupled with the reduction in cross-links observed in osteoarthritic bone tissue[15] and the overhydroxylation of lysine in collagen fibrils[73] could explain the reduction in bone mineralization.

As osteoarthritic osteoblasts show increased osteocalcin and alkaline phosphatase levels in vitro,[16,78] as observed in situ,[77] this implies that the in vivo alterations are due to abnormal cellular metabolism, not to alterations in systemic regulation. Osteoarthritic osteoblasts are also partially resistant to parathyroid hormone (PTH) stimulation[16] due to a decreased expression of PTH receptors,[79] a situation that could favor collagen synthesis because PTH inhibits collagen synthesis.[80,81] Whether this situation is also linked to abnormal degradation of collagen remains unknown. The activities of two matrix metalloproteinases (MMP-2 and MMP-9) are elevated in proximal cancellous bone tissue isolated from the femoral head of osteoarthritic patients,[15] a situation possibly linked with abnormal collagen matrix deposition.

The exact mechanism(s) responsible for abnormal osteoblast function in osteoarthritic individuals remains unknown. However, it is of note that adipocytes share a common mesenchymal stem cell precursor with osteoblasts, chondrocytes, tenocytes, and myoblasts (all cells affected by osteoarthritis) and that osteoblast maturation from bone marrow stromal cells in osteoarthritic patients is enhanced and that of adipocytes and chondrocytes is blunted.[82] This suggests a possible link between abnormal lipid metabolism and connective tissues in osteoarthritis. Hence, osteoarthritis may be a metabolic disease in which systemic and/or local factors induce changes in all skeletal tissues by modifying the formation and activity of mesenchymal precursor cells.[83]

This abnormal subchondral bone osteoblast metabolism may be linked with leptin, a key factor in adipocyte maturation.[84,85] Leptin, the product of the obese (ob) gene, is a 16-kDa secreted protein produced by white adipocytes and placenta that functions as an afferent signal to influence energy homeostasis through effects on energy intake and expenditure.[86,87] Leptin levels are increased in osteoarthritic cartilage,[88] and leptin injections into the joints of normal rats can mimic osteoarthritic features.[89] Indeed, leptin enhances alkaline phosphatase activity, osteocalcin release, and the production of collagen 1 α1 chains, IGF-1, and TGF-β1 levels by approximately 40%.[90] All these features are increased in osteoarthritic subchondral osteoblasts compared to normal.[12,16,78,79] Leptin is also associated with inflammatory states[91-93] and stimulates prostaglandin E$_2$ (PGE$_2$)[94] and leukotriene (LT) production.[95] Of note, we previously observed that osteoarthritic subchondral osteoblasts produced high levels of PGE$_2$ and/or LTB$_4$.[12,13] Leptin signaling contributes to the mechanisms of joint inflammation in antigen-induced arthritis by regulating both humoral and cell-mediated immune responses.[91]

Evidence that osteocalcin knockout mice had an increased mineralization pattern without significant effects on bone resorption[96] suggests that the elevated osteocalcin levels in osteoarthritis may contribute to the abnormal mineralization pattern in these patients. Moreover, in the osteoarthritic hip cancellous bone compartment a combination of increased MMP-2 and alkaline phosphatase activity (indicating increased collagen turnover) has been observed.[15]

Bone sclerosis noted in osteoarthritic subchondral bone may be linked to an abnormal regulation of the urokinase (uPA)/plasmin system, IGF-1/IGFBPs, TGF-β, IL-6, and PGE$_2$.[12,13,16] These may all influence the production of collagenases and other proteolytic pathways, and ultimately promote matrix remodeling/degradation. In osteoarthritic subchondral osteoblasts, uPA was found to regulate its own activity via a positive feedback loop wherein plasmin generated by uPA-dependent plasminogen hydrolysis can stimulate uPA activity directly.[78] Interestingly, in these osteoarthritic osteoblasts IGF-1 can block this positive feedback loop while showing no such effect on normal cells. If these in vitro data reflect the in vivo situation, this mechanism could retard bone remodeling in osteoarthritis and ultimately favor the development of bone sclerosis.

IGFs are among the most important growth factors regulating bone formation.[97] IGF-1 and -2 and TGF-β levels are higher in iliac crest bone of patients with osteoarthritis,[18] and hence at a site distant from weight-bearing joints, suggesting a generalized bone metabolic dysfunction in this disease. Indeed, IGF-1 is an important actor in the changes observed in bone and cartilage in osteoarthritis. Subchondral osteoblasts produce more IGF-1 and fewer IGFBPs compared to normal,[16,98] leading to enhanced free IGF-1 levels, which could promote bone remodeling[99] and secondarily increase bone stiffness, a situation exacerbating cartilage matrix degradation.

TGF-β and IGF-1 are both involved in matrix deposition and turnover, and osteoarthritic osteoblasts produce more of these factors than normal.[18] TGF-β stimulates matrix synthesis[100] and collagenase activity, whereas IGF-1 inhibits the expression of MMPs in bone cells.[101] Thereby, the combined increase of these growth factors could favor matrix deposition in bone and overall limit degradation. To that effect, a study in murine knee joint demonstrated that intraarticular injections of TGF-β into the joint induce osteoarthritic changes[62] and that blocking endogenous TGF-β production during experimental osteoarthritis prevents osteophyte formation.[102] The local role of both TGF-β and IGF-1 may itself be linked to an abnormal response

to leptin of osteoarthritic subchondral osteoblasts, as leptin is able to stimulate both TGF-β and IGF-1 expression in joint tissues.[89]

Among the cytokines and eicosanoids produced by bone cells, IL-1β, IL-6, PGE$_2$, and LTB$_4$ are the most important regulators of the turnover of the extracellular matrix. Interestingly, the analysis of subchondral bone cells from osteoarthritic patients with similar clinical disease profiles can discriminate two groups based on the low or high level of PGE$_2$ and IL-6.[12] In turn, the production of PGE$_2$ by osteoblasts was inversely correlated with the synthesis of LTB$_4$.[13] PGE$_2$ stimulates bone formation at low concentrations, but can exert inhibitory activity at high concentrations while stimulating collagen synthesis and promoting the proliferation of osteoblasts.[103-105] Conversely, LTB$_4$ stimulates osteoclast differentiation and bone resorption.[106] Therefore, conditions in which a high ratio of PGE$_2$/LTB$_4$ is present could promote subchondral bone formation.

### Bone Genetic Factors Involved in Osteoarthritis

One proposal for the alteration of the subchondral bone is that a bone genetic disorder leads to osteoarthritis. Indeed, it has recently been postulated that a vitamin D receptor (VDR) gene locus, the TaqI polymorphism (which has previously been shown to be associated with a high bone mass), was responsible for the observed difference in bone density in osteoarthritic patients.[107] However, recent data indicated the unlikeliness of this association. Similarly, other gene polymorphisms, such as the genes encoding the α1 chain of type I collagen (COL1A1), the COL2A1, the IL-6, and the estrogen receptor gene, have recently been studied.[108-110] However, none of them could be clearly associated with osteoarthritis. Linkage analysis revealed suggestive evidence for association of the IL-1 gene cluster on chromosome 2q13 in affected sibling pairs with knee osteoarthritis,[111] but no such evidence could be found for hip osteoarthritis.

## SUBCHONDRAL BONE/CARTILAGE CROSS-TALK

Healthy cartilage is avascular and aneural (see Fig. 2.2). This suggests that nutrients must enter articular cartilage either from the surface via the synovial fluid or from the underlying subchondral bone. For a long period of time, synovial fluid was believed to be the single route because there is no anatomic barrier and the cartilage cannot survive in its absence.[112] However, in a number of circumstances cartilage degenerates despite being in contact with normal synovial fluid.

We now know that nutrition of articular cartilage by subchondral bone is an obvious route, although it was

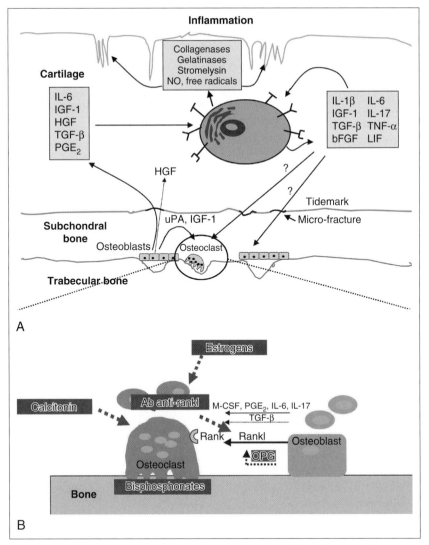

**Fig. 2.2** Illustration of the major pathophysiological pathways involved in osteoarthritis: (A) at the cartilage and subchondral bone interface and (B) in subchondral bone tissue remodelling. In B, potential therapeutic interventions that could modulate these pathways are identified in blue rectangles. Definitions: bFGF (basic fibroblast growth factor), LIF (leukemia inhibitory factor), IGF-1 (insulin-like growth factor 1), IL-1/IL-6/IL-17 (interleukin-1, -6, -17), M-CSF (macrophage colony stimulating factor), NO (nitric oxide), OPG (osteoprotegerin), $PGE_2$ (prostaglandin $E_2$), RANK (receptor activator of NF-κB), RANKL (receptor activator of NF-κB ligand), TGF-β (transforming growth factor β), TNF-α (tumor necrosis factor α), uPA (urokinase plasminogen activator). (See Color Plate 2.)

objected that the dense calcifications in the basal zone of normal articular cartilage could be an insurmountable barrier to solute and fluid diffusion.[40,113] Various researcher groups demonstrated the existence of channels between the subchondral region and the uncalcified cartilage.[114,115] To better understand the concept of a cross-talk between these two tissues, a brief review of cartilage structure during normal and osteoarthritis conditions is outlined.

## Normal Cartilage

Articular cartilage is a remarkably durable tissue that provides almost frictionless motion between the articulating surfaces of diarthrodial joints while protecting the underlying bones from mechanical stresses of normal joint use. Cartilage is composed of a single type of highly specialized cells termed chondrocytes. Chondrocytes are of mesenchymal stem cell origin and are responsible for synthesizing the cartilage extracellular matrix. In a hypoxic environment, such as in articular cartilage, chondrocytes are mainly anaerobic. Their low turnover rate and sparse distribution allow for little cell-to-cell contact.[116] Chondrocytes constitute only 2% of the total volume of adult articular cartilage. The survival of these cells depends on the proper chemical and mechanical environment, including growth factors, mechanical loads, hydrostatic pressures, and piezoelectric forces.[117]

Chondrocytes maintain the cartilage extracellular matrix composed of collagen (10 to 20%), proteoglycans (10 to 20%), and water (65 to 80%). Type II collagen is the major collagen (90%) found in cartilage and belongs to the fibrillar collagens. It is composed of three identical polypeptide chain $\alpha_1$ (II) synthesized and secreted as procollagen precursors before undergoing maturation by protease and lysyloxidase activities and leading to cross-linked fibril formation in the extracellular matrix.[118] The network of type II collagen fibrils provides the tensile strength and is essential for maintaining both the volume and the shape of the tissue.[119] Three other genetically different collagens (types VI, IX, and XI) are also found in cartilage. Although present in low abundance, they also play a major role in the structural and functional properties of the extracellular matrix. For example, type IX collagen is a bridging molecule between type II collagen fibrils.[120,121]

Proteoglycans are another major component of the extracellular matrix. They are composed of a core protein, which is glycosylated with numerous glycosaminoglycan (GAG) chains. Aggrecan represents 90% of proteoglycans in cartilage. Its non-covalent interaction with hyaluronic acid, which is a linear high-molecular-weight GAG, gives rise to aggregates.[118] This non-covalent interaction is stabilized by a link protein. In addition, other proteoglycans (termed small non-aggregating proteoglycans)—such as biglycan, decorin, and fibromodulin—constitute the cartilage extracellular matrix. Proteoglycans are entrapped in collagen fibril network. The negative charges of their GAGs confer highly hydrophilic properties that give articular cartilage its ability to undergo reversible deformation. Other proteins (such as anchorin, cartilage oligomeric matrix protein [COMP], fibronectin, and GP-39) are also of importance and have shown some functions in the cartilage extracellular matrix.[122]

Articular cartilage composition and architecture are organized in zones.[116] The superficial zone consists of tightly packed collagen fibers parallel to the articular surface and a cellular layer of flattened chondrocytes. Preservation of this superficial layer is critical to protect the deeper zones. Type IX collagen is found in this layer between type II bundles that provide resistance to shear. It is thought that this layer limits passage of large molecules between synovial fluid and cartilage. The transitional layer (or intermediate zone) is composed of spherical chondrocytes, proteoglycans, and obliquely oriented collagen fibers that primarily resist compressive forces but also serve as a transition between the shearing forces on the surface and the compressive forces placed on the deeper layers. The deep zone consists of collagen fibers and chondrocytes oriented perpendicularly to the articular surface, which resist compressive loads.[123] Deep into the articular cartilage, and separated from it by the tidemark, is a layer of calcified cartilage.[124] The proteoglycan content increases in the matrix from the articular surface to the tidemark.[125]

## Osteoarthritic Cartilage

The complex structure and function of normal articular cartilage can be disrupted even by minor injuries.[123] Circumstances that impair chondrocyte function can disrupt the balance of synthesis and catabolism in favor of cartilage degradation, which over time can lead to osteoarthritis. The response to the injury depends on the severity and depth of the injury. A seemingly trivial low-energy superficial injury may disrupt or damage cells and matrix and initiate a cascade toward degeneration in the absence of visible changes to the surface. Larger macro-disruption injuries may result in visible chondral fissures or partial-thickness loss. Full-thickness injuries result when the subchondral bone is violated, often resulting in an osteochondral fracture.

The highly specific microscopic anatomy and interdependent physiology of articular cartilage can be disrupted by small, superficial injuries, even without immediate cartilage loss. Superficial damage will injure chondrocytes, limit their metabolic capacity for repair, and lead to decreased proteoglycan concentration, increased hydration, and altered fibrillar organization of collagen.[126-128] Proteoglycan loss, increased water content, decreased cartilage stiffness, and increased hydraulic permeability lead to increased force transmission to the underlying subchondral bone, which increases its stiffness and in turn causes impact loads to be more readily transmitted to the partially damaged cartilage. This vicious cycle is thought to contribute to the progression of partial-thickness articular cartilage injuries.[129]

The biochemical changes in early osteoarthritis seem to indicate increased synthesis rather than destruction.[130,131] Evidence of a strong anabolic component is even more obvious in experimental osteoarthritis. The first change observed is cell division at the site of the future osteophyte, followed by cloning of chondrocytes in the matrix.[132,133] Osteophytes may be identifiable early in the process.[134] These unequivocally anabolic changes are soon followed by evidence of catabolism,[135] but it is now known that the anabolism remains dominant for a long period.[136-138] This early anabolic dominance is reflected in the biochemical changes.[139]

Further in the disease, an imbalance between synthesis and degradation of the extracellular matrix occurs, leading to cartilage component degradation under matrix metalloproteinase activities. Several cytokines, such as interleukins, secreted by the synovial membrane were shown to be implicated in the clinical phase of osteoarthritis. In the osteoarthritis-inflamed synovium, the proinflammatory cytokines stimulate the production of proteases such as metalloproteinases.

Among the different metalloproteinases, collagenase-3 (MMP-13) plays a major role in cartilage degradation.[140-142] This protease has a high level of activity on type II collagen, and in osteoarthritis is predominantly localized in the lower intermediate and deep layers of cartilage.[143] This is of great importance because it is well known that the collagen network destruction is a key step in the progression of osteoarthritis. Moreover, in the intermediate and deep cartilage layers type II collagen fibers are of the largest size and chondrocytes are most efficient in reconstituting qualitative as well as quantitative extracellular matrix.[144] These and other data have led to the conclusion that this enzyme is involved in the remodeling of the cartilage. MMP-13 also showed activities against other cartilage extracellular matrix, including the aggrecan and some proteoglycan families.[145]

The damage occurring at the superficial layer of cartilage in osteoarthritis is easy to identify even macroscopically (i.e., fibrillations and changes in cartilage color [turns yellowish]). In turn, modifications in the deep layer of cartilage are more difficult to discriminate. However, histological data reveal the existence of micro-cracks in the deep layers of cartilage. More importantly, the probability of obtaining micro-injuries due to overloading within the calcified layer (more rigid) is much higher than in uncalcified cartilage and subchondral bone. Then, fibrovascular tissue could grow into calcified cartilage and build new bone.

This process is accompanied by continuous advancement of the mineralization zone into the uncalcified cartilage. In severe injuries, repair advancement is so fast that a new mineralization zone develops and builds a new tidemark, leaving behind zones of non-calcified cartilage. Data from the duplication or even triplication of tidemark show the presence of micro-injuries to the subchondral bone.[146-148] During osteoarthritis, angiogenesis occurs at the osteochondral junction. The blood vessels formed may penetrate the calcified cartilage within fibrovascular channels. With increasing severity of osteoarthritis, these vascular channels breach the tidemark and blood vessels may be found more superficially in the uncalcified articular cartilage.[149] These new vessels may also be associated with new sensory nerves.[150]

## Chondrocyte Phenotype Alterations During Osteoarthritis

Evidence supports the view that articular chondrocytes are susceptible to phenotypic destabilization during osteoarthritis.[151] The metabolic modifications of chondrocytes are both related to new stimuli (proinflammatory cytokines, growth factors, and so on) and changes in the extracellular cartilage matrix composition.[152] Cell phenotype deteriorates and chondrocytes express traits of transient growth plate chondrocytes such as hypertrophy, alkaline phosphatase, type X collagen, and mineralization.[153,154] At a certain stage, the chondrocytes reduce their expression of aggrecan and collagen type II, although they are still very active cells and start expressing collagen types I, III, and V.[155-157] Osteoarthritic chondrocytes also express type IIA collagen, which is a marker of prechondrocyte phenotype. This clearly demonstrates the implication of phenotypic alterations of chondrocytes despite potentially high synthetic activity. Therefore, phenotypic alteration represents another potential reason for the anabolic failure of chondrocytes in osteoarthritic cartilage.

During the progression of osteoarthritis, clusters of chondrocytes appear in the cartilage upper zone. These cells express collagen types not normally found in normal cartilage: types I and III and their proteoglycans lose some properties.[156] Interestingly, a reversion to a fetal-like phenotype and the reinitiation of fetal skeletal developmental processes also occur in the deepest zones of osteoarthritic cartilage. At this location, the cells start to express type X collagen,[158] which is a specific marker for hypertrophy of growth plate chondrocytes,[159,160] and apoptosis occurs.[161] Other developmental genes, such as annexins II and V,[162,163] MMP-13,[141,164] osteopontin,[165] and galectin-3,[152] are also reexpressed throughout osteoarthritic cartilage, and some at the deep zone.

## Evidence for a Cross-talk Between Subchondral Bone and Cartilage

As discussed in the previous sections, although the initiating event responsible for the degradation of cartilage in osteoarthritic patients is still elusive the concept of a key role of the subchondral bone tissue in this disease is gaining strong support.[16-18,166] A plausible hypothesis could be that cytokines, growth factors, and eicosanoids produced locally by subchondral bone tissue seep through the bone/cartilage interface and induce changes in the cartilage metabolism. Although it was previously thought that the calcified cartilage layer was an impenetrable structure, two independent groups demonstrated the presence of many channels between the subchondral region and the uncalcified cartilage (Fig. 2.2A). Moreover, Sokoloff[146] previously demonstrated the presence of micro-cracks in the calcified layer of aging articular cartilage. These micro-cracks and the vascularization in the subchondral bone plate could facilitate the transfer of humoral information from the subchondral bone region to the basal layer of cartilage.

25

The sources of angiogenic signals to the subchondral bone remain poorly understood. Osteoarthritic chondrocytes within the deeper layers of articular cartilage produce angiogenic factors such as vascular endothelial growth factor (VEGFs).[167] With the disruption of the tidemark, angiogenic factors may also reach the osteochondral junction by mass transport and diffusion from the synovium through synovial fluid and the cartilage matrix. The synovial fluid from patients with osteoarthritis stimulates endothelial tube formation in vitro,[168] and synovial tissues and fluid from patients with osteoarthritis contain a variety of angiogenic factors. The subchondral bone could itself contribute or support angiogenic stimuli within the osteoarthritic joint through expression of angiogenic factors by osteoblasts.[149,169,170]

There are several factors produced by subchondral bone cells that are known to be capable of inducing cartilage catabolic changes. For instance, TGF-β has the capacity to induce MMP-13 synthesis by chondrocytes and therefore could be responsible for the increased level of this enzyme found in the intermediate and deep layers of the disease cartilage.[143] This enzyme (as well as the cathepsin K, which are synthesized by bone cells) has been demonstrated to be involved both in endochondral ossification and in osteoarthritic cartilage degradation.[171,172] Moreover, the abnormal osteoarthritic osteoblast production of pro-inflammatory cytokines and $PGE_2/LTB_4$ has a significant influence on the metabolism of the overlying cartilage. This situation would then concur with the observations made by Westacott et al.,[17] which showed that factor(s) produced by osteoarthritic subchondral osteoblasts can promote the breakdown of normal cartilage.

We recently showed that a factor first identified in the liver, the hepatocyte growth factor (HGF), could be an important candidate for such a cross-talk between the subchondral bone and cartilage.[169] HGF was found to be preferentially located in the deep layers of osteoarthritic cartilage.[173,174] We further showed that surprisingly chondrocytes did not express or produce this factor. However, HGF production was also recently demonstrated in cells isolated from the trabecular bone.[175,176] Subchondral osteoblasts also produce HGF, and higher levels are found in osteoarthritic osteoblasts compared to normal.[169]

Since HGF induces MMP-13 synthesis in chondrocytes[177] and in situ MMP-13 is located mainly at the deep zone of osteoarthritic cartilage,[143] altogether these data suggested that following its synthesis by subchondral osteoblasts HGF can reach the deep layers of articular cartilage via local vascularization and/or channels (where it promotes cartilage breakdown and/or enhances matrix remodeling). This intimate link between articular cartilage and subchondral bone is further reflected by the observation that autologous chondrocyte implantation for cartilage repair is less effective than osteochondral cylinder transplantation: the former produced fibrocartilage, whereas the latter retained its hyaline character.[178]

## SUBCHONDRAL BONE CHANGES AND DISEASE SYMPTOMS

### Bone Marrow Edema

Recent studies by Felson et al.,[52,179] which have explored the subchondral bone marrow changes in osteoarthritis, have brought an interesting new perspective into the disease symptoms and risk for its progression. In a first cross-sectional study of knee osteoarthritic patients, the authors found a strong correlation between the bone marrow edema on MRI (defined as the area of increased signal adjacent to the subcortical bone) and the presence of pain but not pain severity.

This is further supported by a recent study by Raynauld et al.[51] Felson et al. in a second longitudinal study found in knee osteoarthritic patients that the presence of bone marrow edema was largely related to limb alignment. Medial bone marrow lesions were seen mainly in patients with varus limbs, and lateral lesions were seen primarily in patients with valgus limbs. However, even after adjustment for mal-alignment there was a substantial residual association of bone marrow edema lesions with radiographic progression of osteoarthritic cartilage lesions.

### Therapeutic Approaches

The ultimate goal in the treatment of osteoarthritis is to improve or preserve the patient's joint structure by preventing the destruction of the articular tissue, including cartilage and bone. Thus, it is tempting to hypothesize that bone rather than cartilage may be the site of the causally most significant pathophysiologic events. Therefore, therapies that interfere with bone remodeling could block or at least attenuate the progression not only of tissue changes but of cartilage alterations. The rationale in a number of pre-clinical models of osteoarthritis was based on data showing that subchondral bone changes are mainly resorptive in nature within the time schedule set for the treatment study, and that anti-resorptive agents could reduce its progression.

Using the experimental dog ACL model of osteoarthritis, Manicourt et al.[180] demonstrated that treatment with calcitonin simultaneously reduced the level of urinary bone resorption biomarkers (pyridinium crosslinks), the severity of cartilage lesions, and the size of osteophytes. Howell et al.[181] reported that the severity of microscopic cartilage lesions and osteophyte formation in the same animal model was reduced by treatment with the bisphosphonate etidronate. Interestingly, although Myers et al.[182] demonstrated that treatment with a bisphosphonate (NE-10055) reduced the formation and resorption of cancellous subchondral bone and improved the biochemical changes of the osteoarthritis cartilage this treatment had no effect on the pathologic changes of the cartilage or on osteophyte formation.

A recent study by Hayami[70] in the rat ACL model indicated that treatment with alendronate reduced the appearance of cartilage lesions and osteophyte formation as well as the resorption of the subchondral bone. The effect of alendronate was linked to its action at reducing the local release in the bone of active TGF-β, and inhibition of the expression levels of MMP-9 in bone and MMP-13 in cartilage. The findings from this latter study are also well in line with the study of Pelletier et al.[183] in the dog ACL model, in which licofelone (a dual inhibitor of 5-lipoxygenase and cyclooxygenase activities) inhibited the development of cartilage lesions and subchondral bone resorption by reducing the synthesis of MMP-13 and cathepsin K in subchondral bone cells and cartilage chondrocytes.

The reduction of the subchondral bone remodeling and resorption in this model was also reduced by an NSAID (inhibitors of cyclooxygenase activity), carprofen.[71] This effect was associated with a reduction in the level of synthesis of several proteolytic enzymes, including uPA, and growth factors known to be involved in bone remodeling. These two sets of data are concordant with the demonstration of the key role played by the eicosanoids $PGE_2$ and $LTB_4$ in mediating the abnormal synthetic activity of human osteoarthritic subchondral osteoblasts.[13]

Altogether, these data strengthen the notion that therapeutic interventions that specifically inhibit bone resorption could have the potential to be used as disease-modifying osteoarthritic drugs (DMOADs). It is often very difficult to extrapolate the data from preclinical studies for clinical assessment. A recent study by Carbone et al.[184] has brought forth new information that may help better understand the potential role of anti-resorptive drugs in the treatment of osteoarthritis. The results for this cross-sectional study in knee osteoarthritic patients showed that treatment with alendronate reduces the severity of knee pain. In addition, patients treated with both alendronate and estrogen showed a reduction of the subchondral bone attrition and bone marrow edema-like abnormalities as assessed by MRI. However, no significant association was found in patients treated with these anti-resorptive drugs and osteoarthritis radiographic changes. Due to the nature of the study, the information provided on the effect of such treatment on disease progression is very limited.

Only longitudinal studies with appropriate imaging technology would be able to answer the question in regard to structural subchondral bone and cartilage changes. Results from a phase II clinical trial demonstrated that risedronate could significantly reduce the symptoms as well as the progression of cartilage degradation as assessed by X-rays. These changes were also correlated with a reduction in the level of biomarkers of cartilage degradation (CTX-II) and bone remodeling/resorption (CTX-I).[185]

The mechanisms by which anti-resorptive drugs could reduce the progression of osteoarthritis are most likely related to the inhibition of subchondral bone remodeling. The inhibition of the activity of osteoblasts could lead to a reduction in the synthesis of cytokines and growth factors, thus decreasing their diffusion into the cartilage. Bisphosphonates could also inhibit the synthesis and secretion of a number of MMPs, including MMP-9 and MMP-13,[186,187] providing a rationale to the hypothesis that these drugs could have DMOAD effects.

The most recent knowledge of the underlying molecular pathologic mechanisms leading to bone remodeling/resorption in arthritic diseases such as osteoarthritis will help bring new therapeutic strategies to clinical practice.[72] For instance, three factors (RANK, RANKL, and OPG) have been clearly demonstrated to be key elements involved in bone resorption (Fig. 2.2B). In brief, RANKL belongs to the TNF superfamily and is an essential mediator of osteoclastogenesis. It is produced from osteoblasts, synovial fibroblasts, chondrocytes, and activated T lymphocytes.[188,189] RANKL binds directly to the receptor RANK on pre-osteoclasts and osteoclasts, resulting in the differentiation of osteoclast progenitors as well as an activation of mature osteoclasts. It is therefore implicated in the osteoclastogenic process.[189,190]

The biological activity of RANKL is regulated by the soluble decoy receptor osteoprotegerin (OPG), another TNF-receptor superfamily member secreted by osteoblasts.[191] OPG competitively inhibits RANKL binding to RANK on the cell surface of osteoclast precursor cells and mature osteoclasts, thus inhibiting the osteoclastogenic actions of RANKL. The levels of OPG and RANKL are often reciprocally regulated by bone active cytokines and hormones. Excessive production of RANKL and/or deficiency of OPG may therefore contribute to increased bone resorption. Clinical trials are already under way using OPG and RANKL antibodies to test their efficacy in the treatment of osteoporosis and of bone erosions in rheumatoid arthritic patients. The potential of these agents as DMOAD is very appealing in the context of the subchondral bone remodeling taking place in osteoarthritis and its likely role in the pathophysiology of cartilage degradation.

Only appropriate clinical trials will be able to provide the information most needed to answer this important question.

## SUMMARY

The preservation of a joint structure is dependent, to a great extent, on the ability to keep intact the architecture of the main supportive structures (cartilage and bone). Osteoarthritis is a result of alterations in these tissue materials that lead to pain, loss of motion, and instability. Data suggests that those changes are caused by a disturbance in the articular joint remodeling process. The strength and function of bone depend on the properties of the tissue (the material) and on their structural parameters (i.e., geometric arrangement). The subchondral bone remodeling in degenerating osteoarthritis is the end result from several distinct biological processes operating temporally within the articulation. In short, there is an increase in the metabolism of subchondral bone with an imbalance that may lead to resorption or bone deposition depending on the stage of the disease process.

The occurrence of the subchondral bone changes, and more particularly of the osteoblast metabolism, is now well established, and there is emerging evidence to suggest that changes in bone may precede changes in cartilage. Bone, rather than cartilage, may be the site of the causally most significant pathophysiologic events. The ultimate goal in the treatment of osteoarthritis is to improve or preserve the patient's joint structure by preventing the destruction of cartilage and bone. This changed view of the pathogenesis of osteoarthritis from cartilage to the involvement of the entire articular joint and the recognition of early changes in the subchondral bone provide the potential for new approaches to the understanding and treatment of this painful and debilitating disease.

The subchondral bone changes in osteoarthritis are numerous and seem to be predictive not only of disease symptoms but of the progression of osteoarthritic lesions. In a large number of both pre-clinical and clinical studies, the presence of structural changes indicative of bone resorption is clearly linked to disease progression. Therapeutic strategies that reduce bone remodeling and resorption could improve the symptoms related to osteoarthritis and reduce the progression of the disease, more particularly by preventing the progression of cartilage degeneration.

There is both greater turnover and greater subchondral bone volume in osteoarthritis. Thus, although the tissue material stiffness is less (hypomineralized) the structural stiffness of the bone is greater. Therefore, restraining collagen deposition and mineral removal and/or improving mineral deposition could provide a better and more mineralized bone matrix in osteoarthritic patients. With the new biological findings in bone metabolism during pathologic conditions, further approaches to target bone resorption/mineralization represent an interesting rationale of therapy for this disease.

## REFERENCES

1. Radin EL, Paul IL, Rose RM. Role of mechanical factors in pathogenesis of primary osteoarthritis. Lancet 1972;1:519.
2. Oehler S, Neureiter D, Meyer-Scholten C, et al. Subtyping of osteoarthritic synoviopathy. Clin Exp Rheumatol 2002;20:633.
3. Carlson CS, Loeser RF, Purser CB, et al. Osteoarthritis in cynomolgus macaques. III: Effects of age, gender, and subchondral bone thickness on the severity of disease. J Bone Miner Res 1996; 11:1209.
4. Grynpas MD, Alpert B, Katz I, et al. Subchondral bone in osteoarthritis. Calcif Tissue Int 1991;49:20.
5. Radin EL, Rose RM. Role of subchondral bone in the initiation and progression of cartilage damage. Clin Orthop 1986;213:34.
6. Pastoureau PC, Chomel AC, Bonnet J. Evidence of early subchondral bone changes in the meniscectomized guinea pig: A densitometric study using dual-energy X-ray absorptiometry subregional analysis. Osteoarthritis Cartilage 1999;7:466.
7. Burr DB, Schaffler MB. The involvement of subchondral mineralized tissues in osteoarthrosis: Quantitative microscopic evidence. Microsc Res Tech 1997;37:343.
8. Brandt KD. Insights into the natural history of osteoarthritis provided by the cruciate-deficient dog: An animal model of osteoarthritis. Ann NY Acad Sci 1994;732:199.
9. Bettica P, Cline G, Hart DJ, et al. Evidence for increased bone resorption in patients with progressive knee osteoarthritis: Longitudinal results from the Chingford study. Arthritis Rheum 2002;46:3178.
10. Dedrick DK, Goldstein SA, Brandt KD, et al. A longitudinal study of subchondral plate and trabecular bone in cruciate-deficient dogs with osteoarthritis followed up for 54 months. Arthritis Rheum 1993;36:1460.
11. Lajeunesse D, Martel-Pelletier J, Fernandes JC, et al. Treatment with licofelone prevents abnormal subchondral bone cell metabolism in experimental dog osteoarthritis. Ann Rheum Dis 2004;63:78.
12. Massicotte F, Lajeunesse D, Benderdour M, et al. Can altered production of interleukin 1β, interleukin-6, transforming growth factor-β and prostaglandin E2 by isolated human subchondral osteoblasts identify two subgroups of osteoarthritic patients? Osteoarthritis Cartilage 2002;10:491.
13. Paredes Y, Massicotte F, Pelletier JP, et al. Study of role of leukotriene B4 in abnormal function of human subchondral osteoarthritis osteoblasts: Effects of cyclooxygenase and/or 5-lipoxygenase inhibition. Arthritis Rheum 2002;46:1804.
14. Pelletier JP, Lajeunesse D, Hilal G, et al. Carprofen reduces the structural changes and the abnormal subchondral bone metabolism of experimental osteoarthritis. Osteoarthritis Cartilage 1999;7:327.
15. Mansell JP, Bailey AJ. Abnormal cancellous bone collagen metabolism in osteoarthritis. J Clin Invest 1998;101:1596.
16. Hilal G, Martel-Pelletier J, Pelletier JP, et al. Osteoblast-like cells from human subchondral osteoarthritic bone demonstrate an altered phenotype in vitro: Possible role in subchondral bone sclerosis. Arthritis Rheum 1998;41:891.

17. Westacott CI, Webb GR, Warnock MG, et al. Alteration of cartilage metabolism by cells from osteoarthritic bone. Arthritis Rheum 1997;40:1282.

18. Dequeker J, Mohan R, Finkelman RD, et al. Generalized osteoarthritis associated with increased insulin-like growth factor types I and II and transforming growth factor beta in cortical bone from the iliac crest: Possible mechanism of increased bone density and protection against osteoporosis. Arthritis Rheum 1993;36:1702.

19. Evans RG, Collins C, Miller P, et al. Radiological scoring of osteoarthritis progression in STR/ORT mice. Osteoarthritis Cartilage 1994;2:103.

20. Bailey AJ, Mansell JP. Do subchondral bone changes exacerbate or precede articular cartilage destruction in osteoarthritis of the elderly? Gerontology 1997;43:296.

21. Watson PJ, Hall LD, Malcolm A, et al. Degenerative joint disease in the guinea pig: Use of magnetic resonance imaging to monitor progression of bone pathology. Arthritis Rheum 1996;39:1327.

22. Watson PJ, Carpenter TA, Hall LD, et al. Cartilage swelling and loss in a spontaneous model of osteoarthritis visualized by magnetic resonance imaging. Osteoarthritis Cartilage 1996;4:197.

23. Carlson CS, Loeser RF, Jayo MJ, et al. Osteoarthritis in cynomolgus macaques: A primate model of naturally occurring disease. J Orthop Res 1994;12:331.

24. Newberry WN, Zukosky DK, Haut RC. Subfracture insult to a knee joint causes alterations in the bone and in the functional stiffness of overlying cartilage. J Orthop Res 1997;15:450.

25. Nakashima K, de Crombrugghe B. Transcriptional mechanisms in osteoblast differentiation and bone formation. Trends Genet 2003;19:458.

26. Ornitz DM, Marie PJ. FGF signaling pathways in endochondral and intramembranous bone development and human genetic disease. Genes Dev 2002;16:1446.

27. DeLise AM, Fischer L, Tuan RS. Cellular interactions and signaling in cartilage development. Osteoarthritis Cartilage 2000;8:309.

28. Erlebacher A, Filvaroff EH, Gitelman SE, et al. Toward a molecular understanding of skeletal development. Cell 1995;80:371.

29. Reddi AH. Role of morphogenetic proteins in skeletal tissue engineering and regeneration. Nat Biotechnol 1998;16:247.

30. Wozney JM, Rosen V. Bone morphogenetic protein and bone morphogenetic protein gene family in bone formation and repair. Clin Orthop 1998;346:26.

31. Valentin-Opran A, Wozney J, Csimma C, et al. Clinical evaluation of recombinant human bone morphogenetic protein-2. Clin Orthop 2002;395:110.

32. Roberts AB, Sporn MB. The transforming growth factor-βs. In MB Sporn and AB Roberts (eds.), *Peptide Growth Factors and Their Receptors*. Berlin: Springer-Verlag 1991.

33. Joyce ME, Roberts AB, Sporn MB, et al. Transforming growth factor-beta and the initiation of chondrogenesis and osteogenesis in the rat femur. J Cell Biol 1990;110:2195.

34. Noda M, Camilliere JJ. In vivo stimulation of bone formation by transforming growth factor-beta. Endocrinology 1989;124:2991.

35. Erlebacher A, Derynck R. Increased expression of TGF-beta 2 in osteoblasts results in an osteoporosis-like phenotype. J Cell Biol 1996;132:195.

36. Alliston T, Choy L, Ducy P, et al. TGF-beta-induced repression of CBFA1 by Smad3 decreases cbfa1 and osteocalcin expression and inhibits osteoblast differentiation. EMBO J 2001;20:2254.

37. Imhof H, Sulzbacher I, Grampp S, et al. Subchondral bone and cartilage disease: A rediscovered functional unit. Invest Radiol 2000;35:581.

38. Dequeker J, Aerssens J, Luyten FP. Osteoarthritis and osteoporosis: Clinical and research evidence of inverse relationship. Aging Clin Exp Res 2003;15:426.

39. Malinin T, Ouellette EA. Articular cartilage nutrition is mediated by subchondral bone: A long-term autograft study in baboons. Osteoarthritis Cartilage 2000;8:483.

40. Imhof H, Breitenseher M, Kainberger F, et al. Importance of subchondral bone to articular cartilage in health and disease. Top Magn Reson Imaging 1999;10:180.

41. Li B, Aspden RM. Mechanical and material properties of the subchondral bone plate from the femoral head of patients with osteoarthritis or osteoporosis. Ann Rheum Dis 1997;56:247.

42. Brown TD, Radin EL, Martin RB, et al. Finite element studies of some juxtarticular stress changes due to localized subchondral stiffening. J Biomech 1984;17:11.

43. Fazzalari NL, Parkinson IH. Femoral trabecular bone of osteoarthritic and normal subjects in an age and sex matched group. Osteoarthritis Cartilage 1998;6:377.

44. Crane GJ, Fazzalari NL, Parkinson IH, et al. Age-related changes in femoral trabecular bone in arthrosis. Acta Orthop Scand 1990;61:421.

45. Buckland-Wright JC, Lynch JA, Macfarlane DG. Fractal signature analysis measures cancellous bone organisation in macroradiographs of patients with knee osteoarthritis. Ann Rheum Dis 1996;55:749.

46. Dieppe P, Cushnaghan J, Young P, et al. Prediction of the progression of joint space narrowing in osteoarthritis of the knee by bone scintigraphy. Ann Rheum Dis 1993;52:557.

47. McCarthy C, Cushnaghan J, Dieppe P. The predictive role of scintigraphy in radiographic osteoarthritis of the hand. Osteoarthritis Cartilage 1994;2:25.

48. Sharif M, George E, Dieppe PA. Correlation between synovial fluid markers of cartilage and bone turnover and scintigraphic scan abnormalities in osteoarthritis of the knee. Arthritis Rheum 1995;38:78.

49. Majumdar S, Genant HK, Grampp S, et al. Correlation of trabecular bone structure with age, bone mineral density, and osteoporotic status: In vivo studies in the distal radius using high resolution magnetic resonance imaging. J Bone Miner Res 1997;12:111.

50. Majumdar S, Genant HK. Assessment of trabecular structure using high resolution magnetic resonance imaging. Stud Health Technol Inform 1997;40:81.

51. Raynauld J-P, Martel-Pelletier J, Berthiaume M-J, et al. Long term evaluation of disease proression through the quantitative magnetic resonance imaging of symptomatic knee osteoarthritis patients: Correlation with clinical symptoms and radiographic changes. Arthritis Res Ther 2005;8:R21.

52. Felson DT, McLaughlin S, Goggins J, et al. Bone marrow edema and its relation to progression of knee osteoarthritis. Ann Intern Med 2003;139:330.

53. Guermazi A, Zaim S, Taouli B, et al. MR findings in knee osteoarthritis. Eur Radiol 2003;13:1370.

54. Beuf O, Ghosh S, Newitt DC, et al. Magnetic resonance imaging of normal and osteoarthritic trabecular bone structure in the human knee. Arthritis Rheum 2002;46:385.

55. Blumenkrantz G, Lindsey CT, Dunn TC, et al. A pilot, two-year longitudinal study of the interrelationship between trabecular bone and articular cartilage in the osteoarthritic knee. Osteoarthritis Cartilage 2004;12:997.

56. Lajeunesse D, Busque L, Ménard P, et al. Demonstration of an osteoblast defect in two cases of human malignant osteopetrosis: Correction of the phenotype after bone marrow transplant. J Clin Invest 1996;98:1835.

57. Li B, Marshall D, Roe M, et al. The electron microscope appearance of the subchondral bone plate in the human femoral head in osteoarthritis and osteoporosis. J Anat 1999;195:101.

58. Li B, Aspden RM. Composition and mechanical properties of cancellous bone from the femoral head of patients with osteoporosis or osteoarthritis. J Bone Miner Res 1997;12:641.

59. Gevers G, Dequeker J, Martens M, et al. Biomechanical characteristics of iliac crest bone in elderly women, according to osteoarthritis grade at the hand joints. J Rheumatol 1989;16:660.

60. Sowers M, Zobel D, Weissfeld L, et al. Progression of osteoarthritis of the hand and metacarpal bone loss: A twenty-year followup of incident cases. Arthritis Rheum 1991;34:36.

61. Seibel MJ, Duncan A, Robins SP. Urinary hydroxy-pyridinium crosslinks provide indices of cartilage and bone involvement in arthritic diseases. J Rheumatol 1989;16:964.

62. van Beuningen HM, van der Kraan PM, Arntz OJ, et al. Transforming growth factor-beta 1 stimulates articular chondrocyte proteoglycan synthesis and induces osteophyte formation in the murine knee joint. Lab Invest 1994;71:279.

63. Moskowitz RW. Bone remodeling in osteoarthritis: Subchondral and osteophytic responses. Osteoarthritis Cartilage 1999;7:323.

64. Radin EL, Paul IL, Tolkoff MJ. Subchondral changes in patients with early degenerative joint disease. Arthritis Rheum 1970;13:400.

65. McKinley TO, Bay BK. Trabecular bone strain changes associated with subchondral stiffening of the proximal tibia. J Biomech 2003;36:155.

66. Brown AN, McKinley TO, Bay BK. Trabecular bone strain changes associated with subchondral bone defects of the tibial plateau. J Orthop Trauma 2002;16:638.

67. McKinley TO, Callendar PW, Bay BK. Trabecular bone strain changes associated with subchondral comminution of the distal tibia. J Orthop Trauma 2002;16:709.

68. Matsui H, Shimizu M, Tsuji H. Cartilage and subchondral bone interaction in osteoarthrosis of human knee joint: A histological and histomorphometric study. Microsc Res Tech 1997;37:333.

69. Shimizu M, Tsuji H, Matsui H, et al. Morphometric analysis of subchondral bone of the tibial condyle in osteoarthrosis. Clin Orthop 1993;293:229.

70. Hayami T, Pickarski M, Wesolowski GA, et al. The role of subchondral bone remodeling in osteoarthritis: Reduction of cartilage degeneration and prevention of osteophyte formation by alendronate in the rat anterior cruciate ligament transection model. Arthritis Rheum 2004;50:193.

71. Pelletier JP, Lajeunesse D, Jovanovic DV, et al. Carprofen simultaneously reduces progression of morphological changes in cartilage and subchondral bone in experimental dog osteoarthritis. J Rheumatol 2000;27:2893.

72. Gravallese EM, Goldring SR. Cellular mechanisms and the role of cytokines in bone erosions in rheumatoid arthritis. Arthritis Rheum 2000;43:2143.

73. Bailey AJ, Sims TJ, Knott L. Phenotypic expression of osteoblast collagen in osteoarthritic bone: Production of type I homotrimer. Int J Biochem Cell Biol 2002;34:176.

74. Zysset PK, Sonny M, Hayes WC. Morphology-mechanical property relations in trabecular bone of the osteoarthritic proximal tibia. J Arthroplasty 1994;9:203.

75. Fazzalari NL, Kuliwaba JS, Forwood MR. Cancellous bone microdamage in the proximal femur: Influence of age and osteoarthritis on damage morphology and regional distribution. Bone 2002;31:697.

76. Dequeker J. The relationship between osteoporosis and osteoarthritis. Clin Rheum Dis 1985;11:271.

77. Gevers G, Dequeker J. Collagen and non-collagenous protein content (osteocalcin, sialoprotein, proteoglycan) in the iliac crest bone and serum osteocalcin in women with and without hand osteoarthritis. Coll Relat Res 1987;7:435.

78. Hilal G, Martel-Pelletier J, Pelletier JP, et al. Abnormal regulation of urokinase plasminogen activator by insulin-like growth factor 1 in human osteoarthritic subchondral osteoblasts. Arthritis Rheum 1999;42:2112.

79. Hilal G, Massicotte F, Martel-Pelletier J, et al. Endogenous prostaglandin E2 and insulin-like growth factor 1 can modulate the levels of parathyroid hormone receptor in human osteoarthritic osteoblasts. J Bone Miner Res 2001;16:713.

80. Beresford JN, Gallagher JA, Poser JW, et al. Production of osteocalcin by human bone cells in vitro: Effects of 1,25(OH)2D3, 24,25(OH)2D3, parathyroid hormone, and glucocorticoids. Metab Bone Dis Relat Res 1984;5:229.

81. Dietrich JW, Canalis EM, Maina DM, et al. Hormonal control of bone collagen synthesis in vitro: Effects of parathyroid hormone and calcitonin. Endocrinology 1976;98:943.

82. Murphy JM, Dixon K, Beck S, et al. Reduced chondrogenic and adipogenic activity of mesenchymal stem cells from patients with advanced osteoarthritis. Arthritis Rheum 2002;46:704.

83. Aspden RM, Scheven BAA, Hutchison JD. Osteoarthritis as a systemic disorder including stromal cell differentiation and lipid metabolism. The Lancet 2001;357:1118.

84. Shimabukuro M, Koyama K, Chen G, et al. Direct antidiabetic effect of leptin through triglyceride depletion of tissues. Proc Natl Acad Sci USA 1997;94:4637.

85. Bai Y, Zhang S, Kim KS, et al. Obese gene expression alters the ability of 30A5 preadipocytes to respond to lipogenic hormones. J Biol Chem 1996;271:13939.

86. Campfield LA, Smith FJ, Guisez Y, et al. Recombinant mouse OB-protein: Evidence for a peripheral signal linking adiposity and central neural networks. Science 1995;269:546.

87. Zhang Y, Procenca R, Maffei M, et al. Positional cloning of the mouse *obese* gene and its human homologue. Nature 1994;372:425.

88. Lajeunesse D, Delalandre A, Fernandes JC. Subchondral osteoblasts from osteoarthritic patients show abnormal expression and production of leptin: Possible role in cartilage degradation. J Bone Miner Res 2004;19:S149.

89. Dumond H, Presle N, Terlain B, et al. Evidence for a key role of leptin in osteoarthritis. Arthritis Rheum 2003;48:3118.

90. Gordeladze JO, Drevon CA, Syversen U, et al. Leptin stimulates human osteoblastic cell proliferation, de novo collagen synthesis, and mineralization: Impact on differentiation markers, apoptosis, and osteoclastic signaling. J Cell Biochem 2002;85:825.

91. Busso N, So A, Chobaz-Péclat V, et al. Leptin signaling deficiency impairs humoral and cellular immune responses and attenuates experimental arthritis. J Immunol 2002;168:875.

92. Matarese G. Leptin and the immune system: How nutritional status influences the immune response. Eur Cytokine Network 2000;11:7.

93. Fantuzzi G, Faggioni R. Leptin in the regulation of immunity, inflammation, and hematopoiesis. J Leukoc Biol 2000;68:437.

94. Raso GM, Pacilio M, Esposito E, et al. Leptin potentiates IFN-gamma-induced expression of nitric oxide synthase and cyclo-oxygenase-2 in murine macrophage J774A.1. Br J Pharmacol 2002;137:799.

95. Mancuso P, Gottschalk A, Phare SM, et al. Leptin-deficient mice exhibit impaired host defense in gram-negative pneumonia. J Immunol 2002;168:4018.

96. Ducy P, Desbois C, Boyce B, et al. Increased bone formation in osteocalcin-deficient mice. Nature 1996;382:448.

97. Hock JM, Centrella M, Canalis E. Insulin-like growth factor I has independent effects on bone matrix formation and cell replication. Endocrinology 1988;122:254.

98. Massicotte F, Martel-Pelletier J, Pelletier J-P, et al. Abnormal modulation of insulin-like growth factor 1 levels in human osteoarthritic bone osteoblasts. Arthritis Rheum 2000;43:S206.

99. Martel-Pelletier J, Di Battista JA, Lajeunesse D, et al. IGF/IGFBP axis in cartilage and bone in osteoarthritis pathogenesis. Inflamm Res 1998;47:90.

100. Palcy S, Goltzman D. Protein kinase signalling pathways involved in the up-regulation of the rat alpha1(I) collagen gene by transforming growth factor beta1 and bone morphogenetic protein 2 in osteoblastic cells. Biochem J 1999;343:21.

101. Rydziel S, Delany AM, Canalis E. Insulin-like growth factor I inhibits the transcription of collagenase 3 in osteoblast cultures. J Cell Biochem 1997;67:176.

102. Scharstuhl A, Glansbeek HL, van Beuningen HM, et al. Inhibition of endogenous TGF-beta during experimental osteoarthritis prevents osteophyte formation and impairs cartilage repair. J Immunol 2002;169:507.

103. Kaneki H, Takasugi I, Fujieda M, et al. Prostaglandin E2 stimulates the formation of mineralized bone nodules by a cAMP-independent mechanism in the culture of adult rat calvarial osteoblasts. J Cell Biochem 1999;73:36.

104. Raisz LG, Fall PM. Biphasic effects of prostaglandin E2 on bone formation in cultured fetal rat calvariae: Interaction with cortisol. Endocrinology 1990;126:1654.

105. Hakeda Y, Nakatani Y, Kurihara N, et al. Prostaglandin E2 stimulates collagen and non-collagen protein synthesis and prolyl hydroxylase activity in osteoblastic clone MC3T3-E1 cells. Biochem Biophys Res Commun 1985;126:340.

106. Gallwitz WE, Mundy GR, Lee CH, et al. 5-Lipoxygenase metabolites of arachidonic acid stimulate isolated osteoclasts to resorb calcified matrices. J Biol Chem 1993;268:10087.

107. Morrison NA, Qi JC, Tokita A, et al. Prediction of bone density from vitamin D receptor alleles. Nature 1994;367:284.

108. Murray RE, McGuigan F, Grant SF, et al. Polymorphisms of the interleukin-6 gene are associated with bone mineral density. Bone 1997;21:89.

109. Grant SF, Reid DM, Blake G, et al. Reduced bone density and osteoporosis associated with a polymorphic Sp1 binding site in the collagen type I alpha 1 gene. Nat Genet 1996;14:203.

110. Kobayashi S, Inoue S, Hosoi T, et al. Association of bone mineral density with polymorphism of the estrogen receptor gene. J Bone Miner Res 1996;11:306.

111. Loughlin J, Dowling B, Mustafa Z, et al. Association of the interleukin-1 gene cluster on chromosome 2q13 with knee osteoarthritis. Arthritis Rheum 2002;46:1519.

112. Maroudas A, Bullough P, Swanson SA, et al. The permeability of articular cartilage. J Bone Joint Surg Br 1968;50:166.

113. Duncan H, Jundt J, Riddle JM, et al. The tibial subchondral plate: A scanning electron microscopic study. J Bone Joint Surg Am 1987;69:1212.

114. Milz S, Putz R. Quantitative morphology of the subchondral plate of the tibial plateau. J Anat 1994;185:103.

115. Mital MA, Millington PF. Osseous pathway of nutrition to articular cartilage of the human femoral head. Lancet 1970;1:842.

116. Buckwalter JA, Mankin HJ. Articular cartilage: tissue design and chondrocyte-matrix interactions. Instr Course Lect 1998;47:477.

117. Buckwalter JA, Hunziker E, Rosenberg LC, Coutts RD, Adams M, Eyre D. Articular cartilage: Composition and structure. In SLY Woo, JA Buckwalter (eds.), Injury and Repair of the Musculoskeletal Soft Tissues. Rosemont, IL: American Academy of Orthopaedic Surgeons 1987.

118. Thonar EJ, Masuda K, Manicourt DH, Kuettner KE. Structure and function of normal adult articular cartilage. In JY Reginster, JP Pelletier, J Martel-Pelletier, Y Henrotin (eds.), Osteoarthritis. Clinical and Experimental Aspects. Berlin: Springer-Verlag 1999.

119. Hunziker EB. Articular cartilage structure in humans and experimental animals. In Kuettner KE, Schleyerbach R, Peyron JG, Hascall VC (eds.), Articular Cartilage and Osteoarthritis. New York: Raven Press 1992,183–199.

120. Wu JJ, Eyre DR. Covalent interactions of type IX collagen in cartilage. Connect Tissue Res 1989;20:241.

121. Muller-Glauser W, Humbel B, Glatt M, et al. On the role of type IX collagen in the extracellular matrix of cartilage: Type IX collagen is localized to intersections of collagen fibrils. J Cell Biol 1986;102:1931.

122. Heinegard D, Lorenzo P, Sommarin Y. Articular cartilage matrix proteins. In KE Kuettner, VE Goldberg (eds.), Osteoarthritic Disorders. Rosemont, IL: American Academy of Orthopedic Surgeons 1995.

123. Alford JW, Cole BJ. Cartilage restoration, part 1: Basic science, historical perspective, patient evaluation, and treatment options. Am J Sports Med 2005;33:295.

124. Weiss C, Rosenberg L, Helfet AJ. An ultrastructural study of normal young adult human articular cartilage. J Bone Joint Surg Am 1968;50:663.

125. O'Connor P, Orford CR, Gardner DL. Differential response to compressive loads of zones of canine hyaline articular cartilage: Micromechanical, light and electron microscopic studies. Ann Rheum Dis 1988;47:414.

126. Mankin HJ. The response of articular cartilage to mechanical injury. J Bone Joint Surg Am 1982;64:460.

127. Lohmander LS, Dahlberg L, Ryd L, et al. Increased levels of proteoglycan fragments in knee joint fluid after injury. Arthritis Rheum 1989;32:1434.

128. Mankin HJ, Brandt KD. Biochemistry and metabolism of articular cartilage in osteoarthritis. In RW Moskowitz, DS Howell, VC Goldberg, et al. (eds.), Osteoarthritis: Diagnosis and Management. Philadelphia: W. B. Saunders 1992.

129. Mow VC, Rosenwasser MP. Articular cartilage: Biomechanics. In SLY Woo, JA Buckwalter (eds.), Injury and Repair of the Musculoskeletal Soft Tissues. Rosemont, IL: American Academy of Orthopaedic Surgeons 1988.

130. Shinmei M, Kobayashi T, Yoshihara Y, et al. Significance of the levels of carboxy terminal type II procollagen peptide, chondroitin sulfate isomers, tissue inhibitor of metalloproteinases, and metalloproteinases in osteoarthritis joint fluid. J Rheumatol Suppl 1995;43:78.

131. Thompson RC Jr., Oegema TR Jr. Metabolic activity of articular cartilage in osteoarthritis: An in vitro study. J Bone Joint Surg Am 1979;61:407.

132. Gilbertson EM. Development of periarticular osteophytes in experimentally induced osteoarthritis in the dog: A study using microradiographic, microangiographic, and fluorescent bone-labelling techniques. Ann Rheum Dis 1975;34:12.

133. Marshall JL, Olsson SE. Instability of the knee: A long-term experimental study in dogs. J Bone Joint Surg Am 1971;53:1561.

134. Langenskiold A, Michelsson JE, Videman T. Osteoarthritis of the knee in the rabbit produced by immobilization: Attempts to achieve a reproducible model for studies on pathogenesis and therapy. Acta Orthop Scand 1979;50:1.

135. Pelletier JP, Martel-Pelletier J. Protective effects of corticosteroids on cartilage lesions and osteophyte formation in the Pond-Nuki dog model of osteoarthritis. Arthritis Rheum 1989;32:181.

136. Adams ME, Brandt KD. Hypertrophic repair of canine articular cartilage in osteoarthritis after anterior cruciate ligament transection. J Rheumatol 1991;18:428.

137. Moskowitz RW, Goldberg VM. Studies of osteophyte pathogenesis in experimentally induced osteoarthritis. J Rheumatol 1987;14:311.

138. Mankin HJ. The reaction of articular cartilage to injury and osteoarthritis (first of two parts). N Engl J Med 1974;291:1285.

139. McDevitt CA, Muir H. Biochemical changes in the cartilage of the knee in experimental and natural osteoarthritis in the dog. J Bone Joint Surg Br 1976;58:94.

140. Otterness IG, Bliven ML, Eskra JD, et al. Cartilage damage after intraarticular exposure to collagenase 3. Osteoarthritis Cartilage 2000;8:366.

141. Reboul P, Pelletier JP, Tardif G, et al. The new collagenase, collagenase-3, is expressed and synthesized by human chondrocytes but not by synoviocytes: A role in osteoarthritis. J Clin Invest 1996;97:2011.

142. Billinghurst RC, Wu W, Ionescu M, et al. Comparison of the degradation of type II collagen and proteoglycan in nasal and articular cartilages induced by interleukin-1 and the selective inhibition of type II collagen cleavage by collagenase. Arthritis Rheum 2000;43:664.

143. Moldovan F, Pelletier JP, Hambor J, et al. Collagenase-3 (matrix metalloprotease 13) is preferentially localized in the deep layer of human arthritic cartilage in situ: In vitro mimicking effect by transforming growth factor beta. Arthritis Rheum 1997;40:1653.

144. Aydelotte MB, Kuettner KE. Differences between sub-populations of cultured bovine articular chondrocytes. I. Morphology and cartilage matrix production. Connect Tissue Res 1988;18:205.

145. Fosang AJ, Last K, Knauper V, et al. Degradation of cartilage aggrecan by collagenase-3 (MMP-13). FEBS Lett 1996; 380:17.

146. Sokoloff L. Microcracks in the calcified layer of articular cartilage. Arch Pathol Lab Med 1993;117:191.

147. Hulth A. Does osteoarthrosis depend on growth of the mineralized layer of cartilage? Clin Orthop 1993;287:19.

148. Lane LB, Bullough PG. Age-related changes in the thickness of the calcified zone and the number of tidemarks in adult human articular cartilage. J Bone Joint Surg Br 1980;62:372.

149. Bonnet CS, Walsh DA. Osteoarthritis, angiogenesis and inflammation. Rheumatology (Oxford) 2005;44:7.

150. Stephens RW, Ghosh P, Taylor TK. The pathogenesis of osteoarthrosis. Med Hypotheses 1979;5:809.

151. Kuettner KE. Biochemistry of articular cartilage in health and disease. Clin Biochem 1992;25:155.

152. Guevremont M, Martel-Pelletier J, Boileau C, et al. Galectin-3 surface expression on human adult chondrocytes: A potential substrate for collagenase-3. Ann Rheum Dis 2004;63:636.

153. von der Mark K, Kirsch T, Nerlich A, et al. Type X collagen synthesis in human osteoarthritic cartilage: Indication of chondrocyte hypertrophy. Arthritis Rheum 1992;35:806.

154. Hoyland JA, Thomas JT, Donn R, et al. Distribution of type X collagen mRNA in normal and osteoarthritic human cartilage. Bone Miner 1991;15:151.

155. Quarto R, Dozin B, Bonaldo P, et al. Type VI collagen expression is upregulated in the early events of chondrocyte differentiation. Development 1993;117:245.

156. Benya PD, Padilla SR, Nimni ME. The progeny of rabbit articular chondrocytes synthesize collagen types I and III and type I trimer, but not type II. Verifications by cyanogen bromide peptide analysis. Biochemistry 1977;16:865.

157. von der Mark K, Gauss V, von der Mark H, et al. Relationship between cell shape and type of collagen synthesised as chondrocytes lose their cartilage phenotype in culture. Nature 1977;267:531.

158. Girkontaite I, Frischholz S, Lammi P, et al. Immunolocalization of type X collagen in normal fetal and adult osteoarthritic cartilage with monoclonal antibodies. Matrix Biol 1996;15:231.

159. Reichenberger E, Aigner T, von der Mark K, et al. In situ hybridization studies on the expression of type X collagen in fetal human cartilage. Dev Biol 1991;148:562.

160. Schmid TM, Linsenmayer TF. Type X collagen. In R Mayne, RE Burgeson (eds.), Structure and Functions of Collagen Types. New York: Academic Press 1987.

161. Sandell LJ, Aigner T. Articular cartilage and changes in arthritis. An introduction: Cell biology of osteoarthritis. Arthritis Res 2001;3:107.
162. Mollenhauer J, Mok MT, King KB, et al. Expression of anchorin CII (cartilage annexin V) in human young, normal adult, and osteoarthritic cartilage. J Histochem Cytochem 1999;47:209.
163. Kirsch T, Swoboda B, Nah H. Activation of annexin II and V expression, terminal differentiation, mineralization and apoptosis in human osteoarthritic cartilage. Osteoarthritis Cartilage 2000;8:294.
164. Mitchell PG, Magna HA, Reeves LM, et al. Cloning, expression, and type II collagenolytic activity of matrix metalloproteinase-13 from human osteoarthritic cartilage. J Clin Invest 1996;97:761.
165. Pullig O, Weseloh G, Gauer S, et al. Osteopontin is expressed by adult human osteoarthritic chondrocytes: Protein and mRNA analysis of normal and osteoarthritic cartilage. Matrix Biol 2000;19:245.
166. Mansell JP, Tarlton JF, Bailey AJ. Biochemical evidence for altered subchondral bone collagen metabolism in osteoarthritis of the hip. Br J Rheumatol 1997;36:16.
167. Pufe T, Petersen W, Tillmann B, et al. The splice variants VEGF121 and VEGF189 of the angiogenic peptide vascular endothelial growth factor are expressed in osteoarthritic cartilage. Arthritis Rheum 2001;44:1082.
168. Semble EL, Turner RA, McCrickard EL. Rheumatoid arthritis and osteoarthritis synovial fluid effects on primary human endothelial cell cultures. J Rheumatol 1985;12:237.
169. Guévremont M, Martel-Pelletier J, Massicotte F, et al. Human adult chondrocytes express hepatocyte growth factor (HGF) isoforms but not HGF: Potential implication of osteoblasts for the HGF presence in cartilage. J Bone Miner Res 2003;18:1073.
170. Deckers MM, van Bezooijen RL, van der Horst G, et al. Bone morphogenetic proteins stimulate angiogenesis through osteoblast-derived vascular endothelial growth factor A. Endocrinology 2002;143:1545.
171. Konttinen YT, Mandelin J, Li TF, et al. Acidic cysteine endoproteinase cathepsin K in the degeneration of the superficial articular hyaline cartilage in osteoarthritis. Arthritis Rheum 2002;46:953.
172. Nakase T, Kaneko M, Tomita T, et al. Immunohistochemical detection of cathepsin D, K, and L in the process of endochondral ossification in the human. Histochem Cell Biol 2000;114:21.
173. Feuerherm AJ, Borset M, Seidel C, et al. Elevated levels of osteoprotegerin (OPG) and hepatocyte growth factor (HGF) in rheumatoid arthritis. Scand J Rheumatol 2001;30:229.
174. Pfander D, Cramer T, Weseloh G, et al. Hepatocyte growth factor in human osteoarthritic cartilage. Osteoarthritis Cartilage 1999;7:548.
175. Blanquaert F, Pereira RC, Canalis E. Cortisol inhibits hepatocyte growth factor/scatter factor expression and induces c-met transcripts in osteoblasts. Am J Physiol Endocrinol Metab 2000;278:E509.
176. Skrtic S, Ohlsson C. Cortisol decreases hepatocyte growth factor levels in human osteoblast-like cells. Calcif Tissue Int 2000;66:108.
177. Reboul P, Pelletier JP, Tardif G, et al. Hepatocyte growth factor induction of collagenase 3 production in human osteoarthritic cartilage: Involvement of the stress-activated protein kinase/c-Jun N-terminal kinase pathway and a sensitive p38 mitogen-activated protein kinase inhibitor cascade. Arthritis Rheum 2001;44:73.
178. Horas U, Pelinkovic D, Herr G, et al. Autologous chondrocyte implantation and osteochondral cylinder transplantation in cartilage repair of the knee joint: A prospective, comparative trial. J Bone Joint Surg Am 2003;85-A:185.
179. Felson DT, Chaisson CE, Hill CL, et al. The association of bone marrow lesions with pain in knee osteoarthritis. Ann Intern Med 2001;134:541.
180. Manicourt DH, Altman RD, Williams JM, et al. Treatment with calcitonin suppresses the responses of bone, cartilage, and synovium in the early stages of canine experimental osteoarthritis and significantly reduces the severity of the cartilage lesions. Arthritis Rheum 1999;42:1159.
181. Howell DS, Altman RD, Pelletier J-P, Martel-Pelletier J, Dean DD. Disease modifying anti-rheumatic drugs: Current status of their application in animal models of osteoarthritis. In KE Keuttner, VM Goldberg (eds.), Osteoarthritis Disorders. Rosemont, IL: American Academy of Orthopaedic Surgeons 1995.
182. Myers SL, Brandt KD, Burr DB, et al. Effects of a bisphosphonate on bone histomorphometry and dynamics in the canine cruciate deficiency model of osteoarthritis. J Rheumatol 1999;26:2645.
183. Pelletier JP, Boileau C, Brunet J, et al. The inhibition of subchondral bone resorption in the early phase of experimental dog osteoarthritis by licofelone is associated with a reduction in the synthesis of MMP-13 and cathepsin K. Bone 2004;34:527.
184. Carbone LD, Nevitt MC, Wildy K, et al. The relationship of antiresorptive drug use to structural findings and symptoms of knee osteoarthritis. Arthritis Rheum 2004;50:3516.
185. Spector TD, Conaghan PG, Buckland-Wright JC, et al. Effect of risedronate on joint structure and symptoms of knee osteoarthritis: Results of the BRISK randomized, controlled trial. Arthritis Res Ther 2005;7:R625.
186. Heikkila P, Teronen O, Moilanen M, et al. Bisphosphonates inhibit stromelysin-1 (MMP-3), matrix metalloelastase (MMP-12), collagenase-3 (MMP-13) and enamelysin (MMP-20), but not urokinase-type plasminogen activator, and diminish invasion and migration of human malignant and endothelial cell lines. Anticancer Drugs 2002;13:245.
187. Teronen O, Heikkila P, Konttinen YT, et al. MMP inhibition and downregulation by bisphosphonates. Ann NY Acad Sci 1999;878:453.
188. Takayanagi H, Iizuka H, Juji T, et al. Involvement of receptor activator of nuclear factor kappaB ligand/osteoclast differentiation factor in osteoclastogenesis from synoviocytes in rheumatoid arthritis. Arthritis Rheum 2000;43:259.
189. Burgess TL, Qian Y, Kaufman S, et al. The ligand for osteoprotegerin (OPGL) directly activates mature osteoclasts. J Cell Biol 199;145:527.
190. Jones DH, Kong YY, Penninger JM. Role of RANKL and RANK in bone loss and arthritis. Ann Rheum Dis 2002;61(2):ii32.
191. Simonet WS, Lacey DL, Dunstan CR, et al. Osteoprotegerin: A novel secreted protein involved in the regulation of bone density. Cell 1997;89:309.

# 3

# The Impact of Mechanical Stress on the Pathophysiology of Osteoarthritis

George Nuki and Donald Salter

Movement and mechanical stimulation are essential during embryonic development and morphogenesis of the skeleton[1] and normal joints.[2,3] Movement and mechanical forces are also crucial for tissue remodeling and the maintenance of healthy articular cartilage,[4] bone,[5] muscles,[6] and tendons.[7] Paradoxically, mechanical stresses also play a critical role in the pathophysiology and progression of osteoarthritis (OA).

OA is not a single disease or process but rather the clinical and pathologic outcome of a range of processes and disorders that lead to pain, loss of function, and eventually structural failure of one or more of the diarthrodial joints. Structural failure in OA can involve all tissues of the joint, including the capsule, synovial membrane and subchondral bone, extra-articular and intra-articular ligaments, the fibrocartilaginous menisci in joints such as the knee, and the articular cartilage. To a variable extent, the pathophysiology of OA is a dynamic process that involves some regeneration and increased turnover of cartilage matrix components, new bone formation and joint remodeling, and degeneration of articular tissues.

Structural failure occurs when joint remodeling, new bone formation, and synthesis of articular cartilage matrix molecules fail to keep pace with catabolic processes.[8-10] Although OA is conventionally defined as primary (idiopathic) or secondary,[11] it is becoming increasingly clear that the development of most phenotypic patterns of OA involves multiple etiologic factors. Although some of these[12] (such as age, gender, race, certain genetic determinants,[13] and bone density,[14,15] identified as risk factors for *susceptibility* to OA) may operate at least in part as *systemic* risk factors, others (such as injury,[16] joint mal-alignment,[17] skeletal dysplasias,[18] obesity,[19] and subchondral bone mineral density[20]) exert their effects predominantly through local biomechanical effects important in determining the site and severity of the disease.[21]

Nevertheless, mechanical stress is likely to be involved in the evolution and pathogenesis of all types of "primary" and secondary OA. Joint failure results from an imbalance between the *combined* effects of mechanical forces and catabolic mediators and the anabolic capacity of the articular tissues to resist and repair the damage. In broad terms, structural failure of articular cartilage, bone, and periarticular tissues in OA may result from either abnormal mechanical stresses damaging initially normal tissues or from the failure of pathologically impaired articular cartilage, bone, or ligaments in response to physiologically normal mechanical stress[22,23] (Fig. 3.1).

Risk factors for the *progression* of OA may be distinct from risk factors for *incident* OA.[24] Obesity, low bone mineral density, chondrocalcinosis, knee effusions, and low intakes of vitamins C and D (as well as biomechanical factors such as joint instability and varus/valgus mal-alignment) have been shown to be risk factors for the *progression* of knee OA.[25]

## JOINT ALIGNMENT AND OBESITY

Joint alignment influences the distribution of load on the articular cartilage and other tissues of weight-bearing joints. The external knee adduction moment generated during walking pushes the knee into the varus, with resulting compression of the medial joint compartment. It has been found that the magnitude of the baseline adduction moment is a strong predictor of progression of medial compartment knee OA,[26] whereas an increased abduction moment at the hip is associated with protection against progression of medial compartment tibiofemoral OA.[27] Intrinsic and acquired changes in alignment are important independent risk factors for the development, localization, and progression of knee OA[17] (with obesity adding significantly to the risk[28,29]). Varus/valgus alignment has been associated with fourfold increases in the progression of medial and lateral compartment knee OA over 18 months.[17] Varus/valgus alignment also influences the development of patellofemoral OA, with lateral patellofemoral OA changes occurring most frequently in association with valgus knees.[30]

After many years of uncertainty, it is now well established that obesity is an important risk factor for

**Fig. 3.1** Mechanical stress and the development of osteoarthritis.[23]

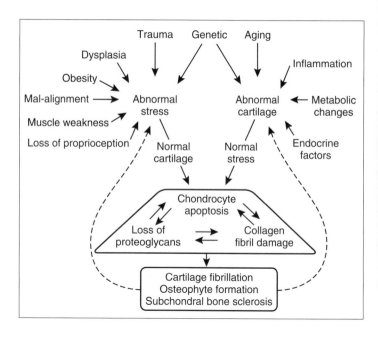

symptomatic and radiographically defined knee OA affecting all compartments of the joint.[31] Cross-sectional data from the U.S. National Health and Nutrition Examination survey shows that men and women with a body mass index of 30 to 35 have a fourfold increase in knee OA compared with normal weight controls.[12] Data from the Framingham study show that obesity precedes the development of knee OA, with a 40% increase in risk (RR 1.4: 95% CI 1.1 to 1.8) for every 5 kg gain in weight.[32] Observations over 8 years in this study showed commensurate decreases in incident knee OA for every 5-kg loss in weight, demonstrating that obesity is a modifiable risk factor. Whereas one recent clinical study has confirmed that weight loss alone can be associated with reduced pain and improved function in overweight patients with knee OA,[33] another emphasized that diet-induced weight loss needs to be combined with exercise to be an effective therapeutic strategy.[34]

## INJURIES AND OCCUPATIONAL RISKS

Meniscus injuries,[35] mal-aligned fractures, and post-traumatic articular cartilage surface defects are important causes of premature localized OA in the knee, and the risk of developing OA is increased more than threefold following major knee injury.[36] Nearly 50% of patients develop knee OA 21 years after open meniscectomy,[37] and the average time to develop secondary hip OA severe enough to warrant hip arthroplasty following fracture dislocation is 7 years.[38] There are cross-sectional epidemiologic studies linking previous injury

with OA of the knee[39,40] and hand,[40] and a longitudinal study with a median follow-up of 36 years confirmed increased risk of knee (RR 5.17, 95% CI 3.07 to 8.71) and hip (RR 3.50, 95% CI 0.84 to 14.69) OA following previous injury.[41] Instability of the knee secondary to cruciate ligament injury leads to premature OA in orthopaedic[42] and veterinary[43] practice, as well as to experimentally induced OA in the stifle joint of dogs.[44,45] It is suggested that joint instability and articular surface incongruity following injury cause repetitive increased contact stress on articular surfaces that can initiate OA or accelerate its progression.[46]

Although it is clear that previous meniscus injury and surgery are the main predisposing causes of knee OA in ex-professional soccer players,[47] the role of sports-related exercise in the absence of defined injury is more controversial. Although there is some evidence for an increase in the prevalence of knee OA in former elite runners, soccer players, weightlifters, and tennis players,[48,49] recreational running seems to be free from this risk[50] and no increase in hip OA was found after 20 years of running marathons.[51] There is some evidence, however, for an increased prevalence of hip OA in professional soccer players,[52] high jumpers, and javelin throwers[53] despite their not having sustained notable hip injuries. There is also evidence that osteophytes may develop in response to some sporting activities in the absence of articular cartilage loss and that joint dysplasia, muscle weakness, neurologic deficits, and increased weight may be confounding risk factors in many reports of OA in athletes.[54]

Evidence that occupations involving repetitive mechanical stress are associated with the development of OA has come from a variety of sources. Industrial surveys in Scotland in the 1960s revealed that OA of the elbows, knees, and spine was a significant clinical problem in miners working at the coalface[55] and that the risk of developing knee OA was increased in dockyard workers involved in heavy manual labor.[56] Subsequent epidemiologic surveys identified occupational risks for the development of OA in the hips and knees in farmers, firefighters, and construction workers.[57] Case-control studies by Croft et al. have shown that farmers are 10 times more likely to develop radiographic evidence of hip OA after 10 years than controls employed in sedentary occupations.[58] Other case-control studies have shown a twofold increase in the risk of developing hip OA in occupations associated with increases in hip joint compression.[59]

Knee OA has been associated with occupations involving knee bending,[12,60,61] squatting,[62] kneeling,[62] and heavy lifting,[12,61,63] with obesity[62] adding considerably to the risk. Lawrence's early studies demonstrating an increase in hand OA in cotton-mill workers in Lancashire[64] were followed by Hadler's seminal investigation of hand OA and job-related activities in three groups of workers in a Virginia textile mill.[65] Women working as burlers or spinners—occupations that involve the use of a repetitive pinch grip, associated with increased mechanical stress through the distal interphalangeal (DIP) joints—developed more OA in the DIPs than those employed as winders (an occupation involving repetitive use of a power grip, which does not impart as much mechanical stress through the DIPs).

## SUBCHONDRAL BONE AND BONE MINERAL DENSITY

The biomechanical properties of the cortical and subchondral bone play a critical role in protecting articular cartilage following impulsive (impact) loading. Tissues of the cortical and subchondral bone and the joint capsule are each 30 times more effective than articular cartilage in attenuating force through joints and synovial fluid, despite its viscoelastic properties, plays no significant role[66] (Table 3.1). The presence of subchondral bone limits the radial deformation of articular cartilage under load and the undulating structure of the tidemark and osteochondral junction helps to transform potentially damaging sheer stresses into less harmful tensile and compressive stresses in the articular cartilage.[67]

Radin and Rose[67] have suggested that the athogenesis of OA is initiated by an increase in density and stiffness in the subchondral bone, allowing microfractures caused by unprotected impulsive loading of joints.

| TABLE 3.1  FORCE ATTENUATION IN JOINTS[66] | |
|---|---|
| Tissue | Attenuation (%) |
| Joint capsule/synovium | 35 |
| Synovial fluid | 0 |
| Articular cartilage | 1–3 |
| Subchondral bone | 30 |
| Cortical bone | 30–35 |

The hypothesis is that loss of bone viscoelasticity results in steep stiffness gradients in the bone, stretching the overlying reticular cartilage to cause cartilage fibrillation. Although the development of subchondral bone sclerosis in OA is associated with loss of up to 50% of the shock-absorbing capacity of normal joints,[68] finite element mathematical models suggest that continued impulsive loading of the stiffened subchondral bone plate could not generate sufficient mechanical strains in the articular cartilage to cause progressive cartilage loss.[69] Nevertheless, support for the hypothesis that the athogenesis of OA may be initiated by changes in bone stiffness has come from studies of bone mineral density (BMD) in patients with OA. Following the critical observation that severe OA changes were seldom observed in femoral heads removed after femoral neck fractures, Foss and Byers showed that BMD was increased in patients with hip OA.[70] It is now well established that people with hip and knee OA do have increased bone mass compared with age-matched controls,[71,72] and this is the case in some[73] but not all[74] studies of patients with hand OA.

Prospective studies of changes in BMD in patients with lower limb OA have also shown contradictory results. Whereas one study showed that women with knee OA maintained or increased heir BMD over three years when compared to a control population,[75] another community-based retrospective study showed that women with hip or knee OA who had 3 to 8% higher femoral neck MD than those without OA lost BMD more rapidly over 2 years than those without OA (possibly as a result of a reduction in physical activity).[76]

Although clinical evidence is beginning to emerge to show that increased subchondral bone density can predict future cartilage loss in patients with knee OA,[20] trabecular bone structure and BMD in the subchondral bone are likely to be important factors determining the transmission of load and mechanical stresses to the articular cartilage in weight-bearing joints. Studies of the relationship between loss of articular cartilage in animal models of mechanically induced OA and subchondral bone density and structure have produced some apparently contradictory results. Using microscopic computed axial tomography (micro CT) in a guinea pig model, Layton and colleagues showed initial loss of trabecular bone volume fraction with thinning of subchondral bone trabeculae followed by thickening of the trabeculae and increases in trabecular bone volume in the femoral heads as the OA advanced.[77]

Using a guinea pig hind limb myectomy OA model, the same group demonstrated micro-CT-detectable changes in the subchondral trabecular bone as early as histologic changes in the articular cartilage.[78] The thickness of the subchondral plate in the medial tibial plateau was also seen to increase with increasing severity of articular cartilage lesions in male and female cynomolgous monkeys with spontaneous knee OA.[79] However, Dedrick et al. showed loss of subchondral trabecular bone in the unstable knee throughout a 54-month longitudinal micro CT study of the subchondral plate and trabecular bone of dogs with experimental stifle joint OA following anterior cruciate ligament transaction (ACLT), suggesting that subchondral bone thickness increase is not a prerequisite for the development of progressive OA lesions in the articular cartilage in this model.[80] Recent experimental studies in female rabbits, in which knee OA was induced by section of the anterior cruciate ligaments and partial medial meniscectomy, have shown that the severity of the articular cartilage damage was increased by prior induction of osteoporosis by ovariectomy and corticosteroids.[81]

Studies of bone texture in macroradiographs of normal and OA knees by analysis of fractal signatures has shown that in OA there are changes in the horizontal structure of the subchondral bone of the tibia, whose height and position match the visual assessment of joint space change.[82] In addition, a recent study has suggested that fractal signature analysis of trabecular bone is a more sensitive marker of structural disease status in knee OA than BMD.[83] High-resolution magnetic resonance imaging (MRI) of trabecular bone adjacent to the knee also shows promise for the noninvasive assessment of trabecular bone volume, trabecular number, and trabecular separation (as well as trabecular thicknesss in patients with knee OA).[84]

## THE MECHANICAL PROPERTIES OF ARTICULAR CARTILAGE

When external loads are applied to joints during movement and weight bearing, shear, tensile, and compressive stresses are generated in the articular cartilage as it changes in shape and the congruence and contact areas of opposing cartilage surfaces are increased. The mechanical functions of articular cartilage and its ability to withstand loading are critically dependent on the structural integrity of its extracellular matrix proteins. In general, the collagen network (predominantly composed of type II collagen) imparts tensile strength, and the negatively charged proteoglycan aggrecan within it resists compression.[85]

When articular cartilage is stretched or loaded in tension, the collagen fibers and aggrecan molecules stretch along the axis of loading.[86,87] The stress/strain relationship follows a sigmoid curve. With minor deformation of the cartilage there is a nonlinear increase in stress as the matrix molecules disentangle and realign. With greater deformation, the fibers stretch and generate a greater linear increase in tensile stress (following Young's modulus), and this has been shown to be dependent on the concentration of the collagen fibrils and cross-links, the type of collagen cross-links, and the strength of the ionic bonds and interactions between the collagen and aggrecan networks.[88-90] In addition to type II collagen and aggrecan, articular cartilage contains small amounts of collagens VI, IX, and XI and a number of other matrix proteins.

Among these, two families of leucine-rich small proteoglycans appear to be important in the assembly of collagen fibers and in their interactions.[91] Collagens IX and XI play a role in determining the diameter of collagen II fibers,[92] whereas decorin and biglycan promote the assembly of collagen VI[93,94] (which is abundant in the pericellular matrix of the chondrocytes). Decorin also inhibits fibrillogenesis.[95] Electron histochemical studies have recently shown that there are proteoglycan bridges between collagen fibrils in cartilage[96] (similar to those previously demonstrated in tendon and other extracellular matrices[97]) that are composed of anionic glycosaminoglycans attached to decorin. Scott suggests that these "shape modules"[98] play a vital mechanical cohesive role in cartilage,[96] resisting pulling forces orthogonal to the collagen fibrils. They may also add to the elasticity of cartilage through the intrinsic intramolecular concertina-like elastic property of the l-iduronate (containing decorin), which has been demonstrated in vitro by atomic force microscopy on stretched single molecules of this small proteoglycan.[99]

When cartilage is loaded in compression, however, it behaves as a viscoelastic material that is predominantly flow dependent.[100] Static compression results in structural deformation that is accompanied by changes in volume as interstitial fluid is lost and redistributed, and by changes in fixed-charge density,[101] mobile ion concentrations,[102] and osmotic pressure.[103] Recovery of shape and volume is time dependent and is accompanied by creep and dissipation of energy.[100] Dynamic compression is associated with physical deformation of the chondrocyte and its nucleus,[104] as well as by hydrostatic pressurization, pressure gradients, and fluid flow (which generate streaming potentials and currents).[105] However, interstitial fluid pressurization provides a mechanism for stress shielding that protects the cells and matrix of cartilage to some extent.[106]

Within the articular cartilage, chondrocytes are enclosed in localized regions of specialized pericellular matrix ("chondrons"[107])—which differ from the interterritorial matrix of the articular cartilage in their biochemical,[108] ultrastructural,[109,110] and biomechanical properties.[111-113] In a series of studies on isolated chondrons, Poole and colleagues demonstrated that the pericellular matrix in these structures is composed of a compacted filamentous capsule containing collagens VI[108] and IX[114] (as well as relatively high concentrations of aggrecan and decorin).[115] They have suggested that the type VI collagen provides a substratum (for functional interaction between the chondrocyte and the pericelluar capsule) that resists the hydrodynamic distention of the chondrons during compressive loading of the cartilage, and that both collagens VI and IX serve to tether and stabilize the chondrocytes within the cartilage matrix.[108,114]

Others have also postulated that the chondron as a whole may function as a mechanical transducer.[116-118] The Young's modulus of the pericellular matrix (approximately 40 kPa) and its permeability (approximately $4 \times 10^{-17}$ m$^4$/Ns)[119] are an order of magnitude lower than those of the extracellular matrix of normal articular cartilage (approximately 1 MPa[119] and $9 \times 10^{-16}$ m$^4$/Ns[121]). In chondrons from osteoarthritic cartilage, Young's modulus is 40% lower still, and permeability is 2.5 times greater.[119] These findings support the hypothesis that the pericellular matrix has a significant influence on the mechanical environment of chondrocytes in articular cartilage.[122,123] Using a biphasic finite element model it has been calculated that the differences in the Young's moduli of the pericellular and interterritorial matrix will result in amplification of strain in the vicinity of the chondrocyte by 50%.[122]

Because the Young's modulus of articular cartilage increases with depth,[124] the ratio of the moduli in the pericellular versus extracellular matrix decreases in the lower zone of the cartilage and the amplification of strain is more pronounced. The reduced permeability of the pericellular matrix, compared with that of the interterritorial matrix, results in a thirtyfold reduction in fluid flow in the vicinity of the chondrocyte. The reduction in the Young's modulus and the permability of the pericellular matrix in OA leads to a further 66% increase in compressive strain and higher fluid flux in the vicinity of chondrocytes in OA articular cartilage.[113]

# PHYSIOLOGIC RESPONSES TO LOADING OF ARTICULAR CARTILAGE

The exact range of mechanical strains experienced by chondrocytes in vivo in normal or osteoarthritic articular cartilage during normal or abnormal physical activities is difficult to determine. Using force plates and gait analyses, Paul[125] showed that forces up to seven times body weight were generated at the hip during rapid walking (2 m/sec) and that forces of three to four times body weight at the hip and knee were generated during walking at normal speeds (1.5 m/sec). A few measurements with implanted pressure transducers have shown that peak contact pressures of 10 to 20 MPa are generated in the hip during standing or climbing stairs.[126]

Using X-ray arthrography and MRI it has been shown that articular cartilage may be compressed by 13 to 44% following prolonged physiologic static loads,[127,128] with up to 3% absolute deformation within the first minute of loading.[128] Static loading is generally associated with depression of matrix synthesis, whereas dynamic high-frequency cyclical loading is associated with increases of up to 50% in proteoglycan synthesis.[129,130] Cyclical compression of articular cartilage can have variable effects on proteoglycan synthesis, depending on the nature of the loading and whether measurements of synthesis are made during or following compression.[130] In general, loads that raise hydrostatic pressure and cause fluid movement without significant fluid loss lead to an increase in matrix synthesis (whereas loading conditions that lead to fluid loss decrease synthesis).

# THE EFFECTS OF EXERCISE AND JOINT IMMOBILIZATION ON ARTICULAR CARTILAGE MATRIX

Overloading[131] and unloading[132] of articular cartilage are both associated with proteoglycan depletion, whereas proteoglycan synthesis and cartilage thickness are increased by mechanical stresses associated with physiologic exercise.[133] Matrix atrophy of articular cartilage following joint immobilization is not always completely restored with normal ambulation, and recovery can be inhibited by exercise. Palmoski and Brandt showed that Safranin O staining, uronic acid content, and net PG synthesis (markedly reduced in articular cartilage following six weeks of immobilization of stifle joints of dogs) recovered to levels in control knees 3 weeks after the removal of the splints. However, matrix PGs remained depleted in dogs run on a treadmill daily for a similar period.[134] Kiviranta found that glycosaminoglycan (GAG) concentrations were reduced by 20 to 48% in canine articular cartilage after splinting the stifle joints in flexion for 11 weeks.[135] GAG concentrations were restored to normal in some parts of the articular cartilage 15 weeks after remobilization[136] but remained reduced in the superficial zone of the cartilage covering the lateral tibial condyle after nearly a year of normal physical activity.[137]

Treadmill running was shown to result in depletion of GAGs in the articular cartilage of rabbits[138] and dogs.[139] Kiviranta and colleagues showed that although treadmill running of 4 km/day five days/week for 15 weeks resulted in increased femoral articular cartilage thickness and PG content in beagles[140] more intensive running for 20 or 40 km/day was associated with increased water content and depletion of GAGs and collagen in the articular cartilage[141,142] (as well as with extensive subchondral bone remodeling).[143] Radin had previously observed a reduction in hexosamine in the distal femoral articular cartilage of sheep (in association with cartilage fibrillation and changes in the trabecular pattern and thickness of the subchondral bone) following 2½ years of daily walking exercise on concrete.[144] Others have shown that moderate exercise exacerbated the histopathologic lesions of OA in the knees of sheep following meniscectomy,[145] although the PG content was increased.[146]

## STUDIES IN CARTILAGE EXPLANTS AND THREE-DIMENSIONAL CHONDROCYTE CULTURES

Because of the difficulties in studying the mechanisms by which chondrocytes respond to mechanical stimulation in vivo, the effects of various regimes of mechanical stress on matrix metabolism and chondrocyte gene expression have been extensively studied in vitro in cartilage explants, or in agarose[147] or alginate[148] 3D chondrocyte cell culture systems in which many of the phenotypic characteristics of chondrocytes are maintained. Inhibition of proteoglycan synthesis following static pressurization or loading[149] occurs within an hour of compression of cartilage explants.[150] However, 50% compression of calf articular cartilage explants was followed by an initial increase in aggrecan and type II collagen mRNA after 30 minutes' compression with only a later decrease in gene expression.[151] Others showed a dose-dependent increase in aggrecan mRNA between 0.1 and 0.25 MPa in bovine cartilage explants following 1 hour of compression with a time-dependent return to normal levels, and a reversal of the stimulatory effect at higher loads (0.5 MPa).[152] Stimulation of PG synthesis by dynamic cyclical loading in cartilage explants[150,153,154] is influenced by the zone of the articular cartilage from which the explant is obtained,[155] as well as by fluid flow[154] and the frequency

and amplitude of compression.[150,156] GAG synthesis was inhibited in chondrocytes from bovine articular cartilage subjected to 15% static or low-frequency (0.3 to 3 Hz) compressive strains in agarose constructs, whereas a frequency of 1 Hz stimulated synthesis[157] with maximal stimulation after 12 hours of intermittent compression.[158] Others have shown that the GAG accumulates in chondrocyte/agarose constructs subjected to 10% intermittent compressive strains at a frequency of 1 Hz over 21 days.[159]

PG synthesis following cyclical compression of cartilage explants is further augmented by the stimulation of matrix transport/release of growth factors such as insulin-like growth factor 1 (IGF-1).[160] In addition to its effects on PG synthesis, cyclical compression of cartilage explants increases the synthesis of fibronectin and cartilage oligomeric matrix protein (COMP)[161] and influences the orientation of the collagen fibers in the superficial zone of the articular cartilage.[162] PG synthesis is also increased by 25 to 50%, and collagen synthesis is stimulated, following dynamic *shear* loading of bovine articular cartilage explants at physiologically relevant strain amplitudes (1 to 3%) and a wide range of frequencies (0.01 to 1.0 Hz), which are associated with matrix and chondrocyte deformation without significant fluid flow.[163]

## MECHANO-TRANSDUCTION

To respond appropriately to applied mechanical forces, chondrocytes need to be able to receive information from their environment and modify that environment appropriately to the mechanical stresses to which they are exposed. This process involves mechano-coupling (where the forces at the macroscopic tissue level are translated into local action at the surface of the chondrocyte) and mechano-transduction, whereby the forces are transduced from the outside of the sensor cell into biochemical signals leading to altered gene expression and protein production.[164]

The responses of cells to mechanical stimuli may be acute or rapid, occurring within seconds to minutes or as longer-term changes that occur over hours. The rapid responses are due to the activation of a variety of intracellular signaling pathways, and include changes in intracellular calcium concentrations and cAMP levels, specific tyrosine phosphorylation events, and activation of signaling molecules [including PLC and protein kinase C (PKC)]. Effects on tissue structure and architecture, subsequent to tissue modeling and remodeling, will take longer to manifest. Such changes are seen in young rabbits (where chondrocytes are enlarged following exercise)[165] and in beagles, where cartilage stiffness and proteoglycan content are increased following a regime of non-strenuous exercise.[140]

In cartilage, mechano-coupling is performed by the extracellular matrix surrounding the chondrocytes. The nature and distribution of the ECM components help distribute the load applied across the tissue and absorb some of the force applied.

Chondrocytes are potentially exposed to a variety of mechanical forces, including stretch, shear, and compressive forces in vivo.[166-168] To recognize and respond to at least some, if not all, of these forms of mechanical stimulation chondrocytes must express cell membrane mechano-receptors that transduce the mechanical stimulus into intracellular biochemical signals. This function may be carried out by a range of transmembrane receptors, including both extracellular matrix receptors and mechanical sensitive ion channels.

A number of model systems are being used to investigate chondrocyte and cartilage responses to mechanical stimuli in vitro. These include monolayer cultures as well as 3D cultures in agarose or alginate, cartilage explants, and explant cultures. The studies using cartilage explants and 3D cultures most closely replicate the in vivo situation, with chondrocytes being surrounded by a specialized pericellular matrix that is likely to be important in transmission of mechanical signals to the cell surface.

Such studies are beginning to provide important information on chondrocyte mechano-transduction, but there is great diversity in the model systems used, differences in source of articular cartilage, animal species, and application of different forms of dynamic stimuli that make comparison difficult. Furthermore, the intrinsic complexity of 3D culture systems and explants and the technical difficulty of analyzing what are often transient biochemical signaling events limit the type of analysis that can be undertaken using such models. Monolayer culture systems, especially those that attempt to minimize the influence of chondrocyte de-differentiation, can provide important information on early signaling events and molecules involved in mechano-transduction.

## BIOLOGICAL RESPONSES TO MECHANICAL STIMULATION

Studies exploring the effects of different forms of mechanical stimulation on cartilage and chondrocytes have analyzed a variety of tissue and cellular responses. Proliferation, measured by radioactive thymidine uptake and glycosaminoglycan or proteoglycan production assessed by radioactive sulfate incorporation, has been widely used as a marker of a biological response of chondrocytes. In general, these studies show that dynamic stimulation of cartilage explants and 3D and monolayer chondrocyte cultures leads to increased proliferation of chondrocytes as well as increased glycosaminoglycan synthesis[150,157,160,169,170] (resulting in an anabolic protective response).

In contrast, static loading of cartilage explants suppresses proliferation as well as GAG synthesis[149,150,170-173] and may be thought of as being catabolic or at least non-anabolic. Studies using molecular methodology have confirmed dynamic mechanical stimulation as anabolic, increasing expression of a number of cellular and cartilage matrix proteins (including aggrecan, type II collagen, and cartilage oligomeric matrix protein).[174-176] In contrast, static, injurious, or high-magnitude mechanical stimuli inhibit aggrecan and type II collagen gene expression and induce expression of genes and activity of catabolic molecules [including MMP-1, MMP-3, MMP-9, IL-1β, and TNF-α].[151,177-179]

## CHONDROCYTE MECHANO-RECEPTORS

Compression of cartilage results in complex changes within the tissue, which include matrix and cell deformation, hydrostatic pressure gradients, fluid flow and altered matrix water content, osmotic pressure, ion concentration, and fixed-charge density. Chondrocytes probably have the capacity to recognize most or all of these physico-chemical changes, and activation of cell signaling cascades subsequent to stimulation of the appropriate cell receptor for that stimulus will most likely be the initial step in chondrocyte mechano-transduction. Therefore, molecules or molecular complexes that recognize physico-chemical changes (including changes in cell shape, cell membrane deformation, local ion concentration, and fluid flow) have been identified as candidate chondrocyte mechano-receptors and include integrins[180] and mechano-sensitive ion channels.[181]

### Integrins

Integrins are heterodimeric transmembrane glycoproteins that comprise an α and a β subunit. There are at least 16 α and 8 β subunits, combining to form more than 20 specific integrin receptors.[182] The combination of α and β subunits determines the ligand specificity of the receptor. Some of these receptors are specific for a particular ligand: α5β1 and αVβ1 bind fibronectin, whereas α6β1 and α6β4 are laminin receptors. Other integrin dimers are able to interact with multiple ligands. αVβ3 binds both vitronectin and osteopontin. α1β1, α2β1, and α11β1 each bind to type II and type VI collagen. Each α and β subunit consists of a large extracellular domain, a single transmembrane region, and a cytoplasmic tail. The extracellular domain provides the ligand-binding site for its extracellular matrix protein ligand. The cytoplasmic tail interacts with intracellular signaling molecules and the actin cytoskeleton, enabling the integrin receptor to transduce mechanical signals into biochemical responses within the cell.[182,183]

Identifying roles for integrins and other potential mechanoreceptors in chondrocytes is dependent on showing that the molecules are present both in vivo and in the in vitro model system being tested. Chondrocytes are known to de-differentiate following passage in monolayer culture, and this is associated with changes in integrin expression (which may influence mechanical signaling). $\alpha_1\beta_1$, $\alpha_5\beta_1$, $\alpha_{10}\beta_1$, and $\alpha V\beta_5$ appear to be the major integrins expressed in normal adult human articular cartilage, although expression alters in OA with increased expression of other subunits such as $\alpha_2$ integrin.[184-186] Roles for integrins in chondrocyte mechano-transduction have been investigated predominantly in monolayer and more recently 3D culture systems.

Oligopeptides and specific integrin subunit function-blocking antibodies are available for study of integrin function and have been used to identify roles for integrins in a variety of mechanical induced responses in chondrocytes. Short peptides such as GRGDSP are known to interfere competitively with integrin binding to a common RGD sequence in a number of ligands, including fibronectin and vitronectin.[182] As a number of integrin dimers (including $\alpha_5\beta_1$, $\alpha V\beta_3$, and $\alpha V\beta_5$) may interact with a variety of ligands in an RGD-dependent manner (studies with RGD peptides are indicative of integrin involvement but do not show specific function). Specific integrin involvement in a mechanical response is more readily identified by the use of subunit-specific function-modulating antibodies.

Studies on short-term primary monolayer culture of human chondrocytes extracted from human knee and hip joint articular cartilage have demonstrated that RGD peptides and function-modifying antibodies against $\alpha_5$ and $\beta_1$ integrin prevent a number of cellular responses to 0.33-Hz mechanical stimulation, including changes in membrane potential, tyrosine phosphorylation, and PKC activation and increases in aggrecan gene expression and GAG production[187-189] (Fig. 3.2). These results suggest that $\alpha_5\beta_1$ integrin is the prime mechano-receptor for this specific form of mechanical stimulus but do not rule out the possibility that other integrins may act as mechano-receptors for other frequencies or forms of mechanical stimulation that may regulate different cell responses. It is known that normal human chondrocytes show different electrophysiologic responses when mechanically stimulated in monolayer at 0.104 Hz and 0.33 Hz. 0.104-Hz stimulation results in a tetrodotoxin-sensitive membrane depolarization, whereas 0.33-Hz stimulation induces an apamin-sensitive hyperpolarization response.[190,191]

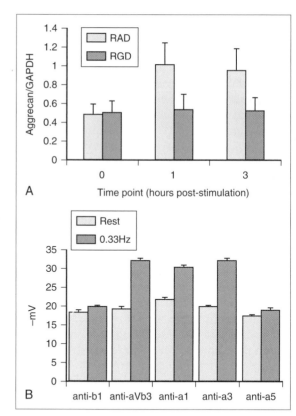

**Fig. 3.2** Effects of blockade of integrin function on (A) the increase of aggrecan gene expression and (B) the membrane hyperpolarization response of chondrocytes to 0.33-Hz mechanical stimulation.

Although it is unclear which specific receptors are involved in the 0.104-Hz response in chondrocytes, similar studies have demonstrated that in human bone cells the 0.104-Hz depolarization is dependent on a Vb5 integrin in addition to a 5b1, the 0.33-Hz response being dependent only on $\alpha_5\beta_1$ integrin.[192] Consistent with the results of studies on chondrocytes in monolayer culture, experiments using 3D culture systems and cartilage explants show roles for integrins in chondrocyte mechano-transduction. RGD peptides block inhibition of NO production and the up-regulation of cell proliferation and proteoglycan synthesis of bovine chondrocytes in 3D agarose culture.[193]

Dynamic compression of explants of calf articular cartilage and cylindrical alginate/chondrocyte constructs results in increased COMP expression, which is abolished by $\beta_1$ integrin antibodies.[194] It remains unclear how mechanical stimulation activates integrin-dependent cascades. As RGD-containing peptides block chondrocyte responses it is broadly accepted that interactions between integrins and their extracellular ligands are necessary for cellular mechano-transduction. $\alpha_5\beta_1$ is the classical fibronectin receptor,[182] and RGD-dependent interactions between the chondrocyte and this extracellular matrix molecule preferentially expressed in a pericellular situation in normal articular cartilage would appear to be an important bridge between the extracellular matrix and the chondrocyte through which mechanical forces can be transferred and converted into biochemical responses.[180]

Integrins are linked to the actin cytoskeleton at specialized sites termed focal adhesions.[183] At focal adhesions, integrin cytoplasmic domains interact with a number of signaling molecules and link to the actin cytoskeleton.[195] The actin cytoskeleton plays an important role in the link between compression of the extracellular matrix and deformation of chondrocyte nuclei.[104] An intact actin cytoskeleton is required for normal human articular mechano-transduction,[187] and mechanical stimulation of chondrocytes results in the transient activation of focal adhesion proteins (including paxillin and focal adhesion kinase).[189] Both static and cyclic compressive strain and hydrostatic pressure induce remodeling of actin cytoskeleton,[196] characterized by a change from a uniform to a more punctuate distribution of cortical actin around the cell periphery.

## Stretch-activated Ion Channels

Stretch-activated ion channels (SACs) are also likely candidates as chondrocyte mechano-receptors/mechano-sensors.[181] SACs are believed to respond to mechanical forces along the plane of the cell membrane (membrane tension), but not to hydrostatic pressure perpendicular to it.[181,197] Mechanical stimulation of chondrocytes by fluid flow and micropipette indentation, osmotic pressure, and hydrostatic pressure[198-201] leads to a rapid increase in intracellular calcium levels.

This elevation of intracellular calcium, which may be seen after only one cycle of compression in 3D agarose constructs,[202] will allow activation of calcium-dependent intracellular signaling pathways. Alternatively, SACs may interact with the integrins (forming an integrated signaling complex),[203] although ion-channel-based mechano-sensory complexes may have different roles in regulation of cell responses from integrin and focal-adhesion-dependent complexes.[204] Gadolinium, a blocker of SACs, has been used to identify the possible role of SACs in chondrocyte mechano-transduction. Gadolinium blocks membrane hyperpolarization, tyrosine phosphorylation of FAK and paxillin, and the increase in aggrecan gene expression that follows 0.33-Hz mechanical stimulation of human chondrocytes in monolayer culture[191,187-189] (Fig. 3.3).

As gadolinium has been shown to abolish proliferation of chick embryonic chondrocytes, but did not affect the up-regulation of cartilage matrix protein mRNA by mechanical stretch,[205] the likelihood is that stretch-activated ion channels are important regulators of

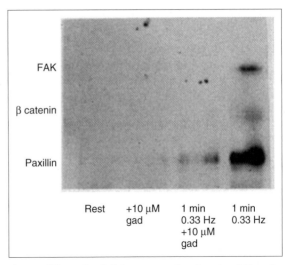

**Fig. 3.3** Effects of gadolinium on tyrosine phosphorylation of focal adhesion kinase (FAK), β catenin, and paxillin following 1-minute 0.33-Hz mechanical stimulation of normal human articular chondrocytes.

the differential response of cells to mechanical stimuli. The effect of gadolinium on mechanically induced proliferation of chicken chondrocytes appears to be through blockade of a mechano-transduction pathway involving Indian hedgehog (and, further downstream, bone morphogenic) protein 2/4.[206]

In addition to SACs, a number of other ion channels appear to show mechano-sensitivity (including voltage or ligand-gated channels, such as the Shaker-IR K+ channel,[207] N-type Ca2+ channels,[208] the NMDA receptor channel,[209] and Ca2+-dependent BK channels).[210] Potential roles for these molecules in chondrocyte mechano-transduction have been suggested. β1-integrins have been shown to co-localize with Na, K-ATPase, epithelial sodium channels, and voltage-activated calcium channels—possibly in mechano-receptor complexes of mouse limb-bud chondrocytes.[203]

Roles for NMDA receptor function in chondrocyte mechano-transduction have been assessed by establishing effects of pharmacologic inhibition of glutamate receptors on the electrophysiologic response of normal chondrocytes to mechanical stimulation.[211] The membrane hyperpolarization of normal chondrocytes to 20-minute 0.33-Hz mechanical stimulation is inhibited by preincubation of the cells with either 30 μM CPP (a competitive NMDA receptor antagonist) or 1-μM MK801 (a noncompetitive NMDA receptor antagonist), whereas AMPA/kainate glutamate receptor antagonists and metabotropic receptor antagonists had no effect on the electrophysiologic response of normal or osteoarthritic chondrocytes.

# MECHANICALLY STIMULATED ACTIVATION OF INTRACELLULAR SIGNAL CASCADES

Following recognition of the mechanical stimulus by the chondrocyte, there is activation of a number of cascades of downstream intracellular signaling pathways with generation of secondary messenger molecules that regulate a range of mechano-sensitive physiologic responses. These include activation of G-proteins, protein kinases, transcription factors, and signaling molecules involved in the generation of death and cell survival pathways.

## G-protein-coupled Receptor Signal Transduction Pathways

Heterotrimeric guanine nucleotide binding proteins (G proteins) are associated with cell surface receptors. G-protein-coupled receptors play an important role in cartilage development.[212,213] G proteins are associated with a number of different intracellular signal cascades, depending on the subclass. Gs proteins interact with adenyl cyclase, which catalyzes the synthesis of the second-messenger cAMP and activation of the protein kinase A signaling pathway. Gq and Go activate phospholipase C (PLC). Activated PLC hydrolyzes phosphatidylinositol-bis-phosphate ($PIP_2$) into inositol-triphosphate ($IP_3$) and diacylglycerol (DAG), which act as second messengers and cause calcium release from intracellular storage sites and PKC activation, respectively.

Studies of the role of G proteins in chondrocyte mechano-transduction are limited. G proteins appear to be involved in the hyper-osmotic stress-induced volume change and calcium transients and shear-induced stimulation of matrix metalloprotease-9 in rabbit chondrocytes.[199] Roles for signaling molecules downstream of G proteins have, however, been investigated further.

### Cyclic AMP and Protein Kinase A

Cyclic AMP, formed from ATP by the action of adenylate cyclase, is increased in chondrocytes following mechanical stimulation. Cyclic AMP is involved in the regulation of gene expression in statically compressed bovine cartilage explants.[177] Cyclic AMP activates protein kinase A and it is likely that this molecule and downstream mediators are important in regulating at least some of the responses of chondrocytes to mechanical stimulation.[177]

### Phospholipase C and Protein Kinase C

In chondrocytes, mechanical stimulation activates PLC, with a subsequent increase of intracellular inositol 1,4,5-triphosphate (which may lead to an increase in intracellular calcium and/or PKC activation).

Compressive stress of 0.1 MPa for 1 hour of bovine articular cartilage explants results in stimulation of aggrecan mRNA levels.[214] This stimulation is inhibited by antagonists of the phosphoinositol, Ca(2+)/calmodulin signaling, indicating a requirement for IP3- and Ca(2+)/calmodulin-dependent signaling processes. PKC is transiently activated in human articular chondrocytes following cyclical mechanical stimulation,[215] but similar studies (albeit with different loading parameters) have shown an inhibition of PKC activity following mechanical stimulation of bovine chondrocytes.[216]

The studies with monolayer cultures of human chondrocytes indicate that both PLC and PKC are required for the integrin-dependent electrophysiologic response of normal and OA chondrocytes, suggesting that activation is downstream of integrin stimulation. PKC activation occurs rapidly after the onset of mechanical stimulation, translocation to the cell membrane of PKCα being seen within 30 to 60 seconds of stimulation.[215] This translocation involves both RACK1 (a PKC regulatory protein) and β1 integrin. PKC activation is believed to be a permissive link in integrin-dependent cytokine signaling[217] and has roles in control of mitogen-activated protein kinase (MAPK) signaling pathways activated in chondrocytes subjected to mechanical stimulation.[218,219]

## The Phosphoinositide3-kinase Akt and Protein Kinase B Pathway

Protein kinase B (PKB) is a 57-kDa serine/threonine kinase, originally identified as an inactivator of glycogen synthase (GSK3β) in response to insulin-like growth factor.[220] PKB, when activated by phosphorylation on amino acids Thr308 and Ser473 by phosphoinositide3-kinase (PI3-kinase), has several important effects (including inhibition of apoptosis by phosphorylation and inactivation of pro-apoptotic factors Bad and caspase-9).[221] PI3-kinase may be activated via integrin stimulation, receptor tyrosine kinases, and cytokines.[222,223] It would be expected that in cartilage optimal or physiologic loading would provide pro-survival signals and injurious mechanical loads might produce death signals in cells.

There is now extensive in vitro work to support the in vivo observations that excess mechanical loads induce chondrocyte cell death,[224] and this may involve PKB signaling. The probable mechanisms of PKB activation in response to mechanical stimulation are yet to be fully explored, but mechanical-stimulation-induced activation of PKB in monolayer cultures of human ankle joint chondrocytes appears to be integrin dependent.[225] High shear forces applied to chondrocytes are also known to suppress PI3-K, which by repressing antioxidant capacity can contribute to apoptosis.[226]

## The NF-κβ Pathway

NF-κβ is a key element of many chondrocyte signaling pathways, including responses to pro-inflammatory cytokines[227] and matrix fragments[228] adopting a pro- or anti-apoptotic role.[229,230] Mechanical stimuli may interact with the NF-κβ pathway to block or augment activity. Dynamic mechanical stimulation of low amplitude has shown to have an inhibitory effect on IL1β–dependent NF-κβ nuclear translocation and thereby have an anti-catabolic effect.[227] Conversely, high-amplitude dynamic stimulation (which may induce catabolic activities) can induce rapid nuclear translocation of NF-κβ subunits p65 and p50 in a similar manner to IL1β.[227]

## Mitogen-activated Protein Kinases

The MAPK signaling pathways are of critical importance for cell survival, cell differentiation, and chondrogenesis. These pathways are involved in a broad range of cellular responses that lead to activation of transcription factors and gene expression in response to growth factors, cytokines, and a wide variety of environmental stresses (including mechanical stresses).[231] Both static and dynamic compression of cartilage explants results in activation of members of the MAPK signaling pathway.[232] Dynamic compression of bovine and porcine cartilage explants results in ERK activation.[233,234]

The response to static compression appears to be magnitude dependent (with greater than 25% static compression activating ERK), whereas lesser degrees of compression do not lead to a significant ERK response.[233,235] Indeed, static compression of cartilage explants (which would be expected to inhibit proteoglycan production) has been shown to result in the phosphorylation of several of the MAPK family (including ERK 1 and 2, p38 mitogen-activated protein kinase (p38), and *c*-Jun).[232] ERK activation by fluid strain in bovine chondrocytes is associated with a decrease in aggrecan gene expression.[235]

The results from these studies are not what one might expect, as growth factors such as IGF-1 (which are anabolic) are also known to induce ERK activation (albeit with a different temporal pattern).[232] However, IGF-1 stimulation of human articular chondrocyte proteoglycan production is through the PI3K signaling pathway rather than the ERK/MAPK pathway.[236] Indeed, ERK activity may serve as a negative regulator of proteoglycan synthesis.[236]

In vivo studies have indicated that functional cartilage loading induces the AP-1 and Runx2 transcription factors through the JNK and ERK/MAPK cascades.[237] As MAPKs may be activated through a number of pathways by stimuli that induce anabolic or catabolic activity, more work needs to be undertaken in this field to provide greater understanding of the interplay between mechanical stimulation and growth factors in the regulation of chondrocyte function.

## Growth Factors and Autocrine/Paracrine Signaling Events in Chondrocyte Mechano-transduction

Chondrocytes express receptors for a large number of soluble mediators, including growth factors, cytokines, and neuropeptides. The interactions between signals generated by ligand ligation of these receptors and mechanical-stimuli-generated signals are likely to be complex. As the cellular responses to mechanical stimuli and soluble mediators activate similar signal cascades (inducing either anabolic or catabolic responses), it would be expected that together they may be antagonistic, additive, or synergistic. This idea is supported by a variety of studies that show that anabolic cytokines and growth factors enhance mechanically induced production of matrix molecules by chondrocytes and tissue-engineered cartilage constructs.[238,239] Similarly, anabolic dynamic mechanical stimuli can counteract the effects of catabolic cytokines such as IL1β,[240-243] and there are synergistic effects on proteoglycan loss with injurious mechanical stimuli and catabolic cytokines.[244]

Changes in the cytokine milieu of joints and cartilage will have important effects on mechanical signaling events. Integrin mechano-receptor expression and integrin-matrix affinity are modulated by growth factors and cytokines, which may alter integrin signaling. This may occur through the alteration of matrix protein production[245] or through stimulation of MMPs and aggrecanase[246,247] matrix degradation (and thereby the composition of the matrix with which the integrin receptors interact).[228] Similarly, a variety of growth factors and cytokines have been shown to be important in the regulation of integrin expression and function.[183,248,249] Both IGF-1 and tissue growth factor (TGF) beta stimulate chondrocyte cell surface expression of the alpha-3/alpha-5 integrin subunit and stimulate adhesion of chondrocytes to fibronectin and type II collagen.[249] Connective tissue growth factor (CTGF) enhances chondrocyte adhesion to fibronectin via α5β1 integrin through direct interaction of its C-terminal domain.

Cytokine and cytokine-activated signaling pathways, including the JAK-STAT pathway, are also heavily influenced by integrin activation following adhesion to the matrix molecules[250] and presumably also following mechanical stimulation. The ability of a cytokine or growth factor to activate at least some intracellular signal cascades is dependent on cell binding to matrix molecules and integrin ligation. Integrin-mediated adhesion to extracellular matrix is necessary for the optimal activation of growth factor receptors,[251] and the proliferative response of rabbit sternal chondrocytes to fibroblast growth factor is dependent on the cells binding to fibronectin via α5β1 integrin.[252] IGF-1 and tissue growth factor β are capable of up-regulating protein and proteoglycan synthesis in chondrocytes without the requirement of additional factors.

When coupled with dynamic mechanical stimulation, but not static stimulation, the up-regulation of proteoglycan is increased.[160,253] In the case of IGF, this increase is additive rather than synergistic, suggesting that mechanical compression and IGF-1 act via different pathways.[160,254] Dynamic compression accelerates the rate at which IGF-1 shows an effect in cartilage explants, raising the possibility that the mechanical compression increased the transport into the tissue of soluble factors present in the surrounding medium. There is also accumulating evidence that production of soluble mediators by chondrocytes or from cartilage in response to mechanical stimulation may be intrinsic to mechano-transduction pathways.

Mechanical forces, including stretch and compression, are known to induce the secretion of soluble mediators (including cytokines, growth factors, and prostaglandins) in a number of mechano-sensitive cell types (including cardiac myocytes, osteoblasts, endothelial cells, and fibroblasts) that may be necessary for tissue modeling and remodeling responses. Similar autocrine/paracrine mechanisms are stimulated when articular chondrocytes are exposed to mechanical stimuli. These soluble factors, which include a number of anabolic and catabolic molecules [such as IL1β[255] and NO],[256] may also have effects on other cells within joints, such as synovial cells, cells of the underlying bone, and neurons.

In vitro studies with monolayer cultures of normal human articular chondrocytes have identified roles for interleukin 4 (IL4) and the neuropeptide substance P in the integrin-dependent response to 0.33-Hz stimulation[174,257,258] (Fig. 3.4). IL4 and substance P are secreted relatively early in the chondrocyte mechano-transduction cascade, activity being demonstrated within 20 minutes of mechanical stimulation (suggesting release from preformed stores). Both IL4 and substance P are necessary for changes in gene expression induced by the mechanical stimulus, suggesting cross-talk with other integrin-dependent signaling pathways activated by the mechanical stimulation.

The mechanisms by which integrin-dependent mechano-transduction results in the production of these autocrine/paracrine signaling molecules and how they influence chondrocyte responses are unclear. Substance P release is upstream of IL4 in the signal cascade and acts through the NK1 receptor to induce IL4 release.[258]

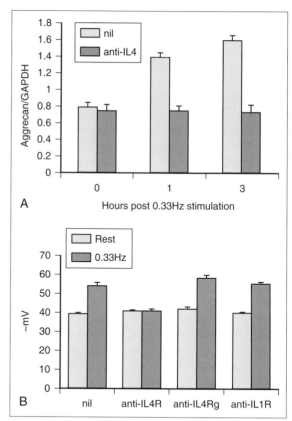

**Fig. 3.4** Effect of blockade of IL4 activity by function-blocking antibodies on (A) the increase of aggrecan mRNA and (B) the hyperpolarization response of normal human articular chondrocytes mechanically stimulated at 0.33 Hz.

The observation that substance P can also modulate integrin-mediated cell adhesion to fibronectin, through up-regulation of α5 integrin expression,[259] raises the possibility of roles for this molecule in feedback control mechanisms of chondrocyte mechano-transduction. Chondrocytes from normal and OA human articular cartilage express components of both the type I (IL4Rα and γc subunits) and type II (IL4Rα and IL13Rα1 subunits) IL4 receptor, and downstream signaling appears to be predominantly through the type II receptor.[260] Mechanical stimulation of chondrocytes results in IL4-dependent phosphorylation of Tyk2, a member of the JAK/STAT transcription pathway.[260]

In addition to IL4, parathyroid-related protein (PTH-RH), TGF, vascular endothelial growth factor (VEGF), and IL1 have been shown to be produced by chondrocytes following mechanical stimulation. Each of these molecules, when secreted by the chondrocyte, will have the potential to influence cartilage and chondrocyte structure and function. PTH-RH and TGF appear to be involved in the effects of mechanical stimulation on the growth plate. Parathyroid-related protein is up-regulated in rat proliferating growth plate chondrocytes by a mechanism that involves a nifedipine-sensitive calcium channel rather than a gadolinium-sensitive stretch-activated ion channel.[261] Terminal differentiation and mineralization of growth plate chondrocytes is negatively regulated by mechanical stimulation through a signal pathway involving TGF.[262]

VEGF, on the other hand, seems to be involved in the response of articular chondrocytes to injurious mechanical stimuli and as such may contribute to OA.[263] VEGF, an important angiogenesis factor, has recently been shown to be expressed in osteoarthritic cartilage. Absent in normal bovine cartilage, mechanical stimulation of VEGF is induced by mechanical overload and appears to be necessary for mechanically induced MMP-1, -3, and -13 expression.[264] Mechanical-compression-induced proteoglycan loss in cartilage explants is inhibited by IL 1 receptor antagonist (IL 1ra), supporting a role for the IL 1 receptor in the pathway linking static compression to reduced proteoglycan synthesis.[265]

Mechanical stimulation may also induce release or activation of growth factors from cartilage matrix, which will then act on nearby resident chondrocytes. Basic fibroblast growth factor (bFGF) has been implicated as a possible mediator of mechanical signaling in cartilage through such a mechanism.[234,266] Dynamic compression of porcine cartilage results in activation of the ERK/MAP kinase, which is dependent on release of the bFGF. In this system, bFGF induces synthesis and secretion of tissue inhibitor of metalloproteinases 1 (TIMP-1). In contrast, bFGF production by bovine cartilage is inhibited by 1 hour of compressive stress of 20 MPa.[267] This mechanically induced suppression of bFGF is blocked by IL 4, indicating further roles for this pleiotropic cytokine in the regulation of chondrocyte responses to mechanical stimulation.

## INFLUENCE OF JOINT SOURCE AND DISEASE ON CHONDROCYTE MECHANICAL SIGNALING AND MECHANO-TRANSDUCTION

Studies on chondrocyte mechanical signaling primarily use cells derived from either bovine articular cartilage or human articular cartilage. Bovine cartilage is often obtained from skeletally immature animals, whereas human cartilage is frequently obtained from aged individuals whose joints may show features of OA. Studies from a number of groups have now demonstrated clearly that chondrocytes from different joints and diseased cartilage show significant differences in cell phenotype, response to catabolic factors, and recently responses to mechanical stimuli. Unlike normal knee joint chondrocytes, ankle joint chondrocytes do not show an increase in relative levels of

aggrecan mRNA when mechanically stimulated at 0.33 Hz in monolayer culture.

Similarly, chondrocytes derived from osteoarthritic cartilage show different cellular responses to mechanical stimulation in monolayer culture when compared to cells from normal joints. The major differences are production of the catabolic cytokines IL1β and IL6 and absence of the anabolic rise in relative levels of aggrecan mRNA following mechanical stimulation.[174,268,269] The reasons for these differences are unclear but raise the possibility that normal and osteoarthritic cartilage-derived cells have modified mechano-transduction cascades as a result of altered recognition and transduction of mechanical signals. Osteoarthritic chondrocytes show a depolarization response to 0.33-Hz stimulation in contrast to the hyperpolarization response of normal chondrocytes.[188]

The mechano-transduction pathway in chondrocytes derived from normal and osteoarthritic cartilage involves recognition of the mechanical stimulus by integrins and activation of integrin signaling pathways leading to generation of a cytokine loop.[269] Normal and osteoarthritic chondrocytes show differences at multiple stages of the mechano-transduction cascade. Early events are similar, involve α5β1 integrin and stretch-activated ion channels, and are associated with similar rapid tyrosine phosphorylation events.[188] The actin cytoskeleton is required for the integrin-dependent mechano-transduction, leading to changes in membrane potential in normal but not osteoarthritic chondrocytes.[188]

Matrix composition in OA is altered as a result of changes in synthetic activity by chondrocytes and the production of proteases, which will digest preexisting matrix molecules. The decrease in proteoglycan content, disruption of the collagen II fiber network, increase in a variety of glycoproteins (including fibronectin, tenascin, and decorin), up-regulation of collagen type VI expression, and altered integrin expression may all result in changes in cell/matrix interactions that will influence how a chondrocyte perceives and responds to a mechanical load. Chondrocytes in osteoarthritic cartilage may have adapted to an altered mechanical environment, and responses may be dependent on an altered threshold of stimulus being required before cellular activation events are stimulated.

## PROSPECTS AND CONCLUSIONS

Mechanical stresses play a critical role in the development and maintenance of healthy joint tissues and in the degenerative and regenerative processes associated with OA. Our understanding of the mechanisms whereby mechanical stresses influence the pathophysiology of OA, joint tissue matrix metabolism, and the cell biology of chondrocytes in articular cartilage has advanced considerably in the past two decades but remains far from complete.

In particular, the way in which genes that predispose to susceptibility to or progression of OA interact with mechanical stress has hardly begun to be explored. Recent linkage studies have, however, identified associations between mutations in frizzled-related protein 3 (FRZB),[270] asporin (ASPN),[13] and calmodulin 1 (CALM 1)[271] with some populations with OA hip in the United Kingdom and Japan and have led to the hypothesis that polymorphism in signal transduction proteins may be a major route through which susceptibility to OA is acting.[272]

Recent developments in microsurgical techniques have also made it possible to induce mechanically determined experimental OA in the knees of mice. In a recent landmark paper, Glasson et al.[273] have shown that deletion of active ADAMTS5 (aggrecanase II) inhibited the development of mechanically induced OA in the knockout mice. With approaches such as these, there are excellent prospects that the next decade will not only see dramatic advances in our understanding of the mechano-biology of joints and the pathogenesis of OA but will lead to novel targets for therapeutic intervention to inhibit structural progression in this disorder.

## REFERENCES

1. Carter DR, Orr TE, Fyhrie DP, Schurman DJ. Influences of mechanical stress on prenatal and postnatal skeletal development. Clin Orthop 1987;219:237–50.
2. Drachman DB, Sokoloff L. The role of movement in embryonic joint development. Dev Biol 1966;14:410–20.
3. Mikic B, Johnson TL, Chhabra AB, Schalet BJ, Wong M, Hunziker EB. Differential effects of embryonic immobilization on the development of fibrocartilaginous skeletal elements. J Rehabil Res Dev 2000;37(2):127–33.
4. Helminen HJ, Kiviranta I, Saamanen AM, et al. In KE Kuettner, R Schleyerbach, JG Peyron, VC Hascall (eds.), Articular Cartilage and Osteoarthritis. New York: Raven Press 1991:501–10.
5. Lanyon LE. Functional strain in bone tissue as an objective, and controlling stimulus for adaptive bone remodelling. J Biomech 1987;20:1083–93.
6. Kjaer M. Role of extracellular matrix in adaptation of tendon and skeletal muscle to mechanical loading. Physiol Rev 2003;84:649–98.
7. Wang JH. Mechanobiology of tendon. J Biomech 2006;39(9):1563–82.
8. Meachim G. Ways of cartilage breakdown in human and experimental osteoarthritis. In G Nuki (ed.), The Aetiopathogenesis of Osteoarthrosis. London: Pitman Medical 1980:16–28.
9. Nuki G. Osteoarthritis: a problem of joint failure. Z Rheumatol 1999;58(3):142–47.
10. Brandt KD, Lohmander S, Doherty M. Pathogenesis of osteoarthritis. Introduction: The concept of osteoarthritis as failure of the diarthrodial joint. In KD Brandt, M Doherty, S Lohmander (eds.), Osteoarthritis, Second Edition. Oxford: Oxford University Press 2003:69–71.
11. Altman RD. The classification of osteoarthritis. J Rheumatol Suppl 1995;43:42–43.
12. Anderson JJ, Felson DT. Factors associated with osteoarthritis of the knee in the first national Health and Nutrition Examination Survey (HANES I): Evidence for an association with overweight, race, and physical demands of work. Am J Epidemiol 1988;128(1):179–89.
13. Kizawa H, Kou I, Lida A, et al. An aspartic acid repeat polymorphism in asporin inhibits chondrogenesis and increases susceptibility to osteoarthritis. Nat Genet 2005;37:138–44.
14. Zhang Y, Hannan MT, Chaisson CE, et al. Bone mineral density and risk of incident and progressive radiographic knee osteoarthritis in women: The Framingham study. J Rheumatol 2000;27:1032–37.
15. Hart DJ, Mootoosamy I, Doyle DV, Spector TD. The relationship between osteoarthritis and osteoporosis in the general population: The Chingford Study. Ann Rheum Dis 1994;53:158–62.
16. Hart DJ, Doyle DV, Spector TD. Incidence and risk factors for radiographic knee osteoarthritis in middle-aged women: The Chingford Study. Arthritis Rheum 1999;42:17–24.
17. Sharma L, Song J, Felson DT, et al. The role of knee alignment in disease progression and functional decline in knee osteoarthritis. JAMA 2001;286:188–95.
18. Lane NE, Lin P, Christiansen L, et al. Association of mild acetabular dysplasia with increased risk of incident hip osteoarthritis in elderly white women: The Study of Osteoporotic Fractures. Arthritis Rheum 2000;43:400–04.
19. Felson DT, Anderson JJ, Naimark A, et al. Obesity and knee osteoarthritis: The Framingham Study. Ann Intern Med 1988;109:18–24.
20. Bruyere O, Dardenne C, Lejeune E, et al. Subchondral tibial bone mineral density predicts future joint space narrowing at the medial femoral-tibial compartment in patients with knee osteoarthritis. Bone 2003;32(5):541–45.
21. Sharma L. Local factors in osteoarthritis. Curr Opin Rheumatol 2002;13(5):441–46.
22. Stockwell RA. A pre-clinician's view of osteoarthritis. JR Coll Surg Edinb 1986;31(6):333–44.
23. Nuki G. Osteoarthritis: Risk factors and pathogenesis. ARC Reports on the Rheumatic Diseases 2005;4:53–63.
24. Hochberg MC. Do risk factors for incident hip osteoarthritis (OA) differ from those for the progression of hip OA? J Rheumatol Suppl 2004;70:6–9.
25. Doherty M. Risk factors for progression of knee osteoarthritis. Lancet 2001;358(9284):775–76.
26. Miyazaki T, Wada M, Kawahara H, et al. Dynamic load at baseline can predict radiographic disease progression in medial compartment knee osteoarthritis. Ann Rheum Dis 2002;61:617–22.
27. Chang A, Hayes K, Dunlop D, et al. Thrust during ambulation and progression of knee osteoarthritis. Arthritis Rheum. 2004;50:3897–3909.
28. Sharma L, Lou C, Cahue S, Dunlop DD. The mechanism of the effect of obesity in knee osteoarthritis: The mediating role of malalignment. Arthritis Rheum 2000;43(3):568–75.
29. Felson DT, Goggins J, Niu J, et al. The effect of body weight on progression of knee osteoarthritis is dependent on alignment. Arthritis Rheum 2004;50:3904–09.
30. Elahi S, Cahue S, Felson DT, Engelman L, Sharma L. The association between varus-valgus alignment and patellofemoral osteoarthritis. Arthritis Rheum 2000;43(8):1874–80.
31. Felson DT, Chaisson CE. Understanding the relationship between body weight and osteoarthritis. Baillieres Clin Rheumatol 1997;11(4):671–81.
32. Felson DT, Zhang Y, Hannan MT, et al. Risk factors for incident radiographic knee osteoarthritis in the elderly: The Framingham Study. Arthritis Rheum 1997;40(4):728–33.
33. Christensen R, Astrup A, Bliddal H. Weight loss: The treatment of choice for knee osteoarthritis? A randomized trial. Osteoarthritis and Cartilage 2005;13:20–27.

34. Messier SP, Loeser RF, Miller GD, et al. Exercise and dietary weight loss in overweight and obese older adults with knee osteoarthritis: The Arthritis, Diet and Activity Promotion Trial. Arthritis Rheum 2004;50:1501–10.

35. Roos H, Adalberth T, Dahlberg L, Lohmander LS. Osteoarthritis of the knee after injury to the anterior cruciate ligament or meniscus: The influence of time and age. Osteoarthritis Cartilage 1995;3(4):261–67.

36. Felson DT. The epidemiology of knee osteoarthritis: Results from the Framingham Osteoarthritis Study. Semin Arthritis Rheum 1990;20(3/1):42–50.

37. Roos H, Lauren M, Adalberth T, Roos EM, Jonsson K, Lohmander LS. Knee osteoarthritis after meniscectomy: Prevalence of radiographic changes after twenty-one years, compared with matched controls. Arthritis Rheum 1998;41(4):687–93.

38. Harris WH. Traumatic arthritis of the hip after dislocation and acetabular fractures: Treatment by mold arthroplasty. An end-result study using a new method of result evaluation. J Bone Joint Surg Am 1969;51(4):737–55.

39. Davis MA, Ettinger WH, Neuhaus JM, Cho SA, Hauck WW. The association of knee injury and obesity with unilateral and bilateral osteoarthritis of the knee. Am J Epidemiol 1989;130(2):278–88.

40. Sowers M, Hochberg M, Crabbe JP, Muhich A, Crutchfield M, Updike S. Association of bone mineral density and sex hormone levels with osteoarthritis of the hand and knee in premenopausal women. Am J Epidemiol 1996;143(1):38–47.

41. Gelber AC, Hochberg MC, Mead LA, Wang NY, Wigley FM, Klag MJ. Joint injury in young adults and risk for subsequent knee and hip osteoarthritis. Ann Intern Med 2000;133(5):321–28.

42. Jacobsen K. Osteoarthrosis following insufficiency of the cruciate ligaments in man: A clinical study. Acta Orthop Scand 1977;48(5):520–26.

43. Tirgari M, Vaughan LC. Arthritis of the canine stifle joint. Vet Rec 1975;96(18):394–99.

44. Pond MJ, Nuki G. Experimentally-induced osteoarthritis in the dog. Ann Rheum Dis 1973;32(4):387–88.

45. Hardingham T, Venn G, Bayliss MT. Chondrocyte responses in cartilage and in experimental osteoarthritis. Br J Rheumatol 1991;30(1):32–7.

46. Buckwalter JA, Brown TD. Articular cartilage injury, repair and remodeling: Roles in post-traumatic osteoarthritis. Clin Orthop Relat Res 2004;427:S96–103.

47. Roos H, Lindberg H, Gardsell P, Lohmander LS, Wingstrand H. The prevalence of gonarthrosis and its relation to meniscectomy in former soccer players. Am J Sports Med 1994;22(2):219–24.

48. Kujala UM, Kettunen J, Paananen H, et al. Knee osteoarthritis in former runners, soccer players, weight lifters, and shooters. Arthritis Rheum 1995;38(4):539–46.

49. Spector TD, Harris PA, Hart DJ, et al. Risk of osteoarthritis associated with long-term weight-bearing sports: A radiologic survey of the hips and knees in female ex-athletes and population controls. Arthritis Rheum 1996;39(6):988–95.

50. Lane NE, Michel B, Bjorkengren A, et al. The risk of osteoarthritis with running and aging: A 5-year longitudinal study. J Rheumatol 1993;20(3):461–68.

51. Puranen J, Ala-Ketola L, Peltokallio P, Saarela J. Running and primary osteoarthritis of the hip. Br Med J 1975;2(5968):424–25.

52. Shepard GJ, Banks AJ, Ryan WG. Ex-professional association footballers have an increased prevalence of osteoarthritis of the hip compared with age matched controls despite not having sustained notable hip injuries. Br J Sports Med 2003;37(1):80–1.

53. Schmitt H, Brocai DR, Lukoschek M. High prevalence of hip arthrosis in former elite javelin throwers and high jumpers: 41 athletes examined more than 10 years after retirement from competitive sports. Acta Orthop Scand 2004;75(1):34–9.

54. Buckwalter JA, Lane NE. Athletics and osteoarthritis. Am J Sports Med 1997;25(6):873–81.

55. Anderson JA, Duthie JJ, Moody BP. Social and economic effects of rheumatic diseases in a mining population. Ann Rheum Dis 1962;21:342–52.

56. Partridge RE, Duthie JJ. Rheumatism in dockers and civil servants: A comparison of heavy manual and sedentary workers. Ann Rheum Dis 1968;27(6):559–68.

57. Vingard E, Alfredsson L, Goldie I, Hogstedt C. Occupation and osteoarthrosis of the hip and knee: A register-based cohort study. Int J Epidemiol 1991;20(4):1025–31.

58. Croft P, Coggon D, Cruddas M, Cooper C. Osteoarthritis of the hip: An occupational disease in farmers. BMJ 1992;304(6837):1269–72.

59. Roach KE, Persky V, Miles T, Budiman-Mak E. Biomechanical aspects of occupation and osteoarthritis of the hip: A case-control study. J Rheumatol 1994;21(12):2334–40.

60. Felson DT, Hannan MT, Naimark A, et al. Occupational physical demands, knee bending, and knee osteoarthritis: Results from the Framingham Study. J Rheumatol 1991;18(10):1587–92.

61. Maetsel A, Makela M, Hawker G, et al. Osteoarthritis of the hip and knee and mechanical occupational exposure: A systematic overview of the evidence. J Rheumatol 1997;24:1599–1607.

62. Coggon D, Croft P, Kellingray S, Barrett D, McLaren M, Cooper C. Occupational physical activities and osteoarthritis of the knee. Arthritis Rheum 2000;43(7):1443–49.

63. Cooper C, McAlindon T, Coggon D, Egger P, Dieppe P. Occupational activity and osteoarthritis of the knee. Ann Rheum Dis 1994;53(2):90–3.

64. Lawrence JS. Rheumatism in cotton operatives. Br J Ind Med 1961;18(4):270–76.

65. Hadler NM, Gillings DB, Imbus HR, et al. Hand structure and function in an industrial setting. Arthritis Rheum 1978;21(2):210–20.

66. Radin EL, Paul IL, Lowy M. A comparison of the dynamic force transmitting properties of subchondral bone and articular cartilage. J Bone Joint Surg Am 1970;52(3):444–56.

67. Radin EL, Rose RM. Role of subchondral bone in the initiation and progression of cartilage damage. Clin Orthop 1986;(213):34–40.

68. Hoshino A, Wallace WA. Impact-absorbing properties of the human knee. J Bone Joint Surg Br 1987;69(5):807–11.

69. Brown TD, Radin EL, Martin RB, Burr DB. Finite element studies of some juxtarticular stress changes due to localized subchondral stiffening. J Biomech 1984;17(1):11–24.

70. Foss MV, Byers PD. Bone density, osteoarthrosis of the hip, and fracture of the upper end of the femur. Ann Rheum Dis 1972;31(4):259–64.

71. Dequeker J, Johnell O. Osteoarthritis protects against femoral neck fracture: The MEDOS study experience. Bone 1993;14(1):S51–6.

72. Hart DJ, Mootoosamy I, Doyle DV, Spector TD. The relationship between osteoarthritis and osteoporosis in the general population: The Chingford Study. Ann Rheum Dis 1994;53(3):158–62.

73. Sowers M, Zobel D, Weissfeld L, et al. Progression of osteoarthritis of the hand and metacarpal bone loss. Arthritis Rheum 1991;34:36–42.

74. Hochberg MC, Lethbridge-Cejku M, Scott WW Jr., Plato CC, Tobin JD. Appendicular bone mass and osteoarthritis of the hands in women: Data from the Baltimore Longitudinal Study of Aging. J Rheumatol 1994;21(8):1532–36.

75. Sowers M, Lachance L, Jamadar D, et al. The associations of bone mineral density and bone turnover markers with osteoarthritis of the hand and knee in pre- and perimenopausal women. Arthritis Rheum 1999;42(3):483–89.

76. Burger H, van Daele PLA, Odding E, et al. Association of radiographically evident osteoarthritis with higher bone mineral density and increased bone loss with age. Arthritis Rheum 1996;38:81–6.

77. Layton MW, Goldstein SA, Goulet RW, et al. Examination of subchondral bone architecture in experimental osteoarthritis by microscopic computed axial tomography. Arthritis Rheum 1988;31(11):1400–05.

78. Dedrick DK, Goulet R, Huston L, et al. Early bone changes in experimental osteoarthritis using microscopic computed tomography. J Rheumatol Suppl 1991;27:44–5.

79. Carlson CS, Loeser RF, Purser CB, et al. Osteoarthritis in cynomolgous macaques. III: Effects of age, gender, and subchondral bone thickness on the severity of disease. J Bone Miner Res 1996;11(9):1209–17.

80. Dedrick DK, Goldstein SA, Brandt KD, et al. A longitudinal study of subchondral plate and trabecular bone in cruciate-deficient dogs with osteoarthritis followed up for 54 months. Arthritis Rheum 1993;36(10):1460–67.

47

81. Calvo E, Castaneda S, Largo R, et al. Osteoporosis increases the severity of cartilage damage in an experimental model of osteoarthritis in rabbits. Osteoarthritis & Cartilage 2006 (in press).

82. Lynch JA, Hawkes DJ, Buckland-Wright JC. Analysis of texture in macroradiographs of osteoarthritic knees using the fractal signature. Phys Med Biol 1991;36(6):709–22.

83. Messent EA, Buckland-Wright JC, Blake GM. Fractal analysis of trabecular bone in knee osteoarthritis (OA) is a more sensitive marker of disease status than bone mineral density (BMD). Calcif Tissue Int 2005;76(6):419–25.

84. Beuf O, Ghosh S, Newitt DC, et al. Magnetic resonance imaging of normal and osteoarthritic trabecular bone structure in the human knee. Arthritis Rheum 2002;46(2):385–93.

85. Stockwell RA. Cartilage failure in osteoarthritis: Relevance of normal structure and function. A review. Clinical Anatomy 1991;4:161–91.

86. Woo SL-Y, Akeson WH, Jemmott GF. Measurements of non-homogeneous directional mechanical properties of articular cartilage in tension. J Biomech 1976;9:789–91.

87. Roth V, Mow VC. The intrinsic tensile behaviour of the matrix of bovine articular cartilage and its variation with age. J Bone Jt Surg 1980;62(A):785–91.

88. Kempson GE, Muir H, Pollard C, et al. The tensile properties of the cartilage of human femoral condyles related to the content of collagen and glycosaminoglycans. Biochim Biophys Acta 1973;297:456–72.

89. Akizuki S, Mow VC, Muller F, et al. Tensile properties of knee joint cartilage, I, influence of ionic conditions, weight bearing, and fibrillation on the tensile modulus. J Orthop Res 1986;4:379–82.

90. Schmidt MB, Mow VC, Chun LE, et al. Effects of proteoglycan extraction on the tensile behaviour of articular cartilage. J Orthop Res 1990;8:353–63.

91. Heinegard D, Aspberg A, Franzen A, Lorenzo P. Glycosylated matrix proteins. In P Royce, B Steinmann (eds.), Connective Tissue and Its Hereditable Disorders, Second Edition. New York: Wiley-Liss 2002:271–93.

92. Mendler M, Eich Bender SG, Vaughan L, et al. Cartilage contains mixed fibrils of collagen types II, IX and XI. J Cell Biol 1989;108:191–97.

93. Wiberg C, Hedbom E, Khairullina A, et al. Biglycan and decorin bind close to the n-terminal region of the collagen VI triple helix. J Biol Chem 2001;276:18947–52.

94. Wiberg C, Heinegard D, Wenglen C, et al. Biglycan organises collagen VI into hexagonal-like networks resembling tissue structures. J Biol Chem 2002;277(51):49120–26.

95. Vogel KG, Paulsson M, Heinegard D. Specific inhibition of type I and type II collagen fibrillogenesis by the small proteoglycan of tendon. Biochem J 1984;223:587–97.

96. Scott JE, Stockwell RA. Cartilage elasticity resides in shape module decoran and aggrecan sumps of damping fluid: Implications in osteoarthrosis. J Physiol 31 March 2006 [E-pub ahead of print]. DOI: 10.1113/jphysiol.2006.108100.

97. Scott JE. Proteoglycan-fibrillar collagen interactions. Biochem J 1988;252:313–23.

98. Scott JE, Thomlinson AM. The structure of interfibrillar proteoglycan bridges ("shape modules") in extracellular matrix of fibrous connective tissues and their stability in various chemical environments. J Anat 1998;192:391–405.

99. Havercamp RG, Williams MAK, Scott JE. Stretching individual molecules of connective tissue glycans to characterise their shape-maintaining elasticity. Biomacromol 2005;6:1816–18.

100. Mow VC, Kuei SC, Lai WM, et al. Biphasic creep and stress relaxation of articular cartilage in compression: Theory and experiments. J Biomech Eng 1980;102:73–84.

101. Maroudas A. Physicochemical properties of articular cartilage. In MAR Freeman (ed.), Adult Articular Cartilage. Tunbridge Wells: Pitman Medical 1973:131–70.

102. Maroudas A. Physicochemical properties of articular cartilage. In MAR Freeman (ed.), Adult Articular Cartilage, Second Edition. Tunbridge Wells: Pitman Medical 1973:215–90.

103. Urban JP, Hall AC, Gehl KA. Regulation of matrix synthesis rates by the ionic and osmotic environment of articular chondrocytes. J Cell Physiol 1993;154:262–70.

104. Guilak F. Compression-induced changes in the shape and volume of the chondrocyte nucleus. J Biomech 1995;28:1529–41.

105. Kim YJ, Bonasser LJ, Grozinsky AJ. The role of cartilage streaming potential, fluid flow and pressure in the stimulation of chondrocyte biosynthesis during dynamic compression. J Biomech 1995;28:1055–66.

106. Solz MA, Ateshian GA. Experimental verification and theoretical prediction of cartilage interstitial fluid pressurization at the impermeable contact interface in confined compression. J Biomech 1998;31:927–34.

107. Szirmai JA. Structure of cartilage. In A Engel, T Larsson (eds.), Aging of Connective and Skeletal Tissue. Nordiska Bokhandelns 1969:163–84.

108. Poole CA, Ayad S, Schofield JR. Chondrons from articular cartilage. 1. Immunolocalisation of type VI collagen in the pericellular capsule of isolated canine chondrons. J Cell Sci 1988;90:635–45.

109. Meachim G, Roy S. Intracytoplasmic filaments in the cells of adult human articular cartilage. Ann Rheum Dis 1967;26:50–8.

110. Weiss C, Rosenberg L, Helfet AJ. An ultrastructural study of normal young adult human articular cartilage. J Bone Jt Surg 1968;50:663–66.

111. Alexopoulos LG, Haider MA, Vail MA, et al. Alterations in the mechanical properties of the human chondrocyte pericellular matrix with osteoarthritis. J Biomech Eng 2003;125:323–33.

112. Allen DM, Mao DJ. Heterogeneous nanostructural and nano-elastic properties of pericellular and interterritorial matrices of chondrocytes by atomic force microscopy. J Structural Biol 2004;145:196–204.

113. Alexopoulos LG, Setton LA, Guilak F. The biomechanical role of the chondrocyte pericellular matrix in articular cartilage. Acta Biomater. 2005;1(3):317–25.

114. Poole CA, Wotton SF, Duance VC. Localization of type IX collagen in chondrons isolated from porcine articular cartilage and rat chondrosarcoma. Histochem J 1988;20(10):567–74.

115. Poole CA. Articular cartilage chondrons: Form, function and failure. J Anat 1997;191(1):1–13.

116. Smirzai JA. The concept of the chondron as a biomechanical unit. In F Hartmann (ed.), Biopolymer und Biomechanik von Bindegewebssystemen. Berlin: Academic Press 1974:87.

117. Greco F, Specchia N, Falciglia F, et al. Ultrastructural analysis of the adaptation of articular cartilage to mechanical stimulation. Ital J Othopaed & Traumatol 1992;18:311–21.

118. Knight MM, Lee DA, Bader DL. The influence of elaborated pericellular matrix on the deformation of isolated articular chondrocytes cultured in agarose. Biochim Biophys Acta 1998;1505:67–77.

119. Alexopoulos LG, Williams GM, Upton ML, et al. Osteoarthritic changes in the biphasic mechanical properties of the chondrocyte pericellular matrix in articular cartilage. J Biomech. 2005;38:509–17.

120. Athanasiou KA, Agarwal A, Muffoletto A, et al. Biomechanical properties of hip cartilage in experimental animal models. Clin Orthop Relat Res 1995;316:254–66.

121. Athanasiou KA, Rosenwasser MP, Buckwalter JA, et al. Interspecies comparisons of in-situ intrinsic mechanical properties of distal femoral cartilage. J Orthopaed Res 1991;9:330–40.

122. Guilak F, Mow VC. The mechanical environment of the chondrocyte: A biphasic finite element model of cel-matrix interactions in articular cartilage. J Biomech 2000;33:1663–73.

123. Hing WA, Sherwin AF, Poole CA. The influence of the pericellular microenvironment on the chondrocyte response to osmotic challenge. Osteoarthritis & Cartilage 2002;10:297–307.

124. Schinagl RM, Gurskis D, Chen AC, et al. Depth dependent confined compression modulus of full-thickness bovine articular cartilage. J Orthop Res 1997;15:499–506.

125. Paul JP. Joint kinetics. In L Sokoloff (ed.), The Joints and Synovial Fluid, Volume II. New York: Academic Press 1980:140–76.

126. Hodge WA, Fijan RS, Carlson KL, et al. Contact pressures in the human hip joint measured in vivo. Proc Natl Acad Sci USA 1986;2879–83.

127. Armstrong CG, Bahrani AS, Gardner DL. Changes in deformational behaviour of human hip cartilage with age. J Biomech Eng 1980;102:214–20.

128. Herberhold C, Faber S, Stammberger T, et al. In situ measurement of articular cartilage deformation in intact femoropatellar joints under static loading. J Biomech 1999;32:1287–95.

129. Parkkinen JJ, Ikonen J, Lammi MJ, et al. Effects of cyclic hydrostatic pressure on proteoglycan synthesis in cultured chondrocytes and articular cartilage explants. Arch Biochem Biophys 1993;300:458–65.

130. Sah SL, Grodzinsky AJ, Plaas AHK, et al. Effects of static and dynamic compression on matrix metabolism in cartilage explants. In K Kuettner, R Schleyerbach, J Peyron, VC Hascall (eds.), Articular Cartilage and Osteoarthritis. New York: Raven Press 1992:373–92.

131. Hall AC, Urban JPG, Gehl GA. The effects of hydrostatic pressure on matrix synthesis in articular cartilage. J Orthop Res 1991;9:1–10.

132. Saamanen A-M, Tammi J, Jurvelin I, et al. Proteoglycan alterations following immobilisation and remobilisation in the articular cartilage of young canine knee (stifle) joint. J Orthop Res 1990;8:863–73.

133. Kiviranta I, Jurvelin J, Tammi M, et al. Weight bearing controls glycosaminoglycan concentration and thickness of articular cartilage in knee joints of young beagle dogs. Arthritis Rheum 1987;30:801–08.

134. Palmoski MJ, Brandt KD. Running inhibits the reveral of atrophic changes in canine knee cartilage after removal of a leg cast. Arthritis Rheum 1981;24(11):1329–37.

135. Kiviranta I, Jurvelin J, Tammi M, et al. Weight bearing controls glycosaminoglycan concentration and articular cartilage thickness in the knee joint of young beagle dogs. Arthritis Rheum 1987;30:801–09.

136. Tammi M, Paukkonen K, Kiviranta I, et al. Joint loading-induced alterations in articular cartilage. In HJ Helminen, I Kiviranta, A-M Saamanen, et al. (eds.), Joint Loading: Biology and Health of Articular Structures. Bristol: Wright 1986:64–88.

137. Jortikka MO, Inkinen R, Tammi MI, et al. Immobilisation causes longlasting matrix changes both in the immobilized and contralateral joint cartilage. Ann Rheum Dis 1997;56:255–61.

138. Videman T, Eronen I. Effects of treadmill running on glycoaminoglycans in articular cartilage of rabbits. Int J Sports Med 1984;5:320–24.

139. Vasan N. Effects of physical stress on the synthesis and degradation of cartilage matrix. Connect Tissue Res 1983;12:49–58.

140. Kiviranta I, Tammi M, Jurvelin J, et al. Moderate running exercise augments glycosaminoglycans and thickness of articular cartilage in the knee joint of young beagle dogs. J Orthop Res 1988;6:188–95.

141. Kiviranta I, Tammi M, Jurvelin J, et al. Articular cartilage thickness and glycosaminoglycan distribution in the canine knee joint after strenuous (20 km/day) running exercise. Clin Orthop 1992;283:302–08.

142. Saamanen A-M, Kiviranta I, Jurvelin J, et al. Proteoglycan and collagen alterations in canine knee articular cartilage following 20km daily running exercise for 15 weeks. Connect Tissue Res 1994;30:191–201.

143. Oettmeier R, Arokoski J, Roth AJ, et al. Subchondral bone and articular cartilage responses to long distance running training (40km/day) in the beagle knee joint. Eur J Musculoskel Res 1992;1:145–54.

144. Radin EL, Orr RB, Kelman JL, et al. Effect of prolonged walking on concrete on the knees of sheep. J Biomech. 1982;15:487–92.

145. Armstrong SJ, Read RA, Ghosh P, et al. Moderate exercise exacerbates the osteoarthritic lesions produced in cartilage by meniscectomy: A morphological study. Osteoarthritis & Cartilage 1993;1(2):89–96.

146. Ghosh P, Sutherland J, Bellenger C, et al. The influence of weight bearing exercise on articular cartilage of meniscectomized joints: An experimental study in sheep. Clin Orthop Relat Res 1990;252:101–13.

147. Benya PD, Shaffer JD. Dedifferentiated chondrocytes reexpress the differentiated collagen phenotype when cultured in agarose gels. Cell 1982;30:215–24.

148. Hauselmann HJ, Fernandes RJ, Mok SS, et al. Phenotypic stability of bovine articular chondrocytes after long-term culture in alginate beads. J Cell Sci 1994;107:17–27.

149. Larsson T, Aspden RM, Heinegard D. Effects of mechanical load on cartilage matrix biosynthesis in-vitro. Matrix 1991; 11:388–94.

150. Sah RL, Kim YJ, Doong JY, et al. Biosynthetic response of cartilage explants to dynamic compression. J Orthop Res 1989;7:619–36.

151. Ragan P, Badger A, Cook M, et al. Down-regulation of chondrocyte aggrecan and type II collagen gene expression correlates with increases in static compression magnitude and duration. J Orthop Res 1999;17:836–42.

152. Valhmu W, Stazzone E, Bachrach N, et al. Load-controlled compression of articular cartilage induces a transient stimulation of aggrecan gene expression. Arch Biochem Biophys 1998; 353:29–36.

153. Parkkinen JJ, Lammi MJ, Helminen HJ. Local stimulation of proteoglycan synthesis in articular cartilage explants by dynamic compression in-vitro. J Orthop Res 1992;10:610–20.

154. Buschmann MD, Kim YJ, Wong M, et al. Stimulation of aggrecan synthesis in cartilage explants by cyclic loading is localised to regions of high interstitial fluid flow. Arch Biochem Biophys 1999;366:1–7.

155. Korver THV, van der Stadt RJ, Kiljan E, et al. Effects of loading on the synthesis of proteoglycans in different layers of anatomically intact articular cartilage in-vitro. J Rheumatol 1992; 19:905–12.

156. Kim YJ, Sah RL, Grodzinsky AJ, et al. Mechanical regulation of cartilage biosynthetic behaviour: Physical stimuli. Arch Biochem Biophys 1994;311:1–12.

157. Lee DA, Bader DL. Compressive strains at physiological frequencies influence the metabolism of chondrocytes seeded in agarose. J Orthop Res 1997;15(2):181–88.

158. Chowdhury TT, Bader DL, Shelton JC, et al. Temporal regulation of chondrocyte metabolism in agarose constructs subjected to dynamic compression. Arch Biochem Biophys 2003;417: 105–11.

159. Mauck RL, Soltz MA, Wang CC, et al. Functional tissue engineering of articular cartilage through dynamic loading of chondrocyte-seeded agarose gels. J Biomech Eng 2000;122(3): 252–60.

160. Bonassar LJ, Grodzinsky AJ, Frank EH, et al. The effect of dynamic compression on the response of articular cartilage to insulin-like growth factor-1. J Orthop Res 2001;19:11–17.

161. Wong M, Siegrist M, Cao X. Cyclic compression of articular cartilage explants is associated with progressive consolidation and altered expression pattern of extracellular matrix proteins. Matrix Biol 1999;18:391–99.

162. Kiraly K, Hyttinen MM, Parkkinen JJ, et al. Articular cartilage collagen birefringence is altered concurrent with changes in proteoglycan synthesis during dynamic in-vitro loading. Anat Rec 1998;251:28–36.

163. Jin M, Frank EH, Quinn TM, et al. Tissue shear deformation stimulates proteoglycan and protein biosynthesis in bovine cartilage explants. Arch Biochem Biophys 2001;395(1):41–8.

164. Duncan RL, Turner CH. Mechanotransduction and the functional response of bone to mechanical strain. Calcif Tissue Int1995;57:344–58.

165. Paukkonen K, Selkainaho K, Jurvelin J, Helminen HJ. Cells and nuclei of articular cartilage chondrocytes in young rabbits enlarged after nonstrenuous physical exercise. J Anat 1985; 142:13–20.

166. Urban JP. The chondrocyte: A cell under pressure. Br J Rheumatol1994;33:901–08.

167. Grodzinsky AJ, Levenston ME, Jin M, Frank EH. Cartilage tissue remodeling in response to mechanical forces. Annu Rev Biomed Eng 2000;2:691–713.

168. Wilkins RJ, Browning JA, Urban JP. Chondrocyte regulation by mechanical load. Biorheology 2000;37:67–74.

169. Lee DA, Noguchi T, Frean SP, Lees P, Bader DL. The influence of mechanical loading on isolated chondrocytes seeded in agarose constructs. Biorheology 2000;37:149–61.

170. Li KW, Williamson AK, Wang AS, Sah RL. Growth responses of cartilage to static and dynamic compression. Clin Orthop Relat Res 2001;391:S34–48.

171. Palmoski MJ, Brandt KD. Effects of static and cyclic compressive loading on articular cartilage plugs in vitro. Arthritis Rheum 1984;7:675–81.

172. Guilak F, Meyer BC, Ratcliffe A, Mow VC. The effects of matrix compression on proteoglycan metabolism in articular cartilage explants. Osteoarthritis Cartilage 1994;2:91–101.

173. Chen AC, Sah RL. Effect of static compression on proteoglycan biosynthesis by chondrocytes transplanted to articular cartilage in vitro. J Orthop Res 1998;16:542–50.

49

174. Millward-Sadler SJ, Wright MO, Davies LW, Nuki G, Salter DM. Mechanotransduction via integrins and interleukin-4 results in altered aggrecan and matrix metalloproteinase 3 gene expression in normal, but not osteoarthritic, human articular chondrocytes. Arthritis Rheum 2000;43:2091–99.

175. Smith RL, Lin J, Trindade MC, Shida J, Kajiyama G, Vu T, et al. Time-dependent effects of intermittent hydrostatic pressure on articular chondrocyte type II collagen and aggrecan mRNA expression. J Rehabil Res Dev 2000;37:153–61.

176. Toyoda T, Seedhom BB, Kirkham J, Bonass WA. Upregulation of aggrecan and type II collagen mRNA expression in bovine chondrocytes by the application of hydrostatic pressure. Biorheology 2003;40:79–85.

177. Fitzgerald JB, Jin M, Dean D, Wood DJ, Zheng MH, Grodzinsky AJ. Mechanical compression of cartilage explants induces multiple time-dependent gene expression patterns and involves intracellular calcium and cyclic AMP. J Biol Chem 2004;279: 19502–11.

178. Honda K, Ohno S, Tanimoto K, Ijuin C, Tanaka N, Doi T, et al. The effects of high magnitude cyclic tensile load on cartilage matrix metabolism in cultured chondrocytes. Eur J Cell Biol 2000;79: 601–09.

179. Murata M, Bonassar LJ, Wright M, Mankin HJ, Towle CA. A role for the interleukin-1 receptor in the pathway linking static mechanical compression to decreased proteoglycan synthesis in surface articular cartilage. Arch Biochem Biophys 2003; 413:229–35.

180. Ingber D. Integrins as mechanochemical transducers. Curr Opin Cell Biol 1991;3:841–48.

181. Martinac B. Mechanosensitive ion channels: Molecules of mechanotransduction. J Cell Sci 2004;117:2449–60.

182. Hynes RO. Integrins: Versatility, modulation and signaling in cell adhesion. Cell 1992;69:11–25.

183. Giancotti FG, Ruoslahti E. Integrin signaling. Science1999;285: 1028–32.

184. Salter DM, Hughes DE, Simpson R, Gardner DL. Integrin expression by human articular chondrocytes. Br J Rheumatol 1992;31: 231–34.

185. Lapadula G, Iannone F, Zuccaro C, Grattagliano V, Covelli M, Patella V, et al. Integrin expression on chondrocytes: Correlations with the degree of cartilage damage in human osteoarthritis. Clin Exp Rheumatol 1997;15:247–54.

186. Ostergaard K, Salter DM, Petersen J, Bendtzen K, Hvolris J, Andersen CB. Expression of alpha and beta subunits of the integrin superfamily in articular cartilage from macroscopically normal and osteoarthritic human femoral heads. Ann Rheum Dis 1998;57:303–08.

187. Wright MO, Godolphin JL, Dunne E, Bavington C, Jobanputra P, Nuki G, Salter DM. Hyperpolarisation of cultured human chondrocytes following cyclical pressurisation involves α5β1 integrin and integrin-associated intracellular pathways. J Orthop Res 1997;15:742–47.

188. Millward-Sadler SJ, Wright MO, Lee H-S, Caldwell H, Nuki G, Salter DM. Altered electrophysiological responses to mechanical stimulation and abnormal signaling through 5 1 integrin in chondrocytes from osteoarthritic cartilage. Osteoarthritis Cartilage 2000;8:272–78.

189. Lee H-S, Millward-Sadler SJ, Wright MO, Nuki G, Salter DM. Integrin and mechanosensitive ion channel-dependent tyrosine phosphorylation of focal adhesion proteins and catenin in human articular chondrocytes after mechanical stimulation. J Bone Miner Res 2000;15:1501–09.

190. Wright MO, Stockwell RA, Nuki G. Response of plasma membrane to applied hydrostatic pressure in chondrocytes and fibroblasts. Connect Tissue Res 1992;28:49–70.

191. Wright MO, Jobanputra P, Bavington C, et al. Effects of intermittent pressure-induced strain on the electrophysiology of cultured human chondrocytes: Evidence for the presence of stretch-activated ion channels. Clinical Science 1996;90: 61–71.

192. Salter DM, Robb JE, Wright MO. Electrophysiological responses of human bone cells to mechanical stimulation: Evidence for specific integrin function in mechanotransduction. J Bone Miner Res 1997;12(7):1133–41.

193. Chowdhury TT, Appleby RN, Salter DM, Bader DA, Lee DA. Integrin-mediated mechanotransduction in IL-1beta stimulated chondrocytes. Biomech Model Mechanobiol 17 March 2006 [E-pub ahead of print].

194. Giannoni P, Siegrist M, Hunziker EB, Wong M. The mechanosensitivity of cartilage oligomeric matrix protein (COMP). Biorheology 2003;40:101–09.

195. Romer LH, Birukov KG, Garcia JG. Focal adhesions: Paradigm for a signaling nexus. Circ Res 2006;98:606–16.

196. Knight MM, Toyoda T, Lee DA, Bader DL. Mechanical compression and hydrostatic pressure induce reversible changes in actin cytoskeletal organisation in chondrocytes in agarose. J Biomech 2006;39(8):1547–51.

197. Sokabe M, Sachs F, Jing Z. Quantitative video microscopy of patch clamped membranes, stress, strain, capacitance and stretch channel activation. Biophys J 1991;59:722–28.

198. Guilak F, Zell RA, Erickson GR, Grande DA, Rubin CT, McLeod KJ, et al. Mechanically induced calcium waves in articular chondrocytes are inhibited by gadolinium and amiloride. J Orthop Res 1999;7:421–29.

199. Erickson GR, Alexopoulos LG, Guilak F. Hyper-osmotic stress induces volume change and calcium transients in chondrocytes by transmembrane, phospholipid, and G-protein pathways. J Biomech 2001;34:1527–35.

200. Edlich M, Yellowley CE, Jacobs CR, Donahue HJ. Cycle number and waveform of fluid flow affect bovine articular chondrocytes. Biorheology 2004;41:315–22.

201. Chao PG, Tang Z, Angelini E, West AC, Costa KD, Hung CT. Dynamic osmotic loading of chondrocytes using a novel microfluidic device. J Biomech 2005;38:1273–81.

202. Pingguan-Murphy B, Lee DA, Bader DL, Knight MM. Activation of chondrocytes calcium signalling by dynamic compression is independent of number of cycles. Arch Biochem Biophys 2005;444:45–51.

203. Shakibaei M, Mobasheri A. Beta1-integrins co-localize with Na, K-ATPase, epithelial sodium channels (ENaC) and voltage activated calcium channels (VACC) in mechanoreceptor complexes of mouse limb-bud chondrocytes. Histol Histopathol 2003; 18:343–51.

204. Geiger B, Bershadsky A. Exploring the neighborhood: Adhesion-coupled cell mechanosensors. Cell 2002;110:139–42.

205. Wu QQ, Chen Q. Mechanoregulation of chondrocyte proliferation, maturation, and hypertrophy: Ion-channel dependent transduction of matrix deformation signals. Exp Cell Res 2000;156:383–91.

206. Wu Q, Zhang Y, Chen Q. Indian hedgehog is an essential component of mechanotransduction complex to stimulate chondrocyte proliferation. J Biol Chem 2001;276:35290–96.

207. Gu CX, Juranka PF, Morris CE. Stretch-activation and stretch-inactivation of Shaker-IR, a voltage-gated K+ channel. Biophys J 2001;80:2678–93.

208. Calabrese B, Tabarean IV, Juranka P, Morris CE. Mechano-sensitivity of N-type calcium channel currents. Biophys J 2002;83:2560–74.

209. Casado M, Ascher P. Opposite modulation of NMDA receptors by lysophospholipids and arachidonic acid, common features with mechanosensitivity. J Physiol (Lond.) 1998;513:317–30.

210. Kawakubo T, Naruse K, Matsubara T, Hotta N, Masahiro SM. Characterization of a newly found stretch-activated KCa,ATP channel in cultured chick ventricular myocytes. Am J Physiol 1999;276:H1827–38.

211. Salter DM, Wright MO, Millward-Sadler SJ. NMDA receptor expression and roles in human articular chondrocyte mechanotransduction. Biorheology 2004;41:273–81.

212. Sakamoto A, Chen M, Kobayashi T, Kronenberg HM, Weinstein LS. Chondrocyte-specific knockout of the G protein G(s) alpha leads to epiphyseal and growth plate abnormalities and ectopic chondrocyte formation. J Bone Miner Res 2005;20: 663–71.

213. Wang G, Beier F. Rac1/Cdc42 and RhoA GTPases antagonistically regulate chondrocyte proliferation, hypertrophy, and apoptosis. J Bone Miner Res 2005;20:1022–31.

214. Valhmu WB, Raia FJ. Myo-Inositol 1,4,5-trisphosphate and Ca(2+)/calmodulin-dependent factors mediate transduction of compression-induced signals in bovine articular chondrocytes. Biochem J 2002;361(3):689–96.

215. Lee H-S, Millward-Sadler SJ, Wright MO, Nuki G, Salter DM, Al Jamal R. Activation of integrin-RACK1/PKC association

in human articular chondrocyte mechanotransduction. Osteoarthritis Cartilage 2002;10:890–97.

216. Fukuda K, Asada S, Kumano F, Saitoh M, Otani K, Tanaka S. Cyclic tensile stretch on bovine articular chondrocytes inhibits protein kinase C activity. J Lab Clin Med 1997;130:209–15.

217. Ivaska J, Bosca L, Parker PJ. PKC″ is a permissive link in integrin-dependent IFN-signaling that facilitates JAK phosphorylation of STAT1. Nat Cell Biol 2003;5:363–69.

218. Moro L, Venturino M, Bozzo C, Silengo L, Altruda F, Beguinot L, et al. Integrins induce activation of the EGF receptor: Role in MAP kinase induction and adhesion dependent cell survival. EMBO J 1998;17:6622–32.

219. Short SM, Boyer JL, Juliano RL. Integrins regulate the linkage between upstream and downstream events in G-protein-coupled receptor signaling to mitogen-activated protein kinase. J Biol Chem 2000;275:12970–77.

220. Cross DAE, Alessi DR, Cohen P, Andjelkovic M, Hemmings BA. The proto-oncogene PKB/Akt mediates the inhibition of glycogen synthase kinase-3 by insulin in the skeletal muscle cell line L6. Nature 1995;378:785–89.

221. Datta SR, Brunet A, Greenberg ME. Cellular survival: A play in three Akts. Genes Dev 1999;13:2903–27.

222. Delcommene M, Tan C, Gray V, Rue L, Woodgett J, Dedhar S. Phosphoinositide-3-OH kinase-dependent regulation of glycogen synthase kinase 3 and protein kinase B/Akt by the integrin-linked kinase. Proc Natl Acad Sci USA 1998;95:11211–16.

223. Oh CD, Chun JS. Signaling mechanisms leading to the regulation of differentiation and apoptosis of articular chondrocytes by insulin-like growth factor-1. J Biol Chem 2003;278:36563–71.

224. Borrelli J Jr., Ricci WM. Acute effects of cartilage impact. Clin Orthop Relat Res 2004;423:33–9.

225. Orazizadeh M, Lee HS, Groenendijk B, et al. CD47 associates with alpha 5 integrin and regulates mechanical responses in human articular chondrocytes. Osteoarthritis & Cartilage 2006 (submitted).

226. Healy ZR, Lee NH, Gao X, Goldring MB, Talalay P, Kensler TW, et al. Divergent responses of chondrocytes and endothelial cells to shear stress: Cross-talk among COX-2, the phase 2 response, and apoptosis. Proc Natl Acad Sci USA 2005;102:14010–15.

227. Agarwal S, Deschner J, Long P, Verma A, Hofman C, Evans CH, et al. Role of NF-kappaB transcription factors in antiinflammatory and proinflammatory actions of mechanical signals. Arthritis Rheum 2004;50:3541–48.

228. Pulai JI, Chen H, Im HJ, Kumar S, Hanning C, Hegde PS, et al. NF-kappa B mediates the stimulation of cytokine and chemokine expression by human articular chondrocytes in response to fibronectin fragments. J Immunol 2005;174:5781–88.

229. Relic B, Bentires-Alj M, Ribbens C, Franchimont N, Guerne PA, Benoit V, et al. TNF-alpha protects human primary articular chondrocytes from nitric oxide-induced apoptosis via nuclear factor-kappaB. Lab Invest 2002;82:1661–72.

230. Kim SJ, Chun JS. Protein kinase C alpha and zeta regulate nitric oxide-induced NF-kappa B activation that mediates cyclooxygenase-2 expression and apoptosis but not dedifferentiation in articular chondrocytes. Biochem Biophys Res Commun 2003;28(303):206–11.

231. Ip YT, Davis RJ. Signal transduction by the c-Jun N-terminal kinase (JNK): From inflammation to development. Curr Opin Cell Biol 1998;10:205–19.

232. Fanning PJ, Emkey G, Smith RJ, Grodzinsky AJ, Szasz N, Trippel SB. Mechanical regulation of mitogen-activated protein kinase signaling in articular cartilage. J Biol Chem 2003;278:50940–48.

233. Li KW, Williamson AK, Wang AS, Sah RL. Growth responses of cartilage to static and dynamic compression. Clin Orthop Relat Res 2001;391:S34–48.

234. Vincent TL, Hermansson MA, Hansen UN, Amis AA, Saklatvala J. Basic fibroblast growth factor mediates transduction of mechanical signals when articular cartilage is loaded. Arthritis Rheum 2004;50:526–33.

235. Hung CT, Henshaw DR, Wang CC, Mauck RL, Raia F, Palmer G, et al. Mitogen-activated protein kinase signaling in bovine articular chondrocytes in response to fluid flow does not require calcium mobilization. J Biomech 2000;33:73–80.

236. Starkman BG, Cravero JD, Delcarlo M, Loeser RF. IGF-I stimulation of proteoglycan synthesis by chondrocytes requires activation

237. Papachristou DJ, Pirttiniemi P, Kantomaa T, Papavassiliou AG, Basdra EK. JNK/ERK-AP-1/Runx2 induction "paves the way" to cartilage load-ignited chondroblastic differentiation. Histochem Cell Biol 2005;124:215–23.

238. Jin M, Emkey GR, Siparsky P, Trippel SB, Grodzinsky AJ. Combined effects of dynamic tissue shear deformation and insulin-like growth factor I on chondrocyte biosynthesis in cartilage explants. Arch Biochem Biophys 2003;414:223–31.

239. Mauck RL, Nicoll SB, Seyhan SL, Ateshian GA, Hung CT. Synergistic action of growth factors and dynamic loading for articular cartilage tissue engineering. Tissue Eng 2003;9: 597–611.

240. Gassner RJ, Buckley MJ, Studer RK, Evans CH, Agarwal S. Interaction of strain and interleukin-1 in articular cartilage: Effects on proteoglycan synthesis in chondrocytes. Int J Oral Maxillofac Surg 2000;29:389–94.

241. Xu Z, Buckley MJ, Evans CH, Agarwal S. Cyclic tensile strain acts as an antagonist of IL-1 beta actions in chondrocytes. J Immunol 2000;165:453–60.

242. Chowdhury TT, Bader DL, Lee DA. Dynamic compression inhibits the synthesis of nitric oxide and PGE(2) by IL-1beta-stimulated chondrocytes cultured in agarose constructs. Biochem Biophys Res Commun 2001;285:1168–74.

243. Chowdhury TT, Bader DL, Lee DA. Dynamic compression counteracts IL-1 beta-induced release of nitric oxide and PGE2 by superficial zone chondrocytes cultured in agarose constructs. Osteoarthritis Cartilage 2003;11:688–96.

244. Patwari P, Cook MN, DiMicco MA, Blake SM, James IE, Kumar S, et al. Proteoglycan degradation after injurious compression of bovine and human articular cartilage in vitro: Interaction with exogenous cytokines. Arthritis Rheum 2003;48(5):1292–1301.

245. Darling EM, Athanasiou KA. Growth factor impact on articular cartilage subpopulations. Cell Tissue Res 2005;322:463–73.

246. Sylvester J, Liacini A, Li WQ, Zafarullah M. Interleukin-17 signal transduction pathways implicated in inducing matrix metalloproteinase-3, -13 and aggrecanase-1 genes in articular chondrocytes. Cell Signal 2004;16:469–76.

247. Barksby HE, Hui W, Wappler I, Peters HH, Milner JM, Richards CD, et al. Interleukin-1 in combination with oncostatin M up-regulates multiple genes in chondrocytes: Implications for cartilage destruction and repair. Arthritis Rheum 2006;54:540–50.

248. Jobanputra PL, Hong K, Jenkins C, Bavington FR, Brennan G, Nuki JL, et al. Modulation of human chondrocyte integrins by inflammatory synovial fluid. Arthritis Rheum 1996;39:1430–32.

249. Loeser RF. Growth factor regulation of chondrocyte integrins: Differential effects of insulin-like growth factor 1 and transforming growth factor beta on alpha 1 beta 1 integrin expression and chondrocyte adhesion to type VI collagen. Arthritis Rheum 1997;40:270–76.

250. Schwartz MA, Baron V. Interactions between mitogenic stimuli, or a thousand and one connections. Curr Opin Cell Biol 1999;11:197–202.

251. Schneller M, Vuori K, Ruoslahti E. αVβ3 integrin associates with activated insulin and PDGFb receptors and potentiates the biological activity of PDGF. EMBO J 1997;16:5600–07.

252. Enomoto-Iwamoto M, Iwamoto M, Nakashima K, Mukudai Y, Boettiger D, Pacifici M, et al. Involvement of alpha5beta1 integrin in matrix interactions and proliferation of chondrocytes. J Bone Miner Res 1997;12:1124–32.

253. Bonassar LJ, Grodzinsky AJ, Srinivasan A, Davila SG, Trippel SB. Mechanical and physicochemical regulation of the action of insulin-like growth factor-I on articular cartilage. Arch Biochem Biophys 2000;379:57–63.

254. Gooch KJ, Blunk T, Courter DL, Sieminski AL, Bursac PM, Vunjak-Novakovic G, et al. IGF-I and mechanical environment interact to modulate engineered cartilage development. Biochem Biophys Res Commun 2001 7;286:909–15.

255. Fujisawa T, Hattori T, Takahashi K, Kuboki T, Yamashita A, Takigawa M. Cyclic mechanical stress induces extracellular matrix degradation in cultured chondrocytes via gene expression of matrix metalloproteinases and interleukin-1. J Biochem (Tokyo) 1999;125:966–75.

256. Matsukawa M, Fukuda K, Yamasaki K, Yoshida K, Munakata H, Hamanishi C. Enhancement of nitric oxide and proteoglycan

synthesis due to cyclic tensile strain loaded on chondrocytes attached to fibronectin. Inflamm Res 2004;53:239–44.

257. Millward-Sadler SJ, Wright MO, Lee H-S, Nishida K, Caldwell H, Nuki G, Salter DM. Integrin-regulated secretion of interleukin 4: A novel pathway of mechanotransduction in human articular chondrocytes. J Cell Biol 1999;45:183–89.

258. Millward-Sadler SJ, Mackenzie A, Wright MO, Lee H-S, Elliot K, Gerrard L, et al. Tachykinin expression in cartilage and function in human articular chondrocyte mechanotransduction. Arthritis Rheum 2003;48:146–56.

259. Nakamura M, Chikama T, Nishida T. Up-regulation of integrin alpha 5 expression by combination of substance P and insulin-like growth factor-1 in rabbit corneal epithelial cells. Biochem Biophys Res Commun 1998;246:777–82.

260. Millward-Sadler SJ, Khan NS, Bracher MG, Wright MO, Salter DM. Roles for the interleukin-4 receptor and associated JAK/STAT proteins in human articular chondrocyte mechano-transduction. Osteoarthritis Cartilage 5 May 2006 [E-pub ahead of print].

261. Tanaka N, Ohno S, Honda K, Tanimoto K, Doi T, Ohno-Nakahara M, et al. Cyclic mechanical strain regulates the PTHrP expression in cultured chondrocytes via activation of the Ca2+ channel. J Dent Res 2005;84:64–8.

262. Ohno S, Tanaka N, Ueki M, Honda K, Tanimoto K, Yoneno K, et al. Mechanical regulation of terminal chondrocyte differentiation via RGD-CAP/beta ig-h3 induced by TGF-beta. Connect Tissue Res 2005;46:227–34.

263. Tanaka E, Aoyama J, Miyauchi M, Takata T, Hanaoka K, Iwabe T, et al. Vascular endothelial growth factor plays an important autocrine/paracrine role in the progression of osteoarthritis. Histochem Cell Biol 2005;123:275–81.

264. Pufe T, Kurz B, Petersen W, Varoga D, Mentlein R, Kulow S, et al. The influence of biomechanical parameters on the expression of VEGF and endostatin in the bone and joint system. Ann Anat 2005;187:461–72.

265. Murata M, Bonassar LJ, Wright M, Mankin HJ, Towle CA. A role for the interleukin-1 receptor in the pathway linking static mechanical compression to decreased proteoglycan synthesis in surface articular cartilage. Arch Biochem Biophys 2003;413:229–35.

266. Vincent T, Hermansson M, Bolton M, Wait R, Saklatvala J. Basic FGF mediates an immediate response of articular cartilage to mechanical injury. Proc Natl Acad Sci USA 2002; 99:8259–64.

267. Fujiwara Y, Uesugi M, Saito T. Down-regulation of basic fibro-blast growth factor production from cartilage by excessive mechanical stress. J Orthop Sci 2005;10:608–13.

268. Mohtai M, Gupta MK, Donlon B, Ellison B, Cooke J, Gibbons G, et al. Expression of interleukin-6 in osteoarthritic chondrocytes and effects of fluid-induced shear on this expression in normal human chondrocytes in vitro. J Orthop Res 1996; 14:67–73.

269. Salter DM, Millward-Sadler SJ, Nuki G, Wright MO. Differential responses of chondrocytes from normal and osteoarthritic human articular cartilage to mechanical stimulation. Biorheology 2002;39:97–108.

270. Loughlin J, Dowling B, Chapman K, et al. Functional variants within the secreted frizzled-related protein 3 gene are associated with hip osteoarthritis in females. Proc Natl Acad Sci USA 2004;101:9757–62.

271. Mototani H, Mabuchi A, Saito S, et al. A functional single nucleotide polymorphism in the core promoter region of CALM 1 is associated with hip osteoarthritis in Japanese. Hum Mol Genet 2005;14(8):1009–17.

272. Loughlin J. Polymorphism in signal transduction is a major route through which osteoarthritis susceptibility is acting. Curr Opin Rheumatol 2005;17:629–33.

273. Glasson SS, Askew R, Sheppard B, et al. Deletion of active ADAMTS5 prevents cartilage degradation in a murine model of osteoarthritis. Nature 2005;434(7033):644–48.

# 4

# Update on the Chondrocyte Lineage and Implications for Cell Therapy in Osteoarthritis

Mary B. Goldring

## INTRODUCTION

Chondrocytes serve diverse functions during development and postnatal life and are the single cellular component of the articular cartilage of diarthrodial joints. During skeletal development, the chondrocyte arises from mesenchymal progenitors and synthesizes the templates, or cartilage anlagen, for the developing limbs in a process known as chondrogenesis. Following mesenchymal condensation and chondroprogenitor cell differentiation, the chondrocytes undergo proliferation, terminal differentiation to chondrocyte hypertrophy, and apoptosis in a process termed endochondral ossification (whereby the hypertrophic cartilage is replaced by bone).

A similar sequence of events occurs in the postnatal growth plate and leads to rapid growth of the skeleton. In the adult, articular chondrocytes are fully differentiated cells that remain after formation of cartilage matrix during chondrogenesis and growth plate formation and maintain matrix constituents in a low turnover state of equilibrium. Chondrocytes comprise 2 to 5% of the tissue volume and are relatively inactive metabolically due in part to the absence of a vascular supply and innervation in the tissue, although they can respond to mechanical stimuli, growth factors, and cytokines that influence normal homeostasis in a positive or negative manner.

Once the cartilage matrix is degraded by adverse insults such as inflammation or abnormal loading, the adult chondrocyte may attempt to recapitulate phenotypes of early stages of cartilage development, but the precise zonal variations in the cartilage matrix network formed originally cannot be replicated. Thus, the chondrocyte has clinical importance in the context of the pathogenesis of osteoarthritis (OA), where its responses to adverse environmental stimuli promote matrix degradation and prevent cartilage repair.

## ORIGIN AND DIFFERENTIATION OF THE CHONDROCYTE

### Chondrogenesis

Chondrocytes arise during chondrogenesis, which is the earliest phase of skeletal development involving mesenchymal cell recruitment, migration, and condensation and differentiation of the mesenchymal chondroprogenitor cells. This process is controlled by cellular interactions with the surrounding matrix, growth and differentiation factors, and other environmental factors that initiate or suppress cellular signaling pathways and transcription of specific genes in a temporal-spatial manner.[1] Much of our current understanding of chondrogenesis is based on early studies in chicken and later in mice. The development of the joint is divided into two morphologic events: formation of the cartilaginous anlagen that model skeletal elements and subsequent joint formation by cavitation.

The skeletal elements are prefigured in mesenchymal condensations, and common precursor mesenchymal cells divide into chondrogenic, osteogenic, fibroblastic, adipogenic, and myogenic lineages that participate in the formation of various joint structures and surrounding tissues (Fig. 4.1). Interactions with the epithelium determine mesenchymal cell recruitment and migration, proliferation, and condensation.[2-4] The chondroprogenitor cells produce extracellular matrix (ECM) rich in hyaluronan, collagen type I, and type IIA collagen containing the exon 2.[5] The initiation of condensation is associated with increased hyaluronidase activity and the appearance of the cell adhesion molecules, neural cadherin (N-cadherin), and neural cell adhesion molecule (N-CAM), which facilitate cell-to-cell interactions.

Prior to chondrocyte differentiation, the cell/matrix interactions are facilitated by fibronectin binding to syndecan (which down-regulates N-CAM and sets the

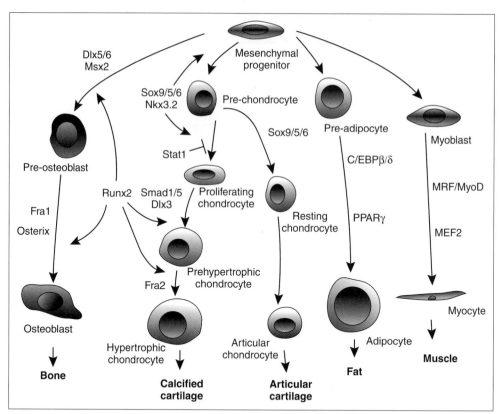

**Fig. 4.1** Scheme of differentiation of mesenchymal stem cells during the formation of muscle, adipose tissue (fat), articular and calcified cartilage (growth plate), and bone. During embryonic development, mesenchymal progenitors differentiate into different lineages depending on cellular interactions with the surrounding matrix and the availability of growth and differentiation factors and other environmental factors that initiate or suppress cellular signaling pathways and transcriptional regulators. Tissue-specific transcription factors involved at the various stages are indicated. Runx = runt domain binding protein; Stat = signal transducer and activator of transcription; Smad, mammalian homologue of *Drosophila* mothers against decapentaplegic (Mad); Dlx = distal-less; Msx = mesh-less; Fra = fos-related antigen; Sox = SRY-related HMG-box protein; C/EBP, CCAAT-enhancer binding protein; PPAR = peroxisome proliferator-activated receptor; MRFs = muscle regulatory factors, including MyoD and myogenin; MEF2, myogenic enhancer factor-2.

condensation boundaries). Increased cell proliferation and ECM remodeling—with the disappearance of type I collagen, fibronectin, and N-cadherin and the appearance of tenascins, matrilins, and thrombospondins (including cartilage oligomeric protein [COMP])—initiate the transition from chondroprogenitor cells to a fully committed chondrocytes.[4,6-8] The differentiated chondrocytes can then proliferate and undergo the complex process of hypertrophic maturation or remain within cartilage elements in articular joints.

Vertebrate limb development is controlled by interacting patterning systems involving fibroblast growth factor (FGF), hedgehog, bone morphogenetic protein (BMP), and Wnt pathways, each of which functions sequentially over time[9,10] (Fig. 4.2). Wnt signaling via β-catenin is required to induce FGFs, such as FGF-10 and FGF-8, which act in positive feedback loops.[11,12] The homeobox (Hox) transcription factors encoded by

the HoxA and HoxD gene clusters are critical for the early events of limb patterning in the undifferentiated mesenchyme, are required for the expression of FGF-8 and Sonic hedgehog (Shh),[13] and modulate the proliferation of cells within the condensations.[2]

Wnt7a is expressed early during limb bud development, where it acts to maintain Shh expression.[9] Shh signaling, which is required for early limb patterning although not for limb formation, is mediated by the Shh receptor Patched (Ptc1), which activates another transmembrane protein Smoothened (Smo) and inhibits processing of the Gli3 transcription factor to a transcriptional repressor.[12,14,15] In coordination, BMP-2, -4, and -7 regulate the patterning of limb elements within the condensations (depending on the temporal and spatial expression of BMP receptors involving SMAD-dependent and -independent signaling and BMP antagonists such as noggin and chordin).[9,16-19] In vitro and in vivo studies have shown that BMP

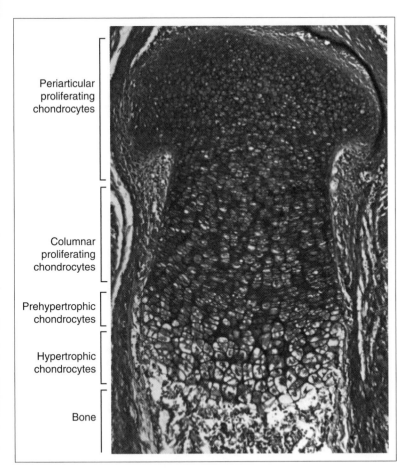

Periarticular proliferating chondrocytes

Columnar proliferating chondrocytes

Prehypertrophic chondrocytes

Hypertrophic chondrocytes

Bone

**Fig. 4.2** Cellular organization of the growth plate of mouse femur at embryonic day 17 of endochondral development. Distinct morphologies are observed in the different zones by histologic staining with hematoxylin and eosin. The periarticular proliferating chondrocytes are also called reserve chondrocytes. (See Color Plate 3.)

signaling is required for the formation of precartilaginous condensations and for the differentiation of precursors into chondrocytes.[19,20]

## Chondrocyte Differentiation and Proliferation

Growth plate formation in the embryonic limb occurs in a highly ordered fashion (Fig. 4.3). Chondrocyte differentiation is characterized by the expression of genes encoding cartilage-specific matrix proteins, including collagens II (COL2A1), IX (COL9), and XI (COL11) and aggrecan. The nuclear transcription factor Sox9, one of the earliest markers expressed in cells undergoing condensation, is required for the expression of COL2A1, COL11A2, and CD-RAP prior to matrix deposition in the cartilage anlagen.[8,21,22] L-Sox5 and Sox6 are not present in early mesenchymal condensations, but are required during overt chondrocyte differentiation[23] in forming heterodimers that induce transcription more efficiently than Sox9 by itself.[24] The expression of SOX proteins is dependent on BMP signaling via BMPR1A and BMPR1B, which are functionally redundant and active in differentiating chondrocyte but not in the perichondrium.[20]

Proliferation of chondrocytes in the embryonic and postnatal growth plate is regulated by multiple mitogenic stimuli, including FGFs, which converge on the cyclin D1 gene.[25] The temporal and spatial balance between BMP and FGF ligands and receptors determines the rate of chondrocyte proliferation during chondrogenesis, thereby adjusting the pace of the differentiation.[26,27] BMP-2, -3, -4, -5, and -7 are expressed primarily in the perichondrium and only BMP-7 is expressed in the proliferating chondrocytes.[26] BMP-6 is found exclusively later in hypertrophic chondrocytes, along with BMP-2.[28] FGFR2 is up-regulated early in condensing mesenchyme and is present later in the periphery of the condensation along with FGFR1, which is expressed in surrounding loose mesenchyme. FGFR3 is associated with proliferation of chondrocytes in the central core of the mesenchymal condensation and may overlap with FGFR2.[27]

During the transition of proliferating chondrocytes to the prehypertrophic stage in the growth plate, FGFR3 serves as a master inhibitor of chondrocyte proliferation via phosphorylation of the Stat1 transcription factor, which increases the expression of the cell cycle inhibitor p21.[29] FGF-18 is the preferred ligand

**Fig. 4.3** Schematic comparison of developmental events during cartilage development that reflects changes in chondrocyte phenotype and matrix remodeling during OA. Regulatory factors involved at each stage are listed to the left of the arrows, and transcription factors are listed to the right.

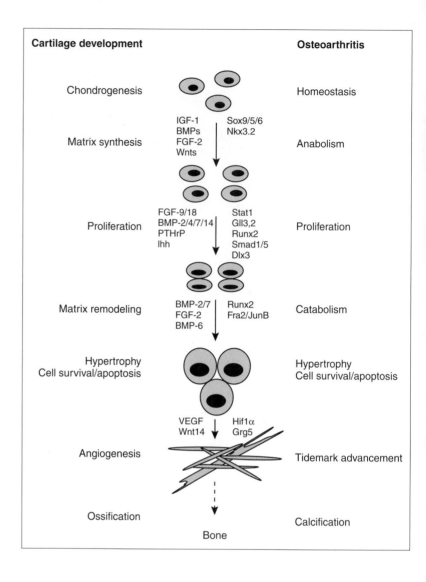

of FGFR3, in that Fgf18-deficient mice have an expanded zone of proliferating chondrocytes similar to that in Fgfr3-deficient mice.[30] FGF18 and FGF9 are expressed in the perichondrium and periosteum and form a functional gradient in the proximal zone of proliferating chondrocytes, where FGF18 acts via FGFR3 to down-regulate proliferation, promoting subsequent maturation.[30,31] As the epiphyseal growth plate develops, FGFR3 disappears and FGFR1 expression is up-regulated in prehypertrophic and hypertrophic chondrocytes, suggesting a role for FGFR1 in the regulation of cell survival and differentiation, and possibly cell death.[27] In the prehypertrophic and hypertrophic zones, both FGF18 and FGF9 interact with FGFR1 and regulate vascular invasion by inducing the expression of VEGF and VEGFR1.

The proliferation of chondrocytes in the lower proliferative and the prehypertrophic zones is also under the control of a local negative feedback loop involving signaling by PTHrP and inhibits Indian hedgehog (Ihh). Ihh expression is restricted to the prehypertrophic zone and PTHrP receptor is expressed in the distal zone of periarticular chondrocytes. The adjacent surrounding perichondrial cells express the hedgehog receptor patched (ptc), which upon Ihh binding (similar to Shh in the mesenchymal condensations) activates Smo and induces Gli transcription factors—which can feedback regulate Ihh target genes in a positive (Gli1 and Gli2) or negative (Gli3) manner.[32-35]

Early work indicated that Ihh induces expression of PTHrP in the perichondrium[36] and that PTHrP signaling then stimulates cell proliferation via its receptor expressed in the periarticular chondrocytes.[37] FGF-18 signaling via FGFR3 can inhibit Ihh expression[30] and BMP signaling up-regulates the expression of Ihh in cells that are beyond the range of the PTHrP-induced signal.[26]

Recent evidence indicates that Ihh acts independently of PTHrP on periarticular chondrocytes to stimulate differentiation of columnar chondrocytes in the proliferative zone, whereas PTHrP acts by preventing premature differentiation into prehypertrophic and hypertrophic chondrocytes (thereby suppressing premature expression of Ihh).[38] Thus, Ihh and PTHrP by transiently inducing proliferation markers and repressing differentiation markers function in a temporo-spatial manner to determine the number of cells that remain in the chondrogenic lineage versus those that enter the endochondral ossification pathway.

## Chondrocyte Hypertrophy and Endochondral Ossification

Endochondral ossification involves terminal differentiation of chondrocytes to the hypertrophic phenotype, cartilage matrix calcification, vascular invasion or angiogenesis, and ossification.[39-42] During chondrocyte hypertrophy, cellular fluid volume can increase by almost 20 times. Ihh (which synchronizes skeletal angiogenesis with perichondrial maturation) is expressed in prehypertrophic chondrocytes as they exit the proliferative phase, enter the hypertrophic phase, and begin to express the hypertrophic chondrocyte markers, type X collagen (Col10a1), and alkaline phosphatase.[43]

The runt-domain transcription factor Runx2 (also known as Core binding factor, or Cbfa1, and Osf2)—which serves as a positive regulatory factor in chondrocyte maturation to the hypertrophic phenotype and subsequent osteogenesis[44-47]—is expressed in the adjacent perichondrium and in prehypertrophic chondrocytes but less in late hypertrophic chondrocytes,[48,49] overlapping with Ihh, Col10a1, and BMP-6.[39,50] BMP-induced Smad1 and interactions between Smad1 and Runx2/Cbfa1 are important for chondrocyte hypertrophy.[44,51,52] Runx2 is required for terminal differentiation[46,47] and for the expression of matrix metalloproteinase (MMP)-13 by hypertrophic chondrocytes.[53-57]

The ECM remodeling that accompanies chondrocyte terminal differentiation induces an alteration in the environmental stress experienced by hypertrophic chondrocytes (which eventually undergo apoptosis)[39,58,59] and is the dominant rate-limiting process for chondrocyte hypertrophy and angiogenesis.[56] MMP-13 appears to cooperate with MMP-9 by degrading non-mineralized matrix in the late hypertrophic zone during primary and secondary ossification.[56,59] The membrane-bound MT1-MMP (MMP-14), which has a broader range of expression than MMP-9, is essential for chondrocyte proliferation and secondary ossification.[60]

Angiogenesis is the process by which the perichondrium and hypertrophic zone are invaded by blood vessels.[50,57] The angiogenic factor VEGF promotes vascular invasion via specifically localized receptors, including Flk expressed in endothelial cells in the perichondrium or surrounding soft tissues, neuropilin (Npn) 1 expressed in late hypertrophic chondrocytes, or Npn2 expressed exclusively in the perichondrium.[40] VEGF is expressed as three different isoforms. VEGF188, a matrix-bound form, is essential for metaphyseal vascularization. The soluble form, VEGF120 (VEGFA), regulates chondrocyte survival and epiphyseal cartilage angiogenesis.[61-63] VEGF164 can be either soluble or matrix bound and may act directly on chondrocytes via Npn2. It has been suggested that VEGF is released from the ECM by MMP-9 and other MMPs expressed by endothelial cells that migrate into the central region of the hypertrophic cartilage coincident with Flk-positive cells.[56] These events of cartilage matrix remodeling and vascular invasion are prerequisite to migration and differentiation of osteoclasts and osteoblasts, which remove mineralized cartilage matrix and replace it with bone.

## Novel Mediators of Chondrogenesis and Endochondral Ossification

Several novel mediators of chondrogenesis are transcription factors that act by promoting or inhibiting gene expression at different stages. Many factors that have been defined by whether they inhibit or enhance the function of Runx2 are able to coordinate chondrocyte and osteoblast differentiation.[64] Because there is no Smad site on the Runx2 promoter, it has been proposed that Hox genes of the Dlx family such as Dlx3 could activate Runx2 signaling in response to BMP-2 during endochondral ossification, whereas Dlx5 and Msx2 are known to inhibit Runx2-mediated activation of genes such as osteocalcin at later stages.[65,66]

In a recent study, we identified GADD45β (which has been implicated in the stress response and cell survival during terminal differentiation of different cell types) as a prominent early response gene induced by BMP-2 through a Smad1/Runx2-dependent pathway that acts as a survival factor in hypertrophic chondrocytes and maintains Mmp13 and Col10a1 expression.[67] The homeodomain protein Nkx3.2, which is an early BMP-induced signal required at the onset of chondrogenesis, is a direct transcriptional repressor of Runx2 promoter activity.[68] The bHLH factor Twist transiently inhibits Runx2 function and prevents premature osteoblast differentiation,[69] whereas cooperation of the Groucho homologue Grg5 or the leucine zipper protein ATF4 with Runx2 promotes chondrocyte maturation[70] or osteoblast differentiation,[71] respectively. Histone deacetylase 4 (HDAC4), which is expressed later in prehypertrophic chondrocytes, prevents premature chondrocyte hypertrophy by interacting with Runx2 and inhibiting its activity.[72]

The hypoxia-inducible factor (HIF) 1α is required for chondrocyte survival during hypertrophic differentiation, partly due to its regulation of VEGF expression.[42,73] A long form of c-Maf interacts with Sox9 at early stages to up-regulate Col2a1 expression,[74] whereas C/EBPβ and γ and AP-2α may inhibit chondrocyte differentiation by blocking transcription of Col2a1, aggrecan, and other cartilage-specific genes by direct or indirect mechanisms.[75-77] Recent reports from several groups indicate that Wnt signaling, via the canonical β-catenin pathway and activation of TCF/Lef transcription factors, functions in a cell autonomous manner to induce osteoblast differentiation and suppress chondrocyte differentiation in early chondroprogenitors.[78-82] During chondrogenesis, Wnt/β-catenin acts at two stages: at low levels to promote chondroprogenitor differentiation and later at high levels to promote chondrocyte hypertrophic differentiation and subsequent endochondral ossification.[78,83]

## Transgenic and Knockout Mouse Models of Defective Chondrogenesis

Mouse models with defects in transcription factors, MMPs, angiogenic factors, or extracellular matrix proteins have provided insight into the mechanisms that control cartilage development and in some cases OA pathology (Table 4.1). In Runx2-deficient mice, the late stages of chondrocyte hypertrophy are blocked and bone formation does not occur.[46,47] Several genetic studies have provided insight into the roles of AP-1 family members.[84] Deficiency or mutation of Fra2,[85] ATF-2,[86] or c-Maf[87] impairs hypertrophic chondrocyte differentiation and delays ossification, whereas overexpression or knockout experiments show that c-Fos, JunB, and Fra1 are important for ossification and osteogenesis.[88-90]

Disruption of TGF-β signaling by dominant-negative overexpression of the type II TGF-β receptor, TgfβRII,[91] or targeted ablation of Smad3[92] results in enhanced chondrocyte hypertrophy and increased Col10a1 expression. Studies in Gadd45β–/– mouse embryos, which have decreased length of the hypertrophic zone and deficient Mmp13 and Col10a1 expression, demonstrate the importance of the survival of hypertrophic chondrocytes long enough to allow matrix synthesis and remodeling.[67] In studies using Mmp13–/– mice, MMP-13 deficiency results in significant interstitial collagen accumulation leading to the

| Gene | Gene Defect or Modification | Features | Reference |
|---|---|---|---|
| **Transcription Factors** | | | |
| Sox9 | Knockout | No cartilage formation | (416, 417) |
| Runx2 | Knockout | Blocked chondrocyte hypertrophy, no bone formation | (45–47) |
| Smad3 | Targeted disruption | Enhanced chondrocyte hypertrophy and OA-like cartilage erosion | (92) |
| Fra2, ATF2, c-Maf | Knockout | Impaired hypertrophic chondrocyte differentiation, delayed ossification | (85–87) |
| c-Fos, JunB, Fra2 | Knockout | Impaired ossification, decreased osteogenesis | (88–90) |
| Gadd45β | Knockout | Compressed hypertrophic zone and decreased Col10a1 and Mmp13 | (67) |
| **Angiogenic Factors** | | | |
| VEGF or VEGFRs | Knockout | Increased length of hypertrophic zone, delayed ossification | (58, 61) |
| **Proteinases** | | | |
| Mmp9 | Knockout | Increased length of hypertrophic zone, delayed ossification | (59) |
| Mmp13 | Knockout | Increased length of hypertrophic zone, delayed ossification | (93, 94) |
| Mmp13 | Postnatal transgenic | Increased susceptibility to OA | (120) |
| Adamts5 | Knockout | Decreased susceptibility to OA | (118, 119) |

TABLE 4.1 MOUSE MODELS FOR STUDYING SKELETAL DEVELOPMENT AND OSTEOARTHRITIS

| | TABLE 4.1 MOUSE MODELS FOR STUDYING SKELETAL DEVELOPMENT AND OSTEOARTHRITIS—cont'd | | |
|---|---|---|---|
| Gene | Gene Defect or Modification | Features | Reference |
| **Collagens** | | | |
| Col10a1 | Knockout or transgenic dominant-negative mutation | Compressed proliferative and hypertrophic zones and altered mineral deposition | (96) |
| Col2a1 | Transgenic internal deletion | Mild chondrodysplasia, OA | |
| Col2a1 | Transgenic overexpression or deficiency | OA-like changes during aging | |
| Col2a1 | Del1, 150-bp deletion | Early-onset OA | |
| Col2a1 | Dmm/+, spontaneous deletion | Early-onset OA | |
| Col9a1 | Transgenic truncation | Mild chondrodysplasia, OA | (108) |
| Col9a1 | Knockout | Early-onset OA | (107) |
| Col11a1 | Cho/+, spontaneous deletion | OA-like changes during aging | (103, 104) |
| **Proteoglycans** | | | |
| Aggrecan | Cmd/+, spontaneous deletion | OA-like changes during aging | (110) |
| Fibromodulin | Knockout | Tendon mineralization, OA | (113, 114) |
| Fibromodulin + biglycan | Double knockout | Ectopic mineralization, early-onset OA | (113, 114) |
| **Other Proteins** | | | |
| α1 integrin | Knockout | Accelerated cartilage degradation | (112) |
| βmpR1a | Postnatal conditional knockout | OA-like cartilage degeneration | (117) |
| TgfβRII | Transgenic dominant-negative truncation | Enhanced chondrocyte hypertrophy and progressive skeletal degeneration with OA | (91) |
| Ank | ank/ank, homozygous truncation mutation | Early-onset OA associated with crystal deposition | (115) |
| Npp1 | Knockout | OA associated with crystal deposition | (116) |
| Matrilin-3 | Knockout | OA-like changes with aging | (111) |

delay of endochondral ossification in the growth plate and increased length of the hypertrophic zone.[93,94] Removal of angiogenic stimuli by ablating VEGF[58] or VEGF receptors[61] results in increased length of the hypertrophic zone.

*Mmp9*–/– mice have a similar phenotype.[59] On the other hand, cleavage by MMPs or aggrecanases is not required for the removal of aggrecan from growth plate cartilage.[95] In contrast to *Mmp13*–/– mice[93,94] but similar to *Gadd45β*–/– mice,[67] both *Col10a1* knockout mice and transgenic mice with a dominant interference *Col10a1* mutation have subtle growth plate phenotypes with compressed proliferative and hypertrophic zones and altered mineral deposition.[96] The dwarfism observed in human chondrodysplasias with *Col10a1* mutations involves skeletal elements that are under great mechanical stress due to disruption in the pericellular matrix in the hypertrophic zone, although a role for defective vascularization has been proposed.[97]

The chondrodysplasia (*cho/cho*) mouse embryo, which carries a loss of function mutation in the *Col11a1* gene and is perinatal lethal, has wider long bones with shorter length possibly because type XI collagen influences the formation of type II collagen fibrils at early stages of chondrogenesis.[98] In contrast, mice with targeted knockout of *Col2a1* survive and develop intramembranous and periosteal bone but cannot undergo endochondral ossification.[99] Thus, the loss or mutation of a single gene that is involved in synthesis or remodeling of the cartilage matrix may lead to a cascade of disruption of other genes and activities in chondrocytes, contributing collectively to the pathologic changes in the architecture of the growth plate.[100]

A number of studies have shown that developmental defects in the cartilage matrix lead to degenerative changes in the adult mice[101,102] (see Table 4.1). The haploinsufficient *cho/+* mouse develops OA-like pathology with increased MMP-3 expression and proteoglycan degradation by 3 months and degradation of the collagen network by 6 months due to increased MMP-13 activity stimulated by interaction of DDR2 with exposed collagen fibers.[103,104] Heterozygous *Col2a1+/−* mice have cartilage matrix with altered collagen network that is susceptible to the development of OA-like changes.[105,106] Mutations in *Col9a1*,[107,108] *Col2a1*,[109] or aggrecan[110] also result in osteoarthritic changes in adult mice.

Models with deficiency of matrilin-3,[111] α1 integrin,[112] or biglycan together with fibromodulin or decorin[113,114] also show OA-like pathology. Mutation in the Ank gene encoding a multipass transmembrane protein and knockout of nucleotide pyrophosphatase phosphodiesterase-1 (*Nnp1*), whose gene products control intracellular pyrophosphate levels, cause progressive or early onset OA associated with increased chondrocyte hypertrophy and inappropriate mineralization of the cartilage matrix.[115,116] The While disruption of BMP signaling by ablation of Bmpr1a results in early embryonic death. Postnatal conditional knockout results in OA-like cartilage degeneration.[117]

Loss of TGF-β signaling also increases OA-like pathology in postnatal articular cartilage, associated with increased chondrocyte hypertrophy and expression of *Col10a1*.[91,92] Of the proteinases that degrade aggrecan, only aggrecanase-2 ADAMTS5 is associated with increased susceptibility to OA, as shown in *Adamts5*-deficient mice.[118,119] Postnatal overexpression of constitutively active *Mmp13* also promotes OA in mice.[120] For most of these mouse models, the OA-like changes become more prevalent with aging.[121]

## The Adult Articular Chondrocyte

The adult articular chondrocyte embedded in its extracellular matrix is a resting cell with no detectable mitotic activity and a very low rate of synthetic activity. The expression patterns of matrix proteins in cartilage have been mapped by immunohistochemistry and in situ hybridization to localize protein and mRNA levels, respectively. The markers of mature articular chondrocytes are type II collagen, other cartilage-specific collagens IX and XI, the large aggregating proteoglycan aggrecan, and link protein.

In adult articular cartilage, the synthesis of matrix components is very slow. The turnover of collagen is estimated to occur with a half-life of greater than 100 years.[122,123] In contrast, the glycosaminoglycan constituents on the aggrecan core protein are more readily replaced, and the half-life of aggrecan subfractions is estimated to be in the range of 3 to 24 years.[124] Other cartilage ECM components (including biglycan, decorin, COMP, tenascins, and matrilins) incorporated previously into the matrix during development may also be synthesized by chondrocytes under low turnover conditions. However, there are regional differences in the remodeling activities of chondrocytes and matrix turnover may be more rapid in the immediate pericellular zones.[125-127]

## The Chondrocyte in Physiologic Conditions

Under normal conditions, the chondrocyte maintains a steady-state metabolism resulting from equilibrium between anabolic processes and catabolic processes. Chondrocytes maintain active membrane transport systems for exchange of cations—including Na+, K+, Ca2+, and H+, whose intracellular concentrations fluctuate with load and changes in the composition of the cartilage matrix.[128] Because articular cartilage is not vascularized, the chondrocyte must rely on diffusion from the articular surface or subchondral bone for the exchange of nutrients and metabolites. Glucose serves both as the major energy source for the chondrocytes and as an essential precursor for glycosaminoglycan synthesis.[129-131]

Facilitated glucose transport in chondrocytes is mediated by several distinct glucose transporter proteins (GLUTs) that are either constitutively expressed (GLUT3 and GLUT8) or cytokine-inducible (GLUT1 and GLUT6).[132,133] Chondrocytes do not normally contain abundant mitochondria, and energy requirements may be modulated by mechanical stress.[134] Chondrocyte metabolism operates at low oxygen tension within the cartilage matrix, ranging from 10% at the surface to less than 1% in the deep zones. When cultured in a range of oxygen tensions between severe hypoxia (0.1% $O_2$) and normoxia (21% $O_2$), chondrocytes adapt to low oxygen tensions by up-regulating hypoxia-inducible factor-1α (HIF-1α).

Hypoxia via HIF-1α can stimulate chondrocytes to express GLUTs[135] and angiogenic factors such as VEGF,[136,137] as well as a number of genes associated with cartilage anabolism and chondrocyte differentiation (including Sox9, TGF-β, and connective tissue growth factor).[138,139] In the growth plate, hypoxia and HIF-1α are associated with type II collagen production.[140] HIF-1α is expressed in both normal and OA articular cartilage,[141] where it maintains tonic activity during physiologic hypoxia in the deeper layers associated with increased proteoglycan synthesis. However, unlike in other tissues it is not completely degraded when normoxic conditions are applied.[142]

Long-term systemic hypoxia (13%), on the other hand, may down-regulate collagen and aggrecan gene expression in articular cartilage.[143] Thus, by modulating the intracellular expression of survival factors such as HIF-1α chondrocytes have a high capacity to survive in the avascular cartilage matrix and to respond to environmental changes. Findings that catabolic stress and inflammatory cytokines up-regulate HIF-1α also suggest that it may serve as a survival factor in OA cartilage.[141,144,145]

## The Chondrocyte in Osteoarthritis
### Phenotypic Modulation
Chondrocytes in vivo respond to structural changes in the surrounding cartilage matrix as occurs during the initial stages of OA when increased chondrocyte proliferation and synthesis of matrix proteins, proteinases, and cytokines are observed. However, the capacity of the adult articular chondrocyte to regenerate the normal cartilage matrix architecture is limited and the damage becomes irreversible unless the destructive process is interrupted. The metabolic potential of these cells is also indicated by their capacity to proliferate in culture and synthesize matrix proteins after enzymatic release from the cartilage. Attempts to map the abnormal occurrence and distribution of matrix proteins in OA cartilage and other cartilage pathologies have provided insights into the pathogenesis of joint disease.

The early changes in synthetic activity are viewed as an attempt to regenerate the matrix with cartilage-specific components (types II, IX, and XI collagens and aggrecan), but the resident chondrocytes also undergo phenotypic modulation by synthesizing type I collagen.[146] The increase in pericellular type VI collagen microfibrils also indicates that the chondrocyte is able to respond to changes in its microenvironment.[147] Other phenotypic alterations have been reported, such as the appearance of the chondroprogenitor collagen type IIA, which is the splice variant of the normal cartilage-specific type IIB collagen (COL2A1).[148,149] A recapitulation of embryonic skeletal development also occurs in the deep and calcified zones where the hypertrophic chondrocyte-specific type X collagen is expressed, and in the upper middle zone where type III collagen expression is detected.[150] A general up-regulation of collagen and proteoglycan synthesis has been observed in an animal model of OA.[151]

Genomic and proteomic analyses of global gene expression have confirmed the increased levels of type II collagen mRNA levels in early OA cartilage,[152,153] which may be associated with the increased levels of anabolic factors such as BMP-2 and inhibin βA/activin.[153,154] These and other TGF-β family members may stimulate aggrecan synthesis at the same time as promoting osteophyte formation.[155,156] Sox9 expression, however, does not correlate with COL2A1 expression in articular chondrocytes of adult normal and OA cartilage.[157] Despite the occurrence of phenotypes associated with cartilage development in OA cartilage, the highly ordered developmental processes do not occur in OA. Instead, degenerative processes control matrix remodeling in an uncoordinated fashion[158] (see Fig. 4.2).

### Matrix Remodeling
In contrast to the anabolism and phenotypic modulation, analogies between cartilage catabolism in OA and matrix remodeling during endochondral ossification are more difficult to identify. The proinflammatory cytokines interleukin-1β (IL-1β) and tumor necrosis factor-α (TNF-α) do not seem to be "players" during chondrogenesis in the embryonic or postnatal growth plate, and a mechanism for the disappearance of aggrecan in the hypertrophic zone has not been elucidated.[95] MMPs do play an important role in matrix remodeling in both processes, however. The localization of MMP-13 expression in the deep zone of OA cartilage has led to speculation that the chondrocyte hypertrophy and the associated tidemark advancement and subchondral bone thickening are major features of progression of the disease.

The recent studies identifying OA-associated polymorphisms in the gene encoding asporin (which inhibits cartilage anabolism by binding to TGF-β) and in FRZB (which encodes secreted frizzled-related protein 3 [sFRP3])[159,160] lend support to this concept. Members of the sFRP family, including sFRP3, are glycoproteins that antagonize the signaling of Wnt ligands through frizzled membrane-bound receptors.[161] The soluble inhibitors of the Wnt signaling, such as sFRP1 and LRP5, have been implicated in the maintenance of adult bone density.[162-164] Ectopic Wnt/β-catenin signaling leads to enhanced ossification and suppression of chondrocyte formation during skeletal development,[78] and disruption of Wnt signaling in adult cartilage and bone may have pathologic consequences. For example, sFRP1 inhibits osteoclast formation by binding to RANKL,[165] and sFRP3 inhibits osteoblast proliferation and increases osteoblast differentiation independently of canonical Wnt/β-catenin signaling.[166]

In OA cartilage, sFRP may have a role in chondrocyte apoptosis.[167] Because activation of β-catenin in mature cartilage cells stimulates hypertrophy; matrix mineralization; and expression of VEGF, ADAMTS5, MMP-13 and several other MMPs,[83] defective inhibition of Wnt signaling due to FRZB polymorphisms may disrupt normal homeostasis (resulting in abnormal cartilage and bone metabolism).

### Anabolic Activities
Many of the growth and differentiation factors that regulate cartilage development are positive regulators of homeostasis of mature articular cartilage due to the

capacity to stimulate chondrocyte anabolic activity and in some cases to inhibit catabolic activity. The most well-characterized anabolic factors in the context of their production and action in articular cartilage include insulin-like growth factor-1 (IGF-1), osteogenic protein-1 (OP-1 or BMP-7), TGF-β, BMP-2, FGF-2, cartilage-derived morphogenetic proteins (CDMPs), and human cartilage glycoprotein 39 (HC-gp39).[168-172]

Many of the anabolic factors that support cartilage matrix biosynthesis are expressed at declining levels with aging (a risk factor for OA) or have their activities down-regulated.[173] For example, the capacity of BMP-6 to stimulate proteoglycan synthesis and the production of BMP-7 (OP-1) declines with age.[174,175] Although FGF-2 is a potent mitogen for articular chondrocytes, recent evidence indicates that it inhibits the anabolic activities of IGF-1 and OP-1.[176] In contrast, TGF-β is able to counteract the expression in chondrocytes of a number of IL-1–induced genes involved in OA,[177] but a reduced TGF-β signaling in aging chondrocytes may contribute to a reduced repair capacity.[178]

The anabolic activities of IGF-1, which stimulates proteoglycan synthesis, promote chondrocyte survival and oppose catabolic activities of catabolic cytokines (which also decline with age). Chondrocytes from animals with experimental arthritis and from patients with OA are hypo-responsive to IGF-1 despite normal or increased IGF-1 receptor levels. This has been attributed to increased levels of IGFBPs that may interfere with IGF-1 actions.[179-183] Disturbances in the balance of IGF-1 to IGFBP-3, in particular, that have been reported in OA and RA joints may contribute to defective chondrocyte responses to IGF-1.[184-186] Although IGF-1 can oppose the effects of inflammatory cytokines that promote cartilage degradation and inhibit proteoglycan synthesis,[187] these cytokines also increase the production of IGFBP-3 by chondrocytes.[188]

Overproduction of nitric oxide may also contribute to IGF-1 resistance by chondrocytes through disruption of integrin signaling, reduction of phosphorylation of the IGF-1 receptor, stimulation of cGMP production, or suppression of mitochondrial oxidative metabolism.[189-193] Recent evidence indicates that suppressor of cytokine signaling 3 (SOCS3) acts as a negative feedback regulator during IGF-1 desensitization in the absence of nitric oxide by inhibiting insulin receptor substrate (IRS)-1 phosphorylation.[194]

## Catabolic Activities

The major events in OA pathogenesis are localized within the cartilage itself, and there is also evidence that the chondrocytes participate in this destructive process not only by responding to the catabolic cytokines released from other joint tissues but possibly by being themselves the source of cytokines that contribute to cartilage matrix loss via autocrine or paracrine mechanisms.[195-198] Our understanding of basic cellular mechanisms regulating chondrocyte responses to cytokine mediators has been inferred from numerous studies in vitro using cultures of cartilage fragments or isolated chondrocytes and is supported by studies in animal models.[199,200]

Chondrocytes produce IL-1 at concentrations capable of inducing the expression of MMPs, aggrecanases, and other catabolic genes.[201-203] MMP-13 is elevated in OA joint tissues, particularly in articular cartilage,[204-206] and co-localizes with type II collagen cleavage epitopes in regions of matrix depletion in OA cartilage.[127] This enzyme cleaves the native collagen molecule and is five- to tenfold more active on type II collagen than are MMP-1 and MMP-8, other collagenases also present in this tissue.[207] IL-1β and TNF-α co-localize with MMPs in superficial regions of OA cartilage.[208] Chondrocytes in OA cartilage, especially those in clonal clusters, are positive for IL-1 immunostaining[202,208,209] and produce IL-1β–converting enzyme (caspase-1)[210] and type I IL-1 receptor.[211] Thus, chondrocytes in OA cartilage may be exposed continuously to the autocrine and paracrine effects of IL-1 and other inflammatory mediators at high local concentrations.

In addition to inducing the synthesis of MMPs and other proteinases by chondrocytes, IL-1 and TNF-α increase the synthesis of prostaglandin $E_2$ ($PGE_2$) by stimulating the expression or activities of cyclooxygenase (COX)-2, microsomal PGE synthase-1 (mPGES-1), and soluble phospholipase A2 (sPLA2). They also up-regulate the production of nitric oxide via inducible nitric oxide synthetase (iNOS); other proinflammatory cytokines, such as IL-6, leukemia inhibitory factor (LIF), IL-17, and IL-18; and chemokines, including IL-8.[197,198] IL-17, a T-lymphocyte product, also stimulates the production of proinflammatory cytokines and has effects on chondrocytes similar to IL-1.[212] Many of these factors synergize with one another in promoting chondrocyte catabolic responses. Oncostatin M produces mild catabolic responses in chondrocytes, but synergizes strongly with IL-1 or TNF-α.[213,214]

## Signaling Pathways

Chondrocytes have receptors for responding to mechanical stress[215,216] and can respond to direct biomechanical perturbation by up-regulating synthetic activity or inflammatory cytokines, which are also produced by other joint tissues.[198] Injurious static compression stimulates depletion of proteoglycans and damage to the collagen network and decreases the synthesis of cartilage matrix proteins, whereas dynamic compression increases matrix synthetic activity.[217-220] Degradation products of extracellular matrix components, including fibronectin (FN) fragments, can also stimulate the production of matrix-degrading proteinases in chondrocytes by both IL-1–dependent and –independent mechanisms.[221-224]

Certain types of mechanical stresses and cartilage matrix degradation products are capable of stimulating the same signaling pathways as those induced by IL-1 and TNF-$\alpha$. These pathways involve cascades of kinases, including the stress-activated protein kinases (SAPKs)—also termed c-Jun N-terminal kinases (JNKs)—and p38 MAP kinase, I$\kappa$B kinases, and phosphatidylinositol-3′-kinase (PI-3K) and NF-$\kappa$B.[225-230] Because these pathways may also induce the expression of the genes encoding these cytokines, it remains controversial whether inflammatory cytokines are primary or secondary regulators of the progressive cartilage destruction in OA.

Both IL-1 and TNF-$\alpha$ also inhibit the synthesis of proteoglycans and type II collagen by chondrocytes,[231-235] thereby promoting chondrocyte dedifferentiation and preventing cartilage repair. The early increase in anabolic activity in OA cartilage due to BMP-2 would activate type II collagen and aggrecan gene expression, and permit down-regulation of these matrix genes by cytokine-induced transcription factors.[236] IL-1 differentially regulates inhibitory Smads, up-regulating Smad7 and down-regulating Smad6 in chondrocytes. Cytoplasmic localization of these inhibitors of TGF-$\beta$ and BMP signaling in normal and OA cartilage does not correlate with the expression of anabolic genes.[237]

Cytokine-induced PGE$_2$ may also feedback regulate type II collagen gene transcription in a positive manner,[238,239] whereas nitric oxide inhibits proteoglycan and collagen synthesis.[240,241] The mechanisms of cross-talk between prostaglandins and nitric oxide that regulate chondrocyte function have been reviewed recently.[197] Recent evidence indicates that peroxisome proliferator-activated receptor $\alpha$?(PPAR$\alpha$) agonists may protect chondrocytes against IL-1–induced responses by increasing the expression of the IL-1 receptor antagonist.[242] The accumulation of advanced glycation end products (AGEs) in aging cartilage suggests an additional mechanism whereby feedback regulation of chondrocyte function could occur due to changes in the extracellular matrix. Recent evidence indicates that the receptor for AGEs (RAGE) interacts preferentially with S100A4 (a member of the S100 family of calcium binding proteins) in chondrocytes and stimulates MMP-13 production via phosphorylation of Pyk2, MAP kinases, and NF-$\kappa$B.[243]

### Chemokines

The role of chemokines in the recruitment of leukocytes to inflamed joints is well established, but it is now known that chondrocytes (when activated by proinflammatory cytokines, including IL-1, TNF-$\alpha$, IL-17, IL-18, and OSM) can express several chemokines and also have receptors that enable responses associated with cartilage catabolism. The first report of expression of functional chemokine receptors (CCR1, CCR2, CCR3, CCR5, CXCR1, and CXCR2) on chondrocytes was by Borzi et al.,[244] who showed that interaction of these receptors with their corresponding ligands (MCP-1, RANTES, and GRO$\alpha$) results in up-regulation of MMP-3.

Yuan et al.[245] showed that both normal and OA chondrocytes express the C-C chemokines MCP-1, MIP-1$\alpha$, MIP-1$\beta$, and RANTES (the levels of which are generally increased by IL-1$\beta$ or TNF-$\alpha$), and that RANTES increases expression of its own receptor, CCR5. MCP-1 and RANTES, in addition to increasing MMP-3 expression, inhibit proteoglycan synthesis and enhance proteoglycan release from the chondrocytes.[245]

The RANTES receptors CCR3 and CCR5 (but not CCR1) are expressed in normal cartilage, whereas all three receptors are expressed in OA cartilage or after stimulation of normal chondrocytes by IL-1$\beta$.[246] Furthermore, RANTES induces the expression of iNOS, IL-6, and MMP-1.[246] More recent work has demonstrated the expression of an additional chemokine receptor (CXCR4) by chondrocytes but not synovial fibroblasts, and high levels of its ligand—stromal cell-derived factor 1 (SDF-1)—in RA and OA synovial fluids.[247] SDF-1 also increases the synthesis of MMP-3, but not MMP-1.[247]

## CHONDROCYTE CULTURE MODELS

The development of therapeutic strategies that prevent degradation of cartilage matrix in patients with OA and permit cartilage regeneration and repair has been limited by the availability of reproducible cell culture models of human origin. Primary cultures of articular chondrocytes isolated from various animal and human sources (or explant cultures of articular cartilage where the chondrocytes remain encased within their own extracellular matrix) have been used as in vitro models to study the mechanisms of cartilage degradation and repair,[195,196,248] as well as to determine differences between normal and OA cartilage.[249] However, the source of the cartilage cannot be controlled, large numbers of cells are not readily obtained from random operative procedures, and the phenotypic stability and proliferative capacity in adult human chondrocytes are lost quickly upon expansion in serial monolayer cultures.

Chondrocyte immortalization techniques have had limited success because of poor stability of phenotype associated with the adult articular chondrocyte. Recent studies using mesenchymal stem cells as models of in vitro chondrogenesis to understand mechanisms of differentiation that could be applied to cartilage tissue engineering have yielded promising results. In some cases, chondroprogenitor cell lines have been established, although primarily from non-human mammalian tissues (as described in material following).

## Articular Chondrocytes

The cartilage explant culture system, based on the pioneering work of Fell,[250] has been used for decades to examine cartilage biochemistry and how it is modified by responses of the chondrocyte to the environment. Bovine cartilage and other animal sources were used to characterize the synthesis and degradation of cartilage proteoglycan and collagens in response to serum,[251] proteolytic enzymes,[252] lipopolysaccharides,[253] interleukin-1,[254-256] retinoic acid,[257] and growth factors.[258-260]

Primary chondrocytes isolated from cartilage and grown in high-density monolayer cultures maintain a rounded polygonal morphology and cartilage-specific phenotype until subculture, although type II collagen gene expression is generally more labile than aggrecan.[261-263] This loss of phenotype is termed *de-differentiation*, during which chondrocytes acquire a fibroblast-like morphology and express some but not all characteristics of the fibroblast phenotype (including type I collagen).[264-267] Freshly isolated human articular or costal chondrocytes express cartilage-specific type II collagen and continue to do so for several days to weeks in primary monolayer culture.[232,261] Other markers expressed in primary chondrocyte cultures include chondromodulin, protein S-100, and Sox9.[268-270]

Because the stability of the phenotype of isolated chondrocytes is critically dependent on cell shape and cell density,[266,271] high-density micromass cultures are useful if sufficient numbers of chondrocytes can be obtained.[272,273] Serum-free defined media of varying compositions, but usually including insulin, have also been used to maintain phenotype.[262,274] Phenotype can be maintained, but without proliferative expansion, if the isolated chondrocytes are placed in suspension cultures in spinner flasks[264,275-278] or in dishes coated with substrates that do not support attachment.[279-281] In 3D matrices, freshly isolated or subcultured chondrocytes in solid support matrices such as collagen gels[282] or sponges,[283,284] agarose,[262,285-288] or alginate[289-294] acquire the normal spherical shape, synthesize and secrete abundant cell-associated extracellular matrix components, and maintain phenotypic stability for several months.

Because articular chondrocytes are unable to proliferate in fluid or gel suspension culture, expansion in monolayer culture followed by transfer to alginate or other suspension culture has been used as a strategy to obtain sufficient numbers of differentiated chondrocytes for study.[295] However, after prolonged culture in monolayer de-differentiated chondrocytes may lose irreversibly their chondrogenic potential.[296] The high-density pellet culture system, developed originally to study growth plate hypertrophy,[297] has also been used

as a 3D model because it permits articular chondrocytes to deposit a well-organized extracellular matrix containing type II collagen and aggrecan.[298-300] Isolated chondrons containing one or more chondrocytes within a capsule enclosing pericellular and interterritorial matrix have also been used for in vitro studies of chondrocyte metabolism within a 3D environment.[301]

## Hypertrophic Chondrocytes: Models of the Growth Plate and Terminal Differentiation

Tissues or cells from embryonic or young animals at specific developmental stages or with different developmental fates have been used widely to recapitulate in vitro the transitional stages of chondrogenesis, chondrocyte hypertrophy, and endochondral ossification.[302-308] A common feature of these models is the requirement for deposition of a collagenous matrix by sufficient numbers of cells following cessation of proliferation of chondrogenic cells in high-density monolayer cultures or their entrapment within a gel/suspension culture.

Epiphyseal chondrocytes isolated from the long bones of postnatal immature rats and rabbits and cultured at high density progress through a differentiation pathway that mimics the transition from a type II collagen-producing proliferating chondrocyte phenotype to the terminally differentiated type X collagen-producing hypertrophic phenotype associated with growth plate formation and endochondral ossification. Alkaline phosphatase, osteocalcin, and osteopontin have also been identified as markers of terminal differentiation.[309]

The pellet culture system has been used widely to study terminal differentiation and hypertrophy because it mimics the distribution of cells within the growth plate and is sufficiently organized to permit calcification in situ.[297,310-313] Arrest of cell proliferation and activation of type X collagen expression occurs when the serum concentration is reduced from 10 to 2% or lower. IGF-1 or insulin added in serum-free medium or as a constituent of serum appears to be a universal basal requirement in these culture systems.[274,314-316] Ascorbic acid has also been used to promote terminal differentiation in vitro.[317-319]

A steroid hormone (such as thyroxine, vitamin $D_3$ metabolite, dexamethasone, or retinoic acid) is required for entry into the late hypertrophic stage characterized by onset of type X collagen synthesis and cessation of type II collagen synthesis.[315,316,320-324] Ectopic matrix mineralization may require a phosphate donor such as β-glycerophosphate (BGP).[313] In contrast, certain BMPs alone or in the presence of ascorbic acid can induce hypertrophy in committed progenitor cell populations.[325]

# Chondrocyte Cell Lines

Because primary human chondrocytes in monolayer cultures maintain phenotype only until they are passaged, researchers have attempted to develop chondrocyte cell lines with variable success. Immortalization with viral oncogenes of avian, rabbit, mouse, and rat chondrocytes has produced cell lines with high proliferative capacities and to some extent properties of differentiated articular chondrocyte.[326-330]

Attempts to generate cell lines that can undergo chondrogenesis and terminal differentiation to the hypertrophic phenotype have been more successful due to the availability and plasticity of progenitor cell populations. For example, cells derived from the ribs of transgenic mice harboring the temperature-sensitive mutant of simian virus 40 (SV40) large T antigen (TAg) are able to undergo hypertrophic differentiation,[331,332] and bone-marrow–derived mesenchymal stem cells derived from these mice contain osteogenic, adipogenic, myogenic, and chondrogenic progenitor cells.

Several chondrogenic cell lines from mouse or rat (including ATDC5,[333,334] C3H10T1/2,[335] RCJ3.1,[306] CK2,[336,337] and C1,[338,339]) are now used widely in the field, as reviewed by Johnstone et al.[340] Whereas the addition of β-glycerophosphate and ascorbate generally favors the osteogenic phenotype, inclusion of BMPs or dexamethasone favors the chondrogenic phenotype often accompanied by terminal differentiation to hypertrophy.[341-345]

Human chondrosarcoma cell lines express some aspects of the chondrocyte phenotype but are tumorigenic.[346,347] Stable expression of SV40-TAg using plasmid or retroviral vectors has yielded immortalized human chondrocyte cell lines that are useful for studying the regulation of gene expression under defined conditions but do not produce sufficient amounts of matrix proteins to form cartilage matrix due to high rates of proliferation.[348-351] Human articular chondrocyte cell lines have also been established using the human papilloma virus type 16 (HPV-16) early-function genes E6 and E7[352] and telomerase.[353]

A general observation is that phenotypic stability of immortalized chondrocytes is lost during serial subculture in monolayer but can be restored by transfer to 3D culture in alginate[351] or hyaluronan[352] or to suspension culture in polyHEMA-coated dishes.[353] However, immortalized chondrocytes may continue to proliferate in suspension culture, and if the scaffold cannot be remodeled necrotic clusters will form. The studies to date indicate that mature chondrocytes removed from the ideal cartilage environment in vivo are incapable of replicating normal phenotype in vitro. The perfect chondrocyte culture model that reproduces the human articular chondrocyte has yet to be fabricated, as confirmed by gene profiling studies.[354-359]

# Therapeutic Strategies Targeting Chondrocytes

Current treatment options for cartilage injuries (in addition to the ultimate therapy of total joint replacement) include joint lavage, tissue debridement, microfracture of the subchondral bone, and the transplantation of autologous or allogeneic osteochondral grafts.[360] However, these procedures have variable success rates—leading frequently to the formation of fibrous tissue, chondrocyte death, and further cartilage degeneration.

Among the novel tissue engineering approaches developed to improve cartilage repair is autologous chondrocyte transplantation, which has been used somewhat successfully to repair small cartilage lesions in young adults with sports injuries.[361] However, the donor site (although not load bearing) often undergoes significant morbidity and osteoarthritic changes, and the defect is repaired with fibrocartilage rather than hyaline cartilage.[362-364] Recent randomized controlled trials suggest little difference in efficacy compared to microfracture of the subchondral bone.[365] Scaffolds such as those containing collagen have been employed in the absence or presence of cells to repair full-thickness defects in larger animals such as dogs and rabbits.[360,366-368]

The importance of extending the defect to the subchondral bone, presumably to expose a source of stimulating factors and progenitor cells, has been highlighted by Wakitani. Recent studies have focused on determining the feasibility of genetically engineering the autologous chondrocytes ex vivo to express anabolic factors to promote differentiation before implantation in the defect. The feasibility of using mesenchymal stem cells from bone marrow or other tissue sites is also the subject of current exploration.

## Anabolic Factors

Growth and differentiation factors are obvious tools for enhancing cartilage repair.[369,370] They also may have direct effects on mature articular chondrocytes in vivo and in vitro.[371-376] However, injection of free TGF-β or adenovirus-mediated delivery of TGF-β into joint cavities may have deleterious effects,[156,377] although introduction of liposome-encapsulated TGF-β in a fibrin matrix directly into partial-thickness defects produces healing in adult articular cartilage.[378]

The capacity of several BMPs (including BMP-2, -4, -6, -7, -9, and -13) to stimulate the synthesis of the cartilage matrix constituents, type II collagen, and aggrecan by adult articular chondrocytes provides the basis for their use to promote cartilage repair. For example, injection of BMP-2 into murine knee joints stimulates cartilage proteoglycan synthesis without counteracting the deleterious effects of IL-1 on proteoglycan synthesis and content.[379] The introduction of BMPs into joints via in vivo or ex vivo gene delivery or in injectable or implantable carriers has been investigated for the repair of small defects in animal models.[380]

Delivery of BMPs and other factors in synthetic or natural carrier scaffolds appears to be more successful than direct injection.[378,381] For example, BMP-2 implanted in a collagen carrier promotes the repair of full-thickness defects of articular cartilage in an animal model.[367,382] The transfer of genes encoding anabolic factors to chondrocytes prior to transplantation has been proposed as an additional strategy for promoting cartilage-specific matrix synthesis.[383] Indeed, the induction of the synthesis of IGF-I, TGF-β, BMP-2, and BMP-7 by gene transfer increases the synthesis of cartilage proteoglycans and collagens in cultured chondrocytes.[384-387] However, under some circumstances BMP-2 promotes chondrocyte hypertrophy,[388] consistent with its primary role in vivo to promote endochondral ossification.

A recent in vitro study using other BMP-2, -9, and -13 suggests that they may serve as potent anabolic factors for juvenile cartilage (which contains chondroprogenitors) but not for adult cartilage.[389] Another study on BMP-2 in resorbable collagen sponges produced appositional cartilage growth from perichondrium more easily in cricoid cartilage from juvenile rabbits than that from adults, where calcification occurred in large areas.[390]

### Mesenchymal Stem Cells

Many studies addressing alternative cellular sources for cartilage repair have aimed at exploiting the capacity of bone-marrow–derived mesenchymal stem cells (MSCs) to undergo endochondral ossification whereby a cartilage intermediate is formed.[391,392] Interestingly, the fates of these cells and patterning within tissues are determined by specific cell-to-cell and cell-to-matrix interactions that are controlled by the same growth and differentiation factors that control embryonic development (see Fig. 4.1). Many of these factors (including BMP-2, -6, -7, and -9; TGF-β; and CDMP-1) are able to induce chondrogenic differentiation of mesenchymal progenitor cells in vitro.[341,393-403]

The initial driving force for the application of BMPs to promote cartilage and bone formation arose from the original study in 1965 of Urist,[404] who showed that demineralized bone implanted subcutaneously in muscle resulted in the formation of endochondral bone. The pioneering work of Friedenstein[405] identified bone-forming progenitor cells from rat bone marrow, and more recent studies established that bone-marrow–derived MSCs also have the capacity to differentiate into cartilage, fat, and muscle cells.[399,406,407] Findings that MSCs remain in other adult tissues (including muscle, adipose tissue, and synovium) prompted further investigations to determine the potential of these cells to participate in the repair of skeletal tissues.[408-410]

Success in using adult MSCs to promote cartilage formation in vivo seems to require enrichment of the chondroprogenitor cell population by culture in a defined "chondrogenic" medium, transfer to a 3D environment, and ex vivo delivery of a growth and differentiation factor by gene transduction approaches. A recent study showed that transgene expression of BMP-2 in MSCs derived from bone marrow, perichondrium/periosteum, and to a lesser extent adipose tissue can support cartilage repair in rats.[410]

Although muscle-derived cells retrovirally transduced with BMP-4 induce endochondral bone formation when implanted in muscle[411] or bone,[412] the local delivery of BMP-4 by an enriched population of muscle-derived stem cells enhances chondrogenesis and improves repair of the articular cartilage in rats.[413] Some of these studies used juvenile tissues as sources of MSCs for transplantation into adult tissues. Challenges to application of these approaches in human subjects include accessibility of the tissue source and the influence of age on donor cells and recipient responses, in that bone-marrow–derived MSCs from patients with OA undergoing joint replacement therapy have impaired age-unrelated chondrogenic activity.[414] However, MSCs do avoid allogeneic rejection in humans and in animal models.[415]

## SUMMARY

During chondrogenesis, the interplay of positive and negative factors controls the rate and progression of chondrogenesis. The discovery and elucidation of several novel pathways have increased our knowledge of the complex gene networks during the different stages of chondrocyte differentiation, proliferation, and maturation. In the adult, chondrocytes are the single cellular component of the articular cartilage that maintain matrix constituents in a low-turnover state of equilibrium unless the matrix is degraded due to adverse environmental stimuli such as inflammation or abnormal loading.

In OA, the adult chondrocyte may attempt to recapitulate phenotypes of early stages of cartilage development, but the precise zonal variations in the cartilage matrix network formed originally cannot be replicated easily. Because OA progression cannot be halted if early events are not prevented, the current challenge is to develop cartilage repair strategies as alternatives to joint replacement. Recent understanding of how the adult articular chondrocyte functions within its unique environment and application of knowledge of how the cartilage was formed during chondrogenesis will enable the further development of novel therapeutic approaches involving gene therapy with anabolic factors and mesenchymal stem cells.

# REFERENCES

1. Goldring MB, Tsuchimochi K, Ijiri K. The control of chondrogenesis. J Cell Biochem 2005 (in press).
2. Hall BK, Miyake T. All for one and one for all: Condensations and the initiation of skeletal development. Bioessays 2000;22:138–47.
3. Capdevila J, Izpisua Belmonte JC. Patterning mechanisms controlling vertebrate limb development. Annu Rev Cell Dev Biol 2001;17:87–132.
4. Tuan RS. Biology of developmental and regenerative skeletogenesis. Clin Orthop Relat Res 2004;427 Suppl:S105–17.
5. Sandell LJ, Nalin AM, Reife RA. Alternative splice form of type II procollagen mRNA (IIA) is predominant in skeletal precursors and non-cartilaginous tissues during early mouse development. Dev Dyn 1994;199:129–40.
6. DeLise AM, Fischer L, Tuan RS. Cellular interactions and signaling in cartilage development. Osteoarthritis Cartilage 2000;8:309–34.
7. Olsen BR, Reginato AM, Wang W. Bone development. Annu Rev Cell Dev Biol 2000;16:191–220.
8. Eames BF, de la Fuente L, Helms JA. Molecular ontogeny of the skeleton. Birth Defects Res C Embryo Today 2003;69:93–101.
9. Tickle C. Patterning systems: From one end of the limb to the other. Dev Cell 2003;4:449–58.
10. Tickle C. Molecular basis of vertebrate limb patterning. Am J Med Genet 2002;112:250–55.
11. Tickle C, Munsterberg A. Vertebrate limb development: The early stages in chick and mouse. Curr Opin Genet Dev 2001; 11:476–81.
12. Niswander L. Pattern formation: Old models out on a limb. Nat Rev Genet 2003;4:133–43.
13. Kmita M, Tarchini B, Zakany J, Logan M, Tabin CJ, Duboule D. Early developmental arrest of mammalian limbs lacking HoxA/HoxD gene function. Nature 2005;435:1113–16.
14. Barna M, Pandolfi PP, Niswander L. Gli3 and Plzf cooperate in proximal limb patterning at early stages of limb development. Nature 2005;436:277–81.
15. Liu A, Wang B, Niswander LA. Mouse intraflagellar transport proteins regulate both the activator and repressor functions of Gli transcription factors. Development 2005;132:3103–11.
16. Pizette S, Niswander L. BMPs are required at two steps of limb chondrogenesis: Formation of prechondrogenic condensations and their differentiation into chondrocytes. Dev Biol 2000; 219:237–49.
17. Niswander L. Interplay between the molecular signals that control vertebrate limb development. Int J Dev Biol 2002;46:877–81.
18. Derynck R, Zhang YE. Smad-dependent and Smad-independent pathways in TGF-beta family signalling. Nature 2003;425:577–84.
19. Yoon BS, Lyons KM. Multiple functions of BMPs in chondrogenesis. J Cell Biochem 2004;93:93–103.
20. Yoon BS, Ovchinnikov DA, Yoshii I, Mishina Y, Behringer RR, Lyons KM. Bmpr1a and Bmpr1b have overlapping functions and are essential for chondrogenesis in vivo. Proc Natl Acad Sci USA 2005;102:5062–67.
21. Ng LJ, Wheatley S, Muscat GE, Conway-Campbell J, Bowles J, Wright E, et al. SOX9 binds DNA, activates transcription, and coexpresses with type II collagen during chondrogenesis in the mouse. Dev Biol 1997;183:108–21.
22. Lefebvre V, Behringer RR, de Crombrugghe B. L-Sox5, Sox6 and Sox9 control essential steps of the chondrocyte differentiation pathway. Osteoarthritis Cartilage 2001;9(A):S69–75.
23. Lefebvre V, Li P, de Crombrugghe B. A new long form of Sox5 (L-Sox5), Sox6 and Sox9 are coexpressed in chondrogenesis and cooperatively activate the type II collagen gene. EMBO J 1998; 17:5718–33.
24. Smits P, Li P, Mandel J, Zhang Z, Deng JM, Behringer RR, et al. The transcription factors L-Sox5 and Sox6 are essential for cartilage formation. Dev Cell 2001;1:277–90.
25. Beier F. Cell-cycle control and the cartilage growth plate. J Cell Physiol 2005;202:1–8.
26. Minina E, Kreschel C, Naski MC, Ornitz DM, Vortkamp A. Interaction of FGF, Ihh/Pthlh, and BMP signaling integrates chondrocyte proliferation and hypertrophic differentiation. Dev Cell 2002;3:439–49.
27. Ornitz DM. FGF signaling in the developing endochondral skeleton. Cytokine Growth Factor Rev 2005;16:205–13.
28. Itoh N, Ornitz DM. Evolution of the Fgf and Fgfr gene families. Trends Genet 2004;20:563–69.
29. Sahni M, Ambrosetti DC, Mansukhani A, Gertner R, Levy D, Basilico C. FGF signaling inhibits chondrocyte proliferation and regulates bone development through the STAT-1 pathway. Genes Dev 1999;13:1361–66.
30. Liu Z, Xu J, Colvin JS, Ornitz DM. Coordination of chondrogenesis and osteogenesis by fibroblast growth factor 18. Genes Dev 2002;16:859–69.
31. Ohbayashi N, Shibayama M, Kurotaki Y, Imanishi M, Fujimori T, Itoh N, et al. FGF18 is required for normal cell proliferation and differentiation during osteogenesis and chondrogenesis. Genes Dev 2002;16:870–79.
32. Ingham PW, McMahon AP. Hedgehog signaling in animal development: Paradigms and principles. Genes Dev 2001;15:3059–87.
33. McMahon AP, Ingham PW, Tabin CJ. Developmental roles and clinical significance of hedgehog signaling. Curr Top Dev Biol 2003;53:1–114.
34. Tyurina OV, Guner B, Popova E, Feng J, Schier AF, Kohtz JD, et al. Zebrafish Gli3 functions as both an activator and a repressor in Hedgehog signaling. Dev Biol 2005;277:537–56.
35. Vokes SA, McMahon AP. Hedgehog signaling: Iguana debuts as a nuclear gatekeeper. Curr Biol 2004;14:R668–70.
36. Vortkamp A, Lee K, Lanske B, Segre GV, Kronenberg HM, Tabin CJ. Regulation of rate of cartilage differentiation by Indian hedgehog and PTH-related protein. Science 1996;273:613–22.
37. Lanske B, Karaplis AC, Lee K, Luz A, Vortkamp A, Pirro A, et al. PTH/PTHrP receptor in early development and Indian hedgehog-regulated bone growth. Science 1996;273:663–66.
38. Kobayashi T, Soegiarto DW, Yang Y, Lanske B, Schipani E, McMahon AP, et al. Indian hedgehog stimulates periarticular chondrocyte differentiation to regulate growth plate length independently of PTHrP. J Clin Invest 2005;115:1734–42.
39. Ferguson CM, Miclau T, Hu D, Alpern E, Helms JA. Common molecular pathways in skeletal morphogenesis and repair. Ann NY Acad Sci 1998;857:33–42.
40. Colnot CI, Helms JA. A molecular analysis of matrix remodeling and angiogenesis during long bone development. Mech Dev 2001;100:245–50.
41. Ballock RT, O'Keefe RJ. The biology of the growth plate. J Bone Joint Surg Am 2003;85-A:715–26.
42. Provot S, Schipani E. Molecular mechanisms of endochondral bone development. Biochem Biophys Res Commun 2005;328:658–65.
43. St-Jacques B, Hammerschmidt M, McMahon AP. Indian hedgehog signaling regulates proliferation and differentiation of chondrocytes and is essential for bone formation. Genes Dev 1999;13: 2072–86.
44. Enomoto H, Enomoto-Iwamoto M, Iwamoto M, Nomura S, Himeno M, Kitamura Y, et al. Cbfa1 is a positive regulatory factor in chondrocyte maturation. J Biol Chem 2000;275:8695–8702.
45. Ducy P, Zhang R, Geoffroy V, Ridall AL, Karsenty G. Osf2/Cbfa1: A transcriptional activator of osteoblast differentiation. Cell 1997;89:747–54.
46. Komori T, Yagi H, Nomura S, Yamaguchi A, Sasaki K, Deguchi K, et al. Targeted disruption of Cbfa1 results in a complete lack of bone formation owing to maturational arrest of osteoblasts. Cell 1997;89:755–64.
47. Otto F, Thornell AP, Crompton T, Denzel A, Gilmour KC, Rosewell IR, et al. Cbfa1, a candidate gene for cleidocranial dysplasia syndrome, is essential for osteoblast differentiation and bone development. Cell 1997;89:765–71.
48. Kim IS, Otto F, Zabel B, Mundlos S. Regulation of chondrocyte differentiation by Cbfa1. Mech Dev 1999;80:159–70.
49. Takeda S, Bonnamy JP, Owen MJ, Ducy P, Karsenty G. Continuous expression of Cbfa1 in nonhypertrophic chondrocytes uncovers its ability to induce hypertrophic chondrocyte differentiation and partially rescues Cbfa1-deficient mice. Genes Dev 2001;15:467–81.
50. Colnot C. Cellular and molecular interactions regulating skeletogenesis. J Cell Biochem 2005;95:688–97.
51. Leboy P, Grasso-Knight G, D'Angelo M, Volk SW, Lian JV, Drissi H, et al. Smad-Runx interactions during chondrocyte maturation. J Bone Joint Surg Am 2001;83-A(1):S15–22.

52. Zheng Q, Zhou G, Morello R, Chen Y, Garcia-Rojas X, Lee B. Type X collagen gene regulation by Runx2 contributes directly to its hypertrophic chondrocyte-specific expression in vivo. J Cell Biol 2003;162:833–42.

53. Jimenez MJ, Balbin M, Lopez JM, Alvarez J, Komori T, Lopez-Otin C. Collagenase 3 is a target of Cbfa1, a transcription factor of the runt gene family involved in bone formation. Mol Cell Biol 1999; 19:4431–42.

54. Inada M, Yasui T, Nomura S, Miyake S, Deguchi K, Himeno M, et al. Maturational disturbance of chondrocytes in Cbfa1-deficient mice. Dev Dyn 1999;214:279–90.

55. Porte D, Tuckermann J, Becker M, Baumann B, Teurich S, Higgins T, et al. Both AP-1 and Cbfa1-like factors are required for the induction of interstitial collagenase by parathyroid hormone. Oncogene 1999;18:667–78.

56. Ortega N, Behonick DJ, Werb Z. Matrix remodeling during endochondral ossification. Trends Cell Biol 2004;14:86–93.

57. Colnot C, Lu C, Hu D, Helms JA. Distinguishing the contributions of the perichondrium, cartilage, and vascular endothelium to skeletal development. Dev Biol 2004;269:55–69.

58. Gerber HP, Vu TH, Ryan AM, Kowalski J, Werb Z, Ferrara N. VEGF couples hypertrophic cartilage remodeling, ossification and angiogenesis during endochondral bone formation. Nat Med 1999;5:623–28.

59. Vu TH, Shipley JM, Bergers G, Berger JE, Helms JA, Hanahan D, et al. MMP-9/gelatinase B is a key regulator of growth plate angiogenesis and apoptosis of hypertrophic chondrocytes. Cell 1998;93: 411–22.

60. Zhou Z, Apte SS, Soininen R, Cao R, Baaklini GY, Rauser RW, et al. Impaired endochondral ossification and angiogenesis in mice deficient in membrane-type matrix metalloproteinase I. Proc Natl Acad Sci USA 2000;97:4052–57.

61. Maes C, Carmeliet P, Moermans K, Stockmans I, Smets N, Collen D, et al. Impaired angiogenesis and endochondral bone formation in mice lacking the vascular endothelial growth factor isoforms VEGF164 and VEGF188. Mech Dev 2002;111:61–73.

62. Maes C, Stockmans I, Moermans K, Van Looveren R, Smets N, Carmeliet P, et al. Soluble VEGF isoforms are essential for establishing epiphyseal vascularization and regulating chondrocyte development and survival. J Clin Invest 2004;113:188–99.

63. Zelzer E, Olsen BR. Multiple roles of vascular endothelial growth factor (VEGF) in skeletal development, growth, and repair. Curr Top Dev Biol 2005;65:169–87.

64. Komori T. Regulation of skeletal development by the Runx family of transcription factors. J Cell Biochem 2005;95:445–53.

65. Balint E, Lapointe D, Drissi H, van der Meijden C, Young DW, van Wijnen AJ, et al. Phenotype discovery by gene expression profiling: Mapping of biological processes linked to BMP-2-mediated osteoblast differentiation. J Cell Biochem 2003;89:401–26.

66. Hassan MQ, Javed A, Morasso MI, Karlin J, Montecino M, van Wijnen AJ, et al. Dlx3 transcriptional regulation of osteoblast differentiation: Temporal recruitment of Msx2, Dlx3, and Dlx5 homeodomain proteins to chromatin of the osteocalcin gene. Mol Cell Biol 2004;24:9248–61.

67. Ijiri K, Zerbini LF, Peng H, Correa RG, Lu B, Walsh N, et al. A novel role for GADD45beta as a mediator of MMP-13 gene expression during chondrocyte terminal differentiation. J Biol Chem 2005 [E-pub ahead of print].

68. Lengner CJ, Drissi H, Choi JY, van Wijnen AJ, Stein JL, Stein GS, et al. Activation of the bone-related Runx2/Cbfa1 promoter in mesenchymal condensations and developing chondrocytes of the axial skeleton. Mech Dev 2002;114:167–70.

69. Bialek P, Kern B, Yang X, Schrock M, Sosic D, Hong N, et al. A twist code determines the onset of osteoblast differentiation. Dev Cell 2004;6:423–35.

70. Wang W, Wang YG, Reginato AM, Glotzer DJ, Fukai N, Plotkina S, et al. Groucho homologue Grg5 interacts with the transcription factor Runx2-Cbfa1 and modulates its activity during postnatal growth in mice. Dev Biol 2004;270:364–81.

71. Xiao G, Jiang D, Ge C, Zhao Z, Lai Y, Boules H, et al. Cooperative interactions between ATF4 and Runx2/Cbfa1 stimulate osteoblast-specific osteocalcin gene expression. J Biol Chem 2005.

72. Vega RB, Matsuda K, Oh J, Barbosa AC, Yang X, Meadows E, et al. Histone deacetylase 4 controls chondrocyte hypertrophy during skeletogenesis. Cell 2004;119:555–66.

73. Schipani E, Ryan HE, Didrickson S, Kobayashi T, Knight M, Johnson RS. Hypoxia in cartilage: HIF-1alpha is essential for chondrocyte growth arrest and survival. Genes Dev 2001; 15:2865–76.

74. Huang W, Lu N, Eberspaecher H, De Crombrugghe B. A new long form of c-Maf cooperates with Sox9 to activate the type II collagen gene. J Biol Chem 2002;277:50668–75.

75. Davies SR, Sakano S, Zhu Y, Sandell LJ. Distribution of the transcription factors Sox9, AP-2, and [delta] EF1 in adult murine articular and meniscal cartilage and growth plate. J Histochem Cytochem 2002;50:1059–65.

76. Huang Z, Xu H, Sandell L. Negative regulation of chondrocyte differentiation by transcription factor AP-2alpha. J Bone Miner Res 2004;19:245–55.

77. Imamura T, Imamura C, Iwamoto Y, Sandell LJ. Transcriptional co-activators CREB-binding protein/p300 increase chondrocyte Cd-rap gene expression by multiple mechanisms including sequestration of the repressor CCAAT/enhancer-binding protein. J Biol Chem 2005;280:16625–34.

78. Day TF, Guo X, Garrett-Beal L, Yang Y. Wnt/beta-catenin signaling in mesenchymal progenitors controls osteoblast and chondrocyte differentiation during vertebrate skeletogenesis. Dev Cell 2005;8:739–50.

79. Gaur T, Lengner CJ, Hovhannisyan H, Bhat RA, Bodine PV, Komm BS, et al. Canonical WNT signaling promotes osteogenesis by directly stimulating RUNX2 gene expression. J Biol Chem 2005.

80. Glass DA II, Bialek P, Ahn JD, Starbuck M, Patel MS, Clevers H, et al. Canonical Wnt signaling in differentiated osteoblasts controls osteoclast differentiation. Dev Cell 2005;8:751–64.

81. Hill TP, Spater D, Taketo MM, Birchmeier W, Hartmann C. Canonical Wnt/beta-catenin signaling prevents osteoblasts from differentiating into chondrocytes. Dev Cell 2005;8:727–38.

82. Hu H, Hilton MJ, Tu X, Yu K, Ornitz DM, Long F. Sequential roles of Hedgehog and Wnt signaling in osteoblast development. Development 2005;132:49–60.

83. Tamamura Y, Otani T, Kanatani N, Koyama E, Kitagaki J, Komori T, et al. Developmental regulation of Wnt/beta-catenin signals is required for growth plate assembly, cartilage integrity, and endochondral ossification. J Biol Chem 2005;280:19185–95.

84. Jochum W, Passegue E, Wagner EF. AP-1 in mouse development and tumorigenesis. Oncogene 2001;20:2401–12.

85. Karreth F, Hoebertz A, Scheuch H, Eferl R, Wagner EF. The AP1 transcription factor Fra2 is required for efficient cartilage development. Development 2004;131:5717–25.

86. Reimold AM, Grusby MJ, Kosaras B, Fries JW, Mori R, Maniwa S, et al. Chondrodysplasia and neurological abnormalities in ATF-2-deficient mice. Nature 1996;379:262–65.

87. MacLean HE, Kim JI, Glimcher MJ, Wang J, Kronenberg HM, Glimcher LH. Absence of transcription factor c-maf causes abnormal terminal differentiation of hypertrophic chondrocytes during endochondral bone development. Dev Biol 2003;262: 51–63.

88. Grigoriadis AE, Schellander K, Wang ZQ, Wagner EF. Osteoblasts are target cells for transformation in c-fos transgenic mice. J Cell Biol 1993;122:685–701.

89. Jochum W, David JP, Elliott C, Wutz A, Plenk H Jr., Matsuo K, et al. Increased bone formation and osteosclerosis in mice overexpressing the transcription factor Fra-1. Nat Med 2000;6:980–84.

90. Hess J, Hartenstein B, Teurich S, Schmidt D, Schorpp-Kistner M, Angel P. Defective endochondral ossification in mice with strongly compromised expression of JunB. J Cell Sci 2003;116:4587–96.

91. Serra R, Johnson M, Filvaroff EH, LaBorde J, Sheehan DM, Derynck R, Moses HL. Expression of a truncated, kinase-defective TGF-beta type II receptor in mouse skeletal tissue promotes terminal chondrocyte differentiation and osteoarthritis. J Cell Biol 1997;139:541–52.

92. Yang X, Chen L, Xu X, Li C, Huang C, Deng CX. TGF-beta/Smad3 signals repress chondrocyte hypertrophic differentiation and are required for maintaining articular cartilage. J Cell Biol 2001; 153:35–46.

93. Inada M, Wang Y, Byrne MH, Rahman MU, Miyaura C, Lopez-Otin C, et al. Critical roles for collagenase-3 (Mmp13) in development of growth plate cartilage and in endochondral ossification. Proc Natl Acad Sci USA 2004;101:17192–97.

94. Stickens D, Behonick DJ, Ortega N, Heyer B, Hartenstein B, Yu Y, et al. Altered endochondral bone development in

matrix metalloproteinase 13-deficient mice. Development 2004;131:5883–95.

95. Little CB, Meeker CT, Hembry RM, Sims NA, Lawlor KE, Golub SB, et al. Matrix metalloproteinases are not essential for aggrecan turnover during normal skeletal growth and development. Mol Cell Biol 2005;25:3388–99.

96. Jacenko O, Chan D, Franklin A, Ito S, Underhill CB, Bateman JF, Campbell MR. A dominant interference collagen X mutation disrupts hypertrophic chondrocyte pericellular matrix and glycosaminoglycan and proteoglycan distribution in transgenic mice. Am J Pathol 2001;159:2257–69.

97. Gress CJ, Jacenko O. Growth plate compressions and altered hematopoiesis in collagen X null mice. J Cell Biol 2000;149:983–93.

98. Li Y, Lacerda DA, Warman ML, Beier DR, Yoshioka H, Ninomiya Y, et al. A fibrillar collagen gene, Col11a1, is essential for skeletal morphogenesis. Cell 1995;80:423–30.

99. Li SW, Prockop DJ, Helminen H, Fassler R, Lapvetelainen T, Kiraly K, et al. Transgenic mice with targeted inactivation of the Col2 alpha 1 gene for collagen II develop a skeleton with membranous and periosteal bone but no endochondral bone. Genes Dev 1995;9:2821–30.

100. So CL, Kaluarachchi K, Tam PP, Cheah KS. Impact of mutations of cartilage matrix genes on matrix structure, gene activity and chondrogenesis. Osteoarthritis Cartilage 2001;9(A):S160–73.

101. Li Y, Olsen BR. Murine models of human genetic skeletal disorders. Matrix Biol 1997;16:49–52.

102. Reginato AM, Olsen BR. The role of structural genes in the pathogenesis of osteoarthritic disorders. Arthritis Res 2002;4:337–45.

103. Xu L, Flahiff CM, Waldman BA, Wu D, Olsen BR, Setton LA, et al. Osteoarthritis-like changes and decreased mechanical function of articular cartilage in the joints of mice with the chondrodysplasia gene (cho). Arthritis Rheum 2003;48:2509–18.

104. Xu L, Peng H, Wu D, Hu K, Goldring MB, Olsen BR, Li Y. Activation of the discoidin domain receptor 2 induces expression of matrix metalloproteinase 13 associated with osteoarthritis in mice. J Biol Chem 2005;280:548–55.

105. Hyttinen MM, Toyras J, Lapvetelainen T, Lindblom J, Prockop DJ, Li SW, et al. Inactivation of one allele of the type II collagen gene alters the collagen network in murine articular cartilage and makes cartilage softer. Ann Rheum Dis 2001;60:262–68.

106. Lapvetelainen T, Hyttinen M, Lindblom J, Langsjo TK, Sironen R, Li SW, et al. More knee joint osteoarthritis (OA) in mice after inactivation of one allele of type II procollagen gene but less OA after lifelong voluntary wheel running exercise. Osteoarthritis Cartilage 2001;9:152–60.

107. Fassler R, Schnegelsberg PN, Dausman J, Shinya T, Muragaki Y, McCarthy MT, et al. Mice lacking alpha 1 (IX) collagen develop noninflammatory degenerative joint disease. Proc Natl Acad Sci USA 1994;91:5070–74.

108. Kimura T, Nakata K, Tsumaki N, Miyamoto S, Matsui Y, Ebara S, et al. Progressive degeneration of articular cartilage and intervertebral discs. An experimental study in transgenic mice bearing a type IX collagen mutation. Int Orthop 1996;20:177–81.

109. Pace JM, Li Y, Seegmiller RE, Teuscher C, Taylor BA, Olsen BR. Disproportionate micromelia (Dmm) in mice caused by a mutation in the C-propeptide coding region of Col2a1. Dev Dyn 1997;208:25–33.

110. Watanabe H, Kimata K, Line S, Strong D, Gao LY, Kozak CA, et al. Mouse cartilage matrix deficiency (cmd) caused by a 7 bp deletion in the aggrecan gene. Nat Genet 1994;7:154–57.

111. van der Weyden L, Wei L, Luo J, Yang X, Birk DE, Adams DJ, et al. Matrilin-3 is required for modulating chondrocyte differentiation, maintaining bone mineral density, and preventing osteoarthritis. Am J Pathol 2005 (in press).

112. Zemmyo M, Meharra EJ, Kuhn K, Creighton-Achermann L, Lotz M. Accelerated, aging-dependent development of osteoarthritis in alpha1 integrin-deficient mice. Arthritis Rheum 2003;48:2873–80.

113. Young MF, Bi Y, Ameye L, Chen XD. Biglycan knockout mice: New models for musculoskeletal diseases. Glycoconj J 2002;19:257–62.

114. Ameye L, Young MF. Mice deficient in small leucine-rich proteoglycans: Novel in vivo models for osteoporosis, osteoarthritis, Ehlers-Danlos syndrome, muscular dystrophy, and corneal diseases. Glycobiology 2002;12:107R–16R.

115. Ho AM, Johnson MD, Kingsley DM. Role of the mouse ank gene in control of tissue calcification and arthritis. Science 2000;289:265–70.

116. Johnson K, Terkeltaub R. Upregulated ank expression in osteoarthritis can promote both chondrocyte MMP-13 expression and calcification via chondrocyte extracellular PPi excess. Osteoarthritis Cartilage 2004;12:321–35.

117. Rountree RB, Schoor M, Chen H, Marks ME, Harley V, Mishina Y, et al. BMP receptor signaling is required for postnatal maintenance of articular cartilage. PLoS Biol 2004;2:e355.

118. Glasson SS, Askew R, Sheppard B, Carito B, Blanchet T, Ma HL, et al. Deletion of active ADAMTS5 prevents cartilage degradation in a murine model of osteoarthritis. Nature 2005;434:644–48.

119. Stanton H, Rogerson FM, East CJ, Golub SB, Lawlor KE, Meeker CT, et al. ADAMTS5 is the major aggrecanase in mouse cartilage in vivo and in vitro. Nature 2005;434:648–52.

120. Neuhold LA, Killar L, Zhao W, Sung ML, Warner L, Kulik J, et al. Postnatal expression in hyaline cartilage of constitutively active human collagenase-3 (MMP-13) induces osteoarthritis in mice. J Clin Invest 2001;107:35–44.

121. Helminen HJ, Saamanen AM, Salminen H, Hyttinen MM. Transgenic mouse models for studying the role of cartilage macromolecules in osteoarthritis. Rheumatology (Oxford) 2002;41:848–56.

122. Maroudas A, Palla G, Gilav E. Racemization of aspartic acid in human articular cartilage. Connect Tissue Res 1992;28:161–69.

123. Verzijl N, DeGroot J, Thorpe SR, Bank RA, Shaw JN, Lyons TJ, et al. Effect of collagen turnover on the accumulation of advanced glycation end products. J Biol Chem 2000;275:39027–31.

124. Maroudas A, Bayliss MT, Uchitel-Kaushansky N, Schneiderman R, Gilav E. Aggrecan turnover in human articular cartilage: Use of aspartic acid racemization as a marker of molecular age. Arch Biochem Biophys 1998;350:61–71.

125. Hollander AP, Pidoux I, Reiner A, Rorabeck C, Bourne R, Poole AR. Damage to type II collagen in aging and osteoarthritis starts at the articular surface, originates around chondrocytes, and extends into the cartilage with progressive degeneration. J Clin Invest 1995;96:2859–69.

126. Chambers MG, Cox L, Chong L, Suri N, Cover P, Bayliss MT, Mason RM. Matrix metalloproteinases and aggrecanases cleave aggrecan in different zones of normal cartilage but colocalize in the development of osteoarthritic lesions in STR/ort mice. Arthritis Rheum 2001;44:1455–65.

127. Wu W, Billinghurst RC, Pidoux I, Antoniou J, Zukor D, Tanzer M, Poole AR. Sites of collagenase cleavage and denaturation of type II collagen in aging and osteoarthritic articular cartilage and their relationship to the distribution of matrix metalloproteinase 1 and matrix metalloproteinase 13. Arthritis Rheum 2002;46:2087–94.

128. Wilkins RJ, Browning JA, Ellory JC. Surviving in a matrix: Membrane transport in articular chondrocytes. J Membr Biol 2000;177:95–108.

129. Stockwell RA. Metabolism of cartilage. In BK Hall (ed.), Cartilage: Structure, Function and Biochemistry, Volume 1. New York: Academic Press 1983:253–80.

130. Kim JJ, Conrad HE. Kinetics of mucopolysaccharide and glycoprotein synthesis by chick embryo chondrocytes: Effect of D-glucose concentration in the culture medium. J Biol Chem 1976;251:6210–17.

131. Mason RM, Sweeney C. The relationship between proteoglycan synthesis in Swarm chondrocytes and pathways of cellular energy and UDP-sugar metabolism. Carbohydr Res 1994;255:255–70.

132. Mobasheri A, Neama G, Bell S, Richardson S, Carter SD. Human articular chondrocytes express three facilitative glucose transporter isoforms: GLUT1, GLUT3 and GLUT9. Cell Biol Int 2002;26:297–300.

133. Shikhman AR, Brinson DC, Valbracht J, Lotz MK. Cytokine regulation of facilitated glucose transport in human articular chondrocytes. J Immunol 2001;167:7001–08.

134. Lee RB, Wilkins RJ, Razaq S, Urban JP. The effect of mechanical stress on cartilage energy metabolism. Biorheology 2002;39:133–43.

135. Mobasheri A, Richardson S, Mobasheri R, Shakibaei M, Hoyland JA. Hypoxia inducible factor-1 and facilitative glucose transporters GLUT1 and GLUT3: Putative molecular components of the

oxygen and glucose sensing apparatus in articular chondrocytes. Histol Histopathol 2005;20:1327–38.

136. Pufe T, Lemke A, Kurz B, Petersen W, Tillmann B, Grodzinsky AJ, et al. Mechanical overload induces VEGF in cartilage discs via hypoxia-inducible factor. Am J Pathol 2004;164:185–92.

137. Lin C, McGough R, Aswad B, Block JA, Terek R. Hypoxia induces HIF-1alpha and VEGF expression in chondrosarcoma cells and chondrocytes. J Orthop Res 2004;22:1175–81.

138. Grimshaw MJ, Mason RM. Modulation of bovine articular chondrocyte gene expression in vitro by oxygen tension. Osteoarthritis Cartilage 2001;9:357–64.

139. Robins JC, Akeno N, Mukherjee A, Dalal RR, Aronow BJ, Koopman P, Clemens TL. Hypoxia induces chondrocyte-specific gene expression in mesenchymal cells in association with transcriptional activation of Sox9. Bone 2005;37:313–22.

140. Pfander D, Cramer T, Schipani E, Johnson RS. HIF-1alpha controls extracellular matrix synthesis by epiphyseal chondrocytes. J Cell Sci 2003;116:1819–26.

141. Coimbra IB, Jimenez SA, Hawkins DF, Piera-Velazquez S, Stokes DG. Hypoxia inducible factor-1 alpha expression in human normal and osteoarthritic chondrocytes. Osteoarthritis Cartilage 2004;12:336–45.

142. Brucker PU, Izzo NJ, Chu CR. Tonic activation of hypoxia-inducible factor 1alpha in avascular articular cartilage and implications for metabolic homeostasis. Arthritis Rheum 2005;52:3181–91.

143. Hofstaetter JG, Wunderlich L, Samuel RE, Saad FA, Choi YH, Glimcher MJ. Systemic hypoxia alters gene expression levels of structural proteins and growth factors in knee joint cartilage. Biochem Biophys Res Commun 2005;330:386–94.

144. Martin G, Andriamanalijaona R, Grassel S, Dreier R, Mathy-Hartert M, Bogdanowicz P, et al. Effect of hypoxia and reoxygenation on gene expression and response to interleukin-1 in cultured articular chondrocytes. Arthritis Rheum 2004;50:3549–60.

145. Yudoh K, Nakamura H, Masuko-Hongo K, Kato T, Nishioka K. Catabolic stress induces expression of hypoxia-inducible factor (HIF)-1alpha in articular chondrocytes: Involvement of HIF-1alpha in the pathogenesis of osteoarthritis. Arthritis Res Ther 2005;7:R904–14.

146. Aigner T, Gluckert K, von der Mark K. Activation of fibrillar collagen synthesis and phenotypic modulation of chondrocytes in early human osteoarthritic cartilage lesions. Osteoarthritis Cartilage 1997;5:183–89.

147. Soder S, Hambach L, Lissner R, Kirchner T, Aigner T. Ultrastructural localization of type VI collagen in normal adult and osteoarthritic human articular cartilage. Osteoarthritis Cartilage 2002;10:464–70.

148. Aigner T, Zhu Y, Chansky HH, Matsen FA, 3rd, Maloney WJ, Sandell LJ. Reexpression of type IIA procollagen by adult articular chondrocytes in osteoarthritic cartilage. Arthritis Rheum 1999;42:1443–50.

149. Sandell LJ, Aigner T. Articular cartilage and changes in arthritis. An introduction: Cell biology of osteoarthritis. Arthritis Res 2001;3:107–13.

150. Aigner T, Dudhia J. Phenotypic modulation of chondrocytes as a potential therapeutic target in osteoarthritis: A hypothesis. Ann Rheum Dis 1997;56:287–91.

151. Young AA, Smith MM, Smith SM, Cake MA, Ghosh P, Read RA, et al. Regional assessment of articular cartilage gene expression and small proteoglycan metabolism in an animal model of osteoarthritis. Arthritis Res Ther 2005;7:R852–61.

152. Bau B, Gebhard PM, Haag J, Knorr T, Bartnik E, Aigner T. Relative messenger RNA expression profiling of collagenases and aggrecanases in human articular chondrocytes in vivo and in vitro. Arthritis Rheum 2002;46:2648–57.

153. Hermansson M, Sawaji Y, Bolton M, Alexander S, Wallace A, Begum S, et al. Proteomic analysis of articular cartilage shows increased type II collagen synthesis in osteoarthritis and expression of inhibin betaA (activin A), a regulatory molecule for chondrocytes. J Biol Chem 2004;279:43514–21.

154. Fukui N, Zhu Y, Maloney WJ, Clohisy J, Sandell LJ. Stimulation of BMP-2 expression by pro-inflammatory cytokines IL-1 and TNF-α in normal and osteoarthritic chondrocytes. J Bone Joint Surg Am 2003;85-A(3):59–66.

155. Bakker AC, van de Loo FA, van Beuningen HM, Sime P, van Lent PL, van der Kraan PM, et al. Overexpression of active TGF-beta-1 in

the murine knee joint: Evidence for synovial-layer-dependent chondro-osteophyte formation. Osteoarthritis Cartilage 2001; 9:128–36.

156. van Beuningen HM, Glansbeek HL, van der Kraan PM, van den Berg WB. Osteoarthritis-like changes in the murine knee joint resulting from intra-articular transforming growth factor-β injections. Osteoarthritis Cart. 2000;8:25–33.

157. Aigner T, Gebhard PM, Schmid E, Bau B, Harley V, Poschl E. SOX9 expression does not correlate with type II collagen expression in adult articular chondrocytes. Matrix Biol 2003;22:363–72.

158. Aigner T, Bartnik E, Sohler F, Zimmer R. Functional genomics of osteoarthritis: On the way to evaluate disease hypotheses. Clin Orthop Relat Res 2004:S138–43.

159. Loughlin J, Dowling B, Chapman K, Marcelline L, Mustafa Z, Southam L, et al. Functional variants within the secreted frizzled-related protein 3 gene are associated with hip osteoarthritis in females. Proc Natl Acad Sci USA 2004;101:9757–62.

160. Lane NE, Lian K, Nevitt MC, Zmuda JM, Lui L, Li J, et al. Frizzled related protein variants are risk factors for hip osteoarthritis. Arthritis Rheum 2006 (in press).

161. Jones SE, Jomary C. Secreted Frizzled-related proteins: Searching for relationships and patterns. Bioessays 2002;24:811–20.

162. Gong Y, Slee RB, Fukai N, Rawadi G, Roman-Roman S, Reginato AM, et al. LDL receptor-related protein 5 (LRP5) affects bone accrual and eye development. Cell 2001;107:513–23.

163. Bodine PV, Zhao W, Kharode YP, Bex FJ, Lambert AJ, Goad MB, et al. The Wnt antagonist secreted frizzled-related protein-1 is a negative regulator of trabecular bone formation in adult mice. Mol Endocrinol 2004;18:1222–37.

164. Mizuguchi T, Furuta I, Watanabe Y, Tsukamoto K, Tomita H, Tsujihata M, et al. LRP5, low-density-lipoprotein-receptor-related protein 5, is a determinant for bone mineral density. J Hum Genet 2004;49:80–6.

165. Hausler KD, Horwood NJ, Chuman Y, Fisher JL, Ellis J, Martin TJ, et al. Secreted frizzled-related protein-1 inhibits RANKL-dependent osteoclast formation. J Bone Miner Res 2004;19: 1873–81.

166. Chung YS, Baylink DJ, Srivastava AK, Amaar Y, Tapia B, Kasukawa Y, et al. Effects of secreted frizzled-related protein 3 on osteoblasts in vitro. J Bone Miner Res 2004;19:1395–1402.

167. James IE, Kumar S, Barnes MR, Gress CJ, Hand AT, Dodds RA, et al. FrzB-2: A human secreted frizzled-related protein with a potential role in chondrocyte apoptosis. Osteoarthritis Cartilage 2000;8:452–63.

168. Trippel SB. Growth factor inhibition: Potential role in the etiopathogenesis of osteoarthritis. Clin Orthop Relat Res 2004:S47–52.

169. van der Kraan PM, Buma P, van Kuppevelt T, van den Berg WB. Interaction of chondrocytes, extracellular matrix and growth factors: Relevance for articular cartilage tissue engineering. Osteoarthritis Cartilage 2002;10:631–37.

170. Chubinskaya S, Kuettner KE. Regulation of osteogenic proteins by chondrocytes. Int J Biochem Cell Biol 2003;35:1323–40.

171. Bobacz K, Gruber R, Soleiman A, Graninger WB, Luyten FP, Erlacher L. Cartilage-derived morphogenetic protein-1 and -2 are endogenously expressed in healthy and osteoarthritic human articular chondrocytes and stimulate matrix synthesis. Osteoarthritis Cartilage 2002;10:394–401.

172. Recklies AD, Ling H, White C, Bernier SM. Inflammatory cytokines induce production of chitinase-3-like protein 1 by articular chondrocytes. J Biol Chem 2005.

173. Loeser RF Jr. Aging cartilage and osteoarthritis: What's the link? Sci Aging Knowledge Environ 2004;2004:pe31.

174. Bobacz K, Gruber R, Soleiman A, Erlacher L, Smolen JS, Graninger WB. Expression of bone morphogenetic protein 6 in healthy and osteoarthritic human articular chondrocytes and stimulation of matrix synthesis in vitro. Arthritis Rheum 2003;48:2501–08.

175. Chubinskaya S, Kumar B, Merrihew C, Heretis K, Rueger DC, Kuettner KE. Age-related changes in cartilage endogenous osteogenic protein-1 (OP-1). Biochim Biophys Acta 2002;1588: 126–34.

176. Loeser RF, Chubinskaya S, Pacione C, Im HJ. Basic fibroblast growth factor inhibits the anabolic activity of insulin-like growth factor 1 and osteogenic protein 1 in adult human articular chondrocytes. Arthritis Rheum 2005;52:3910–17.

177. Takahashi N, Rieneck K, van der Kraan PM, van Beuningen HM, Vitters EL, Bendtzen K, et al. Elucidation of IL-1/TGF-beta interactions in mouse chondrocyte cell line by genome-wide gene expression. Osteoarthritis Cartilage 2005;13:426–38.

178. Blaney Davidson EN, Scharstuhl A, Vitters EL, van der Kraan PM, van den Berg WB. Reduced transforming growth factor-beta signaling in cartilage of old mice: Role in impaired repair capacity. Arthritis Res Ther 2005;7:R1338–47.

179. Middleton JF, Tyler JA. Upregulation of insulin-like growth factor I gene expression in the lesions of osteoarthritic human articular cartilage. Ann Rheum Dis 1992;51:440–47.

180. Dore S, Pelletier JP, DiBattista JA, Tardif G, Brazeau P, Martel-Pelletier J. Human osteoarthritic chondrocytes possess an increased number of insulin-like growth factor 1 binding sites but are unresponsive to its stimulation: Possible role of IGF-1-binding proteins. Arthritis Rheum 1994;37:253–63.

181. Chevalier X, Tyler JA. Production of binding proteins and role of the insulin-like growth factor I binding protein 3 in human articular cartilage explants. Br J Rheumatol 1996; 35:515–22.

182. Tardif G, Reboul P, Pelletier JP, Geng C, Cloutier JM, Martel-Pelletier J. Normal expression of type 1 insulin-like growth factor receptor by human osteoarthritic chondrocytes with increased expression and synthesis of insulin-like growth factor binding proteins. Arthritis Rheum 1996;39:968–78.

183. Fernihough JK, Billingham ME, Cwyfan-Hughes S, Holly JM. Local disruption of the insulin-like growth factor system in the arthritic joint. Arthritis Rheum 1996;39:1556–65.

184. Whellams EJ, Maile LA, Fernihough JK, Billingham ME, Holly JM. Alterations in insulin-like growth factor binding protein-3 proteolysis and complex formation in the arthritic joint. J Endocrinol 2000;165:545–56.

185. Morales TI. The insulin-like growth factor binding proteins in uncultured human cartilage: Increases in insulin-like growth factor binding protein 3 during osteoarthritis. Arthritis Rheum 2002;46:2358–67.

186. Loeser RF, Shanker G, Carlson CS, Gardin JF, Shelton BJ, Sonntag WE. Reduction in the chondrocyte response to insulin-like growth factor 1 in aging and osteoarthritis: Studies in a non-human primate model of naturally occurring disease. Arthritis Rheum 2000;43:2110–20.

187. Tyler JA. Insulin-like growth factor 1 can decrease degradation and promote synthesis of proteoglycan in cartilage exposed to cytokines. Biochem J 1989;260:543–48.

188. Olney RC, Wilson DM, Mohtai M, Fielder PJ, Smith RL. Interleukin-1 and tumor necrosis factor-alpha increase insulin-like growth factor-binding protein-3 (IGFBP-3) production and IGFBP-3 protease activity in human articular chondrocytes. J Endocrinol 1995;146:279–86.

189. Clancy R. Nitric oxide alters chondrocyte function by disrupting cytoskeletal signaling complexes. Osteoarthritis Cartilage 1999;7:399–400.

190. van den Berg WB, van de Loo F, Joosten LA, Arntz OJ. Animal models of arthritis in NOS2-deficient mice. Osteoarthritis Cartilage 1999;7:413–15.

191. Studer RK, Decker K, Melhem S, Georgescu H. Nitric oxide inhibition of IGF-1 stimulated proteoglycan synthesis: Role of cGMP. J Orthop Res 2003;21:914–21.

192. Johnson K, Jung A, Murphy A, Andreyev A, Dykens J, Terkeltaub R. Mitochondrial oxidative phosphorylation is a downstream regulator of nitric oxide effects on chondrocyte matrix synthesis and mineralization. Arthritis Rheum 2000; 43:1560–70.

193. Loeser RF, Carlson CS, Del Carlo M, Cole A. Detection of nitrotyrosine in aging and osteoarthritic cartilage: Correlation of oxidative damage with the presence of interleukin-1beta and with chondrocyte resistance to insulin-like growth factor 1. Arthritis Rheum 2002;46:2349–57.

194. Smeets RL, Veenbergen S, Arntz OJ, Bennink LAB, Joosten LA, van den Berg WB, et al. A novel role for SOCS3 in cartilage destruction via induction of chondrocyte desensitization towards IGF-1. Arthritis Rheum 2006 (in press).

195. Goldring MB. Osteoarthritis and cartilage: The role of cytokines. Curr Rheumatol Rep 2000;2:459–65.

196. Goldring MB. The role of the chondrocyte in osteoarthritis. Arthritis Rheum 2000;43:1916–26.

197. Goldring MB, Berenbaum F. The regulation of chondrocyte function by proinflammatory mediators: Prostaglandins and nitric oxide. Clin Orthop 2004:S37–46.

198. Goldring SR, Goldring MB, Buckwalter J. The role of cytokines in cartilage matrix degeneration in osteoarthritis. Clin Orthop 2004:S27–36.

199. Goldring MB. The role of cytokines as inflammatory mediators in osteoarthritis: Lessons from animal models. Connect Tissue Res 1999;40:1–11.

200. van den Berg WB. Lessons from animal models of osteoarthritis. Curr Opin Rheumatol 2001;13:452–56.

201. Middleton J, Manthey A, Tyler J. Insulin-like growth factor (IGF) receptor, IGF-I, interleukin-1b (IL-1b), and IL-6 mRNA expression in osteoarthritic and normal human cartilage. J Histochem Cytochem 1996;44:133–41.

202. Moos V, Fickert S, Muller B, Weber U, Sieper J. Immunohistological analysis of cytokine expression in human osteoarthritic and healthy cartilage. J Rheumatol 1999;26:870–79.

203. Attur MG, Dave M, Cipolletta C, Kang P, Goldring MB, Patel IR, et al. Reversal of autocrine and paracrine effects of interleukin 1 (IL-1) in human arthritis by type II IL-1 decoy receptor: Potential for pharmacological intervention. J Biol Chem 2000;275:40307–15.

204. Mitchell PG, Magna HA, Reeves LM, Lopresti-Morrow LL, Yocum SA, Rosner PJ, et al. Cloning, expression, and type II collagenolytic activity of matrix metalloproteinase-13 from human osteoarthritic cartilage. J Clin Invest 1996;97:761–68.

205. Reboul P, Pelletier JP, Tardif G, Cloutier JM, Martel-Pelletier J. The new collagenase, collagenase-3, is expressed and synthesized by human chondrocytes but not by synoviocytes: A role in osteoarthritis. J Clin Invest 1996;97:2011–19.

206. Stahle-Backdahl M, Sandstedt B, Bruce K, Lindahl A, Jimenez MG, Vega JA, et al. Collagenase-3 (MMP-13) is expressed during human fetal ossification and re-expressed in postnatal bone remodeling and in rheumatoid arthritis. Lab Invest 1997;76:717–28.

207. Knauper V, Lopez-Otin C, Smith B, Knight G, Murphy G. Biochemical characterization of human collagenase-3. J Biol Chem 1996;271:1544–50.

208. Tetlow LC, Adlam DJ, Woolley DE. Matrix metalloproteinase and proinflammatory cytokine production by chondrocytes of human osteoarthritic cartilage. Arthritis Rheum 2001;44:585–94.

209. Towle CA, Hung HH, Bonassar LJ, Treadwell BV, Mangham DC. Detection of interleukin-1 in the cartilage of patients with osteoarthritis: A possible autocrine/paracrine role in pathogenesis. Osteoarthritis Cartilage 1997;5:293–300.

210. Saha N, Moldovan F, Tardif G, Pelletier JP, Cloutier JM, Martel-Pelletier J. Interleukin-1b-converting enzyme/caspase-1 in human osteoarthritic tissues: Localization and role in the maturation of interleukin-1b and interleukin-18. Arthritis Rheum 1999;42:1577–87.

211. Martel-Pelletier J, McCollum R, DiBattista J, Faure MP, Chin JA, Fournier S, et al. The interleukin-1 receptor in normal and osteoarthritic human articular chondrocytes: Identification as the type I receptor and analysis of binding kinetics and biologic function. Arthritis Rheum 1992;35:530–40.

212. Lubberts E, Koenders MI, van den Berg WB. The role of T cell interleukin-17 in conducting destructive arthritis: Lessons from animal models. Arthritis Res Ther 2005;7:29–37.

213. Catterall JB, Carrere S, Koshy PJ, Degnan BA, Shingleton WD, Brinckerhoff CE, et al. Synergistic induction of matrix metalloproteinase 1 by interleukin-1a and oncostatin M in human chondrocytes involves signal transducer and activator of transcription and activator protein 1 transcription factors via a novel mechanism. Arthritis Rheum 2001;44:2296–2310.

214. Cawston TE, Milner JM, Catterall JB, Rowan AD. Cytokine synergy, collagenases and cartilage collagen breakdown. Biochem Soc Symp 2003:125–33.

215. Millward-Sadler SJ, Wright MO, Davies LW, Nuki G, Salter DM. Mechanotransduction via integrins and interleukin-4 results in altered aggrecan and matrix metalloproteinase 3 gene expression in normal, but not osteoarthritic, human articular chondrocytes. Arthritis Rheum 2000;43:2091–99.

216. Patwari P, Cook MN, DiMicco MA, Blake SM, James IE, Kumar S, et al. Proteoglycan degradation after injurious compression of bovine and human articular cartilage in vitro: Interaction with exogenous cytokines. Arthritis Rheum 2003;48:1292–1301.

217. Gray ML, Pizzanelli AM, Grodzinsky AJ, Lee RC. Mechanical and physiochemical determinants of the chondrocyte biosynthetic response. J Orthop Res 1988;6:777–92.

218. Blain EJ, Gilbert SJ, Wardale RJ, Capper SJ, Mason DJ, Duance VC. Up-regulation of matrix metalloproteinase expression and activation following cyclical compressive loading of articular cartilage in vitro. Arch Biochem Biophys 2001;396:49–55.

219. Li KW, Williamson AK, Wang AS, Sah RL. Growth responses of cartilage to static and dynamic compression. Clin Orthop 2001: S34–48.

220. Fitzgerald JB, Jin M, Dean D, Wood DJ, Zheng MH, Grodzinsky AJ. Mechanical compression of cartilage explants induces multiple time-dependent gene expression patterns and involves intracellular calcium and cyclic AMP. J Biol Chem 2004;279:19502–11.

221. Homandberg GA, Hui F. Association of proteoglycan degradation with catabolic cytokine and stromelysin release from cartilage cultured with fibronectin fragments. Arch Biochem Biophys 1996;334:325–31.

222. Forsyth CB, Pulai J, Loeser RF. Fibronectin fragments and blocking antibodies to $\alpha2\beta1$ and $\alpha5\beta1$ integrins stimulate mitogen-activated protein kinase signaling and increase collagenase 3 (matrix metalloproteinase 13) production by human articular chondrocytes. Arthritis Rheum 2002;46:2368–76.

223. Yasuda T, Poole AR. A fibronectin fragment induces type II collagen degradation by collagenase through an interleukin-1-mediated pathway. Arthritis Rheum 2002;46:138–48.

224. Stanton H, Ung L, Fosang AJ. The 45 kDa collagen-binding fragment of fibronectin induces matrix metalloproteinase-13 synthesis by chondrocytes and aggrecan degradation by aggrecanases. Biochem J 2002;364:181–90.

225. Geng Y, Valbracht J, Lotz M. Selective activation of the mitogen-activated protein kinase subgroups c-Jun NH2 terminal kinase and p38 by IL-1 and TNF in human articular chondrocytes. J Clin Invest 1996;98:2425–30.

226. Ding GJ, Fischer PA, Boltz RC, Schmidt JA, Colaianne JJ, Gough A, et al. Characterization and quantitation of NF-kappaB nuclear translocation induced by interleukin-1 and tumor necrosis factor-alpha: Development and use of a high capacity fluorescence cytometric system. J Biol Chem 1998;273:28897–905.

227. Mengshol JA, Vincenti MP, Coon CI, Barchowsky A, Brinckerhoff CE. Interleukin-1 induction of collagenase 3 (matrix metalloproteinase 13) gene expression in chondrocytes requires p38, c-Jun N-terminal kinase, and nuclear factor kB. Arthritis Rheum 2000;43:801–11.

228. Liacini A, Sylvester J, Li WQ, Zafarullah M. Inhibition of interleukin-1-stimulated MAP kinases, activating protein-1 (AP-1) and nuclear factor kB (NF-kB) transcription factors down-regulates matrix metalloproteinase gene expression in articular chondrocytes. Matrix Biol 2002;21:251–62.

229. Thomas B, Thirion S, Humbert L, Tan L, Goldring MB, Bereziat G, Berenbaum F. Differentiation regulates interleukin-1b-induced cyclo-oxygenase-2 in human articular chondrocytes: Role of p38 mitogen-activated protein kinase. Biochem J 2002;362:367–73.

230. Fan Z, Bau B, Yang H, Aigner T. IL-1beta induction of IL-6 and LIF in normal articular human chondrocytes involves the ERK, p38 and NFkappaB signaling pathways. Cytokine 2004;28:17–24.

231. Saklatvala J. Tumour necrosis factor $\alpha$ stimulates resorption and inhibits synthesis of proteoglycan in cartilage. Nature 1986;322:547–49.

232. Goldring MB, Birkhead J, Sandell LJ, Kimura T, Krane SM. Interleukin 1 suppresses expression of cartilage-specific types II and IX collagens and increases types I and III collagens in human chondrocytes. J Clin Invest 1988;82:2026–37.

233. Goldring MB, Birkhead J, Sandell LJ, Krane SM. Synergistic regulation of collagen gene expression in human chondrocytes by tumor necrosis factor-$\alpha$ and interleukin-1$\beta$. Ann NY Acad Sci 1990;580:536–39.

234. Goldring MB, Fukuo K, Birkhead JR, Dudek E, Sandell LJ. Transcriptional suppression by interleukin-1 and interferon-$\gamma$ of type II collagen gene expression in human chondrocytes. J Cell Biochem 1994;54:85–99.

235. Reginato AM, Sanz-Rodriguez C, Diaz A, Dharmavaram RM, Jimenez SA. Transcriptional modulation of cartilage-specific collagen gene expression by interferon gamma and tumour necrosis factor alpha in cultured human chondrocytes. Biochem J 1993;294:761–69.

236. Tan L, Peng H, Osaki M, Choy BK, Auron PE, Sandell LJ, et al. Egr-1 mediates transcriptional repression of COL2A1 promoter activity by interleukin-1b. J Biol Chem 2003;278:17688–700.

237. Kaiser M, Haag J, Soder S, Bau B, Aigner T. Bone morphogenetic protein and transforming growth factor beta inhibitory Smads 6 and 7 are expressed in human adult normal and osteoarthritic cartilage in vivo and are differentially regulated in vitro by interleukin-1beta. Arthritis Rheum 2004;50:3535–40.

238. Goldring MB, Sohbat E, Elwell JM, Chang JY. Etodolac preserves cartilage-specific phenotype in human chondrocytes: Effects on type II collagen synthesis and associated mRNA levels. Eur J Rheumatol Inflamm 1990;10:10–21.

239. Goldring MB, Suen LF, Yamin R, Lai WF. Regulation of collagen gene expression by prostaglandins and interleukin-1$\beta$ in cultured chondrocytes and fibroblasts. Am J Ther 1996;3:9–16.

240. Hauselmann HJ, Oppliger L, Michel BA, Stefanovic-Racic M, Evans CH. Nitric oxide and proteoglycan biosynthesis by human articular chondrocytes in alginate culture. FEBS Lett 1994;352:361–64.

241. Cao M, Westerhausen-Larson A, Niyibizi C, Kavalkovich K, Georgescu HI, Rizzo CF, et al. Nitric oxide inhibits the synthesis of type-II collagen without altering Col2A1 mRNA abundance: Prolyl hydroxylase as a possible target. Biochem J 1997;324(1):305–10.

242. François M, Richette P, Tsagris L, Fitting C, Lemay C, Corvol MT. Peroxisome proliferator-activated receptor-$\alpha$-activation pathway potentiates interleukin-1 receptor antagonist production in cytokine-treated chondrocytes. Arthritis Rheum 2006 (in press).

243. Yammani RR, Carlson CS, Bresnick AR, Loeser RF. S100A4 activates receptor for advanced glycation end-products (RAGE) signaling and stimulates matrix metalloproteinase-13 production in human articular chondrocytes. Arthritis Rheum 2006 (in press).

244. Borzi RM, Mazzetti I, Cattini L, Uguccioni M, Baggiolini M, Facchini A. Human chondrocytes express functional chemokine receptors and release matrix-degrading enzymes in response to C-X-C and C-C chemokines. Arthritis Rheum 2000;43:1734–41.

245. Yuan GH, Masuko-Hongo K, Sakata M, Tsuruha J, Onuma H, Nakamura H, et al. The role of C-C chemokines and their receptors in osteoarthritis. Arthritis Rheum 2001;44:1056–70.

246. Alaaeddine N, Olee T, Hashimoto S, Creighton-Achermann L, Lotz M. Production of the chemokine RANTES by articular chondrocytes and role in cartilage degradation. Arthritis Rheum 2001;44:1633–43.

247. Kanbe K, Takagishi K, Chen Q. Stimulation of matrix metalloprotease 3 release from human chondrocytes by the interaction of stromal cell-derived factor 1 and CXC chemokine receptor 4. Arthritis Rheum 2002;46:130–37.

248. Hauselmann HJ, Hedbom E. In vitro models of cartilage metabolism. In MJ Seibel, SP Robins, JP Bilezekian (eds.), Dynamics of Bone and Cartilage Metabolism. New York: Academic Press 1999:325–38.

249. Martel-Pelletier J, Pelletier JP. New insights into the major pathophysiological processes responsible for the development of osteoarthritis. Semin Arthritis Rheum 2005;34:6–8.

250. Poole AR. Honor Bridgett Fell, Ph.D., D.Sc. F.R.S., D.B.E., 1900–1986: The scientist and her contributions. In Vitro Cell Dev Biol 1989;25:450–53.

251. Hascall VC, Handley CJ, McQuillan DJ, Hascall GK, Robinson HC, Lowther DA. The effect of serum on biosynthesis of proteoglycans by bovine articular cartilage in culture. Arch Biochem Biophys 1983;224:206–23.

252. Bartholomew JS, Lowther DA, Handley CJ. Changes in proteoglycan biosynthesis following leukocyte elastase treatment of bovine articular cartilage in culture. Arthritis Rheum 1984;27:905–12.

253. Morales TI, Wahl LM, Hascall VC. The effect of bacterial lipopolysaccharides on the biosynthesis and release of proteoglycans from calf articular cartilage cultures. J Biol Chem 1984;259:6720–29.

254. Campbell MA, Handley CJ, Hascall VC, Campbell RA, Lowther DA. Turnover of proteoglycans in cultures of bovine articular cartilage. Arch Biochem Biophys 1984;234:275–89.

255. Tyler JA. Chondrocyte-mediated depletion of articular cartilage proteoglycans in vitro. Biochemical Journal 1985;225:493–507.

256. Sandy JD, Neame PJ, Boynton RE, Flannery CR. Catabolism of aggrecan in cartilage explants: Identification of a major cleavage

site within the interglobular domain. J Biol Chem 1991;266: 8683–85.

257. Handley CJ, Winter GM, Ilic MZ, Ross JM, Anthony Poole C, Clem Robinson H. Distribution of newly synthesized aggrecan in explant cultures of bovine cartilage treated with retinoic acid. Matrix Biol 2002;21:579–92.

258. Luyten FP, Hascall VC, Nissley SP, Morales TI, Reddi AH. Insulin-like growth factors maintain steady-state metabolism of proteoglycans in bovine articular cartilage explants. Arch Biochem Biophys 1988;267:416–25.

259. Barone-Varelas J, Schnitzer TJ, Meng Q, Otten L, Thonar EJ. Age-related differences in the metabolism of proteoglycans in bovine articular cartilage explants maintained in the presence of insulin-like growth factor I. Connect Tissue Res 1991;26:101–20.

260. Morales TI. Transforming growth factor-β and insulin-like growth factor-1 restore proteoglycan metabolism of bovine articular cartilage after depletion by retinoic acid. Arch Biochem Biophys 1994;315:190–98.

261. Goldring MB, Sandell LJ, Stephenson ML, Krane SM. Immune interferon suppresses levels of procollagen mRNA and type II collagen synthesis in cultured human articular and costal chondrocytes. J Biol Chem 1986;261:9049–56.

262. Aulthouse AL, Beck M, Friffey E, Sanford J, Arden K, Machado MA, Horton WA. Expression of the human chondrocyte phenotype in vitro. In Vitro Cell Devel Biol 1989;25:659–68.

263. Kolettas E, Buluwela L, Bayliss MT, Muir HI. Expression of cartilage-specific molecules is retained on long-term culture of human articular chondrocytes. J Cell Sci 1995;108(5):1991–99.

264. Holtzer J, Abbott J, Lash J, Holtzer A. The loss of phenotypic traits by differentiated cells in vitro. I. Dedifferentiation of cartilage cells. Proc Natl Acad Sci USA 1960;46:1533–42.

265. Sokoloff L, Malemud CJ, Srivastava VM, Morgan WD. In vitro culture of articular chondrocytes. Fed Proc 1973;32:1499–1502.

266. von der Mark K, Gauss V, von der Mark H, Muller P. Relationship between cell shape and type of collagen synthesised as chondrocytes lose their cartilage phenotype in culture. Nature 1977;267:531–32.

267. Benya PD, Padilla SR, Nimni ME. Independent regulation of collagen types by chondrocytes during the loss of differentiated function in culture. Cell 1978;15:1313–21.

268. Hiraki Y, Mitsui K, Endo N, Takahashi K, Hayami T, Inoue H, et al. Molecular cloning of human chondromodulin-I, a cartilage-derived growth modulating factor, and its expression in Chinese hamster ovary cells. Eur J Biochem 1999;260:869–78.

269. Tetlow LC, Woolley DE. Expression of vitamin D receptors and matrix metalloproteinases in osteoarthritic cartilage and human articular chondrocytes in vitro. Osteoarthritis Cartilage 2001;9:423–31.

270. Schnabel M, Marlovits S, Eckhoff G, Fichtel I, Gotzen L, Vecsei V, Schlegel J. Dedifferentiation-associated changes in morphology and gene expression in primary human articular chondrocytes in cell culture. Osteoarthritis Cartilage 2002;10:62–70.

271. Watt FM. Effect of seeding density on stability of the differentiated phenotype of pig articular chondrocytes in culture. J Cell Sci 1988;89(3):373–78.

272. Kuettner KE, Pauli BU, Gall G, Memoli VA, Schenk RK. Synthesis of cartilage matrix by mammalian chondrocytes in vitro: I. Isolation, culture characteristics, and morphology. J Cell Biol 1982;93: 743–50.

273. Bassleer C, Gysen P, Foidart JM, Bassleer R, Franchimont P. Human chondrocytes in tridimensional culture. In Vitro Cell Devel Biol 1986;22:113–19.

274. Adolphe M, Froger B, Ronot X, Corvol MT, Forest N. Cell multiplication and type II collagen production by rabbit articular chondrocytes cultivated in a defined medium. Exp Cell Res 1984; 155:527–36.

275. Ham RG, Sattler GL. Clonal growth of differentiated rabbit cartilage cells. J Cell Physiol 1968;72:109–14.

276. Green WT Jr. Behavior of articular chondrocytes in cell culture. Clin Orthopaed Rel Res 1971;75:248–60.

277. Deshmukh K, Kline WH. Characterization of collagen and its precursors synthesized by rabbit-articular-cartilage cells in various culture systems. Eur J Biochem 1976;69:117–23.

278. Norby DP, Malemud CJ, Sokoloff L. Differences in the collagen types synthesized by lapine articular chondrocytes in spinner and monolayer culture. Arthritis Rheum 1977;20:709–16.

279. Glowacki J, Trepman E, Folkman J. Cell shape and phenotypic expression in chondrocytes. Proc Soc Exp Biol Med 1983;172: 93–8.

280. Castagnola P, Moro G, Descalzi-Cancedda F, Cancedda R. Type X collagen synthesis during in vitro development of chick embryo tibial chondrocytes. J Cell Biol 1986;102:2310–17.

281. Reginato AM, Iozzo RV, Jimenez SA. Formation of nodular structures resembling mature articular cartilage in long-term primary cultures of human fetal epiphyseal chondrocytes on hydrogel substrate. Arthritis Rheum 1994;37:1338–49.

282. Gibson GJ, Schor SL, Grant ME. Effects of matrix macromolecules on chondrocyte gene expression: Synthesis of a low molecular weight collagen species by cells cultured within collagen gels. J Cell Biol 1982;93:767–74.

283. Mizuno S, Allemann F, Glowacki J. Effects of medium perfusion on matrix production by bovine chondrocytes in three-dimensional collagen sponges. J Biomed Mater Res 2001;56:368–75.

284. Wu QQ, Chen Q. Mechanoregulation of chondrocyte proliferation, maturation, and hypertrophy: Ion-channel dependent transduction of matrix deformation signals. Exp Cell Res 2000;256:383–91.

285. Benya PD, Shaffer JD. Dedifferentiated chondrocytes reexpress the differentiated collagen phenotype when cultured in agarose gels. Cell 1982;30:215–24.

286. Aydelotte MB, Kuettner KE. Differences between sub-populations of cultured bovine articular chondrocytes: I. Morphology and cartilage matrix production. Conn Tiss Res 1988;18:205–22.

287. Aydelotte MB, Greenhill RR, Kuettner KE. Differences between sub-populations of cultured bovine articular chondrocytes: II. Proteoglycan metabolism. Conn Tiss Res 1988;18:223–34.

288. Buschmann MD, Gluzband YA, Grodzinsky AJ, Kimura JH, Hunziker EB. Chondrocytes in agarose culture synthesize a mechanically functional extracellular matrix. J Orthop Res 1992;10:745–58.

289. Guo J, Jourdian GW, MacCallum DK. Culture and growth characteristics of chondrocytes encapsulated in alginate beads. Conn Tiss Res 1989;19:277–97.

290. Hauselmann HJ, Aydelotte MB, Schumacher BL, Kuettner KE, Gitelis SH, Thonar EJ-MA. Synthesis and turnover of proteoglycans by human and bovine adult articular chondrocytes cultured in alginate beads. Matrix 1992;12:116–29.

291. Hauselmann HJ, Fernandes RJ, Mok SS, Schmid TM, Block JA, Aydelotte MB, et al. Phenotypic stability of bovine articular chondrocytes after long-term culture in alginate beads. J Cell Sci 1994;107(1):17–27.

292. Liu H, Lee YW, Dean MF. Re-expression of differentiated proteoglycan phenotype by dedifferentiated human chondrocytes during culture in alginate beads. Biochim Biophys Acta 1998; 1425:505–15.

293. Bonaventure J, Kadhom N, Cohen-Solal L, Ng KH, Bourguignon J, Lasselin C, et al. Reexpression of cartilage-specific genes by dedifferentiated human articular chondrocytes cultured in alginate beads. Exp Cell Res 1994;212:97–104.

294. Lemare F, Steimberg N, Le Griel C, Demignot S, Adolphe M. Dedifferentiated chondrocytes cultured in alginate beads: restoration of the differentiated phenotype and of the metabolic responses to interleukin-1beta. J Cell Physiol 1998;176:303–13.

295. Srivastava VM, Malemud CJ, Sokoloff L. Chondroid expression by lapine articular chondrocytes in spinner culture following monolayer growth. Connect Tissue Res 1974;2:127–36.

296. Schulze-Tanzil G, de Souza P, Villegas Castrejon H, John T, Merker HJ, Scheid A, et al. Redifferentiation of dedifferentiated human chondrocytes in high-density cultures. Cell Tissue Res 2002;308:371–79.

297. Kato Y, Iwamoto M, Koike T, Suzuki F, Takano Y. Terminal differentiation and calcification in rabbit chondrocyte cultures grown in centrifuge tubes: Regulation by transforming growth factor beta and serum factors. Proc Natl Acad Sci USA 1988;85:9552–56.

298. Xu C, Oyajobi BO, Frazer A, Kozaci LD, Russell RG, Hollander AP. Effects of growth factors and interleukin-1 alpha on proteoglycan and type II collagen turnover in bovine nasal and articular chondrocyte pellet cultures. Endocrinology 1996;137:3557–65.

299. Stewart MC, Saunders KM, Burton-Wurster N, Macleod JN. Phenotypic stability of articular chondrocytes in vitro: The effects of culture models, bone morphogenetic protein 2, and serum supplementation. J Bone Miner Res 2000;15:166–74.

300. Croucher LJ, Crawford A, Hatton PV, Russell RG, Buttle DJ. Extracellular ATP and UTP stimulate cartilage proteoglycan and collagen accumulation in bovine articular chondrocyte pellet cultures. Biochim Biophys Acta 2000;1502:297–306.

301. Lee GM, Poole CA, Kelley SS, Chang J, Caterson B. Isolated chondrons: A viable alternative for studies of chondrocyte metabolism in vitro. Osteoarthritis Cartilage 1997;5:261–74.

302. Gibson GJ, Beaumont BW, Flint MH. Synthesis of a low molecular weight collagen by chondrocytes from the presumptive calcification region of the embryonic chick sterna: The influence of culture with collagen gels. J Cell Biol 1984;99:208–16.

303. Solursh M, Jensen KL, Reiter RS, Schmid TM, Linsenmayer TF. Environmental regulation of type X collagen production by cultures of limb mesenchyme, mesectoderm, and sternal chondrocytes. Dev Biol 1986;117:90–101.

304. Franzen A, Heinegard D, Solursh M. Evidence for sequential appearance of cartilage matrix proteins in developing mouse limbs and in cultures of mouse mesenchymal cells. Differentiation 1987;36:199–210.

305. Boyan BD, Schwartz Z, Swain LD, Carnes DL, Jr., Zislis T. Differential expression of phenotype by resting zone and growth region costochondral chondrocytes in vitro. Bone 1988;9:185–94.

306. Grigoriadis AE, Heersche JN, Aubin JE. Differentiation of muscle, fat, cartilage, and bone from progenitor cells present in a bone-derived clonal cell population: Effect of dexamethasone. J Cell Biol 1988;106:2139–51.

307. Adams SL, Pallante KM, Niu Z, Leboy PS, Golden EB, Pacifici M. Rapid induction of type X collagen gene expression in cultured chick vertebral chondrocytes. Exp Cell Res 1991;193:190–97.

308. Gerstenfeld LC, Kelly CM, Von Deck M, Lian JB. Comparative morphological and biochemical analysis of hypertrophic, non-hypertrophic and $1,25(OH)_2D_3$ treated non-hypertrophic chondrocytes. Conn Tiss Res 1990;24:29–39.

309. Lian JB, McKee MD, Todd AM, Gerstenfeld LC. Induction of bone-related proteins, osteocalcin and osteopontin, and their matrix ultrastructural localization with development of chondrocyte hypertrophy in vitro. J Cell Biochem 1993;52:206–19.

310. Kato Y, Nakashima K, Iwamoto M, Murakami H, Hiranuma H, Koike T, et al. Effects of interleukin-1 on syntheses of alkaline phosphatase, type X collagen, and 1,25-dihydroxyvitamin D3 receptor, and matrix calcification in rabbit chondrocyte cultures. J Clin Invest 1993;92:2323–30.

311. Jikko A, Aoba T, Murakami H, Takano Y, Iwamoto M, Kato Y. Characterization of the mineralization process in cultures of rabbit growth plate chondrocytes. Dev Biol 1993;156:372–80.

312. Ballock RT, Heydemann A, Wakefield LM, Flanders KC, Roberts AB, Sporn MB. TGF-beta 1 prevents hypertrophy of epiphyseal chondrocytes: Regulation of gene expression for cartilage matrix proteins and metalloproteases. Dev Biol 1993;158:414–29.

313. Alini M, Carey D, Hirata S, Grynpas MD, Pidoux I, Poole AR. Cellular and matrix changes before and at the time of calcification in the growth plate studied in vitro: Arrest of type X collagen synthesis and net loss of collagen when calcification is initiated. J Bone Miner Res 1994;9:1077–87.

314. Glaser JH, Conrad HE. Properties of chick embryo chondrocytes grown in serum-free medium. J Biol Chem 1984;259:6766–72.

315. Ballock RT, Reddi AH. Thyroxine is the serum factor that regulates morphogenesis of columnar cartilage from isolated chondrocytes in chemically defined medium. J Cell Biol 1994;126:1311–18.

316. Bohme K, Conscience-Egli M, Tschan T, Winterhalter KH, Bruckner P. Induction of proliferation or hypertrophy of chondrocytes in serum-free culture: The role of insulin-like growth factor-I, insulin, or thyroxine. J Cell Biol 1992;116:1035–42.

317. Habuchi H, Conrad HE, Glaser JH. Coordinate regulation of collagen and alkaline phosphatase levels in chick embryo chondrocytes. J Biol Chem 1985;260:13029–34.

318. Tacchetti C, Quarto R, Nitsch L, Hartmann DJ, Cancedda R. In vitro morphogenesis of chick embryo hypertrophic cartilage. J Cell Biol 1987;105:999–1006.

319. Leboy PS, Vaias L, Uschmann B, Golub E, Adams SL, Pacifici M. Ascorbic acid induces alkaline phosphatase, type X collagen, and calcium deposition in cultured chick chondrocytes. J Biol Chem 1989;264:17281–86.

320. Quarto R, Campanile G, Cancedda R, Dozin B. Thyroid hormone, insulin, and glucocorticoids are sufficient to support chondrocyte differentiation to hypertrophy: A serum-free analysis. J Cell Biol 1992;119:989–95.

321. Alini M, Kofsky Y, Wu W, Pidoux I, Poole AR. In serum-free culture thyroid hormones can induce full expression of chondrocyte hypertrophy leading to matrix calcification. J Bone Miner Res 1996;11:105–13.

322. Pacifici M, Golden EB, Iwamoto M, Adams SL. Retinoic acid treatment induces type X collagen gene expression in cultured chick chondrocytes. Exp Cell Res 1991;195:38–46.

323. Iwamoto M, Shapiro IM, Yagami K, Boskey AL, Leboy PS, Adams SL, et al. Retinoic acid induces rapid mineralization and expression of mineralization-related genes in chondrocytes. Exp Cell Res 1993;207:413–20.

324. Ballock RT, Zhou X, Mink LM, Chen DH, Mita BC. Both retinoic acid and 1,25(OH)2 vitamin D3 inhibit thyroid hormone-induced terminal differentiaton of growth plate chondrocytes. J Orthop Res 2001;19:43–9.

325. Leboy PS, Sullivan TA, Nooreyazdan M, Venezian RA. Rapid chondrocyte maturation by serum-free culture with BMP-2 and ascorbic acid. J Cell Biochem 1997;66:394–403.

326. Alema S, Tato F, Boettiger D. Myc and src oncogenes have complementary effects on cell proliferation and expression of specific extracellular matrix components in definitive chondroblasts. Mol Cell Biol 1985;5:538–44.

327. Gionti E, Pontarelli G, Cancedda R. Avian myelocytomatosis virus immortalizes differentiated quail chondrocytes. Proc Natl Acad Sci USA 1985;82:2756–60.

328. Horton WE Jr., Cleveland J, Rapp U, Nemuth G, Bolander M, Doege K, et al. An established rat cell line expressing chondrocyte properties. Exp Cell Res 1988;178:457–68.

329. Thenet S, Benya PD, Demignot S, Feunteun J, Adolphe M. SV40-immortalization of rabbit articular chondrocytes: Alteration of differentiated functions. J Cell Physiol 1992;150:158–67.

330. Mallein-Gerin F, Olsen BR. Expression of simian virus 40 large T (tumor) oncogene in chondrocytes induces cell proliferation without loss of the differentiated phenotype. Proc Natl Acad Sci USA 1993;90:3289–93.

331. Lefebvre V, Garofalo S, deCrombrugghe B. Type X collagen gene expression in mouse chondrocytes immortalized by a temperature-sensitive simian virus 40 large tumor antigen. J Cell Biol 1995;128:239–45.

332. Mataga N, Tamura M, Yanai N, Shinomura T, Kimata K, Obinata M, et al. Establishment of a novel chondrocyte-like cell line derived from transgenic mice harboring the temperature-sensitive simian virus 40 large T-antigen. J Bone Min Res 1996;11:1646–54.

333. Atsumi T, Miwa Y, Kimata K, Ikawa Y. A chondrogenic cell line derived from a differentiating culture of AT805 teratocarcinoma cells. Cell Differ Dev 1990;30:109–16.

334. Shukunami C, Shigeno C, Atsumi T, Ishizeki K, Suzuki F, Hiraki Y. Chondrogenic differentiation of clonal mouse embryonic cell line ATDC5 in vitro: Differentiation-dependent gene expression of parathyroid hormone (PTH)/PTH-related peptide receptor. J Cell Biol 1996;133:457–68.

335. Taylor SM, Jones PA. Multiple new phenotypes induced in 10T1/2 and 3T3 cells treated with 5-azacytidine. Cell 1979;17:771–79.

336. Bernier SM, Goltzman D. Regulation of expression of the chondrogenic phenotype in a skeletal cell line (CFK2) in vitro. J Bone Miner Res 1993;8:475–84.

337. Seguin CA, Bernier SM. TNFalpha suppresses link protein and type II collagen expression in chondrocytes: Role of MEK1/2 and NF-kappaB signaling pathways. J Cell Physiol 2003;197:356–69.

338. Poliard A, Nifuji A, Lamblin D, Plee E, Forest C, Kellermann O. Controlled conversion of an immortalized mesodermal progenitor cell towards osteogenic, chondrogenic, or adipogenic pathways. J Cell Biol 1995;130:1461–72.

339. Poliard A, Ronziere MC, Freyria AM, Lamblin D, Herbage D, Kellermann O. Lineage-dependent collagen expression and assembly during osteogenic or chondrogenic differentiation of a mesoblastic cell line. Exp Cell Res 1999;253:385–95.

340. Johnstone B, Barthel T, Yoo J. In vitro chondrogenesis with mammalian progenitor cells. In RV Rosier, CH Evans (eds.), Molecular Biology of Orthopaedics. Rosemont, IL: American Academy of Orthopaedic Surgeons 2003:273–87.

341. Shukunami C, Ohta Y, Sakuda M, Hiraki Y. Sequential progression of the differentiation program by bone morphogenetic

protein-2 in chondrogenic cell line ATDC5. Exp Cell Res 1998;241:1–11.

342. Ahrens M, Ankenbauer T, Schroder D, Hollnagel A, Mayer H, Gross G. Expression of human bone morphogenetic proteins-2 or -4 in murine mesenchymal progenitor C3H10T1/2 cells induces differentiation into distinct mesenchymal cell lineages. DNA Cell Biol 1993;12:871–80.

343. Grigoriadis AE, Aubin JE, Heersche JN. Effects of dexamethasone and vitamin D3 on cartilage differentiation in a clonal chondrogenic cell population. Endocrinology 1989;125:2103–10.

344. Denker AE, Haas AR, Nicoll SB, Tuan RS. Chondrogenic differentiation of murine C3H10T1/2 multipotential mesenchymal cells: I. Stimulation by bone morphogenetic protein-2 in high-density micromass cultures. Differentiation 1999;64:67–76.

345. Nifuji A, Miura N, Kato N, Kellermann O, Noda M. Bone morphogenetic protein regulation of forkhead/winged helix transcription factor Foxc2 (Mfh1) in a murine mesodermal cell line C1 and in skeletal precursor cells. J Bone Miner Res 2001;16:1765–71.

346. Block JA, Inerot SE, Gitelis S, Kimura JH. Synthesis of chondrocytic keratan sulphate-containing proteoglycans by human chondrosarcoma cells in long-term cell culture. J Bone Joint Surg Am 1991;73:647–58.

347. Takigawa M, Pan HO, Kinoshita A, Tajima K, Takano Y. Establishment from a human chondrosarcoma of a new immortal cell line with high tumorigenicity in vivo, which is able to form proteoglycan-rich cartilage-like nodules and to respond to insulin in vitro. Int J Cancer 1991;48:717–25.

348. Benoit B, Thenet-Gauci S, Hoffschir F, Penformis P, Demignot S, Adolphe M. SV40 large T antigen immortalization of human articular chondrocytes. In Vitro Cell Dev Biol 1995;31:174–77.

349. Steimberg N, Viengchareun S, Biehlmann F, Guenal I, Mignotte B, Adolphe M, et al. SV40 large T antigen expression driven by col2a1 regulatory sequences immortalizes articular chondrocytes but does not allow stabilization of type II collagen expression. Exp Cell Res 1999;249:248–59.

350. Goldring MB, Birkhead JR, Suen L-F, Yamin R, Mizuno S, Glowacki J, et al. Interleukin-1β-modulated gene expression in immortalized human chondrocytes. J Clin Invest 1994;94: 2307–16.

351. Robbins JR, Thomas B, Tan L, Choy B, Arbiser JL, Berenbaum F, et al. Immortalized human adult articular chondrocytes maintain cartilage-specific phenotype and responses to interleukin-1β. Arthritis Rheum 2000;43:2189–2201.

352. Grigolo B, Roseti L, Neri S, Gobbi P, Jensen P, Major EO, et al. Human articular chondrocytes immortalized by HPV-16 E6 and E7 genes: Maintenance of differentiated phenotype under defined culture conditions. Osteoarthritis Cartilage 2002;10:879–89.

353. Piera-Velazquez S, Jimenez SA, Stokes D. Increased life span of human osteoarthritic chondrocytes by exogenous expression of telomerase. Arthritis Rheum 2002;46:683–93.

354. Vincenti MP, Brinckerhoff CE. Early response genes induced in chondrocytes stimulated with the inflammatory cytokine interleukin-1beta. Arthritis Res 2001;3:381–88.

355. Sironen RK, Karjalainen HM, Torronen K, Elo MA, Kaarniranta K, Takigawa M, et al. High pressure effects on cellular expression profile and mRNA stability: A cDNA array analysis. Biorheology 2002;39:111–17.

356. Karjalainen HM, Sironen RK, Elo MA, Kaarniranta K, Takigawa M, Helminen HJ, et al. Gene expression profiles in chondrosarcoma cells subjected to cyclic stretching and hydrostatic pressure: A cDNA array study. Biorheology 2003;40:93–100.

357. Saas J, Lindauer K, Bau B, Takigawa M, Aigner T. Molecular phenotyping of HCS-2/8 cells as an in vitro model of human chondrocytes. Osteoarthritis Cartilage 2004;12:924–34.

358. Finger F, Schorle C, Soder S, Zien A, Goldring MB, Aigner T. Phenotypic characterization of human chondrocyte cell line C-20/A4: A comparison between monolayer and alginate suspension culture. Cells Tissues Organs 2004;178:65–77.

359. Gebauer M, Saas J, Sohler F, Haag J, Soder S, Pieper M, et al. Comparison of the chondrosarcoma cell line SW1353 with primary human adult articular chondrocytes with regard to their gene expression profile and reactivity to IL-1beta. Osteoarthritis Cartilage 2005;13:697–708.

360. Hunziker EB. Articular cartilage repair: Basic science and clinical progress. A review of the current status and prospects. Osteoarthritis Cartilage 2002;10:432–63.

361. Brittberg M, Lindahl A, Nilsson A, Ohlsson C, Isaksson O, Peterson L. Treatment of deep cartilage defects in the knee with autologous chondrocyte transplantation. N Engl J Med 1994;331:889–95.

362. Nehrer S, Spector M, Minas T. Histologic analysis of tissue after failed cartilage repair procedures. Clin Orthop Relat Res 1999: 149–62.

363. Lee CR, Grodzinsky AJ, Hsu HP, Martin SD, Spector M. Effects of harvest and selected cartilage repair procedures on the physical and biochemical properties of articular cartilage in the canine knee. J Orthop Res 2000;18:790–99.

364. Breinan HA, Hsu HP, Spector M. Chondral defects in animal models: Effects of selected repair procedures in canines. Clin Orthop Relat Res 2001:S219–30.

365. Knutsen G, Engebretsen L, Ludvigsen TC, Drogset JO, Grontvedt T, Solheim E, et al. Autologous chondrocyte implantation compared with microfracture in the knee: A randomized trial. J Bone Joint Surg Am 2004;86-A:455–64.

366. Cook SD, Patron LP, Salkeld SL, Rueger DC. Repair of articular cartilage defects with osteogenic protein-1 (BMP-7) in dogs. J Bone Joint Surg Am 2003;85-A(3):116–23.

367. Sellers RS, Zhang R, Glasson SS, Kim HD, Peluso D, D'Augusta DA, et al. Repair of articular cartilage defects one year after treatment with recombinant human bone morphogenetic protein-2 (rhBMP-2). J Bone Joint Surg Am 2000;82:151–60.

368. Buma P, Pieper JS, van Tienen T, van Susante JL, van der Kraan PM, Veerkamp JH, et al. Cross-linked type I and type II collagenous matrices for the repair of full-thickness articular cartilage defects: A study in rabbits. Biomaterials 2003;24:3255–63.

369. van den Berg WB, van der Kraan PM, Scharstuhl A, van Beuningen HM. Growth factors and cartilage repair. Clin Orthop 2001:S244–50.

370. Lories RJ, Luyten FP. Bone morphogenetic protein signaling in joint homeostasis and disease. Cytokine Growth Factor Rev 2005;16:287–98.

371. Luyten FP, Yu YM, Yanagishita M, Vukicevic S, Hammonds RG, Reddi AH. Natural bovine osteogenin and recombinant human bone morphogenetic protein-2B are equipotent in the maintenance of proteoglycans in bovine articular cartilage explant cultures. Journal of Biological Chemistry 1992;267:3691–95.

372. Chen P, Vukicevic S, Sampath TK, Luyten FP. Bovine articular chondrocytes do not undergo hypertrophy when cultured in the presence of serum and osteogenic protein-1. Biochemical & Biophysical Research Communications 1993;197:1253–59.

373. Luyten FP, Chen P, Paralkar V, Reddi AH. Recombinant bone morphogenetic protein-4, transforming growth factor-beta 1, and activin A enhance the cartilage phenotype of articular chondrocytes in vitro. Experimental Cell Research 1994;210:224–29.

374. Lietman SA, Yanagishita M, Sampath TK, Reddi AH. Stimulation of proteoglycan synthesis in explants of porcine articular cartilage by recombinant osteogenic protein-1 (bone morphogenetic protein-7). J Bone Joint Surg Am 1997;79:1132–37.

375. Erlacher L, Ng CK, Ullrich R, Krieger S, Luyten FP. Presence of cartilage-derived morphogenetic proteins in articular cartilage and enhancement of matrix replacement in vitro. Arthritis & Rheumatism 1998;41:263–73.

376. Valcourt U, Ronziere MC, Winkler P, Rosen V, Herbage D, Mallein-Gerin F. Different effects of bone morphogenetic proteins 2, 4, 12, and 13 on the expression of cartilage and bone markers in the MC615 chondrocyte cell line. Exp Cell Res 1999;251:264–74.

377. Mi Z, Ghivizzani SC, Lechman ER, Glorioso JC, Evans CH, Robbins PD. Adverse effects of adenovirus-mediated gene transfer of human transforming growth factor beta 1 into rabbit knees. Arthritis Res 2003;5:R132–39.

378. Hunziker EB, Driesang IM, Morris EA. Chondrogenesis in cartilage repair is induced by members of the transforming growth factor-beta superfamily. Clin Orthop 2001:S171–81.

379. Glansbeek HL, van Beuningen HM, Vitters EL, Morris EA, van der Kraan PM, van den Berg WB. Bone morphogenetic protein 2 stimulates articular cartilage proteoglycan synthesis in vivo but does not counteract interleukin-1α effects on proteoglycan synthesis and content. Arthritis Rheum 1997;40:1020–28.

380. Seeherman H, Wozney JM. Delivery of bone morphogenetic proteins for orthopedic tissue regeneration. Cytokine Growth Factor Rev 2005;16:329–45.

75

381. Li RH, Wozney JM. Delivering on the promise of bone morphogenetic proteins. Trends Biotechnol 2001;19:255–65.

382. Sellers RS, Peluso D, Morris EA. The effect of recombinant human bone morphogenetic protein-2 (rhBMP-2) on the healing of full-thickness defects of articular cartilage. J Bone Joint Surg 1997;79A:1452–63.

383. Kang R, Marui T, Ghivizzani SC, Nita IM, Georgescu HI, Suh JK, et al. Ex vivo gene transfer to chondrocytes in full-thickness articular cartilage defects: A feasibility study. Osteoarthritis Cartilage 1997;5:139–43.

384. Mi Z, Ghivizzani SC, Lechman ER, Jaffurs D, Glorioso JC, Evans CH, et al. Adenovirus-mediated gene transfer of insulin-like growth factor 1 stimulates proteoglycan synthesis in rabbit joints. Arthritis Rheum 2000;43:2563–70.

385. Shuler FD, Georgescu HI, Niyibizi C, Studer RK, Mi Z, Johnstone B, et al. Increased matrix synthesis following adenoviral transfer of a transforming growth factor beta1 gene into articular chondrocytes. J Orthop Res 2000;18:585–92.

386. Smith P, Shuler FD, Georgescu HI, Ghivizzani SC, Johnstone B, Niyibizi C, et al. Genetic enhancement of matrix synthesis by articular chondrocytes: Comparison of different growth factor genes in the presence and absence of interleukin-1. Arthritis Rheum 2000;43:1156–64.

387. Kaps C, Bramlage C, Smolian H, Haisch A, Ungethum U, Burmester GR, et al. Bone morphogenetic proteins promote cartilage differentiation and protect engineered artificial cartilage from fibroblast invasion and destruction. Arthritis Rheum 2002;46:149–62.

388. Gooch KJ, Blunk T, Courter DL, Sieminski AL, Vunjak-Novakovic G, Freed LE. Bone morphogenetic proteins-2, -12, and -13 modulate in vitro development of engineered cartilage. Tissue Eng 2002;8:591–601.

389. Hills RL, Belanger LM, Morris EA. Bone morphogenetic protein 9 is a potent anabolic factor for juvenile bovine cartilage, but not adult cartilage. J Orthop Res 2005;23:611–17.

390. Tcacencu I, Carlsoo B, Stierna P. Effect of recombinant human BMP-2 on the repair of cricoid cartilage defects in young and adult rabbits: A comparative study. Int J Pediatr Otorhinolaryngol 2005;69:1239–46.

391. Barry FP, Murphy JM. Mesenchymal stem cells: Clinical applications and biological characterization. Int J Biochem Cell Biol 2004;36:568–84.

392. Caplan AI. Review, mesenchymal stem cells: Cell-based reconstructive therapy in orthopedics. Tissue Eng 2005;11:1198–1211.

393. Carrington JL, Chen P, Yanagishita M, Reddi AH. Osteogenin (bone morphogenetic protein-3) stimulates cartilage formation by chick limb bud cells in vitro. Developmental Biology (Orlando) 1991;146:406–15.

394. Chen P, Carrington JL, Hammonds RG, Reddi AH. Stimulation of chondrogenesis in limb bud mesoderm cells by recombinant human bone morphogenetic protein 2B (BMP-2B) and modulation by transforming growth factor beta 1 and beta 2. Experimental Cell Research 1991;195:509–15.

395. Asahina I, Sampath TK, Nishimura I, Hauschka PV. Human osteogenic protein-1 induces both chondroblastic and osteoblastic differentiation of osteoprogenitor cells derived from newborn rat calvaria. J Cell Biol 1993;123:921–33.

396. Rosen V, Nove J, Song JJ, Thies RS, Cox K, Wozney JM. Responsiveness of clonal limb bud cell lines to bone morphogenetic protein 2 reveals a sequential relationship between cartilage and bone cell phenotypes. J Bone Miner Res 1994;9:1759–68.

397. Johnstone B, Hering TM, Caplan AI, Goldberg VM, Yoo JU. In vitro chondrogenesis of bone marrow-derived mesenchymal progenitor cells. Exp Cell Res 1998;238:265–72.

398. Klein-Nulend J, Semeins CM, Mulder JW, Winters HA, Goei SW, Ooms ME, et al. Stimulation of cartilage differentiation by osteogenic protein-1 in cultures of human perichondrium. Tissue Eng 1998;4:305–13.

399. Pittenger MF, Mackay AM, Beck SC, Jaiswal RK, Douglas R, Mosca JD, et al. Multilineage potential of adult human mesenchymal stem cells. Science 1999;284:143–47.

400. Kramer J, Hegert C, Guan K, Wobus AM, Muller PK, Rohwedel J. Embryonic stem cell-derived chondrogenic differentiation in vitro: Activation by BMP-2 and BMP-4. Mech Dev 2000;92:193–205.

401. Majumdar MK, Wang E, Morris EA. BMP-2 and BMP-9 promotes chondrogenic differentiation of human multipotential mesenchymal cells and overcomes the inhibitory effect of IL-1. J Cell Physiol 2001;189:275–84.

402. Gruber R, Mayer C, Bobacz K, Krauth MT, Graninger W, Luyten FP, et al. Effects of cartilage-derived morphogenetic proteins and osteogenic protein-1 on osteochondrogenic differentiation of periosteum-derived cells. Endocrinology 2001;142:2087–94.

403. Sekiya I, Colter DC, Prockop DJ. BMP-6 enhances chondrogenesis in a subpopulation of human marrow stromal cells. Biochem Biophys Res Commun 2001;284:411–18.

404. Urist MR. Bone: Formation by autoinduction. Science 1965;150:893–99.

405. Friedenstein AJ, Piatetzky S, II, Petrakova KV. Osteogenesis in transplants of bone marrow cells. J Embryol Exp Morphol 1966;16:381–90.

406. Bruder SP, Fink DJ, Caplan AI. Mesenchymal stem cells in bone development, bone repair, and skeletal regeneration therapy. J Cell Biochem 1994;56:283–94.

407. Tuan RS. Biology of developmental and regenerative skeletogenesis. Clin Orthop Relat Res 2004:S105–17.

408. Sakaguchi Y, Sekiya I, Yagishita K, Muneta T. Comparison of human stem cells derived from various mesenchymal tissues: Superiority of synovium as a cell source. Arthritis Rheum 2005;52:2521–29.

409. Huang JI, Kazmi N, Durbhakula MM, Hering TM, Yoo JU, Johnstone B. Chondrogenic potential of progenitor cells derived from human bone marrow and adipose tissue: A patient-matched comparison. J Orthop Res 2005;23:1383–9.

410. Park J, Gelse K, Frank S, von der Mark K, Aigner T, Schneider H. Transgene-activated mesenchymal cells for articular cartilage repair: A comparison of primary bone marrow-, perichondrium/periosteum- and fat-derived cells. J Gene Med 2005;8:112–25.

411. Shen HC, Peng H, Usas A, Gearhart B, Cummins J, Fu FH, Huard J. Ex vivo gene therapy-induced endochondral bone formation: Comparison of muscle-derived stem cells and different subpopulations of primary muscle-derived cells. Bone 2004;34:982–92.

412. Adachi N, Sato K, Usas A, Fu FH, Ochi M, Han CW, et al. Muscle derived, cell based ex vivo gene therapy for treatment of full thickness articular cartilage defects. J Rheumatol 2002;29:1920–30.

413. Kuroda R, Usas A, Kubo S, Corsi K, Peng H, Rose T, et al. Cartilage repair using bone morphogenetic protein 4 and muscle-derived stem cells. Arthritis Rheum 2005;54:433–4.

414. Murphy JM, Dixon K, Beck S, Fabian D, Feldman A, Barry F. Reduced chondrogenic and adipogenic activity of mesenchymal stem cells from patients with advanced osteoarthritis. Arthritis Rheum 2002;46:704–13.

415. Ryan JM, Barry FP, Murphy JM, Mahon BP. Mesenchymal stem cells avoid allogeneic rejection. J Inflamm (Lond) 2005;2:8.

416. Bell DM, Leung KK, Wheatley SC, Ng LJ, Zhou S, Ling KW, et al. SOX9 directly regulates the type-II collagen gene. Nat Genet 1997;16:174–78.

417. Bi W, Deng JM, Zhang Z, Behringer RR, de Crombrugghe B. Sox9 is required for cartilage formation. Nat Genet 1999;22:85–9.

# 5 Aging Cartilage and Osteoarthritis Cartilage: Differences and Shared Mechanisms

Richard F. Loeser

## INTRODUCTION

The strongest risk factor for the development of osteoarthritis (OA) in humans as well as in many animal species is age. Even some of the most severe forms of OA, such as those associated with type II collagen gene mutations, are usually not clinically evident in children but first appear in young adults.[1] The much more common multifactorial forms of OA begin to appear sometime after the age of 40 years in humans, with a striking increase in incidence and prevalence after about age 50.[2,3] By the age of 60, almost 80% of the population will have radiographic evidence of OA in at least one joint.[4] However, the majority of this radiographic disease is osteophyte formation (which is of questionable clinical significance). Perhaps more importantly, clinically defined OA increases directly with age and self-reported activity limitation due to arthritis rises from 3.5% of people aged 45 to 54 years to 18.5% of those 85 years of age or older.[5]

Because OA is so common in the older adult population, it is sometimes mistakenly considered to be a normal part of the aging process. However, the poor correlation of radiographic disease with symptoms and disability as well as the fact that many healthy older adults do not suffer from symptomatic OA indicate that aging and OA are not one and the same.

This chapter reviews the similarities and differences between changes in the articular cartilage that have been described with aging and those noted in OA. The major theme will be that aging-related changes do not directly result in OA but rather make the joints of older adults more susceptible to the development of OA when other "OA factors" are also present. Because OA is a condition that affects the joint as an organ, aging may influence the development of OA due to age-related changes in any of the joint tissues. However, to date the majority of the research on joint aging has centered on the articular cartilage and thus this tissue is the focus of most of the discussion here. Because OA is so common in the older adult population, it is sometimes difficult to determine if an observed change in a particular joint tissue is due to tissue aging or due to early disease. Despite this limitation, it is becoming clear that many of the changes that occur with aging in cartilage are different from those seen in OA.

## AGE AS A RISK FACTOR FOR THE DEVELOPMENT OF OA

The prevalence of OA in susceptible joints increases directly with increasing age whether OA is defined by characteristic joint pathology, radiographic findings, joint pain, or disability (Fig. 5.1). The strong association between age and OA also holds true for animals that develop spontaneous OA.[6,7] Because OA does not usually interfere with physical function until the postreproductive years, there is little evolutionary pressure to select against genes that may predispose older adults to OA. Several studies have shown that OA has a strong genetic component with an estimated contribution to the risk for OA in the range of 40%.[8,9]

In addition to age and genetics, the other major risk factors for OA include obesity, joint injury, occupational overuse, and anatomic factors such as joint shape and alignment.[10] It would appear that the majority of people with OA have one or more risk factors in addition to age. This suggests that to develop OA more than one "hit" is required, similar to the theory behind certain other diseases that become more common with increasing age (such as cancer and neurodegenerative diseases). In this paradigm, age serves as a risk factor for OA because aging changes make it easier for OA to develop when a second risk factor is also present (Fig. 5.2). As one example, it has been shown that having a knee injury due to an anterior ligament or meniscal tear results in

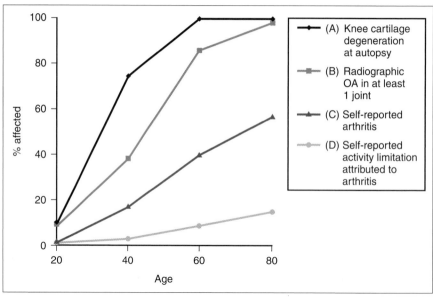

**Fig. 5.1** Effect of age on the prevalence of arthritis. (A) Knee cartilage degeneration at autopsy is the prevalence of significant histologic changes of degeneration. (B) Radiographic evidence of OA (Kellgren and Lawrence grade 2 or greater) present in at least one joint site (hands, feet, spine, knees, and hips) in a population survey in Northern England. (C) Self-reported arthritis and (D) activity limitation attributable to arthritis derived from the National Health Interview Survey (United States, 1989–1991). (Redrawn with permission from Rheumatic Disease Clinics of North America 2000;26:547.)

the appearance of OA approximately three times faster in adults injured past the age of 30 compared to injuries occurring in 17- to 30-year-olds.[11]

This model is not meant to suggest that the OA factors are not active until after the aging changes have been established. Joint injuries that lead to OA later in life most commonly occur in young active adults, anatomic variants such as acetabular dysplasia are present from birth, and obesity often begins in childhood or adolescence. Thus, it is likely that the OA factors are often present before aging changes come into play and that

the OA factors help drive the site and severity of the disease.

The close relationship between aging and the development of OA also suggests that protective mechanisms are in place that prevent the development of OA in youth. If this is true, and if any of these protective mechanisms are genetic, it would mean that some older adults may be better protected against the development of OA than others. This would be an additional explanation for why aging and OA are not one and the same and why not all older adults have OA. In a Danish

**Fig. 5.2** Hypothetical relationship between aging and the development of OA. In this model, aging changes are shown that increase the susceptibility of the musculoskeletal system to the development of OA. However, OA factors acting on the aging joint are necessary for OA to develop.

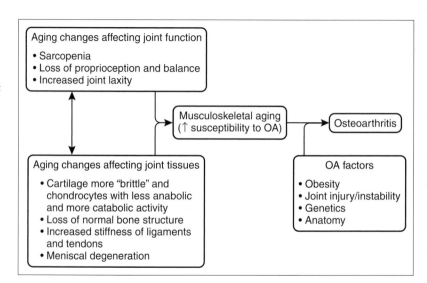

study of centenarians, the prevalence of symptomatic OA of the hip, knee, shoulder, or spine was only 54%.[12] It would certainly be of interest to determine what factors are associated with the lack of OA in the oldest of the old.

## AGE-RELATED CHANGES IN CARTILAGE MACROSTRUCTURE

Age-related changes that occur in cartilage at the macroscopic level include mild thinning, browning, and some surface "wear" or roughening. Browning is probably due to accumulation of advanced glycation end products (discussed further in material following). The surface wear or roughening is particularly common in load-bearing areas[13] and can be found in tissue donors who had no known prior history of arthritis.[14]

The possibility that these minor surface changes might represent early OA cannot be addressed until longitudinal data is available to determine how these changes progress over time. Biomechanical testing of the cartilage surface has shown an association between surface degeneration and decreased indentation stiffness, which was more strongly related to the degree of degeneration than to age.[15] This suggests that some degree of surface damage can affect the biomechanical properties of cartilage and could predispose to further damage but that age alone could be less of a factor than the degree of damage.

By MRI it can be seen that knee cartilage thins with aging, particularly at the femoral side of the joint[16] and at the patella.[17] There are more cartilage defects with aging,[17] and the patellar cartilage in older adults appears to be less deformable.[16] Another MRI study examined the effect of age on patellar cartilage T2 values, which are hypothesized to reflect collagen structure.[18] In that study, asymptomatic women aged 22 to 86 years were studied and an age-related increase in T2 values was noted (which progressed to deeper in the cartilage with age). These findings were interpreted to indicate that age-related changes in collagen structure had occurred that progressed from the surface to deeper cartilage with increasing age.[18] This would be consistent with previous biochemical studies that have shown evidence of type II collagen denaturation that begins in the superficial zone in older adults and with progression to OA involves deeper zones.[19]

## AGE-RELATED CHANGES IN THE CARTILAGE MATRIX

Additional studies have examined the matrix of early cartilage lesions seen with aging that may be "pre-OA" lesions. Evidence of collagenase-mediated collagen cleavage as well as loss of proteoglycan was noted in the areas closest to focal lesions, whereas the cartilage matrix in areas remote from a lesion was more biochemically normal.[20] When macroscopically normal ankle cartilage was examined, there was no age-related change in collagen or proteoglycan content and there was evidence for a low level of continued type II collagen turnover in donors up to 75 years of age.[21] However, when the ratio of cleaved/denatured type II collagen was examined in these samples a striking and highly significant positive correlation ($r = 0.78$, $p < 0.0001$) with age was noted, suggesting a disassociation between cleavage and denaturation with aging. These studies suggest that the matrix changes associated with early cartilage damage are more striking than those seen with aging but that detectable changes are occurring in the matrix with age.

In addition to a continuous low level of type II collagen turnover that persists with age, there is evidence for turnover of aggrecan (the large cartilage proteoglycan that is largely responsible for the resiliency of articular cartilage). When aggrecan is degraded, a fragment that contains the binding region for hyaluronic acid can be left behind. This fragment appears to accumulate in cartilage with aging due to a low turnover rate. Its estimated half-life in cartilage is 25 years.[22] The aggrecan fragment that remains bound to hyaluronic acid can occupy the space where a newly synthesized complete aggrecan molecule would bind and thus result in smaller proteoglycan aggregates being present with increasing age.

Age-related changes in aggrecan are thought to affect cartilage hydration. Because of the hydrophilic nature of aggrecan, articular cartilage is about 70 to 80% water. Age-related changes in the size, structure, and sulfation of aggrecan have been reported.[23-26] These changes are thought to be responsible for an observed decrease in cartilage hydration with age, which is opposite from the increase in hydration noted in early OA.[27]

Another age-related change in the cartilage matrix is an increase in calcification. The prevalence of radiographic chondrocalcinosis has been shown to increase directly with age[28,29] and to be associated with OA.[28,29] The increase in the formation of calcium pyrophosphate crystals may be due to an age-related increase in the activity of transglutaminase (an enzyme involved in the biomineralization process)[30] as well as to an increase in inorganic pyrophosphate production in response to transforming growth factor-β stimulation.[31] Despite a strong association among age, chondrocalcinosis, and the presence of OA, the precise role of cartilage matrix calcification in the development of OA is not clear—in part due to the number of older people with asymptomatic chondrocalcinosis.[32]

An age-related increase in the lipid content of human articular cartilage was reported years ago.[33] Lipids were found to be most abundant in the superficial layer of cartilage. In particular, there was almost a twofold increase in the amount of arachidonic acid in the superficial cartilage between ages 30 and 49 and 60 and 69 and almost a threefold difference from the 10- to 21-year-old age group.[33] Because arachidonic acid is a necessary substrate for the production of inflammatory lipid mediators (including prostaglandins and leukotrienes), an age-related increase could contribute to the increased susceptibility for OA.

## CARTILAGE AGING AND THE FORMATION OF ADVANCED GLYCATION END PRODUCTS

Aging in various connective tissues throughout the body is associated with the accumulation of proteins in the extracellular matrix that have been modified in some way by the environment in which they exist. Because the articular cartilage has a relatively low turnover rate, it is particularly susceptible to these time-dependent processes. The best studied aging-related protein modification in cartilage is the formation of advanced glycation end products (AGEs). AGEs are produced from the spontaneous nonenzymatic glycation of proteins that occurs when reducing sugars such as glucose, fructose, or ribose react with lysine or arginine residues.[34]

Type II collagen is particularly susceptible to AGE modification due to its extremely long half-life, which has been calculated to be over 100 years.[35] The AGE modification of collagen can result in the formation of cross-links, the most common of which is pentosidine (which has been found to be present in cartilage in increasing amounts with age).[35-37] The formation of collagen cross-links due to AGEs has been associated with increased stiffness, which in turn increases the susceptibility of the tissue to fatigue failure.[36] These changes have been hypothesized to be responsible for making cartilage more brittle with age.[38]

In addition to pentosidine, another type of AGE that has been detected in articular cartilage is Nε-(carboxymethyl)lysine (CML).[39] CML can form from glycation as well as glycoxidation and lipid peroxidation and has been associated with aging in a number of tissues.[40] It has been reported in the superficial zone of normal cartilage (age of subjects not provided) and in OA cartilage in areas of damage.[39] It has also been found to be present in intervertebral discs, where the concentration was shown to associate with other age-related changes.[41] Because CML can form under conditions of oxidative damage, its presence suggests that such damage has occurred with aging in cartilage.

Much of the work on cartilage AGE formation has been performed by a Dutch group, which has proposed that the accumulation of AGEs in cartilage may play a role in the development of OA.[34,42] In one study, they

tested this hypothesis by stimulating the formation of AGEs in the joints of young dogs through intra-articular injections of ribose that resulted in AGE formation similar to that seen with aging.[42] They then induced OA by transection of the anterior cruciate ligament, and when the joints were assessed 7 weeks later found that the OA was more severe in the ribose-treated joints. This finding is consistent with the "two-hit" hypothesis for OA in which age-related AGE formation increases the susceptibility to OA when an OA factor (joint injury) is also present.

## THE AGING CHONDROCYTE

### Proliferation and Cell Death

In addition to the low matrix turnover, another important feature of articular cartilage that may promote its susceptibility to age-related changes is the low cellular turnover. It is felt that articular chondrocytes must be very long-lived cells because it is difficult to find evidence of cell division in normal adult articular cartilage.[43] In addition, there does not appear to be a ready supply in cartilage of immature precursor cells that differentiate and replace lost chondrocytes. However, a recent study did provide evidence that limited numbers of chondrocyte precursors may be present (particularly in OA cartilage),[44] and thus the potential exists for stimulating chondrocyte replacement. The low turnover of cells in adult articular cartilage has two important consequences. First, if cells are lost due to cell death they are unlikely to be replaced. Second, an individual chondrocyte has many years in which cellular damage can occur and accumulate.

The loss of chondrocytes due to cell death with aging as well as in OA cartilage has been reported, but the extent of cell death is debated.[45-47] An overall decline in cell numbers would be consistent with the observed cartilage thinning with age described previously. In a study of human hip cartilage, a 30% fall in cell density between the ages of 30 and 70 years was noted.[48] Likewise, a recent study of femoral head cartilage in rats found a 46% decline in cell numbers in old (15- to 18-month-old) rats compared to young adult rats (6 months).[49] However, another study of cell death in aging and OA tissue in the knee found less than 5% cell loss.[43] Although many studies have reported apoptotic chondrocytes in OA cartilage,[47] few examined apoptosis in cartilage with normal aging with the exception of a study in rat cartilage.[50] Currently, the consensus seems to be that cell death likely occurs at some stage in the development of OA but more than likely it is at a later stage and is not an initiating factor.

Although articular chondrocytes appear dormant, they can and do divide when the matrix is damaged. One of the hallmarks of OA is the appearance of clusters or "clones" of chondrocytes that are thought to represent an attempt to repair damaged matrix by increasing the cell number. However, the proliferative capacity of chondrocytes appears to decrease with aging. When compared to cells from young adults, cells from older adults demonstrate a reduced mitogenic response to growth factor stimulation.[51] Whether or not this is related to replicative senescence, where cells lose their capacity to divide further after a certain number of cell divisions, is not known. Replicative senescence is thought in part to be related to shortened telomeres, and evidence of telomere shortening in chondrocytes from older adults has been reported.[52]

Normally, signals that regulate cell proliferation and survival are provided by growth factors that work in concert with signals from the extracellular matrix. It is not clear which growth factors are most active in adult articular cartilage in terms of stimulating proliferation, but the most likely candidates are transforming growth factor-β (TGF-β) and basic fibroblast growth factor (bFGF).[51,53] There is evidence that in adult cartilage insulin-like growth factors and a protein called Gas-6 may function as survival factors.[54,55] Matrix survival signals appear to be provided by type II collagen[56] (as well as by signaling through the α5β1 integrin, which is a receptor for fibronectin).[57] The effect of aging on the ability of growth factors and matrix signals to promote chondrocyte survival has not been well studied. Preliminary results suggest that survival in response to IGF-1 goes down with age (Loeser et al., unpublished observations).

## Anabolic and Catabolic Activity

Although the effects of aging on chondrocyte survival have not been well studied, there is evidence to suggest that the synthetic or anabolic activity goes down with age. In addition to promoting survival, IGF-1 stimulates chondrocyte proteoglycan and collagen synthesis and this response has been shown to decline with increasing age.[58-60] A reduced anabolic response to IGF-1 has also been noted in chondrocytes isolated from OA cartilage.[59,61] Although the anabolic response to TGF-β was maintained in cartilage from aging mice, the ability of TGF-β to counteract the anti-anabolic affects of IL-1 was lost.[62]

In addition to IGF-1 and TGF-β, another key cartilage growth factor is osteogenic protein-1 (OP-1), which is also called bone morphogenetic protein 7 (BMP-7). Although it is not known if the response to OP-1 declines with aging, it has been shown that the expression and amount of OP-1 present in cartilage decline with age.[63] Therefore, the overall effect of aging results in reduced anabolic activity in cartilage. Because OA is characterized by an imbalance in anabolic and catabolic activity, which results in excessive matrix degradation, aging could directly contribute to this imbalance.

There is also some limited evidence to suggest that although anabolic activity may decline with aging catabolic activity may increase, which would further contribute to an anabolic/catabolic imbalance. In support of increased catabolic activity with aging are studies showing an age-related accumulation of collagen neoepitopes representing denatured or cleaved collagen.[19,21] Also in support of this is increased staining for MMP-3 and MMP-13 in cartilage with aging.[64] In these studies, early damage to type II collagen was been noted in cartilage from hip joints of older individuals[19] as well as in "normal-appearing" knee cartilage taken at autopsy.[64] Because these joints are commonly affected by OA, it is not clear if the collagen damage represents aging changes, early OA, or a continuum from aging to OA.

Consistent with an observation of increased collagen cleavage with aging, a recent study examined the response of human articular chondrocytes to two different catabolic stimuli (IL-1β and fibronectin fragments) and found that production of matrix metalloproteinase 13 (MMP-13) was significantly increased with age.[65] This may be important to the increased susceptibility to OA as well in that MMP-13 appears to be a major mediator of type II collagen destruction in OA.[66,67]

The mechanism underlying the age-related change in anabolic and catabolic activity is not clear. Because growth factors such as IGF-1, OP-1, and TGF-β can be anti-catabolic in addition to being anabolic, a decline in responsiveness to them could affect both sets of pathways. A deceased response to growth factors could be due to an increased production of inhibitory binding proteins, other changes in the extracellular matrix that decrease growth factor availability, decreased receptors or receptor activity, or decreased signal transduction. In rat cartilage an age-related increase in the production of an IGF binding protein (IGFBP) was noted,[58] but the lack of response of monkey chondrocytes to a form of IGF-1 that is not blocked by binding proteins suggests that increased production of IGFBPs may not be the mechanism.[59] Another study in rat tissue suggests that an age-related reduction in signal transduction may be more likely.[60]

A matrix change that might alter growth factor responsiveness is the accumulation of AGEs described previously. A very significant age-related decline in serum-stimulated proteoglycan synthesis was closely associated with the amount of pentosidine in cartilage.[68] Whether AGEs directly interfere with the ability of growth factors to stimulate their receptors or have some indirect effect on growth factor activity is not clear. There are receptors for AGEs present on articular chondrocytes, including the receptor for advanced glycation end products (RAGE).[69] The levels of RAGE appear to be increased in cartilage from older adults and in OA cartilage.[69] This latter study showed that stimulation of RAGE signaling increases NF-κB activity and MMP-13 expression, suggesting that RAGE stimulation could also play a role in cartilage destruction in OA.

## Oxidative Stress and Damage

One of the long-held theories of aging has been the free radical theory first put forth by Harman in the 1950s.[70] Oxidative damage from the chronic production of endogenous reactive oxygen species (ROS) or "free radicals" has been associated with aging in various human tissues and in animal studies.[71] Oxidative stress refers to a condition within cells when the amount of ROS exceeds the anti-oxidant capacity of the cell. Excess production of ROS or loss of anti-oxidants can cause oxidative stress, which in turn can result in oxidative damage.

It is well known that human articular chondrocytes can actively produce ROS, including nitric oxide (NO$^\bullet$), the superoxide anion (O$_2^{\bullet -}$), the hydroxyl radical (HO$^\bullet$), and hydrogen peroxide (H$_2$O$_2$).[72-74] Increased levels of intracellular ROS were recently detected in cartilage from old rats when compared to young adults.[49] In chondrocytes isolated from humans it was also recently shown that the ratio of oxidized to reduced glutathione increased with age, which is a sign of oxidative stress.[75] Importantly, age-related oxidative stress was found to make human chondrocytes[75] and rat chondrocytes[49] more susceptible to cell death mediated by oxidants.

Further evidence for oxidative damage in articular cartilage is provided by a study showing increased nitrotyrosine with aging and in OA.[76] When O$_2^{\bullet -}$ and NO$^\bullet$ react, peroxynitrite (ONOO$^-$) is formed (which is a powerful oxidant that can nitrate tyrosine residues present in proteins to form 3-nitrotyrosine).[77] The presence of nitrotyrosine can therefore serve as a marker for oxidative damage. In monkey cartilage, the presence of nitrotyrosine correlated with reduced response to IGF-I (suggesting that oxidative damage may be one mechanism for the reduced growth factor response).[76]

There is also evidence that ROS play a role in OA.[78] Excess production of ROS by chondrocytes could damage both intracellular proteins and the extracellular matrix. Because ROS are also involved in the stimulation of MMP production and activity,[79] they could

| TABLE 5.1  AGING-RELATED CHANGES IN CARTILAGE AND THE RELATIONSHIP TO OSTEOARTHRITIS | |
|---|---|
| Changes Related to Aging | Relationship to OA Changes |
| **Cartilage Structure** | |
| Surface roughening and fibrillation | Progressive fibrillation and erosion into deep zones |
| Superficial zone collagen denaturation | Extensive collagen cleavage and denaturation |
| No change in total collagen and PG content | Progressive loss of collagen and PG |
| Decreased cartilage hydration | Increased hydration in early disease |
| Asymptomatic chondrocalcinosis | Increased cartilage calcification in advanced disease |
| Increased lipid content | Increased production of inflammatory lipid mediators |
| Accumulation of AGE | Increased RAGE expression |
| Increased cartilage stiffness | Loss of tensile strength |
| Oxidative damage in superficial zone | More extensive oxidative damage associated with matrix damage |
| **Chondrocyte Function** | |
| Little to no proliferation | Increased proliferation and clustering |
| Minimal loss of cells | More extensive loss of cells in areas of damage |
| Decreased anabolic activity | Early increase in anabolic activity |
| Increased catabolic responsiveness | Increased catabolic activity that overwhelms anabolic activity |
| Increased oxidative stress | Extensive oxidative damage |

Abbreviations: PG (proteoglycan), AGE (advanced glycation end products), RAGE (receptor for AGE).

play an important role in stimulating cartilage degradation in OA. Age-related oxidative stress that results in excessive ROS activity could therefore be another mechanism by which aging increases the susceptibility of cartilage to the development of OA.

## SUMMARY

There is no disagreement that aging is intimately connected to the development of OA. Table 5.1 summarizes the major changes in articular cartilage that occur with aging and how these changes may relate to the development of OA. Because OA is so common in older adults, it is sometimes difficult to separate what is normal aging from early OA, but the findings to date suggest that they are not one and the same. Rather, a number of aging-related changes in cartilage make the tissue more susceptible to the development of the cartilage matrix damage that is characteristic of OA.

## ACKNOWLEDGMENTS

Dr. Loeser's work was supported by the National Institutes of Health (AG16697 and AR49003) and the American Federation for Aging Research.

## REFERENCES

1. Knowlton RG, Katzenstein PL, Moskowitz RW, et al. Genetic linkage of a polymorphism in the type II procollagen gene (COL2A1) to primary osteoarthritis associated with mild chondrodysplasia. N Engl J Med 1990;322:526.
2. Sowers M, Lachance L, Hochberg M, et al. Radiographically defined osteoarthritis of the hand and knee in young and middle-aged African American and Caucasian women. Osteoarthritis Cartilage 2000;8:69.
3. Oliveria SA, Felson DT, Reed JI, et al. Incidence of symptomatic hand, hip, and knee osteoarthritis among patients in a health maintenance organization. Arthritis Rheum 1995;38:1134.
4. Lawrence JS, Bremner JM, Bier F. Osteo-arthrosis: Prevalence in the population and relationship between symptoms and X-ray changes. Ann Rheum Dis 1966;25:1.
5. Lawrence RC, Helmick CG, Arnett FC, et al. Estimates of the prevalence of arthritis and selected musculoskeletal disorders in the United States. Arthritis Rheum 1998;41:778.
6. Bendele AM, White SL, Hulman JF. Osteoarthrosis in guinea pigs: Histopathologic and scanning electron microscopic features. Lab Anim Sci 1989;39:115.
7. Carlson CS, Loeser RF, Purser CB, et al. Osteoarthritis in cynomolgus macaques. III: Effects of age, gender, and subchondral bone thickness on the severity of disease. J Bone Miner Res 1996;11:1209.
8. Spector TD, Cicuttini F, Baker J, et al. Genetic influences on osteoarthritis in women: A twin study. BMJ 1996;312:940.
9. Felson DT, Couropmitree NN, Chaisson CE, et al. Evidence for a Mendelian gene in a segregation analysis of generalized radiographic osteoarthritis: The Framingham Study. Arthritis Rheum 1998;41:1064.
10. Felson DT, Lawrence RC, Dieppe PA, et al. Osteoarthritis: New insights. Part 1: The disease and its risk factors. Ann Intern Med 2000;133:635.
11. Roos H, Adalberth T, Dahlberg L, et al. Osteoarthritis of the knee after injury to the anterior cruciate ligament or meniscus: The influence of time and age. Osteoarth Cartilage 1995;3:261.
12. Andersen-Ranberg K, Schroll M, Jeune B. Healthy centenarians do not exist, but autonomous centenarians do: A population-based study of morbidity among Danish centenarians. J Am Geriatr Soc 2001;49:900.
13. Meachim G. Cartilage fibrillation on the lateral tibial plateau in Liverpool necropsies. J Anat 1976;121:97.
14. Cole AA, Margulis A, Kuettner KE. Distinguishing ankle and knee articular cartilage. Foot Ankle Clin N Am 2003;8:305.
15. Bae WC, Temple MM, Amiel D, et al. Indentation testing of human cartilage: Sensitivity to articular surface degeneration. Arthritis Rheum 2003;48:3382.
16. Hudelmaier M, Glaser C, Hohe J, et al. Age-related changes in the morphology and deformational behavior of knee joint cartilage. Arthritis Rheum 2001;44:2556.
17. Ding C, Cicuttini F, Scott F, et al. Association between age and knee structural change: A cross sectional MRI based study. Ann Rheum Dis 2005;64:549.
18. Mosher TJ, Liu Y, Yang QX, et al. Age dependency of cartilage magnetic resonance imaging T2 relaxation times in asymptomatic women. Arthritis Rheum 2004;50:2820.
19. Hollander AP, Pidoux I, Reiner A, et al. Damage to type II collagen in aging and osteoarthritis starts at the articular surface, originates around chondrocytes, and extends into the cartilage with progressive degeneration. J Clin Invest 1995;96:2859.
20. Squires GR, Okouneff S, Ionescu M, et al. The pathobiology of focal lesion development in aging human articular cartilage and molecular matrix changes characteristic of osteoarthritis. Arthritis Rheum 2003;48:1261.
21. Aurich M, Poole AR, Reiner A, et al. Matrix homeostasis in aging normal human ankle cartilage. Arthritis Rheum 2002;46:2903.
22. Maroudas A, Bayliss MT, Uchitel-Kaushansky N, et al. Aggrecan turnover in human articular cartilage: Use of aspartic acid racemization as a marker of molecular age. Arch Biochem Biophys 1998;350:61.
23. Buckwalter JA, Roughley PJ, Rosenberg LC. Age-related changes in cartilage proteoglycans: Quantitative electron microscopic studies. Microsc Res Tech 1994;28:398.
24. Dudhia J, Davidson CM, Wells TM, et al. Age-related changes in the content of the C-terminal region of aggrecan in human articular cartilage. Biochem J 1996;313(3):933.
25. Bayliss MT, Osborne D, Woodhouse S, et al. Sulfation of chondroitin sulfate in human articular cartilage: The effect of age, topographical position, and zone of cartilage on tissue composition. J Biol Chem 1999;274:15892.
26. Wells T, Davidson C, Morgelin M, et al. Age-related changes in the composition, the molecular stoichiometry and the stability of proteoglycan aggregates extracted from human articular cartilage. Biochem J 2003;370:69.
27. Grushko G, Schneiderman R, Maroudas A. Some biochemical and biophysical parameters for the study of the pathogenesis of osteoarthritis: A comparison between the processes of ageing and degeneration in human hip cartilage. Connect Tissue Res 1989;19:149.
28. Wilkins E, Dieppe P, Maddison P, et al. Osteoarthritis and articular chondrocalcinosis in the elderly. Ann Rheum Dis 1983;42:280.
29. Felson DT, Anderson JJ, Naimark A, et al. The prevalence of chondrocalcinosis in the elderly and its association with knee osteoarthritis: The Framingham Study. J Rheumatol 1989;16:1241.
30. Rosenthal AK, Derfus BA, Henry LA. Transglutaminase activity in aging articular chondrocytes and articular cartilage vesicles. Arthritis Rheum 1997;40:966.
31. Rosen F, McCabe G, Quach J, et al. Differential effects of aging on human chondrocyte responses to transforming growth factor beta: Increased pyrophosphate production and decreased cell proliferation. Arthritis Rheum 1997;40:1275.
32. Doherty M, Dieppe P. Clinical aspects of calcium pyrophosphate dihydrate crystal deposition. Rheum Dis Clin North Am 1988;14:395.

33. Bonner WM, Jonsson H, Malanos C, et al. Changes in the lipids of human articular cartilage with age. Arthritis Rheum 1975;18:461.

34. Verzijl N, Bank RA, TeKoppele JM, et al. AGEing and osteoarthritis: A different perspective. Curr Opin Rheumatol 2003;15:616.

35. Verzijl N, DeGroot J, Thorpe SR, et al. Effect of collagen turnover on the accumulation of advanced glycation endproducts. J Biol Chem 2000;275:39027.

36. Bank RA, Bayliss MT, Lafeber FP, et al. Ageing and zonal variation in post-translational modification of collagen in normal human articular cartilage: The age-related increase in non-enzymatic glycation affects on biomechanical properties of cartilage. Biochem J 1998;330(1):345.

37. Verzijl N, DeGroot J, Ben ZC, et al. Crosslinking by advanced glycation end products increases the stiffness of the collagen network in human articular cartilage: A possible mechanism through which age is a risk factor for osteoarthritis. Arthritis Rheum 2002;46:114.

38. Chen AC, Temple MM, Ng DM, et al. Induction of advanced glycation end products and alterations of the tensile properties of articular cartilage. Arthritis Rheum 2002;46:3212.

39. Schwab W, Friess U, Hempel U, et al. Immunohistochemical demonstration of (carboxymethyl)lysine protein adducts in normal and osteoarthritic cartilage. Histochem Cell Biol 2002;117:541.

40. Schleicher ED, Wagner E, Nerlich AG. Increased accumulation of the glycoxidation product N(epsilon)-(carboxymethyl)lysine in human tissues in diabetes and aging. J Clin Invest 1997;99:457.

41. Nerlich AG, Schleicher ED, Boos N. 1997 Volvo Award winner in basic science studies: Immunohistologic markers for age-related changes of human lumbar intervertebral discs. Spine 1997; 22:2781.

42. DeGroot J, Verzijl N, Wenting-van Wijk MJ, et al. Accumulation of advanced glycation end products as a molecular mechanism for aging as a risk factor in osteoarthritis. Arthritis Rheum 2004;50:1207.

43. Aigner T, Hemmel M, Neureiter D, et al. Apoptotic cell death is not a widespread phenomenon in normal aging and osteoarthritis human articular knee cartilage: A study of proliferation, programmed cell death (apoptosis), and viability of chondrocytes in normal and osteoarthritic human knee cartilage. Arthritis Rheum 2001;44:1304.

44. Alsalameh S, Amin R, Gemba T, et al. Identification of mesenchymal progenitor cells in normal and osteoarthritic human articular cartilage. Arthritis Rheum 2004;50:1522.

45. Horton WE Jr., Feng L, Adams C. Chondrocyte apoptosis in development, aging and disease. Matrix Biol 1998;17:107.

46. Aigner T, Kim HA, Roach HI. Apoptosis in osteoarthritis. Rheum Dis Clin North Am 2004;30:639.

47. Kuhn K, D'Lima DD, Hashimoto S, et al. Cell death in cartilage. Osteoarthritis Cartilage 2004;12:1.

48. Vignon E, Arlot M, Patricot LM, et al. The cell density of human femoral head cartilage. Clin Orthop 1976;121:303.

49. Jallali N, Ridha H, Thrasivoulou C, et al. Vulnerability to ROS-induced cell death in ageing articular cartilage: The role of antioxidant enzyme activity. Osteoarthritis Cartilage 2005;13:614.

50. Adams CS, Horton WE Jr. Chondrocyte apoptosis increases with age in the articular cartilage of adult animals. Anat Rec 1998;250:418.

51. Guerne PA, Blanco F, Kaelin A, et al. Growth factor responsiveness of human articular chondrocytes in aging and development. Arthritis Rheum 1995;38:960.

52. Martin JA, Buckwalter JA. Telomere erosion and senescence in human articular cartilage chondrocytes. J Gerontol A Biol Sci Med Sci 2001;56:B172.

53. Jones KL, Addison J. Pituitary fibroblast growth factor as a stimulator of growth in cultured rabbit articular chondrocytes. Endocrinology 1975;97:359.

54. Loeser RF, Shanker G. Autocrine stimulation by insulin-like growth factor 1 and insulin-like growth factor 2 mediates chondrocyte survival in vitro. Arthritis Rheum 2000;43:1552.

55. Loeser RF, Varnum BC, Carlson CS, et al. Human chondrocyte expression of growth-arrest-specific gene 6 and the tyrosine kinase receptor axl: Potential role in autocrine signaling in cartilage. Arthritis Rheum 1997;40:1455.

56. Yang C, Li SW, Helminen HJ, et al. Apoptosis of chondrocytes in transgenic mice lacking collagen II. Exp Cell Res 1997;235:370.

57. Pulai JI, Del Carlo M Jr., Loeser RF. The alpha5beta1 integrin provides matrix survival signals for normal and osteoarthritic human articular chondrocytes in vitro. Arthritis Rheum 2002;46:1528.

58. Martin JA, Ellerbroek SM, Buckwalter JA. Age-related decline in chondrocyte response to insulin-like growth factor-I: The role of growth factor binding proteins. J Orthop Res 1997;15:491.

59. Loeser RF, Shanker G, Carlson CS, et al. Reduction in the chondrocyte response to insulin-like growth factor 1 in aging and osteoarthritis: Studies in a non-human primate model of naturally occurring disease. Arthritis Rheum 2000;43:2110.

60. Messai H, Duchossoy Y, Khatib A, et al. Articular chondrocytes from aging rats respond poorly to insulin-like growth factor-1: An altered signaling pathway. Mech Ageing Dev 2000;115:21.

61. Dore S, Pelletier JP, DiBattista JA, et al. Human osteoarthritic chondrocytes possess an increased number of insulin-like growth factor 1 binding sites but are unresponsive to its stimulation: Possible role of IGF-1-binding proteins. Arthritis Rheum 1994;37:253.

62. Scharstuhl A, van Beuningen HM, Vitters EL, et al. Loss of transforming growth factor counteraction on interleukin 1 mediated effects in cartilage of old mice. Ann Rheum Dis 2002;61:1095.

63. Chubinskaya S, Kumar B, Merrihew C, et al. Age-related changes in cartilage endogenous osteogenic protein-1 (OP-1). Biochim Biophys Acta 2002;1588:126.

64. Wu W, Billinghurst RC, Pidoux I, et al. Sites of collagenase cleavage and denaturation of type II collagen in aging and osteoarthritic articular cartilage and their relationship to the distribution of matrix metalloproteinase 1 and matrix metalloproteinase 13. Arthritis Rheum 2002;46:2087.

65. Forsyth CB, Cole A, Murphy G, et al. Increased matrix metalloproteinase-13 production with aging by human articular chondrocytes in response to catabolic stimuli. J Gerontol A Biol Sci Med Sci 2005;60:1118.

66. Mitchell PG, Magna HA, Reeves LM, et al. Cloning, expression, and type II collagenolytic activity of matrix metalloproteinase-13 from human osteoarthritic cartilage. J Clin Invest 1996;97:761.

67. Billinghurst RC, Dahlberg L, Ionescu M, et al. Enhanced cleavage of type II collagen by collagenases in osteoarthritic articular cartilage. J Clin Invest 1997;99:1534.

68. DeGroot J, Verzijl N, Bank RA, et al. Age-related decrease in proteoglycan synthesis of human articular chondrocytes: The role of nonenzymatic glycation. Arthritis Rheum 1999;42:1003.

69. Loeser RF, Yammani RR, Carlson CS, et al. Articular chondrocytes express the receptor for advanced glycation end products: Potential role in osteoarthritis. Arthritis Rheum 2005;52:2376.

70. Harman D. Aging: A theory based on free radical and radiation chemistry. J Gerontol 1956;11:298.

71. Finkel T, Holbrook NJ. Oxidants, oxidative stress and the biology of ageing. Nature 2000;408:239.

72. Studer R, Jaffurs D, Stefanovic-Racic M, et al. Nitric oxide in osteoarthritis. Osteoarthritis Cartilage 1999;7:377.

73. Hiran TS, Moulton PJ, Hancock JT. Detection of superoxide and NADPH oxidase in porcine articular chondrocytes. Free Radic Biol Med 1997;23:736.

74. Tiku ML, Shah R, Allison GT. Evidence linking chondrocyte lipid peroxidation to cartilage matrix protein degradation: Possible role in cartilage aging and the pathogenesis of osteoarthritis. J Biol Chem 2000;275:20069.

75. Del Carlo M Jr., Loeser RF. Increased oxidative stress with aging reduces chondrocyte survival: Correlation with intracellular glutathione levels. Arthritis Rheum 2003;48:3419.

76. Loeser RF, Carlson CS, Carlo MD, et al. Detection of nitrotyrosine in aging and osteoarthritic cartilage: Correlation of oxidative damage with the presence of interleukin-1beta and with chondrocyte resistance to insulin-like growth factor 1. Arthritis Rheum 2002;46:2349.

77. Reiter CD, Teng RJ, Beckman JS. Superoxide reacts with nitric oxide to nitrate tyrosine at physiological pH via peroxynitrite. J Biol Chem 2000;275:32460.

78. Henrotin YE, Bruckner P, Pujol JP. The role of reactive oxygen species in homeostasis and degradation of cartilage. Osteoarthritis Cartilage 2003;11:747.

79. Nelson KK, Melendez JA. Mitochondrial redox control of matrix metalloproteinases. Free Radic Biol Med 2004;37:768.

# 6 Adipokines in Osteoarthritis

Nathalie Presle, Pascale Pottie, Didier Mainard, Patrick Netter, and Bernard Terlain

## INTRODUCTION

Osteoarthritis (OA) is the most common joint disease in humans. It is a primary cause of decreased activity in daily living and quality of life after middle age. This pathology affects more than 5% of adults worldwide,[1] and this percentage increases with aging population.

OA has been usually regarded as a disease whose central pathologic feature is hyaline cartilage and the result of age and trauma.[2] However, this concept has evolved. It is now well established that OA is an inflammatory disease that affects also many periarticular tissues such as bone, muscles, ligaments, joint capsule, and synovium. If its exact etiology is not established, some risk factors are well known (including mechanical, biochemical, genetic, and other factors).

Indeed, breakdown and synthesis inhibition of matrix molecules such as proteoglycan and collagen are the pathologic events leading to imbalance of cartilage homeostasis. These involve inflammatory cytokines, metalloproteases, and growth factors with a pivotal role. However, regarding OA as a whole-organ disease it is possible to speculate that several components (structural or not) or disturbed factors could favor or contribute to its progression—suggesting a potential cross-talk between them and cartilage. Thus, many authors suggest that OA is a disease of bone, including osteophyte formation, bony eburnation, entesophytes, abnormal ossification, and so on. They further suggest that bone may be the primary organ triggering OA.[3-5] Concomitant with subchondral bone changes, the loss of cartilage properties in relation with metabolic and biomechanical factors explains the progressive loss of articular function.

This concept of "metabolic disease" is in good accordance with the relationship between a high body mass index (BMI) and an increased risk of OA.[6-8] This positive association between overweight/obesity and OA is observed not only for knee joints but for non weight-bearing joints such as the hands,[9,10] suggesting that systemic or local factors may contribute to OA. These factors may concern cartilage, bone, and fat tissue as a link with obesity. Adipocytes share common mesenchymal stem cell precursors with osteoblasts and chondrocytes, which suggests a link between lipid metabolism and connective tissues.[11]

Today, adipose tissue has been recognized as a real endocrine organ that releases many factors acting in endocrine, autocrine, and paracrine manners.[12] These factors may derive from adipose tissue (subcutaneous, visceral, and so on) and from specific or local sources such as the infrapatellar fat pad in the knee joint.[13] Adipokines are important components of the neuroendocrine-immune network and are molecular links between obesity and several pathologies.[14,15] Their potential contribution as metabolic factors is in good accordance with a recent hypothesis supporting OA as a systemic disorder in relation to lipid metabolism.[16] So far, studies have revealed some fat-derived molecules linking inflammation and arthritis, but no factor involved in degenerative articular disease is known at present. One objective of the material following is to evaluate the relationship between OA and adipokines, particularly in regard to clinically established OA.

## ADIPOSE TISSUE

### A Secretory Organ

Adipose tissue is a specialized connective tissue found in several locations throughout the body. The main cellular components are mature lipid-filled adipocytes, lipid-free preadipocytes, endothelial cells, and additional cells in the form of nerve fibers and monocytes/macrophages.[17] The size of fat cells is variable. Fat cells from lean humans have an average cell diameter of about 70 μm, whereas fat cells from obese subjects can reach a mean diameter of about 120 μm. Adipocyte cellularity is also highly variable, depending on age, gender, body weight, and regional origin. Substantial morphologic differences are seen between the subcutaneous and visceral fat depots.

The omental adipose tissue has more blood vessels and sympathetic nerve fibers than subcutaneous depots,

85

indicating a greater metabolic activity in the former. In addition, omental adipose tissue contains more monocytes/macrophages than subcutaneous fat. This means that each adipose tissue may have particular metabolic impacts and that the distribution of body fat may be even more important than the total amount of fat.[18] Until recently, adipose tissue was considered to serve only as a triglyceride reservoir and was relegated to a passive storage organ for excess energy. In the case of a chronic positive energy balance the excess calories are converted into triglycerides, whereas in the case of undernutrition and high energy demand triglycerides are rapidly mobilized.

This classical view of adipose tissue as a specialized passive storage organ has fully changed with the discovery of leptin,[19] and particularly with explosive expansion of research regarding the prevalence of obesity in developed nations. Adipose tissue is a dynamic endocrine cellular system that is continually active in the highly regulated uptake storage and release of lipids and in the secretion of hormones, cytokines, and growth factors.[20] The concept that adipose tissue is both a dynamic endocrine organ and a highly active metabolic tissue has become fully accepted. Fat produces and secretes many factors in an integrated network that maintains an intensive communication between adipose tissue and other organs.

These different secretions are necessary for normal physiologic homeostasis.[21] However, it is tempting to speculate that an impaired or imbalanced secretion of such factors may be involved in pathophysiologic conditions (such as those linked to obesity-associated complications[17] as metabolic and vascular diseases and as obesity-related articular pathologies).[7,16] To date, more than 100 mediators have been described to be produced and released by adipocytes. These cells secrete not only a variety of peptides and proteins but also prostaglandins, steroid hormones, and low-molecular-weight components. All of these products are released by adipocytes and by other cells of adipose tissue, such as adipocyte precursor cells, endothelial cells, and so on. Preadipocytes and macrophages may thus have an important role in the production of molecules and could contribute to the enhanced release of pro-inflammatory mediators, particularly in the adipose tissue of obese populations.[22,23]

Human pre-adipose cells behave as multipotent mesenchymal stem cells and are obviously capable of developing into other cells types in addition to differentiation into adipocytes. Thus, preadipocytes may be able to differentiate into myocytes, chondrocytes,[24] and osteoblasts,[16] as well as into macrophages, cardiomyocytes, and so on. This new perspective may open a new area of cellular therapy,[17] but also could be regarded in the scope of a local cellular pathologic contribution.

Clinical observations have confirmed the differential behavior of the various adipose tissue depots for their factor secretions. Thus, abdominal fat distribution with increased visceral fat mass is closely associated with the adverse metabolic and cardiovascular consequences of obesity.[25] There is evidence that substantial differences may also exist for the secretory pattern of fat cells from subcutaneous and omental adipose tissue.[26] In addition, specific fat tissue—such as infrapatellar fat pad ("Hoffa ligament") in human knee joint—may release adipokines in the articular cavity.

## Adipokines and Secreted Compounds

As developing pre-adipocytes differentiate to become mature adipocytes, they acquire the ability to synthesize more than a hundred proteins (many of which are released as cytokines, growth factors, and hormones). These protein signals, derived from adipose tissue, were initially referred to as "adipocytokines."[27] The alternative name today is "adipokine,"[28] to describe a protein that is secreted and synthesized by adipocytes rather than by adipose tissue. The main reason for this is that cells (such as macrophages) that also secrete protein signals are found in many organs, as well as in many adipose tissues.[29]

Thus, some differences may be found among the adipokines released by adipose tissue, adipose tissue matrix, and adipocytes.[30] In addition, the term *adipokine* may concern the protein secreted from white and brown adipocytes.[28] Thus, the totality of secreted proteins from adipocytes constitutes the adipokinome, and the totality of the molecules secreted by the adipocytes (adipokinome and other lipid substances) constitutes the secretome of the adipocytes. At the moment, more than 50 adipokines have been documented (their main functional domains are represented in Fig. 6.1).

The earliest adipokine identified was the enzyme lipoprotein lipase, followed by adipsin (a component of the alternative complement pathway). The discovery of leptin in 1994 was a key development that led to our understanding of adipose tissue importance.

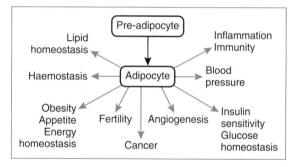

Fig. 6.1 Associated with terminal fat cell differentiation, a simplified classification of functional domains of adipokines.

Figure 6.2 shows the contribution of some adipokines[31] and other adipose-derived proteins in the main functional domains depicted in Fig. 6.1. The last discovered adipokine (visfatin)[32,33] is a new adipose factor involved in fat and sugar metabolism. Three of these hormones (TNF-α, resistin, and IL-6) induce resistance to insulin.

Adiponectin and visfatin act synergistically with insulin to enhance glucose uptake and metabolism in muscle and to inhibit gluconeogenesis in liver. Visfatin is an insulin mimetic, lowering plasma glucose levels in mice. Visfatin binds to the insulin receptor but does not compete with insulin, suggesting that insulin and visfatin bind to different sites. This new adipokine, initially described as pre-B-cell colony-enhancing factor (PBEF), could serve as a model for studying other insulin-mimetic molecules.[34]

Three adipokines (leptin, adiponectin, and resistin) are at the moment the main subjects of investigations.

These "big three" have major biological properties in high emergent pathologies (obesity, atherosclerosis, and diabetes) and may have between them opposite or complementary biological properties.

The contribution of these adipokines to articular degenerative pathologies may be suggested for the following reasons: detection of these three adipokines in the synovial fluid of OA and RA patients,[35] secretory activity of articular fat tissue,[13] leptin relation with obesity and satiety,[36,37] leptin regulatory effects on bone tissue,[38,39] their relation to inflammatory cytokines,[13] their relations to inflammatory or anti-inflammatory processes,[40-42] and their sensitivity to the regulating effect of PPAR.[43,44] In the following, we discuss the biochemical and biological properties of leptin, adiponectin, and resistin. Thereafter, we discuss findings that show the potential contribution of these adipokines to OA pathophysiology.

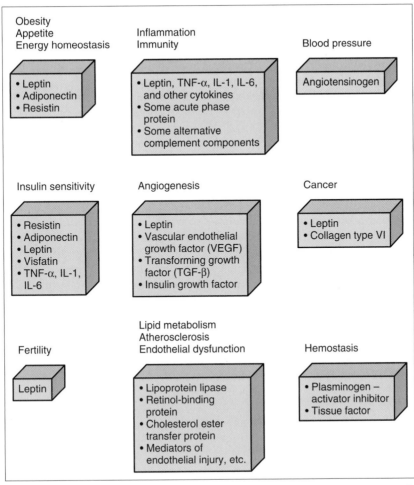

**Fig. 6.2** A simplified view of the involvement of some adipokines and other adipose-derived protein compounds in the main functional domains described in Fig. 6.1.

## Main Adipokines

### Leptin

Evidence for the existence of a physiologic system regulating body weight has accumulated over several decades. It was proposed that the amount of energy stored in adipose tissue represented the balance between ingested calories and energy expenditure.[45,46] This model was supported by studies in rodents in which forced over-feeding resulted in an inhibition of voluntary feeding, whereas food deprivation or surgical removal of adipose tissue stimulated food intake until body weight was restored.[47] Further experiments provided evidence that a factor emanating from adipose tissue signaled the brain to regulate body weight and fat content.[48]

A revolution occurred with the discovery that leptin is a circulating factor[49] related to adipose tissue. Leptin, the product of the ob gene,[19] is a 16-kDa protein monomer that regulates body weight and appetite.[50] A rise in leptin levels was proposed to prevent obesity by decreasing appetite and increasing thermogenesis through action in the brain. However, leptin is not only an anti-obesity hormone but is viewed now as a more complex factor (as an adipokine) acting in an intricate network that links nutrition, metabolism, and immune homeostasis (along with a growing number of other functions).[51] An understanding of the biology of leptin offers significant insights into the complex relationships among adipose tissue (and its other adipokines), the nervous system, and peripheral organs—such as those related to articular pathologies (see Table 6.1).

### Ob Gene and Leptin Production

The mouse ob gene encodes a 4.5-kilobase mRNA transcript with a highly conserved 167-amino-acid open reading frame.[19] Mouse and human ob genes have been localized to chromosomes 6 and 7, respectively.[19] Several regulatory elements have been identified within the ob gene promoter (including cyclic AMP, glucocorticoid-responsive elements, CCATT/enhancer, and SP1 binding sites),[52] suggesting a direct regulation of leptin expression through membrane and transcriptional pathways.[53] Leptin is synthesized mainly by adipose tissue and released into the blood. Leptin is also produced at a lower level in other tissues, such as the stomach,[54] skeletal muscle, placenta, and so on. Leptin is highly conserved among species. For example, human leptin is 84% identical to mouse leptin and 83% identical to rat leptin.[55]

Structural analysis has indicated that leptin is similar to cytokines. In C57 Bl/6J ob/ob mice, a C-to-T substitution results in synthesis of a truncated protein that is not secreted.[19,56] In the ob2J/ob2J mutant, a transposon inserted into the first intron of the gene prevents the synthesis of mature ob mRNA. Both ob/ob mouse mutants are leptin deficient, hyperphagic, hypothermic, and obese.[56] Rare human ob gene mutations have been reported in Pakistani and Turkish families.

Leptin expression is modulated by the level of energy stores in fat, as shown by obese people having higher leptin mRNA and protein than lean individuals.[36] The adipocyte size is also related to leptin synthesis, as larger adipocytes contain more leptin than smaller ones. Leptin levels seem regulated by a constitutive mechanism and by various physiologic states. In fact, leptin level may be a long-term regulator of body adiposity and may limit food intake on a meal-to-meal basis by regulating a central response to short-acting satiety signals.[37]

Some authors propose that forebrain signaling by adiposity signal (such as by leptin) and hindbrain by satiety signals—from cholecystokinin (CCK) and others from the gastrointestinal tract—are partially related to (respectively) the regulation of changes in body fat and food intake. Leptin signaling in the forebrain (adiposity signals) also controls meal size by modulating the hindbrain response to satiety signals such as CCK. This could explain how the response to satiety signals is impaired by the absence of leptin signaling, thereby favoring the consumption of larger meals rather than an increased number of meals.

Many other factors can be implicated in leptin regulation. Some of these (acting on adipose tissue) are outlined in Table 6.2, which emphasizes the importance of insulin and steroid hormones. Leptin increases during acute infection, in response to endotoxin and pro-inflammatory cytokines.[57] In humans, leptin levels are higher in females than in males. This difference may be due to a stimulatory effect of estrogens on adipose tissue in females, and to a suppressive effect of testosterone in males.[58,59] The reverse is seen with rodents. The regulation of leptin gene expression varies according to tissue, with glucosamine as a nutrient-sensing pathway for regulating gene expression in fat and muscle[60] and a hypoxia-induced increase in leptin expression in placenta.[61]

| TABLE 6.1  FACTORS REGULATING LEPTIN IN ADIPOSE TISSUE | |
| --- | --- |
| • Increase of leptin | • Decrease of leptin |
| • Feeding up | • Fasting |
| • High BMI | • Cold exposure |
| • Insulin | • β adrenergic agonists |
| • Glucocorticoids | • Testosterone |
| • Pro-inflammatory cytokines | • PPARγ agonists |

**TABLE 6.2 INFLUENCE OF THIAZOLINEDIONE (TZD), DEXAMETHAZONE (DEX), INSULIN, AND ISOPROTERENOL ON GENE RESISTIN EXPRESSION[a]**

| | Insulin | TZD | DEX | Isoproterenol |
|---|---|---|---|---|
| White adipose tissue | ↓ | ↓ | ↑ | ↓ |
| Brown adipose tissue | ↑ | ↑ | ↓ | ↓ |

[a]↓ = repression, ↑ = induction.

### Leptin Receptors

Leptin acts via transmembrane receptors (obR), which show structural similarity to those of the cytokine families.[62] Leptin receptors are the products of the diabetes (db) gene,[63] which is alternatively spliced to produce at least six isoforms: obRa, obRb, obRc, obRd, obRe, and obRf.

Leptin receptors share a common extracellular leptin-binding domain but differ at the carboxy terminus intracellular domain (Fig. 6.3). Only the long isoform obRb has intracellular motifs necessary for JAK/STAT signaling and activation. ObRa, obRc, obRd, and obRf have transmembrane domains but have shorter C-terminal domains. Short C-terminal receptors may have a role in leptin's access to some regions, such as leptin crossing the blood/brain barrier.[64,65] The affinity of leptin for its binding site is in the nanomolar range. ObRe lacks a transmembrane domain and circulates as a soluble receptor. This isoform does not play a direct role in leptin signaling but is important in determining the amount of bioavailable leptin in the circulation.[66,67] Soluble receptors (which may play key roles in, for example, pregnancy)[69] can be generated by alternative splicing of obR mRNA (obRe) and/or ectodomain shedding of membrane-spanning receptors.[68]

The db/db mutation is produced by insertion of a premature stop codon in the 3′ end of obRb RNA transcript, resulting in synthesis of obRa. Under these conditions, db/db mice are hyperphagic and obese and do not respond to leptin.[70] ObR mutations have also been discovered in rats, producing Zucker fatty (fa/fa) rats[71] with a low binding to leptin and the obese Koletsky rats (SHROB, fak).[72,73]

Mutations of human ob receptors are rare. A single nucleotide substitution in a French family produces an obR lacking both transmembrane and intracellular domains.[74] The mutant receptor circulates at high concentrations bound to leptin and induces obesity and several endocrine dysfunctions.

### Leptin Signaling

As with other class I cytokine receptors—such as IL-6, leukemia inhibitory factor (LIF), oncostatin M (OSM), ciliary neurotrophic factor (CNTF), and others—the leptin signal mainly occurs through the JAK/STAT pathway.[75-78] However, leptin can also signal by alternative pathways.[77,79] Leptin signaling through the JAK2/STAT pathway has been described in several major reviews.[55,67] Briefly, leptin receptors have no intrinsic tyrosine kinase activity and their major signaling events are dependent on association with kinases such as JAK2. Leptin binding to obR and subsequent oligomerization allows juxtaposition of JAKs, which induces phosphorylation and activation of the leptin receptors or other substrates. All of the membrane-bound leptin receptors contain in their cytoplasmic tail a box-1 motif, whereas box-2 and -3 motifs are found only in the long isoform ObRb.

Domains 1 and 2 are involved in the interaction and activation of JAK-2 tyrosine kinase to phosphorylate and activate members of the STAT family of transcription factors, such as STAT 1, 3, and 5. STAT 3 activation has been characterized in the hypothalamus and required a box-3 motif in the receptor intracellular domain.[79,80] Activated JAK-2 phosphorylates tyrosine residues in the intracellular domain of ObRb, supplying binding motifs for SHP-2 and STAT proteins.[81,82] These activated transcription factors translocate to the nucleus, where they transactivate target genes by binding to specific promotor elements.[78,83] Leptin regulates the expression of STAT3-dependent genes in hypothalamic neurons expressing ObRb, which include *c-fos*, *c-jun*, genes encoding many neuropeptides (such as agouti-related peptide, cocaine, and amphetamine-regulated

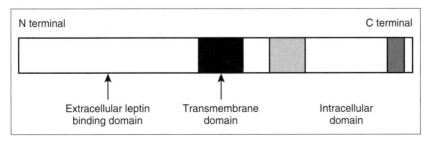

**Fig. 6.3** ObRb receptor domains.

transcript or CART, and so on),[84] and the suppressor of cytokine signaling-3 (SOCS-3).

SOCS proteins induced by leptin and cytokines act as negative feedback regulators.[84,85] Overexpression of SOCS-3 inhibits leptin-mediated tyrosine phosphorylation of JAK-2.[85,86] Protein-tyrosine phosphatase (PTP-1B) is, conversely, a downstream regulator of leptin signal transduction.[87] Overexpression of PTP-1B decreases phosphorylation of JAK-2 and blocks leptin-induced transcription of SOCS-3 when deletion of PTP-1B gene-enhanced leptin sensitivity occurs in mice and thus prevents obesity.[88,89]

These findings suggest an important role of the JAK/STAT pathway in leptin signaling, but some rapid effects of leptin cannot be explained solely by gene expression[90] because leptin inhibits NPY secretion from hypothalamic explants[91] and is able to rapidly regulate glucose-sensitive neurons in the brain and insulin secretion from pancreatic islet.[92] Leptin receptors may use alternative signaling pathways. ObRb stimulates tyrosine phosphorylation of IRS-1, PI3-kinase activity, and SHP-2-dependent ERK-1/2 activation.[83,93] Leptin is also able to induce phosphorylation of P38MAP kinase in human mononuclear cells.[94] Several other signaling pathways have been described.[41,66]

### Biological Activities of Leptin

Leptin circulates partially bound to plasma proteins[95] and to obRe, and the free leptin is increased in serum of obese subjects.[96] The free form of leptin determines its bioavailability to target tissues and thus the biological activity of this adipokine. Investigations on binding of leptin to the soluble form of its receptor obRe may thus provide further information on the potential effects of circulating and local leptin on various tissues.

### Central Effects of Leptin

Leptin enters the rat brain by a saturable transport system,[97] possibly through the short isoforms of leptin receptor. ObRa is highly expressed in the blood/brain barrier and is able to bind and to internalize leptin. Leptin plays various physiologic roles, but it is primarily involved in energy homeostasis and satiety—making a link between the periphery and the brain (serum leptin levels increase with fat mass to convey information to the hypothalamus regarding the amount of energy stored in adipose tissue, suppressing appetite and increasing energy expenditure). Mice deficient in leptin (ob/ob mice[19]) or in leptin receptor (db/db mice[70]) are hyperphagic, hyperinsulinemic, and obese. Chronic administration of leptin to the ob/ob mice induces sustained reduction in body weight and food intake, but has no effect on the db/db mice.

It is well established that food intake and body weight are regulated by interactions between hormonal and neural mechanisms,[98-102] and several hypothalamus sites (such as the arcuate nucleus [ARC]) are the major sites for integration of central and peripheral signals. Briefly, ARC has two opposing sets of neuronal pathways: an appetite-stimulating pathway (orexigenic) and an appetite-inhibiting pathway (anorexigenic). These two pathways send signals mainly to the paraventricular nucleus (PVN) and to other nuclei of the hypothalamus, which then directly modulate feeding behavior.[102]

Orexigenic and anorexigenic pathways are influenced by peripheral hormonal signals capable of crossing the blood/brain barrier with leptin and several others (i.e., insulin, ghrelin, and peptide YY). When activated, the orexigenic pathway produces neuropeptide Y (NPY) and agouti-related peptide (AGRP), which in turn promote appetite. The anorexigenic pathway involves cocaine/amphetamine-regulated transcript (CART) and pro-opiomelanocortin (POMC), which produce α-melanocyte-stimulating hormone (α-MSH).

This latter hormone decreases appetite mainly through the melanocortin type 4 receptor.[100] Leptin triggers the anorexigenic pathway through up-regulation of α-MSH and inhibits the orexigenic pathway by suppressing NPY and AGRP mRNA expressions in the hypothalamus. The appetite-regulating effect of leptin is probably more complex than described, involving many other factors and other neural pathways[103] in the regulation of long-term and short-term[37] satiety signals. It is also more complicated in terms of explaining how the leptin-resistance phenomenon seen in obesity is overcome.[104,105]

### Peripheral Effects of Leptin

In addition to its central effects, leptin also plays several main roles at the periphery.[106]

## Hematopoiesis and Angiogenesis

ObR is expressed in hematopoietic cells, and leptin may be involved in the proliferation and differentiation of hematopoietic precursors.[107,108] High concentrations of human leptin, similar to plasma leptin levels measured in obese individuals, are able to promote platelet aggregation.[109] Vascular endothelium has been shown in rodents and humans to express the long form of leptin receptor, and leptin stimulates angiogenesis through VEGF overexpression.[110,111] A study[112] demonstrated an accelerating effect of leptin on wound repair in diabetic mice after binding to its receptors at the wound site.

## Fertility and Pregnancy

Leptin plays a role in reproduction through central and peripheral effects.[107] Male and female ob/ob mice are sterile, with a reduced level of reproductive hormones in ob/ob females. Repeated administration of human leptin to female ob/ob mice restored ovulation, pregnancy, parturition, and lactation, showing that leptin plays an essential role in the endocrine process controlling fertility.

In vitro studies showed that leptin mRNA expression increases in response to estrogen but is inhibited by testosterone, suggesting that androgens and estrogens modulate leptin expression through a sex steroid receptor-dependent transcriptional mechanism.[113] Human ovary and prostate express mRNA for the leptin receptor,[114] and ObR expression has been demonstrated in human granulosa cells.[115] In addition, a significant increase in circulating leptin occurs during controlled ovarian hyperstimulation.[116]

The importance of leptin in pregnancy is demonstrated by the high expression of leptin and its receptor in placenta and fetus, suggesting a role for leptin as a possible fetal growth factor. Human and animal studies suggest that placental leptin affects maternal, placental, and fetal leptin functions through several mechanisms.

## Leptin and Insulin

Insulin that stimulates uptake of glucose, free fatty acid, and amino acid by tissues is an important regulator of energy homeostasis—suggesting a link between leptin and insulin in this process. Many studies provide evidence for a regulatory role of insulin on leptin gene expression and secretion in adipocytes due to increased glucose transport and metabolism.[117] Conversely, leptin might influence directly β cells[118] through activation of its receptors in pancreatic cells.[119] However, contradictory results have indicated an inhibitory effect of leptin on insulin secretion by pancreatic cells and on insulin binding or insulin effects in adipocytes.[120,121] Regulatory effects between leptin and insulin may also occur in skeletal muscles. In these tissues, there is a large proportion of insulin-stimulated glucose uptake and lipid oxidation. In addition, leptin mRNA and leptin receptors (obRa and obRb) have been found in mouse skeletal muscle.[122-125]

## Additional Major Adipokines

Among adipokines, adiponectin and resistin are more specifically associated with leptin in playing key roles in the regulation of insulin action, inflammation, homeostasis, and some pathologic events associated with their dysregulation (such as diabetes, obesity, cardiovascular diseases, and so on).[126-134]

### Adiponectin

Human adiponectin—also called "gelatine-binding protein" (gbp 28, 28 kDa), "adipocyte complement-related protein" (Acrp30, 30 kDa), and "adipoQ"[135-139]—is a protein of 247 amino acids (30 kDa) and is coded by the gene apM1 (most abundant adipose gene transcript protein). Human adiponectin has four domains: a signal sequence (N terminal), followed by a hypervariable region, a collagen domain, and a C-terminal globular domain with C1q analogy. Its 3D structure is similar to that of TNF-α.[130,137] Endogenous adiponectin is post-translationally modified to result in eight different isoforms.[130]

The globular head appears to be as efficient as full-length adiponectin in some conditions, and forms trimers-dimers and high-molecular-weight complexes in the circulation.[130,135] Different properties have been ascribed to various recombinant or processed forms (globular head) of the protein, and the active form(s) has not yet been fully determined.[135,140] Adiponectin produced by mammalian cells is much more potent than bacterially generated adiponectin (in enhancing insulin sensitivity) in relation to trimers, hexamers, or higher molecular forms.[140]

In contrast to leptin, the levels of adiponectin in plasma are negatively correlated with BMI, body fat, and resting insulin levels.[141-143] Adiponectin seems to be an important hormone in the regulation of lipid metabolism and insulin action, enhancing glucose uptake in muscle and increasing fatty acid oxidation both in muscle and liver and possibly activating signal cascade of insulin in these tissues.

A longitudinal study in type 2 diabetic Rhesus monkeys[147] showed that a strong positive correlation was found between adiponectin and insulin-stimulated glucose uptake.[131,144] A study confirmed the connection between adiponectin levels and insulin resistance.[145] Thiazolinediones (TZD) improve insulin resistance and significantly increase plasma adiponectin concentration, both in humans and rodents.[145-147] Adiponectin gene expression in human visceral adipose tissue is negatively regulated by glucocorticoids and TNF-α, and positively by insulin and IGF-1.[148] Its physiologic role remains to be fully clarified, but experimental data suggest that it may play an important role in modulating insulin action and that it has anti-inflammatory and anti-atherogenic properties.[128-130]

The cloning of human and mouse adiponectin receptors has been reported.[149] These receptors (called AdipoR1 and AdipoR2) are expressed in skeletal muscle and liver (respectively) and can bind both globular and full-length adiponectin. They have seven transmembrane domains, but are very different from G-protein-coupled receptors. They mediate AMP kinase and PPARα activities, producing an increase in fatty acid oxidation and glucose uptake.[150] Both receptors have been found in mouse and human pancreatic B cells. Their expression was shown to increase in response to unsatured free fatty acids, providing a new mechanism modulating the regulatory effects of adiponectin on insulin sensitivity.[130,151] The increase in fatty acid oxidation mediated by adiponectin may also occur through AMPK activation.[130,152,153]

## Resistin

Resistin (also called "adipose-tissue-specific secretory factor,"[154] FIZZ-3[155]) is a 12.5-kDa cysteine-rich peptide secreted from adipocytes and present in the circulation. Its discovery derived from investigations on the stimulatory effect of thiazolidinediones (PPARγ agonists) on glucose uptake in skeletal muscles.[156] It was postulated that thiazolidinediones decrease the production of an unidentified adipose hormone that is able to mediate insulin resistance. Resistin is a protein up-regulated during adipocyte differentiation and down-regulated in mature adipocytes by rosiglitazone (thiazolidinedione PPARγ agonists). Resistin is one of a series of proteins now known as resistin-like molecules.[157]

Human resistin has 108 amino acids and is a disulfide-linked homodimer circulating in human blood as dimeric protein of two 92-amino-acid polypeptides.[158,159] Resistin can also dimerize as heterodimers, through a disulfide bond using or not using the N-terminal-cysteine (CYS-26).[159-162] Resistin was expressed in several tissues, including adrenal cortex of rat,[163] mouse pituitary gland,[164] and rat and human[156,157] hypothalamus and white adipose tissue.[165,166] Resistin is secreted from mature human adipocytes[167] and preadipocytes, and abdominal subcutaneous and omental fats have higher amount of resistin than thigh and mammary fat in human. Resistin is also detected in brown adipose tissue[165,168] and in synovial fluid of patients with rheumatoid arthritis (RA) and OA (discussed in material following).[35]

Resistin production is regulated by various factors, depending on cell type and adipose tissue. Thus, in adipocyte cell lines (3T3-L1) or in vivo (mice, rats) several factors can modulate resistin expression.[164] However, clear differences between promoting or inhibiting properties appear between white and brown adipose tissues.[170] These differences (outlined in Table 6.3) suggest that resistin may have various regulatory effects on energy metabolism and thermogenesis.

For several other factors, conflicting results are obtained on resistin expression in adipocytes, in other cells, or in vivo in response to lipopolysaccharide, TNF-α, IL-6, and gender.[165] The functions of resistin are not fully established.[169] Steppan et al.[156,157] proposed that resistin is increased in type 2 diabetes and thus may be a link between obesity and insulin resistance. The injection of recombinant resistin into mice reduces glucose tolerance and insulin action, when resistin neutralization with antibodies improves insulin action. In addition, resistin increases blood glucose and insulin concentrations, impairing hypoglycemic response to insulin infusion in mice. Some studies demonstrated that obesity (high-fat diet) and mutations of the leptin gene (ob/ob mice) or its receptor (db/db mice) are associated in mice with increased circulating resistin levels.

These results suggest that resistin induces insulin resistance and that its increased level in blood contributes to impaired insulin sensitivity in obese rodents.[170] However, other data do not confirm these results.[171-173] Initial observational and interventional studies in humans failed to support a role for circulating resistin in regulating insulin resistance.[174-176]

## ADIPOKINE CONTRIBUTIONS TO OSTEOARTHRITIS

OA is a degenerative joint disorder and represents one of the most frequent and disabling diseases encountered in elderly people. In the early stages of the disease, the cartilage surface undergoes fibrillations before full-thickness matrix loss. OA changes are not limited to cartilage because remodeling of the underlying bone and development of osteophytes are also observed in osteoarthritic joints. Obesity represents a potent risk factor for the development and the progression of OA. The overload effect may explain most of the increased risk for OA of the knee and hip among overweight persons.

However, the risk factor for developing OA in non weight-bearing joints (such as the hands) was also shown to be associated with increased BMI.[9,10] In addition, if it is accepted that weight loss prevents changes during OA Toda et al. found that the loss of body fat is more closely related to symptomatic benefit than is the loss of body weight.[177] Taken together, these findings suggest that OA may be driven by metabolic disorders and that adipose factors may provide a metabolic link between obesity and OA. This hypothesis is emphasized by the recent concept that obesity is characterized by a chronic low grade of inflammation.[178-182]

More specifically, leptin is an efferent message (from adipose tissue) associated with the "metabolic syndrome."[183] This syndrome is characterized by insulin resistance and dyslipidemia that lead to type 2

| Tissue | Leptin Released During 48 Hours (pg/mg tissue ± sem) |
|---|---|
| Synovium | 14.7 ± 3.55 |
| Fat pad | 14.35 ± 4.59 |
| Meniscus | 1.15 ± 0.28 |
| Osteophytes | 22.05 ± 2.50 |
| Cartilage | 0.54 ± 0.05 |
| Bone | 1.84 ± 0.36 |

**TABLE 6.3  RELEASE OF LEPTIN BY ARTICULAR TISSUES[a]**

[a]From Presle et al.

diabetes, cardiovascular disease, or obesity (all of which are potentially associated with degenerative joint disease). Moreover, adipocytes share a common mesenchymal stem-cell precursor with osteoblasts and chondrocytes, suggesting that similar mechanisms may regulate the production of their respective extracellular matrix. Because leptin was shown to control bone growth, and is thus considered an endocrine bone regulator,[184-188] one can speculate that this adipokine and other adipose-derived proteins may contribute to changes associated with OA.

Based on these data and because of the high prevalence of obesity in most industrialized countries, the role of adipokines in the development of joint disorders has been the aim of increasing investigations. Synovial fluid and articular tissues obtained from patients with OA or RA were analyzed to evaluate the production of leptin, adiponectin, and resistin in the joint space. In addition, the expression of leptin and its receptor in the cartilage from OA-affected joints and the effect of leptin on chondrocytes have been investigated.

## Adipokines in the Synovial Fluid

OA can affect every synovial joint but is more frequent in the hand, knee, hip, and spine. These joints consist of two bone ends covered by articular cartilage. The joint stability is maintained by a fibrous joint capsule that encloses the joint and is covered on its inner surface by a confining sheet of tissue called synovial membrane.

Synovial fluid may be considered mainly as an ultra-filtrate of plasma, generated by capillaries just beneath the synovial surface. Synovial fluid is not a static pool, but is continually being absorbed and replenished by the synovial lining of the joint. Intra-articular fluid pressure is an important factor that affects net flow across synovial interstitium and promotes drainage from whole-joint cavity. Synovial fluid has two main functions. First, by containing lubricating molecules secreted by synovial lining cells (such as hyaluronan and lubricin) it lubricates the cartilaginous and synovial surfaces during joint movement.

Second, it supplies nutrients to (and removes waste products from) the chondrocytes, which have no direct blood supply. Synovial fluid exploration may provide a dynamic indication of the metabolic activity of the whole articular tissues, and local changes in the concentrations of soluble factors in this biological fluid may have important pathophysiologic implications.

Recent studies have been conducted to determine adipokine levels in the synovial fluid obtained from OA- or RA-affected joints, especially for leptin, adiponectin, and resistin.[35,189-191] The three adipose-derived proteins are detected in the synovial fluid obtained from patients with OA or RA with concentrations falling within the range of values measured in serum. As is found in serum, adiponectin is the most abundant adipokine detected in the joint. Leptin levels in synovial fluid from OA patients correlate with BMI,[190] and synovial fluid concentrations of both adiponectin and resistin have been shown to be higher in patients with RA than in those with OA.[35]

When paired samples of synovial fluid and serum obtained from patients with OA are examined, the adipokines exhibit different patterns of distribution between the joint and the circulating compartment. Serum levels of resistin and adiponectin exceed those in the paired synovial fluid.[189] Leptin contrasts with the other adipokines in that synovial fluid concentrations are higher than the serum counterparts in female patients, and are similar to corresponding serum values in male patients. By contrast, a significant decrease of synovial fluid leptin levels is found in RA patients compared with matched plasma samples.[191] The most clear-cut difference in leptin between plasma and synovial fluid is seen in patients with non-erosive RA. The authors suggest that leptin may have a protective effect.

Leptin circulates in free and bound forms, and several works indicate that the soluble isoform of leptin receptor (ObRe) may determine the biological activity of this adipokine.[95,192] ObRe has been detected in the synovial fluid obtained from patients with OA, but at a low level compared to serum values.[189] Interestingly, the difference between synovial fluid and serum leptin levels increases when the molar ratio of leptin/ObRe is used as an index of free leptin or of bioactive leptin. Consequently, the high level of leptin associated with a decline in obRe level in the joint compartment leads to a large rise in the synovial fluid bioavailable leptin. The presence of a high level of bioactive leptin in OA-affected joints may have pathophysiologic implications, particularly because leptin was shown to increase the effects induced by pro-inflammatory cytokines in chondrocytes.[193,194]

All of these findings provide evidence for a specific local metabolism of adipokines in the joint space and suggest that serum levels of adipokines do not represent the situation in the joint. Based on these data, only analysis of adipokine levels in synovial fluid rather than in plasma may account for their local effects or be used to assess disease progression.

Whereas the synovial fluid level of bioactive leptin increases in both male and female OA patients compared to serum, a gender-specific difference is observed (with female OA patients exhibiting the highest level of free leptin in the joint). In addition, adipokines and ObRe levels in serum and synovial fluid correlate more closely in the male group compared to the female group. These data strengthen the hypothesis that obesity and female sex are both risk factors for OA that may be attributable to local rather than systemic turnover of these adipokines.[195]

## Adipokines in Osteoarthritis-affected Joints

The presence of leptin, adiponectin, and resistin in the synovial fluid raises the question of whether articular tissues may be both potential targets and sources of adipokines in the joint cavity. To date, little is known about the contribution of resistin and adiponectin in OA-affected joints. By contrast, further studies provide evidence for a key role of leptin in cartilage homeostasis.

### Production of Adipokines by Articular Tissues

Synovial membrane and cartilage are thought to be the primary sources of cytokines detected in the synovial fluid obtained from patients with OA. However, soluble factors may also originate from infrapatellar fat pad. This adipose tissue is located in the space between the patellar tendon, femoral condyle, and tibial plateau. As its surface is covered by a layer of synovial cells, this structure is both intra-articular and extra-synovial. The infrapatellar fat pad, which may have secretory properties different from other adipose tissues, was shown to be another source of cytokines and growth factors secreted in knee synovial fluids.[13]

Very recently, Presle et al. investigated the production of leptin, adiponectin, and resistin in human OA-affected joints by measuring their concentrations in media of cultured tissues (including synovium, infrapatellar fat pad, meniscus, osteophyte, cartilage, and bone).[189] As outlined in Table 6.3, each joint tissue examined releases leptin—but the production is quite variable depending on the tissue. Synovium and infrapatellar fat pad are the main sources of leptin in the joint. Surprisingly, osteophytes release larger amounts of leptin than do synovium or infrapatellar fat pad.

When samples used for leptin determination are examined for the other adipokines, no resistin is detected, probably because of a low detection limit of the commercial ELISA kit. By contrast, the conditioned media from ex vivo cultured specimens contained large amounts of adiponectin (Table 6.4). As was shown for leptin, synovium and infrapatellar fat pad represent the major sources of adiponectin in human OA-affected joints. However, in contrast to leptin osteophytes produce small amounts of adiponectin—suggesting that this articular structure is a preferential tissue for leptin synthesis in OA joints.

### Expression of Leptin and Its Receptor in Cartilage

To date, no data are available on the expression of adiponectin or resistin in cartilage. By contrast, leptin has been identified in human chondrocytes.[190] In normal cartilage, few chondrocytes in the mid zone exhibit positive immunostaining for leptin. The expression of this adipose-derived protein is strongly up-regulated

| TABLE 6.4  RELEASE OF ADIPONECTIN BY ARTICULAR TISSUES[a] | |
|---|---|
| Tissue | Adiponectin Released During 48 Hours (pg/mg tissue ± sem) |
| Synovium | 325.95 ± 36.53 |
| Fat pad | 522.31 ± 89.72 |
| Meniscus | 128.65 ± 7.63 |
| Osteophytes | 91.58 ± 15.40 |
| Cartilage | 22.65 ± 4.57 |
| Bone | 114.75 ± 33.62 |

[a]From Presle et al.

in cartilage obtained from patients with OA (especially in areas of matrix depletion, fibrillations, and chondrocyte clusters) and is related to the grade of cartilage destruction. In addition to mature cartilage, leptin is also produced in resting and prehypertrophic chondrocytes in growth plate of mice.[196] In agreement with the results found for leptin production, osteophytes obtained from OA patients exhibit strong leptin expression.

Serially cultured human articular chondrocytes possess the leptin receptor present on chondrocytes in native human cartilage.[197] In cultured human chondrocytes, mRNA for the functional isoform of leptin receptor was detected. ObRb is also found in rat cartilage,[190] mouse mandibular condyle,[198] the ATDC5 mouse chondrocytic cell line, porcine chondrocyte, and hypertrophic chondrocytes in mice.[196]

### Effects of Leptin on Chondrocytes

The expression of functional leptin receptor in chondrocyte suggests that leptin may display peripheral effects in joint. This adipokine stimulates both the proliferation and the extracellular matrix synthesis (proteoglycan and collagen) of cultured human chondrocytes, but in a biphasic manner with an optimum between 0.1 and 100 ng/ml.[197] These concentrations range within the synovial fluid level found in OA patients, suggesting that increasing concentrations of leptin in the joint may account for reduced synthesis of extracellular matrix (probably through a negative feedback loop involving SOCS-3). Surprisingly, immunoblotting analysis reveals that leptin triggers intracellular signal transduction through activation of STAT 1 and 5, but not STAT 3.[197]

The stimulatory effect of leptin is also found in rat. When injected into the knee joints, recombinant leptin induces the expression of TGF-β and IGF-1 in cartilage at both mRNA and protein levels, and strongly increases proteoglycan synthesis.[190] The stimulatory effect of leptin on cartilage anabolism is consistent with studies in which leptin was shown to promote bone growth by targeting osteoblasts directly.[184] As was previously shown for IGF-I receptor in leptin-stimulated mandibular condyles,[199] the anabolic effect of leptin may be further increased by the up-regulation of growth factor receptors. However, the biphasic effect of leptin shown in vitro for human chondrocytes is also found in vivo in rat (with a decreased proteoglycan synthesis at the highest concentrations).[190]

Human OA chondrocytes produce both leptin and growth factors in the same topographic localization and to the same extent, depending on the histologic grade of cartilage destruction, suggesting that this adipose-derived protein may be a key regulator of growth factor synthesis in human OA-affected joints.[190] In addition to leptin, synovial fluid obtained from OA patients contains abundant mediators of inflammation and cartilage destruction, implying that adipokines may associate with cytokines to induce and/or enhance damage to cartilage.

Recently, Otero et al. demonstrated in human primary chondrocytes and in the mouse chondrogenic ATDC5 cell line a synergistic effect of leptin on nitric oxide production with both interferon-α and more interestingly with interleukin-1 (IL-1), which plays a key role in the pathogenesis of OA.[193,194] Under these experimental conditions, leptin alone was unable to induce the expression of the nitric oxide synthase. This synergy between IL-1 and leptin occurs through JAK2, PI3K, MEK-1, and p38 kinase.

## Other Links Between Leptin and Osteoarthritis

Although cartilage is often considered the primary target of the degenerative process during OA, the whole joint with all articular structures is involved in changes associated with OA. Hypertrophic bone changes, with osteophyte formation and subchondral bone plate thickening, and synovial inflammation occur during OA. By their various physiologic effects on bone and inflammation, adipokines may contribute to these changes.

### Leptin and Bone

In addition to the hypothalamus, leptin targets a variety of other tissues (as indicated by expression of functional receptors in peripheral cells). It has been shown that primary adult osteoblasts possess functional leptin receptors,[200] and leptin has emerged as a mediator of the protective effects of fat on bone tissue.[201] Bone mass is positively correlated with body fat,[202,203] and there is a positive correlation between bone mass and serum levels of leptin in humans.[204] Leptin administration to ob/ob-deficient mice leads to a significant increase in femoral length, total body area, bone mineral content, and bone density compared to that of vehicle-treated controls.

These findings provide evidence that leptin may be considered an endocrine bone regulator, but it is debated whether bone remodeling is centrally or locally regulated.[205] Some authors suggest that leptin regulates both bone formation by osteoblast and resorption by osteoclast via the sympathetic nervous system,[186] whereas others assign to leptin osteogenic activity with direct stimulatory effect on osteoblast proliferation, collagen synthesis, and bone mineralization.[184] Leptin is also a skeletal growth factor that stimulates endochondral ossification.[206] Longitudinal bone growth involves endochondral ossification in which a scaffold of cartilage develops that is later replaced with bone by the invading osteoblast.

A significant increase in bone turnover and remodeling of the bone/cartilage interface occurs during OA, especially in areas underlying damaged cartilage. Expression and production of leptin were shown to increase in human OA subchondral osteoblasts compared with normal.[207] Metabolic markers of osteoblasts (namely, alkaline phosphatase activity, osteocalcin collagen I α1 chains, and growth factors such as IGF-1 and TGF-β) are stimulated in response to leptin and are increased in OA osteoblasts.[208] Even if it is still a matter of debate which happens first between early cartilage destruction and bony changes, all of these data add further insight into the contribution of leptin to OA pathogenesis.

### Adipokines in Inflammation

Although OA is not a joint disease driven by inflammation, episodic and non-erosive synovial inflammation may occur during OA. However, by contrast to RA synovial inflammation predominantly develops secondarily to pathologic processes in cartilage. The obese state is characterized by what has been called low-grade systemic inflammation,[209] and white adipose tissue is emerging as an active participant in regulating inflammation.[210] Macrophages are components of adipose tissue and actively participate in its activities. Furthermore, cross-talk between lymphocytes and adipocytes may lead to immune regulation. Increasing studies provide evidence for a contribution of adipokines in the inflammatory process. However, pro- or anti-inflammatory activity has been described (depending on the adipokine).

In animals, inflammatory stimuli acutely induce leptin mRNA and increase serum leptin levels. Most of the in vivo studies on the immune-modulating effects of leptin reveal that leptin exerts a pro-inflammatory role, while at the same time protecting against infections. Leptin protects T lymphocytes from apoptosis and regulates T-cell proliferation and activation. Leptin also influences cytokine production from T lymphocytes, generally switching the phenotype toward a $T_H1$ response.

In addition to its effects on T lymphocytes, leptin influences monocyte activation, phagocytosis, and production of cytokines—including interleukin 1 receptor antagonist (IL-1Ra),[42] IL-1,[211] and TNF-α.[212] Extensive studies suggest that leptin may display pro- or anti-inflammatory effects in the joint, depending on the immune response. In an experimental model of arthritis involving T- and B-cells, leptin appears to contribute to the mechanisms of joint inflammation. By contrast, a delayed resolution of joint swelling and severe histologic damage are observed in leptin-deficient mice with zymosan-induced arthritis (a model not dependent on the adaptive immune response).[213]

Adiponectin appears to act as an anti-inflammatory molecule.[143] This adipokine reduces the production and activity of TNF-α and IL-6, and induces the anti-inflammatory cytokines IL-10 and IL-1 receptor antagonist.[214] However, the relationship between adiponectin and inflammation in joint diseases remains unclear. A significant positive correlation between synovial fluid levels of adiponectin and the levels of systemic markers of inflammation such as C-reactive protein is found for patients with OA but not for those with RA.

Although TNF-α is a negative regulator of resistin expression in mouse adipose cells, resistin displays largely pro-inflammatory activities. Recent data indicate that stimulation of macrophages in vitro with endotoxin or pro-inflammatory cytokines leads to a marked increase in resistin production, and administration of endotoxin to human volunteers is associated with dramatically increased circulating resistin levels. In patients with RA, resistin accumulates locally in the inflamed joints, and the synovial resistin levels are positively correlated with markers of inflammation (including IL-6 and white blood cells). This adipokine is able to induce arthritis[215] when injected into mouse joints, and to stimulate the production in PBMC of various pro-inflammatory cytokines (including TNF-α, IL-1, and IL-6). Based on these data, adipokines may modulate the inflammatory process during OA—especially through regulation of pro-inflammatory cytokines.

## Adipokines as Local Effectors in Osteoarthritis?

Recent studies on adipokines in rheumatic diseases provide evidence for their potential contribution to cartilage changes during OA. Although the investigations focused mainly on leptin, and although few data on resistin and adiponectin are to date available, they help to better understand the relationships between systemic and local adipokines in OA. More particularly, they showed that the joint cavity may be considered a special space in which leptin, adiponectin, and resistin undergo specific metabolic pathways and may modulate chondrocyte functions in cartilage.[195,216,217]

Several arguments strengthen the hypothesis that adipokines may have pathophysiologic effects in the joint. Leptin, adiponectin, and resistin are found in synovial fluid from OA-affected joints, but adipokines are individually distinguished by their differing patterns of distribution between the joint space and serum. Resistin and adiponectin (in particular) exhibit low synovial fluid level compared to serum, whereas the opposite is observed for leptin. The difference between both compartments markedly increases when levels of bioactive free leptin are determined. Articular tissues (including synovium, infrapatellar fat pad, meniscus, cartilage, and bone) produce leptin and adiponectin—the synovial membrane and the infrapatellar fat pad being the major sources of adipokines in the joint. Leptin is strongly overexpressed in cartilage, osteophytes, and subchondral bone obtained from OA patients (depending on the histologic grade of cartilage destruction). Finally, functional leptin receptor has been identified in human chondrocytes.

All of these findings suggest that adipokines may be important local effectors involved in cartilage changes associated with OA. Moreover, when compared to normal specimens leptin expression in human OA is up-regulated in various articular tissues that undergo strong structural and biochemical changes during OA (i.e., cartilage, osteophytes, and subchondral bone), and this expression is largely related to the grade of cartilage destruction. Interestingly, these articular tissues also produce growth factors during OA with the same distribution as observed with leptin.

The stimulatory effect of leptin on TGF-β and IGF-1 expression indicates that leptin is a key regulator of growth factor synthesis in the joint and thus may be implicated in OA. High levels of IGF-1 and TGF-β were indeed measured in the synovial fluid of OA patients, and their synthesis was increased in human OA cartilage as well as in animal models of OA.[218] These growth factors are believed to play a beneficial role in the cartilage repair process that may occur during OA.[219] However, in addition to their protective role against cartilage damage they may trigger degeneration of this connective tissue. Excessive and/or prolonged exposure to TGF-β leads to lesions similar to those observed in spontaneous OA mice.

In addition to their effects on chondrocyte functions, growth factors are involved in hypertrophic bone changes that are a prominent feature of OA-affected joints. TGF-β and IGF-1 have been detected in osteophytes, and repeated injections or overexpression of TGF-β in mice knee joints results in osteophyte formation.[220] Leptin (but not adiponectin) is released in large amounts by osteophytes, suggesting that among adipokines leptin may play a special role in osteophyte formation.

The adipose-derived protein may contribute to osteophyte formation either indirectly by stimulating TGF-β expression or directly by inducing endochondral ossification. In addition, OA subchondral bone osteoblasts produce elevated levels of IGF-1, which may promote bone cell growth and bone matrix deposition (subsequently leading to abnormal bone remodeling and subchondral bone sclerosis). Consequently, leptin may have dualistic effects on the joint: variations in levels of locally produced leptin might regulate chondrocyte proliferation and anabolic function, and might induce osteophyte formation and subchondral bone changes during OA.

Leptin displays biological activity on chondrocytes with stimulation of chondrocyte proliferation, collagen, and proteoglycan synthesis through growth factor overexpression. This adipose-derived protein (which is expressed at a low level in healthy cartilage) may thus control cartilage homeostasis under normal conditions. However, leptin exhibits a reduced stimulatory effect at high concentration, suggesting that the elevated level of leptin found in synovial fluid from OA patients may account for a decreased extracellular matrix synthesis. The presence of a high level of bioactive leptin in the joint from OA patients due to a high level of leptin (associated with a decline in obRe level in the joint compartment compared to serum) may further decrease proteoglycan and collagen production during OA.

This elevated bioactive leptin in the joint from OA patients may have many pathophysiologic implications, as leptin was shown to synergize with pro-inflammatory cytokines. Moreover, the adipokine increases nitric oxide production in chondrocytes stimulated with interleukin-1. This free radical is known to interfere with chondrocyte functions, resulting in loss of cartilage matrix through induction of apoptosis, activation of MMPs, inhibition of proteoglycan, and type II collagen synthesis.[194] These findings indicate that the effects of leptin on chondrocytes may be modulated by other cytokines, and that leptin associated with pro-inflammatory cytokines may promote cartilage destruction during OA.

Interestingly, large amounts of free leptin are found in the synovial fluid obtained from female OA patients compared to male patients (whereas no significant difference between males and females is observed with respect to age or BMI). This elevated level of free leptin within the joint represents an important local pool of bioavailable leptin with potential biologic activity. Because obesity and female sex are both risk factors for the development of OA, these data provide further evidence for the contribution of leptin to the pathogenesis of OA and may argue for the gender disparity toward the disease.

These preliminary data on adipokines in human OA are raising considerable questions on the mechanisms by which they may control cartilage homeostasis, especially for leptin. The dose-dependent effect of this adipose-derived protein in human chondrocytes suggests that any variation in locally produced leptin may be a determinant for cartilage homeostasis. Further studies are required to determine whether the high synovial fluid level of leptin is explained solely by local production or may be controlled by other factors found in synovial fluid. Because leptin is able to induce its own expression in chondrocyte, it would be interesting to evaluate how systemic leptin may regulate locally produced leptin.

In addition, pathophysiologic status (such as inflammation of the synovial membrane secondary to cartilage changes or metabolic disorders in the infrapatellar fat pad) may also influence leptin level in the joint. In addition, the level of ObRe in synovial fluid obtained from OA patients is also a determinant for the biologic activity of leptin. ObRe found in the joint space may derive from the circulation. However, the lack of correlation between synovial fluid and serum levels in female OA patients[189] suggests that ObRe undergoes a specific local regulation.[221] Based on these data, it remains to be determined whether ObRe results from an expression in joint tissues or from a proteolytic cleavage of the membrane-associated receptor (especially through activated MMPs).

One of the hallmarks of OA is the loss of cartilage matrix through activation of catabolic processes and inhibition of collagen and proteoglycan synthesis. Given that leptin exhibits a biphasic effect on extracellular matrix synthesis and that an elevated level of leptin is found in synovial fluid from OA patients, it would be interesting to know if leptin resistance occurs in human chondrocytes and contributes to the reduction of extracellular matrix synthesis during OA. In addition, the elevated expression of leptin in markedly damaged cartilage suggests that leptin may be involved in cartilage destruction.

Although the effects of leptin on extracellular matrix synthesis are well established, nothing is known about the contribution of this adipose-derived protein to the catabolic processes. Leptin was shown to enhance the expression of MMPs, including MMP-2 and MMP-9 and their inhibitors TIMP-1 and TIMP-2. Investigations on leptin-mediated effects on MMP and TIMP expression may add further insights on the role of leptin in the equilibrium of anabolic versus catabolic processes, and may characterize the mechanisms underlying osteophyte formation and subchondral bone sclerosis.

In fact, the contribution of leptin to the pathogenesis of OA may not be simply evaluated by investigating its effects when used alone. Studies by Otero et al. indicate rather that leptin may have dualistic effects on chondrocytes, depending on other local factors such as growth factors or pro-inflammatory cytokines.[193] Indeed, this adipokine stimulates extracellular matrix synthesis and chondrocyte proliferation when used alone, but synergizes with IL-1 to induce nitric oxide production. Further understanding of the complex interactions between leptin and other cytokines and growth factors might help in demonstrating the overall contribution of leptin in cartilage changes associated with OA. Moreover, the use of animal models of OA in which pro-inflammatory cytokines and growth factors are locally produced in the joint may provide information on the expression and effects of leptin throughout the course of OA. This would be helpful in defining the role of this adipokine in the onset and progression of the disease.

The effects of adiponectin and resistin on cartilage homeostasis also need to be studied. As was suggested by Schaffler et al.,[35] adiponectin is a signaling molecule with metabolic effects, suggesting that deficiency in adiponectin found in the synovial fluid obtained from OA patients may lead to a reduced extracellular matrix synthesis. Moreover, the molecular ratio between each adipokine in synovial fluid differs from that found in serum. Moreover, the imbalance between adiponectin and leptin (with a decline in the adiponectin synovial fluid level compared to serum and an excess of leptin in the joint) may account for the development and progression of OA. The effects on cartilage of leptin associated with adiponectin require further investigation, particularly in that very recently adiponectin was shown to modulate the biologic activity of several growth factors by controlling their bioavailability at a pre-receptor level.

## SUMMARY

Current studies indicate that adipokines may contribute to the changes associated with OA, and more especially may be involved in the local regulation of articular cartilage metabolism. Leptin, resistin, and adiponectin are detected in the synovial fluid obtained from OA patients. Although little is known about the role of resistin and adiponectin in OA, extensive studies provide evidence for a key role of leptin in the pathophysiology of this rheumatic disease. Leptin is found in both osteophytes and cartilage obtained from patients with OA, with a marked increased expression in areas of matrix depletion, fibrillations, and chondrocyte clusters. This adipokine exhibits biologic activity on chondrocytes through binding on the functional long form of its receptor and activation of STAT 1 and 5.

Leptin induces the expression of growth factors, stimulates proteoglycan and collagen synthesis, and increases the stimulatory effects of pro-inflammatory cytokines on nitric oxide production in chondrocytes. Altogether, these data strengthen the hypothesis that OA is a metabolic disorder in which systemic factors that include altered lipid metabolism induce changes in skeletal tissues by modification of the formation and biosynthetic activity of mesenchymal precursor cells.[16] On this basis, adipokines may be the metabolic link between obesity and OA.

Interestingly, the various patterns of distribution of adipokines between synovial fluid and serum (especially in female OA patients) suggest that the joint is a special space in which leptin, adiponectin, and resistin may each undergo specific metabolic pathways and may have local effects on articular tissues. In addition, the gender-specific difference in this distribution offers an explanation for the gender disparity toward the disease. In this context, adipokines may be considered cytokines and growth factors likely to promote articular damage. It remains to be determined whether adipokines have a physiologic role in cartilage homeostasis and whether any metabolic dysregulation or an imbalance between adipokines may account for the development and/or progression of OA.

## REFERENCES

1. Felson DT, Zhang Y. An update on the epidemiology of knee and hip osteoarthritis with a view to prevention. Arthritis Rheum 1998;41(8):1343–55.
2. Martel-Pelletier J. Pathophysiology of osteoarthritis. Osteoarthritis Cartilage 2004;12(A):S31–33.
3. Felson DT, Neogi T. Osteoarthritis: Is it a disease of cartilage or of bone? Arthritis Rheum 2004;50(2):341–44.
4. Lajeunesse D. The role of bone in the treatment of osteoarthritis. Osteoarthritis Cartilage 2004;12(A):S34–38.
5. Carlson CS, Loeser RF, Jayo MJ, et al. Osteoarthritis in cynomolgus macaques: A primate model of naturally occurring disease. J Orthop Res 1994;12(3):331–39.
6. Marks R, Allegrante JP. Body mass indices in patients with disabling hip osteoarthritis. Arthritis Res 2002;4(2):112–16.
7. Eaton CB. Obesity as a risk factor for osteoarthritis: Mechanical versus metabolic. Med Health R I 2004;87(7):201–04.
8. Felson DT, Goggins J, Niu J, et al. The effect of body weight on progression of knee osteoarthritis is dependent on alignment. Arthritis Rheum 2004;50(12):3904–09.
9. Cicuttini FM, Baker JR, Spector TD. The association of obesity with osteoarthritis of the hand and knee in women: A twin study. J Rheumatol 1996;23(7):1221–26.
10. Oliveria SA, Felson DT, Cirillo P, et al. Body weight, body mass index, and incident symptomatic osteoarthritis of the hand, hip, and knee. Epidemiology 1999;10(2):161–66.
11. Pittenger MF, Mackay AM, Beck SC, et al. Multilineage potential of adult human mesenchymal stem cells. Science 1999;2;284 (5411):143–47.
12. Mohamed-Ali V, Goodrick S, Rawesh A, et al. Subcutaneous adipose tissue releases interleukin-6, but not tumor necrosis factor-alpha, in vivo. J Clin Endocrinol Metab 1997;82(12): 4196–4200.

13. Ushiyama T, Chano T, Inoue K, Matsusue Y. Cytokine production in the infrapatellar fat pad: Another source of cytokines in knee synovial fluids. Ann Rheum Dis 2003;62(2):108–12.

14. Lyon CJ, Law RE, Hsueh WA. Minireview: Adiposity, inflammation, and atherogenesis. Endocrinology 2003;144(6): 2195–2200.

15. Lau DC, Dhillon B, Yan H, et al. Adipokines: Molecular links between obesity and atherosclerosis. Am J Physiol Heart Circ Physiol 2005;288(5):H2031–41.

16. Aspden RM, Scheven BA, Hutchison JD. Osteoarthritis as a systemic disorder including stromal cell differentiation and lipid metabolism. Lancet 2001;7;357(9262):1118–20.

17. Hauner H. The new concept of adipose tissue function. Physiol Behav 2004;30;83(4):653–58.

18. Giorgino F, Laviola L, Eriksson JW. Regional differences of insulin action in adipose tissue: Insights from in vivo and in vitro studies. Acta Physiol Scand 2005;183(1):13–30.

19. Zhang Y, Proenca R, Maffei M, et al. Positional cloning of the mouse obese gene and its human homologue. Nature 1994;372 (6505):425–32.

20. Fruhbeck G, Gomez-Ambrosi J, Muruzabal FJ, et al. The adipocyte: A model for integration of endocrine and metabolic signaling in energy metabolism regulation. Am J Physiol Endocrinol Metab 2001;280(6):E827–47.

21. Moitra J, Mason MM, Olive M. Life without white fat: A transgenic mouse. Genes Dev 1998;15;12(20):3168–81.

22. Wellen KE, Hotamisligil GS. Obesity-induced inflammatory changes in adipose tissue. J Clin Invest 2003;112(12):1785–88.

23. Weisberg SP, McCann D, Desai M, et al. Obesity is associated with macrophage accumulation in adipose tissue. J Clin Invest 2003;112(12):1796–1808.

24. Winter A, Breit S, Parsch D, Benz, et al. Cartilage-like gene expression in differentiated human stem cell spheroids: A comparison of bone marrow-derived and adipose tissue-derived stromal cells. Arthritis Rheum 2003;48(2):418–29.

25. Kissebah AH, Krakower GR. Regional adiposity and morbidity. Physiol Rev 1994;74(4):761–811.

26. Fried SK, Bunkin DA, Greenberg AS. Omental and subcutaneous adipose tissues of obese subjects release interleukin-6: Depot difference and regulation by glucocorticoid. J Clin Endocrinol Metab 1998;83(3):847–50.

27. Funahashi T, Nakamura T, Shimomura I, et al. Role of adipocytokines on the pathogenesis of atherosclerosis in visceral obesity. Intern Med 1999;38(2):202–06.

28. Trayhurn P, Wood IS. Adipokines: Inflammation and the pleiotropic role of white adipose tissue. Br J Nutr 2004;92(3):347–55.

29. Xu H, Barnes GT, Yang Q. Chronic inflammation in fat plays a crucial role in the development of obesity-related insulin resistance. J Clin Invest 2003;112(12):1821–30.

30. Fain JN, Madan AK, Hiler ML, et al. Comparison of the release of adipokines by adipose tissue, adipose tissue matrix, and adipocytes from visceral and subcutaneous abdominal adipose tissues of obese humans. Endocrinology 2004;145(5): 2273–82.

31. Lau DC, Dhillon B, Yan H, et al. Adipokines: Molecular links between obesity and atherosclerosis. Am J Physiol Heart Circ Physiol 2005;288(5):H2031.

32. Hug C, Lodish HF. Visfatin: A new adipokine. Science 2005;21;307 (5708):366–67.

33. Fukuhara A, Matsuda M, Nishizawa M, Segawa K, Visfatin: A protein secreted by visceral fat that mimics the effects of insulin. Science 2005;307(5708):426–30.

34. Zhang B, Salituro G, Szalkowski D, et al. Discovery of a small molecule insulin mimetic with antidiabetic activity in mice. Science 1999;284:974–77.

35. Schaffler A, Ehling A, Neumann E. Adipocytokines in synovial fluid. JAMA 2003;290:1709–10.

36. Considine RV, Sinha MK, Heimann ML. Serum immunoreactive leptin concentrations in normal-weights and obese humans. New England J Med 1996;334:292–95.

37. Morton G, Blevins J, Williams D, et al. Leptin action in the forebrain regulates the hindbrain response to satiety signals. J Clin Invest 2005;115:703–10.

38. Takeda S, Elefteriou F, Karsenty G. Common endocrine control of body weight, reproduction and bone mass. Annu Rev Nutr 2003; 23:403–11.

39. Lenchik L, Register T, Hsu, et al. Adiponectin as a novel determinant of bone mineral density and visceral fat. Bone 2003;33:646–51.

40. Otero M, Lago R, Lago F, et al. Leptin, from fat to inflammation: Old questions and new insights. FEBS Letter 2005;579:295–301.

41. Axelsson J, Heimburger O, Lindholm B, et al. Adipose tissue and its relation to inflammation: The role of adipokines. J Ren Nutr 2005;15(1):131–36.

42. Gabay C, Dreyer M, Pellegrinelli N, et al. Leptin directly induces the secretion of interleukin 1 receptor antagonist in human monocytes. J Clin Endocrinol Metab 2001;86(2):783–91.

43. Bendinelli P, Piccoletti R, Maroni P. Leptin rapidly activates PPARs in C2C12 uscl cells. Biochem Biophys Res Commun 2005;332: 719–25.

44. Erol A. PPAR alpha activators may be good candidates as antiaging agents. Med Hypotheses 2005;65:35–8.

45. Kennedy GC. The role of depot fat in the hypothalamic control of food intake in the rat. Proc R Soc Lond B Biol Sci 1953;140: 578–96.

46. Harris RB. Role of set-point theory in regulation of body weight. FASEB J 1990;4(15):3310–18.

47. Faust IM, Johnson PR, Hirsch J. Surgical removal of adipose tissue alters feeding behavior and the development of obesity in rats. Science 1977;197(4301):393–96.

48. Hervey GR. The effects of lesions in the hypothalamus in parabiotic rats. J Physiol 1959;145(2):336–52.

49. Coleman DL. Effects of parabiosis of obese with diabetes and normal mice. Diabetologia 1973;9:294–98.

50. Friedman JM, Halaas JL. Leptin and the regulation of body weight in mammals. Nature 1998;395(6704):763–70.

51. La Cava A, Matarese G. The weight of leptin in immunity. Nat Rev Immunol 2004;4(5):371–79.

52. Gong DW, Bi S, Pratley RE, Weintraub BD. Genomic structure and promoter analysis of the human obese gene. J Biol Chem 1996;271(8):3971–74.

53. Ahima RS, Osei SY. Leptin signaling. Physiol Behav 2004;81(2): 223–41.

54. Guilmeau S, Buyse M, Bado A. Gastric leptin: A new manager of gastrointestinal function. Curr Opin Pharmacol 2004;4(6):561–66.

55. Ahima RS, Flier JS. Leptin. Annu Rev Physiol 2000;62:413–37.

56. Campfield LA, Smith FJ, Guisez Y, et al. Recombinant mouse OB protein: Evidence for a peripheral signal linking adiposity and central neural networks. Science 1995;269(5223):546–49.

57. Finck BN, Kelley KW, Dantzer R, Johnson RW. In vivo and in vitro evidence for the involvement of tumor necrosis factor-alpha in the induction of leptin by lipopolysaccharide. Endocrinology 1998;139(5):2278–83.

58. Casabiell X, Pineiro V, Peino R, et al. Gender differences in both spontaneous and stimulated leptin secretion by human omental adipose tissue in vitro: Dexamethasone and estradiol stimulate leptin release in women, but not in men. J Clin Endocrinol Metab 1998;83:2149–55.

59. Castracane VD, Kraemer RR, Franken MA, et al. Serum leptin concentration in women: Effect of age, obesity, and estrogen administration. Fertil Steril 1998;70(3):472–77.

60. Wang J, Liu R, Hawkins M, et al. A nutrient-sensing pathway regulates leptin gene expression in muscle and fat. Nature 1998;393(6686):684–88.

61. Mise H, Sagawa N, Matsumoto T, et al. Augmented placental production of leptin in preeclampsia: Possible involvement of placental hypoxia. J Clin Endocrinol Metab 1998;83(9):3225–29.

62. Tartaglia LA. The leptin receptor. J Biol Chem 1997;272(10): 6093–96.

63. Tartaglia LA, Dembski M, Weng X, et al. Identification and expression cloning of a leptin receptor, OB-R. Cell 1995;83(7): 1263–71.

64. Hileman SM, Pierroz DD, Masuzaki H, et al. Characterization of short isoforms of the leptin receptor in rat cerebral microvessels and of brain uptake of leptin in mouse models of obesity. Endocrinology 2002;143:775–83.

65. Golden PL, Maccagnan TJ, Pardridge WM. Human blood-brain barrier leptin receptor: Binding and endocytosis in isolated human brain microvessels. J Clin Invest 1997;99(1):14–8.

66. Fong TM, Huang RR, Tota MR, et al. Localization of leptin binding domain in the leptin receptor. Mol Pharmacol 1998;53(2): 234–40.

67. Sweeney G. Leptin signalling. Cell Signal 2002;14(8):655–63.

68. Yang G, Ge H, Boucher A, et al. Modulation of direct leptin signaling by soluble leptin receptor. Mol Endocrinol 2004;18: 1354–62.

69. Edwards DE, Bohm RP Jr., Purcell J, et al. Two isoforms of the leptin receptor are enhanced in pregnancy-specific tissues and soluble leptin receptor is enhanced in maternal serum with advancing gestation in the baboon. Biol Reprod 2004;71: 1746–52.

70. Chen H, Charlat O, Tartaglia LA, et al. Evidence that the diabetes gene encodes the leptin receptor: Identification of a mutation in the leptin receptor gene in db/db mice. Cell 1996;84(3):491–95.

71. Chua SC Jr., Chung WK, Wu-Peng XS, et al. Phenotypes of mouse diabetes and rat fatty tissue due to mutations in the OB (leptin) receptor. Science 1996;271(5251):994–96.

72. Takaya K, Ogawa Y, Hiraoka J, et al. Nonsense mutation of leptin receptor in the obese spontaneously hypertensive Koletsky rat. Nat Genet 1996;14(2):130–31.

73. Wu-Peng XS, Chua SC Jr., Okada N, et al. Phenotype of the obese Koletsky (f) rat due to Tyr763Stop mutation in the extracellular domain of the leptin receptor (Lepr): Evidence for deficient plasma-to-CSF transport of leptin in both the Zucker and Koletsky obese rat. Diabetes 1997;46(3):513–18.

74. Clement K, Vaisse C, Lahlou N, et al. A mutation in the human leptin receptor gene causes obesity and pituitary dysfunction. Nature 1998;392(6674):398–401.

75. Bahrenberg G, Behrmann I, Barthel A, et al. Identification of the critical sequence elements in the cytoplasmic domain of leptin receptor isoforms required for Janus kinase/signal transducer and activator of transcription activation by receptor het-erodimers. Mol Endocrinol 2002;16(4):859–72.

76. Bates SH, Stearns WH, Dundon TA, et al. STAT3 signalling is required for leptin regulation of energy balance but not repro-duction. Nature 2003;421(6925):856–59.

77. Muraoka O, Xu B, Tsurumaki T, Akira S, et al. Leptin-induced trans-activation of NPY gene promoter mediated by JAK1, JAK2 and STAT3 in the neural cell lines. Neurochem Int 2003;42(7):591–601.

78. Vaisse C, Halaas JL, Horvath CM, et al. Leptin activation of Stat3 in the hypothalamus of wild-type and ob/ob mice but not db/db mice. Nat Genet 1996;14(1):95–7.

79. Waelput W, Verhee A, Broekaert D, et al. Identification and expression analysis of leptin-regulated immediate early response and late target genes. Biochem J 2000;348(1):55–61.

80. Hakansson ML, Meister B. Transcription factor STAT3 in leptin target neurons of the rat hypothalamus. Neuroendocrinology 1998;68(6):420–27.

81. White DW, Kuropatwinski KK, Devos R, et al. Leptin receptor (OB-R) signaling: Cytoplasmic domain mutational analysis and evidence for receptor homo-oligomerization. J Biol Chem 1997;272(7):4065–71.

82. BJorbaek C, Lavery H, Bates S, et al. SOCS3 mediates feedback inhibition of the leptin receptor via Tyr 985. J Biol Chem 2000;275:40649–57.

83. Bjorbaek C, Buchholz RM, Davis SM, et al. Divergent roles of SHP-2 in ERK activation by leptin receptors. J Biol Chem 2001;276:4747–55.

84. Bjorbaek C, El-Hashimi K, Frantz D, et al. The role of SOCS3 in leptin signaling and leptin resistance. J Biol Chem 1999;274: 30059–65.

85. Emilsson V, Arch JR, de Groot RP, et al. Leptin treatment increases suppressors of cytokine signaling in central and peripheral tissues. FEBS Lett 1999;455(1/2):170–74.

86. Bjorbaek C, Elmquist JK, Frantz JD, et al. Identification of SOCS-3 as a potential mediator of central leptin resistance. Mol Cell 1998;1(4):619–25.

87. Zabolotny JM, Bence-Hanulec KK, Stricker-Krongrad A, et al. PTP1B regulates leptin signal transduction in vivo. Dev Cell 2002;2(4):489–95.

88. Cheng A, Uetani N, Simoncic PD, et al. Attenuation of leptin action and regulation of obesity by protein tyrosine phos-phatase 1B. Dev Cell 2002;2(4):497–503.

89. Cowley MA, Smart JL, Rubinstein M, et al. Leptin activates anorexigenic POMC neurons through a neural network in the arcuate nucleus. Nature 2001;411(6836):480–84.

90. Glaum SR, Hara M, Bindokas VP, et al. Leptin, the obese gene product, rapidly modulates synaptic transmission in the hypo-thalamus. Mol Pharmacol 1996;50(2):230–35.

91. Spanswick D, Smith MA, Groppi VE, et al. Leptin inhibits hypo-thalamic neurons by activation of ATP-sensitive potassium channels. Nature 1997;390(6659):521–25.

92. Banks AS, Davis SM, Bates SH, et al. Activation of downstream signals by the long form of the leptin receptor. J Biol Chem 2000;275(19):14563–72.

93. Van den Brink GR, O'Toole T, Hardwick JC, et al. Leptin signal-ing in human peripheral blood mononuclear cells, activation of p38 and p42/44 mitogen-activated protein (MAP) kinase and p70 S6 kinase. Mol Cell Biol Res Commun 2000;4(3):144–50.

94. Zhao AZ, Bornfeldt KE, Beavo JA. Leptin inhibits insulin secre-tion by activation of phosphodiesterase 3B. J Clin Invest 1998;102(5):869–73.

95. Sinha MK, Opentanova I, Ohannesian JP, et al. Evidence of free and bound leptin in human circulation: Studies in lean and obese subjects and during short-term fasting. J Clin Invest 1996;98(6):1277–82.

96. Houseknecht KL, Mantzoros CS, Kuliawat R, et al. Evidence for leptin binding to proteins in serum of rodents and humans: Modulation with obesity. Diabetes 1996;45(11):1638–43.

97. Banks WA, Kastin AJ, Huang W, et al. Leptin enters the brain by a saturable system independent of insulin. Peptides 1996;17(2):305–11.

98. Korner J, Leibel RL. To eat or not to eat: How the gut talks to the brain. N Engl J Med 2003;349(10):926–28.

99. Druce MR, Small CJ, Bloom SR. Gut peptides regulating satiety. Endocrinology 2004;145(6):2660–65.

100. Gale SM, Castracane VD, Mantzoros CS. Energy homeostasis, obesity and eating disorders: Recent advances in endocrinology. J Nutr 2004;134(2):295–98.

101. Bouret SG, Simerly RB. Leptin and development of hypothalamic feeding circuits. Endocrinology 2004;145(6):2621–26.

102. Sahu A. A hypothalamic role in energy balance with special emphasis on leptin. Endocrinology 2004;145:2613–20.

103. Zigman JM, Elmquist JK. From anorexia to obesity: The yin and yang of body weight control. Endocrinology 2003;144(9):3749–56.

104. Mark AL, Correia ML, Rahmouni K, Haynes WG. Loss of leptin actions in obesity: Two concepts with cardiovascular implica-tions. Clin Exp Hypertens 2004;26(7/8):629–36.

105. Montez JM, Soukas A, Asilmaz E, et al. Acute leptin deficiency, leptin resistance, and the physiologic response to leptin with-drawal. Proc Natl Acad Sci USA 2005;102(7):2537–42.

106. Margetic S, Gazzola C, Pegg GG, et al. Leptin: A review of its peripheral actions and interactions. Int J Obes Relat Metab Disord 2002;26(11):1407–33.

107. Cioffi JA, Shafer AW, Zupancic TJ, et al. Novel B219/OB receptor isoforms: Possible role of leptin in hematopoiesis and repro-duction. Nat Med 1996;2(5):585–89.

108. Gainsford T, Willson TA, Metcalf D, et al. Leptin can induce pro-liferation, differentiation, and functional activation of hemo-poietic cells. Proc Natl Acad Sci USA 1996;93(25):14564–68.

109. Nakata M, Yada T, Soejima N, et al. Leptin promotes aggrega-tion of human platelets via the long form of its receptor. Diabetes 1999;48(2):426–29.

110. Sierra-Honigmann MR, Nath AK, Murakami C, et al. Biological action of leptin as an angiogenic factor. Science 1998;281(5383): 1683–86.

111. Bouloumie A, Drexler HC, Lafontan M, et al. Leptin, the product of Ob gene, promotes angiogenesis. Circ Res 1998;83(10):1059–66.

112. Ring BD, Scully S, Davis CR, et al. Systemically and topically administered leptin both accelerate wound healing in diabetic ob/ob mice. Endocrinology 2000;141(1):446–49.

113. Machinal F, Dieudonne M, Leneveu M, et al. In vivo and in vitro ob gene expression and leptin secretion in rat adipocytes: Evidence for a regional specific regulation by sex steroid hor-mones. Endocrinology 1999;140:1567–74.

114. Chehab FF, Lim ME, Lu R. Correction of the sterility defect in homozygous obese female mice by treatment with the human recombinant leptin. Nat Genet 1996;12(3):318–20.

115. Spicer LJ, Francisco CC. Adipose obese gene product, leptin, inhibits bovine ovarian thecal cell steroidogenesis. Biol Reprod 1998;58(1):207–12.

116. Lindheim SR, Sauer MV, Carmina E, Chang PL, Zimmerman R, Lobo RA. Circulating leptin levels during ovulation induction: Relation to adiposity and ovarian morphology. Fertil Steril 2000;73(3):493–98.

117. Kieffer TJ, Habener JF. The adipoinsular axis: Effects of leptin on pancreatic beta-cells. Am J Physiol Endocrinol Metab 2000;278(1).

118. Kieffer TJ, Heller RS, Habener JF. Leptin receptors expressed on pancreatic beta-cells. Biochem Biophys Res Commun 1996;224(2):522–27.

119. Walder K, Filippis A, Clark S, et al. Leptin inhibits insulin binding in isolated rat adipocytes. J Endocrinol 1997;155(3):R5–7.

120. Seufert J, Kieffer TJ, Leech CA, et al. Leptin suppression of insulin secretion and gene expression in human pancreatic islets: Implications for the development of adipogenic diabetes mellitus. J Clin Endocrinol Metab 1999;84(2):670–76.

121. Wang J, Liu R, Hawkins M, Barzilai N, et al. A nutrient-sensing pathway regulates leptin gene expression in muscle and fat. Nature 1998;393(6686):684–88.

122. Ghilardi N, Ziegler S, Wiestner A, et al. Defective STAT signaling by the leptin receptor in diabetic mice. Proc Natl Acad Sci USA 1996;93(13):6231–35.

123. Murakami T, Yamashita T, Iida M, et al. A short form of leptin receptor performs signal transduction. Biochem Biophys Res Commun 1997;231(1):26–9.

124. Ceddia RB, William WN Jr., Curi R. Comparing effects of leptin and insulin on glucose metabolism in skeletal muscle: Evidence for an effect of leptin on glucose uptake and decarboxylation. Int J Obes Relat Metab Disord 1999;23(1):75–82.

125. Considine RV, Cooksey RC, Williams LB, et al. Hexosamines regulate leptin production in human subcutaneous adipocytes. J Clin Endocrinol Metab 2000;85(10):3551–56.

126. Klaus S. Adipose tissue as a regulator of energy balance. Curr Drug Targets 2004;5(3):241–50.

127. Guerre-Millo M. Adipose tissue and adipokines: For better or worse. Diabetes Metab 2004;30(1):13–9.

128. Lau DC, Dhillon B, Yan H, et al. Adipokines: Molecular links between obesity and atherosclerosis. Am J Physiol Heart Circ Physiol 2005;288(5):H2031–41.

129. Nawrocki AR, Scherer PE. The delicate balance between fat and muscle: Adipokines in metabolic disease and musculoskeletal inflammation. Curr Opin Pharmacol 2004;4(3):281–89.

130. Fasshauer M, Paschke R, Stumvoll M. Adiponectin, obesity, and cardiovascular disease. Biochimie 2004;86(11):779–84.

131. Beltowski J. Adiponectin and resistin: New hormones of white adipose tissue. Med Sci Monit 2003;9(2):RA55–61.

132. Diez JJ, Iglesias P. The role of the novel adipocyte-derived hormone adiponectin in human disease. Eur J Endocrinol 2003;148(3):293–300.

133. Gil-Campos M, Canete RR, Gil A. Adiponectin, the missing link in insulin resistance and obesity. Clin Nutr 2004;23(5):963–74.

134. Berg AH, Combs TP, Scherer PE. ACRP30/adiponectin: An adipokine regulating glucose and lipid metabolism. Trends Endocrinol Metab 2002;13(2):84–9.

135. Hu E, Liang P, Spiegelman BM. AdipoQ is a novel adipose-specific gene dysregulated in obesity. J Biol Chem 1996;271(18):10697–703.

136. Maeda K, Okubo K, Shimomura I, et al. cDNA cloning and expression of a novel adipose specific collagen-like factor, apM1 (AdiPose Most abundant Gene transcript 1). Biochem Biophys Res Commun 1996;221(2):286–89.

137. Nakano Y, Tobe T, Choi-Miura NH, et al. Isolation and characterization of GBP28, a novel gelatin-binding protein purified from human plasma. J Biochem 1996;120(4):803–12.

138. Ouchi N, Kihara S, Arita Y, et al. Novel modulator for endothelial adhesion molecules: Adipocyte-derived plasma protein adiponectin. Circulation 1999;100(25):2473–76.

139. Arita Y, Kihara S, Ouchi N, et al. Paradoxical decrease of an adipose-specific protein, adiponectin, in obesity. Biochem Biophys Res Commun 1999;257(1):79–83.

140. Wang Y, Xu A, Knight C, Xu LY, et al. Hydroxylation and glycosylation of the four conserved lysine residues in the collagenous domain of adiponectin: Potential role in the modulation of its insulin-sensitizing activity. J Biol Chem 2002;277(22):19521–29.

141. Hotta K, Funahashi T, Arita Y, et al. Plasma concentrations of a novel, adipose-specific protein, adiponectin, in type 2 diabetic patients. Arterioscler Thromb Vasc Biol 2000;20(6):1595–99.

142. Berg AH, Combs TP, Du X, et al. The adipocyte-secreted protein Acrp30 enhances hepatic insulin action. Nat Med 2001;7(8):947–53.

143. Yang WS, Lee WJ, Funahashi T, et al. Weight reduction increases plasma levels of an adipose-derived anti-inflammatory protein, adiponectin. J Clin Endocrinol Metab 2001;86(8):3815–19.

144. Hotta K, Funahashi T, Bodkin NL, et al. Circulating concentrations of the adipocyte protein adiponectin are decreased in parallel with reduced insulin sensitivity during the progression to type 2 diabetes in rhesus monkeys. Diabetes 2001;50(5):1126–33.

145. Weyer C, Funahashi T, Tanaka S, et al. Hypoadiponectinemia in obesity and type 2 diabetes: Close association with insulin resistance and hyperinsulinemia. J Clin Endocrinol Metab 2001;86(5):1930–35.

146. Yamauchi T, Kamon J, Waki H, et al. The fat-derived hormone adiponectin reverses insulin resistance associated with both lipoatrophy and obesity. Nat Med 2001;7(8):941–46.

147. Maeda N, Takahashi M, Funahashi T, et al. PPARgamma ligands increase expression and plasma concentrations of adiponectin, an adipose-derived protein. Diabetes 2001;50(9):2094–99.

148. Wajchenberg BL. Subcutaneous and visceral adipose tissue: Their relation to the metabolic syndrome. Endocr Rev 2000;21(6):697–738.

149. Yamauchi T, Kamon J, Ito Y, et al. Cloning of adiponectin receptors that mediate antidiabetic metabolic effects. Nature 2003;423(6941):762–69.

150. Yamauchi T, Kamon J, Minokoshi Y, et al. Adiponectin stimulates glucose utilization and fatty-acid oxidation by activating AMP-activated protein kinase. Nat Med 2002;8(11):1288–95.

151. Kharroubi I, Rasschaert J, Eizirik DL, et al. Expression of adiponectin receptors in pancreatic beta cells. Biochem Biophys Res Commun 2003;312(4):1118–22.

152. Yamauchi T, Kamon J, Waki H, et al. Globular adiponectin protected ob/ob mice from diabetes and ApoE-deficient mice from atherosclerosis. J Biol Chem 2003;278(4):2461–68.

153. Fruebis J, Tsao TS, Javorschi S, et al. Proteolytic cleavage product of 30-kDa adipocyte complement-related protein increases fatty acid oxidation in muscle and causes weight loss in mice. Proc Natl Acad Sci USA 2001;98(4):2005–10.

154. Kim KH, Lee K, Moon YS, Sul HS. A cysteine-rich adipose tissue-specific secretory factor inhibits adipocyte differentiation. J Biol Chem 2001;276(14):11252–56.

155. Holcomb IN, Kabakoff RC, Chan B, et al. FIZZ1, a novel cysteine-rich secreted protein associated with pulmonary inflammation, defines a new gene family. EMBO J 2000;19(15):4046–55.

156. Steppan CM, Bailey ST, Bhat S, Brown EJ, et al. The hormone resistin links obesity to diabetes. Nature 2001;409(6818):307–12.

157. Steppan CM, Brown EJ, Wright CM, et al. A family of tissue-specific resistin-like molecules. Proc Natl Acad Sci USA 2001;98(2):502–06.

158. Aruna B, Ghosh S, Singh AK, et al. Human recombinant resistin protein displays a tendency to aggregate by forming intermolecular disulfide linkages. Biochemistry 2003;42:10554–59.

159. Chen J, Wang L, Boeg YS, et al. Differential dimerization and association among resistin family proteins with implications for functional specificity. J Endocrinol 2002;175(2):499–504.

160. Banerjee RR, Lazar MA. Dimerization of resistin and resistin-like molecules is determined by a single cysteine. J Biol Chem 2001;276(28):25970–73.

161. Rea R, Donnelly R. Resistin: An adipocyte-derived hormone. Has it a role in diabetes and obesity? Diabetes Obes Metab 2004;6(3):163–70.

162. Adeghate E. An update on the biology and physiology of resistin. Cell Mol Life Sci 2004;61:2485–96.

163. Nogueiras R, Gallego R, Gualillo O, et al. Resistin is expressed in different rat tissues and is regulated in a tissue- and gender-specific manner. FEBS Lett 2003;548:21–7.

164. Morash BA, Willkinson D, Ur E, et al. Resistin expression and regulation in mouse pituitary. FEBS Lett 2002;526:26–30.

165. McTernan CL, McTernan PG, Harte AL, et al. Resistin, central obesity, and type 2 diabetes. Lancet 2002;359:46–7.

166. Mc Ternan P, Mc Ternan C, Chetty C. Increased resistin gene and protein expression in human abdominal adipose tissue. J Clin Endocrinol Metab 2002;87:2407.

167. Janke J, Engeli S, Gorzelniak K, et al. Resistin gene expression in human adipocytes is not related to insulin resistance. Obes Res 2002;10(1):1–5.

**101**

168. Viengchareun S, Zennaro MC, Pascual-Le Tallec L, et al. Brown adipocytes are novel sites of expression and regulation of adiponectin and resistin. FEBS Lett 2002;532(3):345–50.

169. Meier U, Gressner AM. Endocrine regulation of energy metabolism: Review of pathobiochemical and clinical chemical aspects of leptin, ghrelin, adiponectin, and resistin. Clin Chem 2004;50(9):1511–25.

170. Shuldiner AR, Yang R, Gong DW. Resistin, obesity and insulin resistance: The emerging role of the adipocyte as an endocrine organ. N Engl J Med 2001;345(18):1345–46.

171. Way JM, Gorgun CZ, Tong Q, et al. Adipose tissue resistin expression is severely suppressed in obesity and stimulated by peroxisome proliferator-activated receptor gamma agonists. J Biol Chem 2001;276(28):25651–53.

172. Moore GB, Chapman H, Holder JC, et al. Differential regulation of adipocytokine mRNAs by rosiglitazone in db/db mice. Biochem Biophys Res Commun 2001;286(4):735–41.

173. Le Lay S, Boucher J, Rey A, et al. Decreased resistin expression in mice with different sensitivities to a high-fat diet. Biochem Biophys Res Commun 2001;289(2):564–67.

174. Youn BS, Yu KY, Park HJ, et al. Plasma resistin concentrations measured by enzyme-linked immunosorbent assay using a newly developed monoclonal antibody are elevated in individuals with type 2 diabetes mellitus. J Clin Endocrinol Metab 2004;89(1):150–56.

175. Rea R, Donnelly R. Resistin: An adipocyte-derived hormone. Has it a role in diabetes and obesity? Diabetes Obes Metab 2004;6(3):163–70.

176. Lee JH, Chan JL, Yiannakouris N, et al. Circulating resistin levels are not associated with obesity or insulin resistance in humans and are not regulated by fasting or leptin administration: Cross-sectional and interventional studies in normal, insulin-resistant, and diabetic subjects. J Clin Endocrinol Metab 2003;88(10):4848–56.

177. Toda Y, Toda T, Takemura S, et al. Change in body fat, but not body weight or metabolic correlates of obesity, is related to symptomatic relief of obese patients with knee osteoarthritis after a weight control program. J Rheumatol 1998;25:2181–86.

178. Yudkin JS, Stehouwer CD, Emeis JJ, et al. C-reactive protein in healthy subjects: Associations with obesity, insulin resistance, and endothelial dysfunction: A potential role for cytokines originating from adipose tissue? Arterioscler Thromb Vasc Biol 1999;19(4):972–78.

179. Festa A, D'Agostino R Jr., Williams K, et al. The relation of body fat mass and distribution to markers of chronic inflammation. Int J Obes Relat Metab Disord 2001;25(10):1407–15.

180. Das UN. Is obesity an inflammatory condition? Nutrition 2001; 17(11/12):953–66.

181. Axelsson J, Heimburger O, Lindholm B, et al. Adipose tissue and its relation to inflammation: The role of adipokines. J Ren Nutr 2005;15(1):131–36.

182. Trayhurn P. Adipose tissue in obesity: An inflammatory issue. Endocrinology 2005;146(3):1003–05.

183. Lafontan M. Fat cells: Afferent and efferent messages define new approaches to treat obesity. Annu Rev Pharmacol Toxicol 2005;45:119–46.

184. Gordeladze JO, Drevon CA, Syversen U, et al. Leptin stimulates human osteoblastic cell proliferation, de novo collagen synthesis, and mineralization: Impact on differentiation markers, apoptosis, and osteoclastic signaling. J Cell Biochem 2002;85(4):825–36.

185. Ducy P, Amling M, Takeda S, et al. Leptin inhibits bone formation through a hypothalamic relay: A central control of bone mass. Cell 2000;100(2):197–207.

186. Takeda S, Elefteriou F, Levasseur R, et al. Leptin regulates bone formation via the sympathetic nervous system. Cell 2002; 111(3):305–17.

187. Elefteriou F, Takeda S, Ebihara K, et al. Serum leptin level is a regulator of bone mass. Proc Natl Acad Sci USA 2004;101(9):3258–63.

188. Schett G, Kiechl S, Bonora E, et al. Serum leptin level and the risk of nontraumatic fracture. Am J Med 2004;117(12):952–56.

189. Presle N, Pottie P, Dumond H, Guillame C, Lapicque F, Paullu S, et al. Differential distribution of adipokines between serum and synovial fluid in patients with osteoarthritis: Contribution of joint tissues to their articular production. Osteoarthritis Cartilage 2006;14(7):690–95.

190. Dumond H, Presle N, Terlain B, et al. Evidence for a key role of leptin in osteoarthritis. Arthritis Rheum 2003;48(11):3118–29.

191. Bokarewa M, Bokarew D, Hultgren O, et al. Leptin consumption in the inflamed joints of patients with rheumatoid arthritis. Ann Rheum Dis 2003;62(10):952–56.

192. Huang L, Wang Z, Li C. Modulation of circulating leptin levels by its soluble receptor. J Biol Chem 2001;276:6343–49.

193. Otero M, Gomez Reino JJ, Gualillo O. Synergistic induction of nitric oxide synthase type II: In vitro effect of leptin and interferon-gamma in human chondrocytes and ATDC5 chondrogenic cells. Arthritis Rheum 2003;48:404–09.

194. Otero M, Lago R, Lago F, et al. Signalling pathway involved in nitric oxide synthase type II activation in chondrocytes: Synergistic effect of leptin with interleukin-1. Arthritis Res Ther 2005;7:R581–91.

195. Teichtahl AJ, Wluka AE, Proietto J, et al. Obesity and the female sex, risk factors for knee osteoarthrtitis that may be attributable to systemic or local leptin biosynthesis and its cellular effects. Medical Hypotheses 2005;65:312–15.

196. Kishida Y, Hirao M, Tamai N, et al. Leptin regulates chondrocyte differentiation and matrix maturation during endochondral ossification. Bone 2005 (in press).

197. Figenschau Y, Knutsen G, Shahazeydi S, et al. Human articular chondrocytes express functional leptin receptors. Biochem Biophys Res Commun 2001;287(1):190–97.

198. Morroni M, De Matteis R, Palumbo C, et al. In vivo leptin expression in cartilage and bone cells of growing rats and adult humans. J Anat 2004;205:291–96.

199. Maor G, Rochwerger M, Segev Y, et al. Leptin acts as a growth factor on the chondrocytes of skeletal growth centers. J Bone Miner Res 2002;17:1034–43.

200. Steppan CM, Crawford DT, Chidsey-Frink KL, et al. Leptin is a potent stimulator of bone growth in ob/ob mice. Regul Pept 2000;92:73–8.

201. Thomas T. The complex effects of leptin on bone metabolism through multiple pathways. Curr Opin Pharmacol 2004;4:295–300.

202. Reid IR, Ames R, Evans MC, et al. Determinants of total body and regional bone mineral density in normal postmenopausal women: A key role for fat mass. J Clin Endocrinol Metab 1992;75:45–51.

203. Khosla S, Atkinson EJ, Riggs BL, et al. Relationship between body composition and bone mass in women. J Bone Miner Res 1996;11(6):857–63.

204. Pasco JA, Henry MJ, Kotowicz MA, et al. Serum leptin levels are associated with bone mass in non obese women. J Clin Endocrinol Metab 2001;86:1884–87.

205. Ducy P, Schinke T, Karsenty G. The osteoblast: A sophisticated fibroblast under central surveillance. Science 2000;289:1501–04.

206. Kume K, Satomura K, Nishisho S, et al. Potential role of leptin in endochondral ossification. J Histochem Cytochem 2002;50:159–69.

207. Lajeunesse D, Delalandre H, Fernandez J. Subchondral osteoblasts from osteoarthritic patients show abnormal expression and production of leptin: Possible role in cartilage degradation. J Bone Mineral Research 2004;19(1):S149.

208. Lajeunesse D. The role of bone in the treatment of osteoarthritis. Osteoarthritis Cartilage 2004;12(A):S34–38.

209. Wellen K, Hotamisligil G. Inflammation, stress, and diabetes. J Clin Invest 2005;115:1111–19.

210. Xu H, Barnes GT, Yang Q, et al. Chronic inflammation in fat plays a crucial role in the development of obesity-related insulin resistance. J Clin Invest 2003;112(12):1821–30.

211. Luheshi GN, Gardner JD, Rushforth DA, et al. Leptin actions on food intake and body temperature are mediated by IL-1. Proc Natl Acad Sci USA 1999;96(12):7047–52.

212. Loffreda S, Yang SQ, Lin HZ, et al. Leptin regulates proinflammatory immune responses. FASEB J 1998;12(1):57–65.

213. Bernotiene E, Palmer G, Talabot Ayer D, et al. Delayed resolution of acute inflammation during zymosan-induces arthritis in leptin-deficient mice. Arthritis Research Ther 2004;6:R256–63.

214. Wolf AM, Wolf D, Rumpold H, et al. Adiponectin induces the anti-inflammatory cytokines IL-10 and IL-1 RA. Biochem Biophys Research Commun 2004;323:630–35.

215. Bokarewa M, Nagaev I, Dahlberg I, et al. Resistin, an adipokine with potent pro-inflammatory properties. J Immunol 2005; 174:5789–95.

216. Lajeunesse D, Pelletier JP, Martel-Pelletier J. Osteoarthritis: A metabolic disease induced by local abnormal leptin activity? Curr Rheumatol Rep 2005;7:79–81.

217. Loeser RF. Systemic and local regulation of articular cartilage metabolism: Where does leptin fit in the puzzle? Arthritis Rheum 2003;48:3009–12.

218. Scharstuhl A, Glansbeek HL, van Beuningen HM, Vitters EL, van der Kraan PM, van den Berg WB. Inhibition of endogenous TGF-α during experimental osteoarthritis prevents osteophyte formation and impairs cartilage repair. J Immunol 2002;169:507–601.

219. Grimaud E, Heymann D, Rédini F. Recent advances in TGF-α effects on chondrocyte metabolism: Potential therapeutic roles of TGF-α in cartilage disorders. Cytokine and Growth Factor Reviews 2002;13:241–57.

220. Bakker AC, van de Loo FAJ, van Beuningen HM, Sime P, van Lent PLME, van der Kraan PM, et al. Overexpression of active TGF-beta-1 in the murine knee joint: Evidence for synovial-layer-dependent chondro-osteophyte formation. Osteoarthritis Cartilage 2001;9:128–36.

221. Gallardo N, Arribas C, Villar M, et al. Ob-Ra and Ob-Re are differentially expressed in adipose tissue in aged food restricted rats: Effects on circulating soluble leptin receptor levels. Endocrinology 2005;146:4934-42.

# 7 Pathology and Animal Models of Osteoarthritis

Frank A. Wollheim and L. Stefan Lohmander

## INTRODUCTION

Osteoarthritis (OA), formerly called osteoarthrosis, was once considered a "degenerative" condition of the elderly and was not an attractive field of research.[1] Whereas it is true that OA prevalence increases sharply with age, it is not part of normal aging. Most research of OA has for obvious reasons focused on established cases and the early events are still largely unexplored, although animal models have offered some new insights into the initial pathology.

A recent review concludes: "Osteoarthritis is a disease affecting all joint structures, not just hyaline articular cartilage. It develops as a consequence of injurious activities acting on a vulnerable joint. The correlation between structural changes of the disease and joint symptoms is poor. Risk factors include age, obesity, and joint injury. Risk factors for symptoms include bone marrow edema, synovitis, and joint effusion."[2]

## FUNCTION AND ANATOMY OF THE NORMAL JOINT

Understanding of joint dysfunction requires some knowledge of normality. Normal joint function requires the following.

- The freedom of the opposed articular surfaces to move painlessly over each other within the required range of motion
- The correct distribution of load across joint tissues, which might be altered by mechanical overloading (resulting in damage) or by habitual underloading[2,3] (resulting in disuse atrophy)
- The maintenance of stability

These three interdependent aspects of joint function further depend on three features of joint design. First, the geometry of its opposed articulating surfaces is the most obvious feature of a joint. In general, one articular surface is convex, whereas the other is concave.

These complementary shapes are necessary to permit the range of motion required, to provide stability, and to ensure the most equitable loading during use. It was long thought that precise fit or congruence was a normal feature of a joint.[4] However, many joints are multiaxial and if they were to remain congruent in all positions the opposed surfaces would have to be perfectly spherical. As they are not, no joint can be congruent in all positions, although it may be more congruent in one position than in others (Figs. 7.1 and 7.2).

When loaded, the tissues of the joint surface (particularly the cartilage, but also the bone) undergo elastic deformation. Therefore, as the load is increased the surfaces come into increasing contact. In this way, as the load is increased it is more equally distributed. The deformation of the joint space under load also provides for the circulation and mixing of synovial fluid, essential to the metabolism of the chondrocytes (Fig. 7.3). It should be appreciated that overuse as well as underuse will affect joint structures and potentially cause pathology (Fig. 7.4).

## PATHOLOGY

OA may affect all parts of a joint and the periarticular tissues. The old dogma that OA is primarily and predominantly a cartilage abnormality is no longer true. Release of biomarkers indicate altered bone *and* cartilage metabolism, as well as inflammation in the earliest detectable stage of knee OA. Bone sialoprotein (BSP), cartilage oligomeric matrix protein (COMP), and CRP are all increased in such individuals—with attendant pain but as yet no detectable radiographic abnormality.[5] Some OA pathology features are shown in Table 7.1. Advanced OA in a large joint shows marked heterogeneity, as seen in Fig. 7.5. This is the result of long-standing processes of cartilage damage, bone sclerosis, cyst formation, and osteophyte formation.

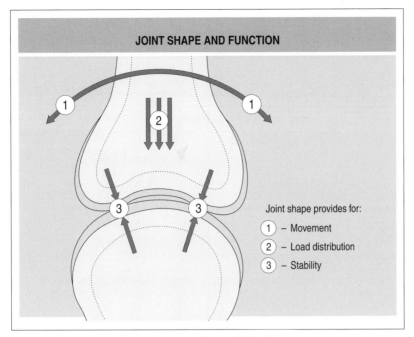

**Fig. 7.1** Joint shape and function.

Gross pathology can be studied radiographically or in specimens obtained at joint surgery, but these features are of limited interest for understanding initiating events in OA. However, even in specimens from advanced large-joint OA one can appreciate that OA gives rise to patchy lesions and that different areas of individual joints show varying degrees of gross pathology (Fig. 7.6). It can be seen that even the "early" changes of cartilage involve chondrocyte clustering and mitosis, fibrillation of the surface, chondrocyte death, and aggrecan loss.

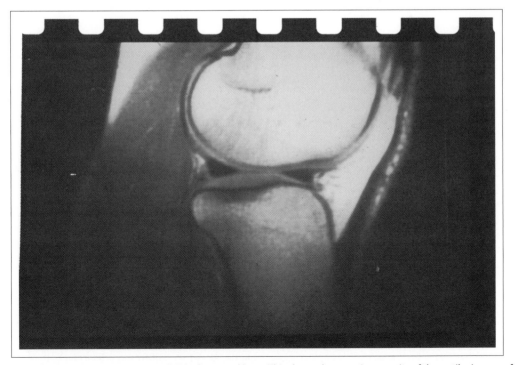

**Fig. 7.2** Sagittal magnetic resonance image (MRI) of a normal knee. This shows the gross incongruity of the cartilaginous surfaces, partially corrected by the interposed meniscus (which acts as load-bearing structure).

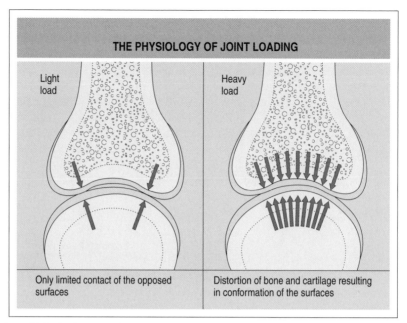

**Fig. 7.3** The physiology of joint loading. Light load: only limited contact of the opposed surfaces. Heavy load: distortion of bone and cartilage resulting in increased incongruity with increased loading of the surfaces.

Early phases of OA development in humans have been examined in few studies. One such study indicated initial changes in the middle zone of the cartilage, with characteristic up-regulation of cartilage intermediate layer protein (CILP).[6] COMP was also up-regulated in this area, whereas collagens were normal. Animal models of OA are a source of more substantial information on early events in OA.

## SPONTANEOUS AND EXPERIMENTALLY INDUCED OSTEOARTHRITIS

OA models have been used widely in attempts to understand the pathogenesis of the disorder and to develop therapeutic strategies for its management. Initially, drastic measures such as injections of noxious substances and mechanical destruction of parts of joints

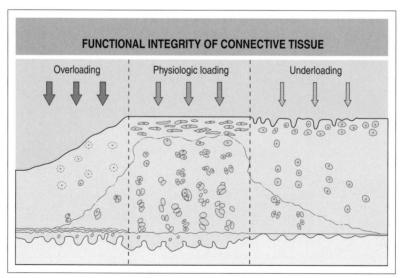

**Fig. 7.4** Functional integrity of connective tissue. The continued optimal functional integrity of connective tissue depends on balanced rates of matrix production and breakdown by the cells. Healthy tissue (center) results from a physiologic range of stress that maintains optimal cell activity and matrix production. If this range of stress is exceeded (left), the result is cell injury and eventual tissue death. If the stress is inadequate (right), disuse atrophy (i.e., lack of adequate matrix production by the cells) may occur. In cartilage, this is associated with increased water content, superficial fibrillation of the collagen, altered organization of collagen fibrils, and increased ease of dissociation of proteoglycan from the collagen framework.

**TABLE 7.1 PATHOLOGIC FEATURES OF OSTEOARTHRITIS**

| Tissue | Activity | Early Progression | Advanced Progression |
|---|---|---|---|
| Cartilage | Matrix edema<br>Proteoglycan depletion<br>Chondrocyte apoptosis, necrosis<br>Perichondrocyte proteoglycan<br>Chondrocyte hypertrophy with<br>intracellular proteoglycans<br>Tidemark active calcification | Fibrillation, superficial zone<br>Perichondral collagen condensation<br>Chondrocyte proliferation<br>Tidemark advancement | Fissures (clefts), midzone<br>Matrix delamination<br>Matrix erosion<br>Matrix fibrosis<br>Reparative fibrocartilage<br>Articular disruption |
| Bone | Osteoblast/osteoclast activity<br>Decreased mineralization,<br>subchondral plate | Subchondral thickening<br>Capillary penetration through<br>the subchondral plate | Eburnated bone surface<br>Articular plate fractures<br>Corrugated bone surface<br>Osteonecrosis<br>Osteophyte formation<br>Subchondral marrow fibrosis<br>Subchondral cyst formation |
| Synovium | Edema<br>Vascular congestion<br>Infiltration by occasional<br>lymphocytes and plasma cells | Lining cell hyperplasia<br>Increased collagen at surface<br>Focal lymphoid follicles | Subliminal and<br>perivascular fibrosis<br>Fragments of necrotic<br>cartilage and bone |

Source: Brandt KD, Doherty M, and Lohmander LS. *Osteoarthritis, Second Edition*. Oxford, UK: Oxford University Press 2003:51.

were used. Later, Pond and Nuki[7] refined the model of Paatsama[8] of transection of the anterior cruciate ligament in the dog, which has been extensively used as an OA model that closely parallels that resulting from human knee ligament lesions.[9] Most of the older OA models induce injury and study attempted repair.[10] The models listed in Fig. 7.7 are based on induced instability or induction of abnormal loading. Other methods target cells by injection of toxic substances such as colchicine and osmic acid, which cause synovial inflammation or iodoacetamide (which penetrates cartilage and affects chondrocytes). The relevance for human OA of these chemically induced disease models can be questioned.

Perhaps more relevant but more difficult to study are the spontaneous forms of OA in mice, rats, guinea pigs, dogs, horses, rhesus monkeys, and other species. Some mouse strains develop "spontaneous" OA, and in one such strain (STR/1N) evidence of attempted repair, chondrocyte hypertrophy, and increased bone formation have been studied.[11] Another strain (STR/ort) was derived from STR/1N after a period of outbreeding, and in this strain 85% of male animals developed OA by week 35. This model has many features of human OA (Fig. 7.8) and allows precise monitoring of the process on magnetic resonance imaging (MRI), scanning electron microscopy, and by biomarkers.[12] The medial knee joint is generally affected, whereas the lateral parts are spared.

Ankle deformities are not unusual, but it is unclear whether this represents real OA or is a manifestation of joint laxity. Patellar subluxation was originally believed to be of pathogenetic importance, but the correlation is not strong. Soft tissue calcifications are also a feature in the STR/ort strain. As in human OA, net cartilage matrix proteoglycan depletion and metalloproteinase and aggrecanase expression occur. Increased chondrocyte apoptosis is present. Inflammation is not prominent in STR/ort disease. A recent study looked at gene expression of aggrecan and types II, X, and XI collagen in non OA-prone CBA mice in comparison with STR/ort mice.[13] All four genes were expressed in both young and old mice of both species, but were inactive adjacent to OA lesions. Thus, it is unlikely that OA development in this model is caused by failure to synthesize the proteins. However, once the lesions are manifest synthesis may be down-regulated. The molecular basis of this interesting model merits further investigation.

A recent comprehensive review of spontaneous chemically and physically induced animal models emphasized that the only way to validate a model is to show that it is responsive to measures proved to be effective in human OA.[14] Instability is a well-established route to OA in the Pond–Nuki dog OA model. Neurogenic acceleration of joint damage, influence of immobilization and muscle weakness, and evidence against a primary role of subchondral bone stiffening have all been convincingly documented in this model. Therapeutic studies were also reviewed. Cyclo-oxygenase (COX) inhibitors are without effect on joint damage, whereas doxycycline has an inhibiting effect on OA

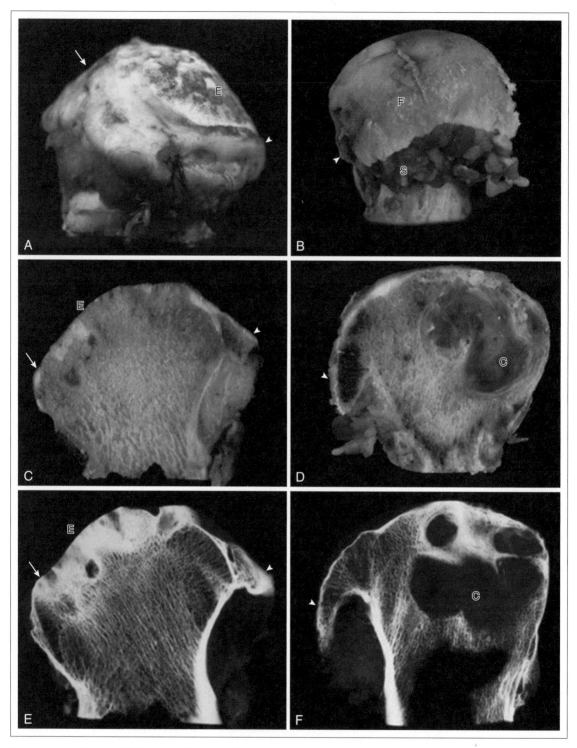

**Fig. 7.5** Gross pathology of OA involving the femoral head. To demonstrate the variability of gross pathology, two femoral heads that have been removed surgically because of OA are illustrated. Both specimens show extensive remodeling. The femoral head is shown in A, B, and C (with extensive eburnation of the surface and articular plate bone sclerosis): 1a (surface), 1b (cut surface), and 1c (specimen X-ray of 1b). Prominent features of OA include cartilage erosion, bone eburnation (E), and osteophyte formation. The femoral head (with a relative preservation of cartilage, extreme subchondral bone cyst formation, and extreme osteophyte formation) is shown in D, E, and F: D (surface), E (cut surface), and F (specimen X-ray of E). Prominent features include cartilage fibrillation (F), synovial hypertrophy (S), osteophyte formation, and cyst formation (C). (From Brandt KD, Doherty M, and Lohmander LS. *Osteoarthritis,* Second Edition. Oxford, UK: Oxford University Press 2003:53, fig. 5.1.)

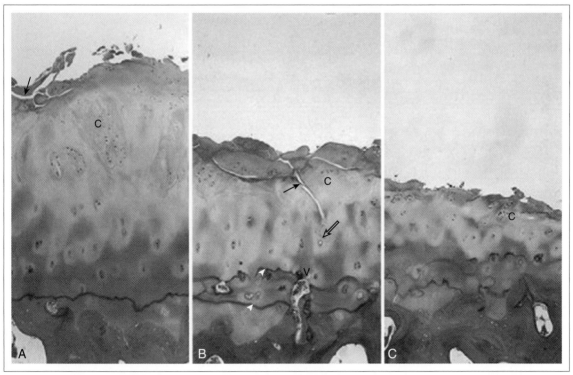

**Fig. 7.6** Microscopic pathology of OA articular cartilage. The photomicrographs are taken from different areas of the same specimen: A (early OA, horizontal fibrillation, and chondrocyte clusters [C]), B (moderate OA, vertical fissure, chondrocyte death, tidemark undulation and duplication, vascular penetration into cartilage [V], and chondrocyte clusters [C]), C (advanced OA, with cartilage erosion; cartilage matrix disorganization; and chondrocyte clusters [C]). Hematoxylin and eosin stain, magnification × 40. (From Brandt KD, Doherty M, and Lohmander LS. *Osteoarthritis,* Second Edition. Oxford, UK: Oxford University Press 2003:54, fig. 5.2.)

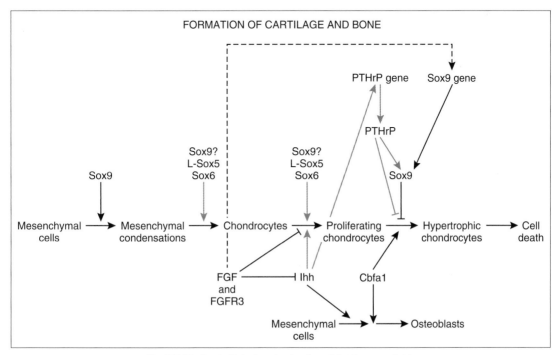

**Fig. 7.7** Mechanically induced animal models of osteoarthritis.

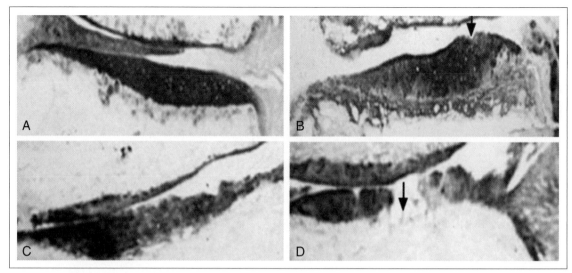

**Fig. 7.8** Medical tibial cartilage of male STR/ort mice with Alcian blue (AB) showing varying stages of histologic OA. (A) Normal cartilage with smooth surface and uniform AB matrix staining. (B) Early OA with loss of AB stain and small surface lesion. (C) Advancing OA with marked loss of AB staining and extensive surface roughening and fibrillation. (D) Severe OA with loss of AB staining and loss of articular cartilage down to the subchondral bone. Original magnification × 10. (From Mason RM, Chambers MG, Flannelly J, et al. The STR/ort mouse and its use as a model of osteoarthritis. Osteoarthritis Cartilage 2001;9:85–91.)

development in the Pond–Nuki model—possibly mediated by matrix metalloproteinase (MMP) inhibition. Co-administration of pentosan sulfate and insulin-like growth factor-1 (IGF-1) is also protective, possibly by lowering MMPs and increasing tissue inhibitor of metalloproteinase (TIMP).

A new generation of animal OA models has been created by means of gene manipulation. Targeted deletions directed at components of the structural collagen network that predispose animals to premature OA confirm the importance of these collagens for cartilage function. An example is the transgenic Del1 mouse that carries a deletion in exon 7 and intron 7 of the COL2a gene, resulting in early OA.[15] A transient up-regulation of the COMP gene at the border to the calcified cartilage and a shift from interterritorial to pericellular location of the COMP compared to non-transgenic control C57B1∞DBA mice closely mimic similar changes in human OA.

In the same model, expression of the Sox9 gene and deposition of embryonic collagen type IIA, characteristic features of early chondrogenesis, were found in some areas (indicative of repair). Expression of metalloproteinases and tissue inhibitors has also been explored in the Dell mouse model. MMP-13 and TIMP-1 were absent in degrading cartilage but were up-regulated in hyperplastic synovial tissue, subchondral bone, and calcified cartilage.[16,17] Neoepitopes of aggrecan (possibly resulting from MMP-13-driven catabolism) were found in the same location.

Another study showed that transgenic postnatal expression of human MMP-13 in articular cartilage chondrocytes of mice induced OA.[18] Other animal experiments have addressed the old question whether OA starts in bone or cartilage and lend support to the early bone involvement.[19]

More recent transgenic mouse models have targeted aggrecan and aggrecanases to clarify their role in OA pathogenesis. These reports show that in the mouse ADAMTS-5 is the protease of primary importance for joint cartilage aggrecan degradation and loss in OA and arthritis models, in that knockout of this gene protects the animals from disease.[20,21] On the other hand, ADAMTS-4 does not appear to be crucial for aggrecan degradation in mouse arthritis because knockout of these genes does not influence arthritis model severity.[22] However, additional work will be needed to confirm the applicability of these findings to other animal OA models or for human OA.[23,24]

Genetic background and variability as well as sex strongly influence OA susceptibility, even in standardized animal OA models. This was shown by the widely varying frequency of OA induced in various inbred mouse strains by a standardized OA model using meniscus destabilization.[25,26]

The role of muscle strength and loading has also been studied, and its role in unstable knee joints is well established. A quadriceps muscle weakness model in cats based on injection of botulinum toxin produced knee joint deterioration even in the absence of joint instability.[27]

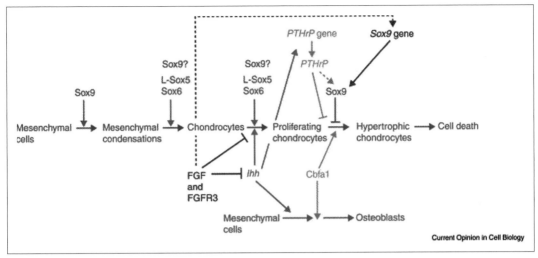

**Fig. 7.9** Chondrocyte reaction pattern. Schematic representation of basic chondrocyte reaction pattern and main factors influencing it. (Redrawn with permission from De Crombrugghe B, Lefebvre V, Nakashima K. Regulatory mechanisms in the pathways of cartilage and bone formation. Curr Opin Cell Biol 2001;13:721–27.)

Animal models thus have great potential for the study of early and later phases of the OA process, for identifying candidate genes, for the identification of biomarkers, and for investigating therapeutic interventions. However, extrapolation from animal to human disease is never straightforward—as evidenced in years of frustrations in drug development for OA.

## SUMMARY

OA in various forms affects the lives of more individuals than any other joint disease. Its pathogenesis involves all joint tissues, but structural changes become manifest mainly in cartilage and bone. Under the influence of mechanical factors, cartilage pathology in OA will result from unbalanced synthesis and catabolism by cells responding to signals from its matrix and to mediators from the outside. Genetic abnormalities of structural matrix components such as collagens, aggrecan, and COMP may lead to premature OA.

Age and genetic predisposition interact with a number of modifying factors, which include obesity, trauma, mechanical overload, crystal deposition, abnormal biomechanics, impaired joint alignment or stability, decreased proprioception, and muscle weakness. Inflammatory and hormonal mechanisms participate in the progression of OA. OA may thus be considered the net result of a number of different processes acting on the joint tissues of a susceptible individual. How and when OA becomes symptomatic is complex and is still poorly understood (Fig. 7.9).

## REFERENCES

1. Dieppe P. Osteoarthritis. In P Dieppe, FA Wollheim, HR Schumacher Jr. (eds.), *Classic Papers in Rheumatology*. London: Martin Dunitz 2002:256–73.
2. Felson DT. An update on the pathogenesis and epidemiology of osteoarthritis. Radiol Clin North Am 2004;42(1):1–9.
3. Palmoski MJ, Colyer RA, Brandt KD. Joint motion in the absence of normal loading does not maintain normal articular cartilage. Arthritis Rheum 1980;23:325–34.
4. Bullough PG. The geometry of diarthrodial joints: Its physiological maintenance and the possible significance of age-related changes in geometry to load distribution and the development of osteoarthritis. Clin Orthop 1981;156:61–6.
5. Petersson IF, Boegard T, Dahlstrom J, Svensson B, Heinegard D, Saxne T. Bone scan and serum markers of bone and cartilage in patients with knee pain and osteoarthritis. Osteoarthritis Cartilage 1998;6(1):33–9.
6. Lorenzo P, Bayliss MT, Heinegard D. Altered patterns and synthesis of extracellular matrix macromolecules in early osteoarthritis. Matrix Biol 2004;23(6):381–91.
7. Pond MJ, Nuki G. Experimentally-induced osteoarthritis in the dog. Ann Rheum Dis 1973;32:387–88.
8. Paatsama S. Ligament injuries in the canine stifle joint: A clinical and experimental study. Ph.D. Thesis, Helsinki, 1952.
9. Brandt KD, Myers SL, Burr D, Albrecht M. Osteoarthritic changes in canine articular cartilage, subchondral bone, and synovium fifty-four months after transection of the anterior cruciate ligament. Arthritis Rheum 1991;34:1560–70.
10. Pritzker KP. Animal models for osteoarthritis: Processes, problems and prospects. Ann Rheum Dis 1994;53:406–20.
11. Benske J, Schunke M, Tillmann B. Subchondral bone formation in arthrosis: Polychrome labeling studies in mice. Acta Orthop Scand 1988;59:536–41.
12. Mason RM, Chambers MG, Flannelly J, et al. The STR/ort mouse and its use as a model of osteoarthritis. Osteoarthritis Cartilage 2001;9:85–91.
13. Chambers MG, Kuffner T, Cowan SK, et al. Expression of collagen and aggrecan genes in normal and osteoarthritic murine knee joints. Osteoarthritis Cartilage 2002;10:51–61.

14. Brandt KD. Animal models of osteoarthritis. Biorheology 2002;39:221–35.

15. Salminen H, Perala M, Lorenzo P, et al. Up-regulation of cartilage oligomeric matrix protein at the onset of articular cartilage degeneration in a transgenic mouse model of osteoarthritis. Arthritis Rheum 2000;43:1742–48.

16. Salminen H, Vuorio E, Samaanen AH. Expression of Sox9 and type IIA procollagen during attempted repair of articular cartilage damage in a transgenic mouse model of osteoarthritis. Arthritis Rheum 2001;44:947–55.

17. Salminen HJ, Saamanen AM, Vankemmelbeke MN, et al. Expression of collagen and aggrecan genes in normal and osteoarthritic murine knee joints. Ann Rheum Dis 2002; 61:591–97.

18. Neuhold LA, Killar L, Zhao W, Sung ML, Warner L, Kulik J, et al. Postnatal expression in hyaline cartilage of constitutively active human collagenase-3 (MMP-13) induces osteoarthritis in mice. J Clin Invest 2001;107(1):35–44.

19. van den Berg WB. Lessons from animal models of osteoarthritis. Curr Opin Rheumatol 2001;13(5):452–56.

20. Stanton H, Rogerson FM, East CJ, Golub SB, Lawlor KE, Meeker CT, et al. ADAMTS5 is the major aggrecanase in mouse cartilage in vivo and in vitro. Nature 2005;434(7033):648–52.

21. Glasson SS, Askew R, Sheppard B, Carito B, Blanchet T, Ma HL, et al. Deletion of active ADAMTS5 prevents cartilage degradation in a murine model of osteoarthritis. Nature 2005;434(7033): 644–48.

22. Glasson SS, Askew R, Sheppard B, Carito BA, Blanchet T, Ma HL, et al. Characterization of osteoarthritis susceptibility in ADAMTS-4-knockout mice. Arthritis Rheum 2004;50(8):2547–58.

23. Lark MW, Bayne EK, Flanagan J, Harper CF, Hoerrner LA, Hutchinson NI, et al. Aggrecan degradation in human cartilage: Evidence for both aggrecanase and matrix metalloproteinase activity in normal, osteoarthritic and rheumatoid joints. J Clin Invest 1997;100:93–106.

24. Struglics A, Larsson S, Pratta MA, Kumar S, Lohmander LS. Human osteoarthritis synovial fluid and joint cartilage contain both aggrecanase and matrix metalloproteinase generated aggrecan fragments. Osteoarthritis Cartilage 2006 Feb;14(2):101–13.

25. Ma H, Blanchet TJ, Morris EA, Glasson SS. Disease progression in surgically induced murine osteoarthritis is strain and sex dependent. Transactions of the Orthopaedic Research Society (Washington) 2005;30:1422.

26. Glasson SS, Blanchet TJ, Morris EA. Less severe OA is observed in IL-1 beta KO mice and more severe OA is observed in MMP-9 and MK2 KO mice in a surgical model of OA. Transactions of the Orthopaedic Research Society (Washington) 2005;30:0251.

27. Herzog W, Longino D, Clark A. The role of muscles in joint adaptation and degeneration. Langenbecks Arch Surg 2003; 388(5):305–15.

# 8 Biochemical Markers of Osteoarthritis

Patrick Garnero

## INTRODUCTION

The major manifestations of osteoarthritis (OA) are abnormal and degraded cartilage, synovial, and bone tissue, changes that may contribute to pain and severe mobility impairment. Consequences of the disease on pain and function are often scored according to questionnaire indices, and although a number of standardized rating systems have been introduced it remains difficult to quantify these parameters. Because inflammation of synovial tissue is present in a substantial proportion of patients with OA, inflammatory parameters such as highly sensitive assay for C-reactive protein (CRP) have been suggested to provide useful information about the general inflammatory process. However, these biologic markers are not joint specific and correlate poorly with cartilage damage at the individual level.

Because measures of symptoms, function, and pathogenic processes cannot capture the extent of joint damage itself, imaging modalities and X-ray in particular remain the mainstay of assessing OA disease severity. Although improvements in positioning and other elements of the radiographic protocol have been achieved in recent years, because of its poor sensitivity and relatively large precision error this technique does not allow early detection of joint tissue damage or an efficient monitoring of the efficacy of treatment aimed at preventing joint destruction. Clearly, for identifying patients at high risk for destructive OA and for monitoring efficacy of novel disease-modifying therapies (DMOADs) there is a need for better approaches than plain radiographs.

Magnetic resonance (MR) imaging (MRI), which provides direct information on the alteration of the different joint structures, is more sensitive than radiography in detecting cartilage loss and its application is currently being optimized in OA. Complementary to developments in imaging, there has recently been a considerable interest in developing specific biologic markers that reflect quantitative and dynamic variations in joint tissue remodeling and that can predict progression ahead of the time required for imaging studies to show change. In this chapter, we briefly review the biochemistry of the extracellular matrix of bone, cartilage, and synovial tissue—which form the molecular rationale for the development of biochemical markers. The chapter also discusses their potential clinical uses in OA.

## BASIC BIOLOGY AND BIOCHEMISTRY OF JOINT TISSUES

Joints are enclosed in a strong fibrous capsule. The inner surfaces of the joint capsule are lined with a metabolically active tissue, the synovium, which secretes the synovial fluid that provides the nutrients required by the tissues within the joint. Each articular bone end within the joint is lined by a thin layer of hydrated soft tissue (i.e., the articular cartilage).

In joint diseases, there is a loss of the normal balance between synthesis and degradation of the macromolecules that provide articular cartilage with its biomechanical and functional properties. Concomitantly, changes occur in the metabolism of the synovium and of the subchondral bone. Consequently, for a comprehensive assessment of the abnormalities of joint metabolism associated with OA it is important to obtain biochemical markers that reflect specifically the turnover of bone, cartilage, and synovial tissue.

### Bone

A thorough review of bone matrix and related biochemical markers is beyond the scope of this chapter, and the reader is referred to two recent detailed reviews.[1,2] The organic component of bone matrix is mainly composed of type I collagen molecules linked by cross-linking molecules (such as pyridinoline, deoxypyridinoline, and pyrolle) in the telopeptide regions. Bone matrix also includes several non-collagenous proteins, some of which are fairly unique to bone tissue (including osteocalcin and bone sialoprotein [BSP]). BSP is a 60- to 70-Kd phosphorylated glycoprotein that could be involved in the mineralization process.

Interestingly, and in contrast to the other bone proteins, BSP has a relatively restricted distribution to the osteocartilaginous interfaces involved early in OA.[3]

## Articular Cartilage

Articular cartilage is a material with two major phases: a fluid phase composed of water and electrolytes and a solid phase composed of collagen, proteoglycans, glycoproteins, other proteins, and the chondrocytes. Each of the phases contributes to the mechanical and physiologic properties of cartilage. Of the organic components, the collagens (largely collagen type II) are quantitatively the major component, followed by proteoglycans (especially aggrecan).[4] Although the other proteins are not major components in terms of the absolute solid phase, they may approach the molar concentration of collagen and aggrecan. Much of the non-collagenous component of articular cartilage has yet to be identified.

### Collagens of the Articular Cartilage

The predominant type of collagen is type II, which is cartilage specific and forms the basic fibrillar structure of the extracellular matrix. Types IX and XI are also cartilage specific, and are present together with type II collagen. There is evidence that many collagens (including types II, IX, and XI in cartilage) exist as hybrid molecules. In contrast, type VI collagen forms distinct microfibrils that appear concentrated in the capsular matrix surrounding individual chondrocytes or groups of chondrocytes. Type II collagen is a homotrimer $(\alpha 1 \, [II])_3$.

In cartilage, the various type II collagen molecules are covalently linked by pyridinoline. In contrast to bone, deoxypyridinoline is virtually absent from cartilage. Type IX collagen contributes only 1% of the total collagen in mature articular cartilage, although it is present at a much higher concentration in fetal tissue. It is present on the surface of type II collagen fibrils in an anti-parallel fashion, and each type IX collagen is covalently linked to at least one type II collagen molecule. Type IX collagen therefore appears to have an important role in stabilizing the 3D organization of the collagen network, and its reduction in function has the potential to contribute to articular cartilage damage.

### Type II Collagen Synthesis

The synthesis of type II collagen proceeds in the same way as the other secreted glycoproteins by chondrocytes. Type II collagen undergoes a series of post-translational modifications. Of importance is the glycosylation of the hydroxylysine. The predominant glycosylation is that by galactose-glucose, which is different from the predominant galactose form found in bone type I collagen.

Only after secretion, as the molecules reach the extracellular space, are the non-helicoidal domains at the end—namely, the N and C type II propeptides (PIINP and PIICP)—cleaved from the helicoidal domain. There are two splicing alternative forms of type II procollagen, which differ by the presence (IIA) or absence (IIB) of a 69-amino-acid sequence coded by exon 2 in the N-propeptide (Fig. 8.1). Procollagen IIA is expressed mainly during development but can be reexpressed in osteoarthritic cartilage,[5] whereas the IIB variant is the major form of adult cartilage. The two forms of PIINP (PIIANP and PIIBNP) and PIICP may thus serve as markers of type II collagen synthesis.

### Type II Collagen Degradation

Type II collagen is degraded by proteolytic enzymes secreted by the chondrocytes and the synoviocytes of

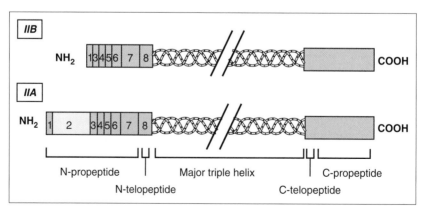

Fig. 8.1 Schematic representation of the two alternative forms of type II procollagen. Type II procollagen is constituted by the type II collagen molecule—comprising the major triple helix $[\alpha 1 \, (II)]_3$ and the linear N- and C-telopeptides—and the N- and C-terminal propeptides at the two extremities. The propeptides are removed by specific proteinases before the mature molecules are incorporated into fibrils in matrix. They are released into biologic fluids and their levels are believed to reflect type II collagen synthesis. Type II procollagen is synthesized in two splice forms: type IIA and type IIB. Type IIA contains an additional 207-base-pair exon (exon-2) encoding the 69-amino-acid cysteine-rich domain of the N-propeptide and is expressed mainly by fetal tissues.

the synovial tissue, including the matrix metalloproteinases (MMP) and the cysteine proteases. Among the MMPs, the collagenases cleave the triple helical region of type II collagen at a single site between residues 778 and 776—generating two fragments representing (respectively) $\frac{3}{4}$ and $\frac{1}{4}$ of the intact collagen molecule. Other MMPs—including the gelatinases and stromelysins, especially stromelysin 1 (also named MMP3)—can cleave denatured collagen within the triple helical domain and the telopeptides. Stomelysin 1, which attacks type II collagen within the telopeptides, may not have a major role in this process[6] but could contribute indirectly to collagen breakdown by activating the other MMPs. MMP13 (whose expression is increased in OA) could be one of the major enzymes involved in the increased type II collagen degradation.[7,8]

Although MMPs are likely to play a major role in degradation of type II collagen in OA, several cysteine proteases have also been suggested to contribute to cartilage destruction. Among them, several reports have shown increased expression of cathepsins B, L, K, and S.[9] Cathepsins B and L have been shown to cleave

type II collagen within the non-helical telopeptide of collagens, whereas cathepsin K is capable of cleaving collagen at multiple sites within the triple helix of type I and type II collagen[10,11] and has recently been suggested to be the major cysteine protease expressed in OA cartilage.[12,13] Cathepsin S has the peculiarity of being the only cysteine protease to be active at neutral and slightly alkaline pH and thus capable of participating in extracellular matrix degradation of articular cartilage. Although cathepsin S has a weak collagenolytic activity, it is very efficient in hydrolyzing aggrecan[14] and thus may play a deleterious role in the integrity of the aggrecan/type-II-collagen network.

### Aggrecan

Aggrecans are proteoglycans composed of a protein (core protein) and glycosaminoglycan (GAG) chains that are covalently attached to the core protein (Fig. 8.2). The core protein of aggrecan has a molecular mass of approximately 230 kDa and consists of three globular domains (G1, G2, and G3) and two GAG attachment domains: the keratan sulfate (KS) and

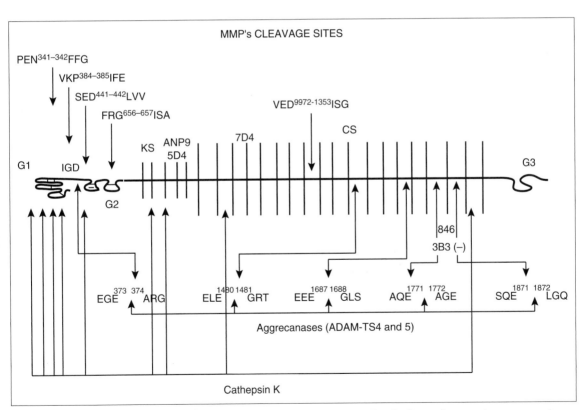

**Fig. 8.2** Schematic illustration of the aggrecan molecule, localization of the epitopes of antibodies used to assess its turnover, and proteolytic cleavage sites. A central core protein is substituted with about 100 glycosaminoglycan chains of chondroitin sulfate (CS) and keratan sulfate (KS). Specific domains include an N-terminal hyaluronate binding domain (G1), a homologous domain (G2), an interglobular domain (IGD), a KS-rich region, a CS-rich region, and a C-terminal domain (G3). This latter may be absent as a result of proteolytic cleavage. Several proteolytic cleavage sites have been identified for matrix-metalloproteases (MMPs), aggrecanases (including members of ADAMTS), and cysteine proteases such as cathepsin K. Antibodies against these various cleavage sites and other motifs (ANP9, 5D4, 7D4, 846, and 3B3 [−]) have been developed and used to investigate aggrecan turnover. (See Color Plate 4.)

the chondroitin sulfate (CS) domains. The total molecular mass can reach approximately 2,200 kDa.[15] The G1 domain has a structure consisting of three disulfide-bonded loops. Loop A has structural characteristics common to members of the IgG family and is involved in the interaction between aggrecan and link protein. Loops B and B′ are involved in binding to hyaluronan (HA).

The interglobular domain (IGD) between the G1 and G2 domains is rod shaped and contains proteolytic cleavage sites susceptible to a variety of proteinases, including MMPs; aggrecanases, including members of the A disintegrin and metalloproteinase with thrombospondin motifs (ADAMTS) family, such as ADMATS-5;[16] serine proteases such as plasmin and leukocyte elastase; and cysteine proteases such as cathepsin B and K[8,14,17] (Fig. 8.2). It is 90 residues long. The G2 domain is unique to aggrecan. This domain shows approximately 67% amino acid homology to that of the B–B′ region of the G1 domain.[15]

The location of the cysteine residues is essential for its ternary structure. After synthesis of the core protein by the chondrocytes, up to 50 KS chains (Gal β[1–4] GlucNAc β[1–3]) and 100 CS chains (GlcA β[1–3] GalNAc β[1–4]) are added during post-transcriptional processing and together these carbohydrates make up more than 90% of the molecular mass. Most of the KS chains are located within the KS domain at the C-terminus of the G2 domain, with the remainder being found in the CS attachment region. The CS domain is the largest domain of aggrecan and consists of approximately 120 serine-glycine (S-G) repeats.

The G3 domain (located at the C-terminus) consists of three modules: an epidermal growth factor (EGF)-like module, a C-type lectin module, and a complement regulatory proteins module. The aggrecan G3 domain may interact with tenascin in the cartilage.[15] With aging, the population of aggrecan without the G3 domain increases compared to that with full length.[18] This is likely to result from the proteolytic cleavage in the cartilage matrix rather than alternative splicing or other intracellular modifications.

## Synovium

The essential elements of synovium are a surface layer of cells (intima, or synovial lining); a superficial microvasculature net, and a connective tissue substratum (subintima, or subsynovium).[19] These elements are variable and at any one point one or more may be absent.

## Synovial Lining

The synovial lining (intima) is only a few cell layers deep, typically about three. It averages about 50 μm in the normal human knee. Most of the cells are macrophages or specialized fibroblasts. Intercellular links are rare in synovium, and the lining cells are mostly separated by spaces of 1 to 2 mm. The extracellular matrix contains elements found in basement membrane such as laminin and collagen type IV, but probably because of the absence of entactin (which links other basement membrane components) no true basement membrane is present. This represents a key importance of the filtering properties of the intima.

The major collagen is represented by microfibrils of type VI collagen, which seem to have a major role in maintaining structural integrity because they bind to hyaluronan and fibronectin. Because type VI collagen is resistant to metalloproteinases released by the inflamed synovium, it may be important for tissue integrity in this situation. Synovium also contains three other collagens that form striated fibrils (types I, III, and V). Type III is extensively distributed in the intimal matrix and in the subsynovium. Type I is also present in the intimal synovium matrix, but it appears less extensively distributed than type III collagen.[20]

## Synovial Fluid

Immediately beneath the synovial lining there is a net of capillaries that promotes rapid transfer of water and lipid-soluble solutes such as electrolytes, glucose, amino acids, and non protein-bound drugs. The passive ultrafiltration of plasma and exit of leukocytes across the walls of the synovial capillarities form the lymphatic component of the synovial tissue.[21] All proteins of plasma are also found in the lymph, but at decreased concentration due to molecular sieving by the capillary wall. Albumin is the predominant protein of the lymph and dominates the colloid osmotic pressure. The components that make the lymph of the synovium unusual are HA and lubricin, two biopolymers actively secreted by cells of the synovial lining.

HA is a high-molecular-weight glycosaminoglycan consisting of alternating units of β(1–4)-linked N-acetyl-β-D-glucosamine and β(1–3)-linked β-D-glucuronic acid. Each HA chain is a long unbranched polysaccharide of variable size ($2 \times 10^5 - 5 \times 10^5$). Its molecular weight in synovial fluid from healthy adults is approximately $0.5 \times 10^6$ daltons, and its concentration range is 0.1 to 5 mg/ml. Lubricin, a product of the gene proteoglycan 4 (PRG4), is a major component of synovial fluid and participates in the boundary lubrication of synovial fluids.[22,23] This protein is an O-linked glycosylated protein that is highly expressed by the synoviocytes.

It should be mentioned, however, that the PRG4 genes also coded the related gene products called superficial zone protein (SZP), megakaryocyte-stimulating growth factor (MSGF), and hemangiopoietin (HAPO). SZP is expressed by superficial zone chondrocytes at the cartilage surface but not in intermediate or deep cartilage.[24] In vitro studies suggest that MSF and HAPO could be involved in hemapoietic functions, but their roles in vivo remain uncertain. In contrast, the critical role of lubricin/SZP in joint homeostasis is demonstrated by the identification of loss-of-function mutations in the *PRG4* gene in patients with camptodactyl-arthropathy-coxa vara-peridicarditis syndrome, a disease characterized by joint failure, synoviocyte hyperplasia, and fibrosis of subsynovium.[25]

### Subsynovium

The synovial lining has no distinct outer border. However, at a depth of about 20 to 50 µm the lining gives way to the subsynovium. Subsynovium varies in composition in different regions of the joint, including loose connective tissue, adipose tissue, and dense fibrous tissues. Subsynovium contains a plexus of fine lymphatic vessels, which are important for synovial fluid regulation because they drain excess fluid from the joint cavity (maintaining a subatmospheric pressure in the joint). These lymphatics are also the unique route by which macromolecules such as plasma protein, hyaluronan, and partly degraded cartilage are removed from the joint.[26]

The only other means of removal of intra-articular macromolecules is by local degradation. Subsynovium extracellular matrix is mainly composed of type I and III collagens, which differ in structure from type I and III collagen by post-translational modifications—including glycosylations of hydroxylysine residues. In addition to collagens, the extracellular matrix of subsynovium is composed of GAG (sulfate GAGs and hyaluronan) and structural glycoproteins (including fibronectin, laminin, entactin [a sulfated glycoprotein with high affinity for laminin], and tenascin). Both chondroitin 4 sulfate (S) and 6S are secreted by synovial cells. The extracellular matrix of the intima of normal synovium contains mainly chondroitin 6S, whereas subsynovium does not. Water accounts for about 60 to 70% of total weight, collagens for 10 to 20%, sulfated GAGs (including both chondroitin and dermatan sulfate) for 4 to 5%, and hyaluronan for 4%.[21]

## CANDIDATE BIOCHEMICAL MARKERS OF JOINT TISSUES IN OSTEOARTHRITIS

### Bone Markers

For bone formation the most specific markers are serum osteocalcin, bone-specific alkaline phosphatase (bone ALP), and the amino-terminal propeptide of type I collagen (PINP) (Table 8.1). The most sensitive markers for bone resorption identified to date are collagen cross-links, including deoxypyridinoline (DPD) and the amino- and carboxy-terminal cross-linked telopeptide of type I collagen (CTX-I, NTX-I). Such markers have been clinically validated in the field of metabolic bone diseases, particularly in regard to osteoporosis.[2] BSP is a non-collagenous protein preferentially distributed at the subchondral bone interface.

The early involvement of this area in OA has led to the suggestion that serum BSP may be a sensitive indicator for alterations of bone turnover. However, available immunoassays require technical improvements, especially in the characterization of the various circulating immunoreactive forms (few studies using this marker in OA have been published in recent years). Although bone turnover markers may reflect the focal abnormalities of bone metabolism in OA, circulating and urinary levels are more likely to reflect the overall skeletal turnover—which may be influenced by a variety of conditions, including age, menopausal status, osteoporosis, and other bone diseases. This may explain the discordant results across various studies in patients with OA.[27] Consequently, most studies have concentrated on the development of specific biochemical markers of cartilage and synovium turnover.

## Cartilage Markers

### Markers of Aggrecan Turnover

Aggrecan synthesis can be evaluated by assaying epitopes located on the chondroitin sulfate chains of the aggrecan, such as the 3-B-3, 7-D-4, and 846 epitope. The 3-B-3 antibody recognizes atypical structures at the nonreducing terminal of the CS glycosaminoglycan side chains of the proteoglycans (Fig. 8.2). The 7-D-4 antibody is directed against another atypical structure (sulfation pattern) in native CS glycosaminoglycans of proteoglycans.[28,29] Epitopes 3-B-3 (−) and 846[30] are present in high concentration in fetal cartilage and are almost absent in mature normal cartilage.[31-33] In contrast, epitope 7-D-4 is frequently found in normal adult cartilage.[32]

Aggrecan degradation can be evaluated by measuring the fragments of the aggrecan protein moiety generated by MMPs, aggrecanases, cathepsins, or keratan sulfate epitopes such as epitopes 5D4[34] and AN9P1[35] (Fig. 8.2). Antibodies detecting these aggrecan epitopes have been mostly used in immunohistochemical experiments to analyze mechanisms of aggrecan turnover in OA.

Currently, the most widely used assay for evaluating aggrecan synthesis is for epitope 846. For cartilage degradation (although several research groups have recently developed assays for the various neoepitopes in the protein portion of aggrecan), it is still unclear which of these epitopes is the most relevant to be

| TABLE 8.1 CANDIDATE BIOCHEMICAL MARKERS OF BONE, CARTILAGE, AND SYNOVIUM TURNOVER | | |
|---|---|---|
| **Area** | **Synthesis** | **Degradation** |
| **Bone** | | |
| • Type I collagen | • N- and C-propeptides (PICP, PINP) | • Pyridinoline (PYD)<br>• Deoxypyridinoline (DPD)<br>• C- and N-telopeptide (CTX-I, NTX-I, ICTP) |
| • Non-collagenous proteins | • Osteocalcin<br>• Bone alkaline phosphatase | • Helical peptide<br>• Bone sialoprotein (BSP)<br>• Tartrate-resistant acid phosphatase (TRAP, 5b isoenzyme)<br>• Cathepsin K |
| **Cartilage** | | |
| • Type II collagen | • N- and C-propeptides (PIICP, PIIANP, PIIBNP) | • PYD<br>• Type II collagen C-telopeptide (CTX-II)<br>• Type II collagen collagenase neoepitope (C2C, C12C, TIINE)<br>• Type II collagen helical fragments (Helix-II and Coll 2-1) |
| • Aggrecan | • Chondroitin sulfate (epitopes 846, 3B3, 7D4) | • Core protein MMPs and aggrecanase neoepitopes<br>• Keratan sulfate (epitopes 5D4, ANP9) |
| • Non-aggrecan and non-collagen proteins | • Chitinase 3-like proteins 1 and 2 (YKL-40, YKL-39) | • Cartilage oligomeric matrix protein (COMP) |
| **Synovium/Synovitis** | | |
| • Type I/III collagen | • Type I/type III N propeptide (PINP/PIIINP) | • PYD<br>• CTX-I, NTX-I<br>• Glucosyl-galactosyl-pyridinoline (Glc-Gal-PYD) |
| • Non-collagenous proteins | • Hyaluronic acid<br>• YKL-40<br>• COMP | |
| • Proteases | • MMP-1, 2, 3, 9 | |
| **Systemic Inflammation** | | |
| | • Ultrasensitive C-reactive protein (CRP) | |

measured in biological fluids and clinical data are still very limited.

## Markers of Type II Collagen Turnover

### Markers of Type II Collagen Synthesis

The major recent achievement in biomarkers for OA is the development of biochemical markers reflecting the synthesis and degradation of type II collagen, the most abundant protein of the tissue. Type II collagen synthesis can be evaluated by measuring the serum concentration of the N- (PIINP) or C-terminal (PIICP) propeptides (Fig. 8.1). An ELISA for PIIANP was developed using a specific polyclonal antibody raised against recombinant exon-2 protein.

Compared to healthy sex- and age-matched controls, increased serum levels of PIIANP were reported in early knee OA,[36] whereas decreased values[37] were found in patients with advanced knee OA. These results obtained from analysis of systemic levels of PIIANP are in agreement with direct measurements of type II collagen in human OA cartilage using hydroxyproline incorporation—showing that type II collagen synthesis increased in early stages of cartilage degeneration but progressively decreased in late stages.[38] Because type IIB collagen is the major form of adult cartilage, the development of an assay for PIIBNP would be very useful in that it may provide different information compared to PIIANP in OA. Such an assay is currently being developed.

## Markers of Type II Collagen Degradation

The recent development of assays specific for type II collagen breakdown represents a breakthrough in the field of biological markers for OA, given that degradation of collagen fibers is associated with irreversible cartilage destruction. Antibodies recognizing different type II collagen fragments have been developed (Fig. 8.3). Those directed against the neoepitopes generated by the collagenases included the so-called COL2-3/4 long mono (C2C, which is specific of type II collagen) and the COL2-3/4C short (C1,2C), which detects cleavages of both type II and type I collagen.[7]

These collagenase neoepitopes have been mainly used to demonstrate increased type II collagen cleavage in OA cartilage explants, although more recently they have been applied in synovial fluid and serum immunoassays both in animal models of OA[39] and in patients with knee OA.[40] More recently, two other type II collagen markers have been identified—including a fragment of the triple helical domain (Helix-II)[41] and fragments of the C-telopeptide (CTX-II)[42] (Fig. 8.2).

Although both Helix-II and CTX-II have been shown to be increased in patients with knee and hip OA and rheumatoid arthritis (RA), in vitro studies indicate that they reflect different enzymatic pathways of type II collagen degradation.[43] Thus, the combination of these two markers may allow a more comprehensive assessment of the complex mechanisms of cartilage degradation. This assumption was supported by clinical data indicating that the combined measurement of Helix-II and CTX-II was more effective than one of these two markers alone to identify patients with a rapidly progressive hip OA[44] and patients with early RA[41] (Fig. 8.4).

## Post-translational Modifications of Type II Collagen

Cartilage matrix molecules (including type II collagen) can undergo post-translational modifications that can be either mediated by an enzymatic process or be spontaneous and age related. Measuring post-translational-modified cartilage matrix proteins may lead to the development of biochemical markers that can give valuable information on altered biological processes related to OA. Chondrocytes can express high levels of inducible and neuronal forms of nitric oxide synthetase that generate nitric oxide. Nitric oxide can then react with superoxide radical to form peroxynitrite, a potent oxidizing radical that can in turn react with tyrosine residues of proteins to form nitrotyrosine.

Two different assays recognizing a sequence—which can be either un-nitrosylated (Coll 2-1) or nitrosylated (Coll 2-1 $NO_2$)—of the triple helix of type II collagen have been recently developed.[45] Increased serum levels of Coll 2-1 and Coll 2-1 $NO_2$ have been reported in patients with knee OA. One-year changes of their urinary levels (but not baseline values) were modestly related to more rapid disease progression of knee OA

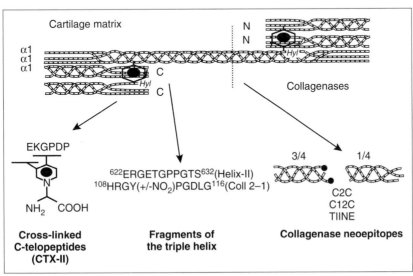

**Fig. 8.3** Type II collagen fragments as specific biologic markers of cartilage degradation. Type II collagen is formed by the association of three identical $\alpha1$ chains in triple helix except at the ends (telopeptides). In the extracellular matrix of cartilage, collagen molecules are cross-linked by pyridinoline (PYD) involving the telopeptide regions. During cartilage degradation, different molecules are released in synovial fluid, serum, and urine. These include neoepitopes generated by the collagenases (e.g., C2C, C12C, and TIINE), fragments of the triple helix (Helix-II and Col 2-1), and C-terminal cross-linking telopeptides (CTX-II). See text for details. (See Color Plate 4.)

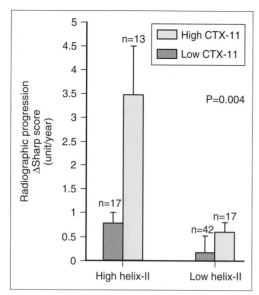

**Fig. 8.4** Combination of biochemical markers of type II collagen helical (Helix-II) and C-telopeptide (CTX-II) breakdown to predict disease progression in early rheumatoid arthritis (RA). Patients with early RA (disease duration <3 years, no previous disease-modifying antiarthritic drugs) were categorized in high and low cartilage degradation according to urinary Helix-II and urinary CTX-II levels at baseline (high = upper tertile and low = tertiles 1 or 2). The bars represent the mean (SE) of radiologic progression assessed by changes of total Sharp score at one year. Progression of the disease was highest in patients who had increased levels of both urinary Helix-II and CTX-II at baseline. [From Charni N, Juillet F, Garnero P. Urinary type II collagen helical peptide (Helix II) as a new biochemical marker of cartilage degradation in patients with osteoarthritis and rheumatoid arthritis. Arthritis Rheum 2005;52:1081–90, with permission.]

over 3 years.[46] It remains unclear from these studies whether there is an additive value of investigating the nitrosylated form of type II collagen fragments in OA.

Another post-translational modification of cartilage matrix molecule is the non-enzymatic glycation, which is the spontaneous condensation of reducing sugars such as glucose with free amino groups in lysine or arginine residues—which gives rise to the formation of advanced glycation end products (AGEs). Because cartilage matrix is characterized by a very low turnover in healthy adults, AGEs accumulate in this tissue with aging and they may affect the biochemical, cellular, and biomechanical properties of cartilage.[47] Pentosidine is one of the most studied AGEs that form a covalent cross-link between adjacent collagen molecules.

Serum pentosidine was increased by 37% in 38 patients with advanced knee OA compared to 38 healthy controls.[48] Whether pentosidine is a valuable biochemical marker for OA remains to be demonstrated because serum and urinary levels were not associated with the extent of radiologic damage[48] and the progression of the disease.[49] One has to remember that pentosidine is not specific for cartilage because it is also found in other aging tissues, including bone. In addition, pentosidine is only one of the multiple AGEs (which are for the vast majority not yet characterized) occurring in aged tissues, and it is currently unknown which of these AGEs is the most relevant for OA.

## Non-aggrecan and Non-collagenous Proteins
### Cartilage Oligomeric Matrix Protein
Among non-collagenous proteins, the most investigated cartilage marker is the protein called cartilage oligomeric matrix protein (COMP). COMP is a 524-kDa homopentameric extracellular matrix glycoprotein (five identical units of 755 amino acids) that belongs to the thrombospondin family. Each monomer is composed of an amino-terminal cysteine-rich domain, four epithelial growth factor (EGF)-like domains, eight calmodulin-like repeats, and a C-terminal globular domain.[50-52] The biologic function of COMP is still unclear.

Bovine and human (but not rat) protein contains an RGD sequence, suggesting that COMP may mediate cell binding. The carboxy-terminal globular domain binds to collagens I, II, and IX—suggesting that COMP may be involved in regulating fibril formation and maintaining integrity of collagen network. The fact that COMP may have important functions is also illustrated by the data showing that two human-dominant skeletal dysplasia, pseudoachondroplasia, and multiple epiphyseal dysplasia[53-55] are associated with a mutation in the potentially Ca-binding domain of COMP gene. However, COMP-deficient mice do not have cartilage abnormalities[56]—suggesting that these human diseases are probably not caused by reduced amounts of COMP but to other mechanisms (such as folding defects or extracellular assembly alterations due to potential dysfunctional mutated COMP).

Originally felt to be cartilage specific, over the last years COMP has been identified in all structures of the joints (including ligaments, meniscus, tendons, and synovium).[57] COMP was also found to be secreted by osteoblasts and vascular smooth muscle. In the cartilage, synovial fluid, and serum of patients with OA COMP has been shown to be present as the intact molecule and several fragments.[58] These fragments are likely to result from the activity of MMPs such as MMP-1, MMP-9, MMP-13, and ADAMTS-4,[59] although it remains unknown which of these enzymes plays the major role of COMP degradation in vivo. A careful epitope mapping is required, and monoclonal antibodies specific for intact molecules and fragments would be very useful—especially for assessing the efficacy of MMP inhibitors in preventing cartilage destruction in patients with OA. Currently, however, available immunoassays based on polyclonal[60] or monoclonal antibodies[61] appear to detect both the intact molecule and fragments in body fluids.

## YKL-40 and YKL-39

Chitinase-3-like protein 1 (YKL-40, also named human cartilage glycoprotein 39) is a mammalian glycoprotein related in sequence to family 18 of bacterial and fungal chitinases.[62] However, it does not exhibit glycosidase activity against chitinase substrates, as the glutamate in the active site Trp-Glu-Tyr-Pro is replaced by another amino acid. It was originally described as a major gene product of chondrocytes and synovial cells.[63] Subsequently, however, mRNA for YKL-40 has also been detected in high amounts in the liver (which may be the main source of circulating YKL-40); weakly in brain, kidney, and placenta; and undetectable in heart, lung, skeletal muscle, mononuclear cells, and skin fibroblasts.[63,64]

The function of YKL-40 is unknown. One hypothesis is that increased expression of this protein by human articular chondrocytes and/or synovial cells in patients with OA/RA could increase the degradative capacity of these cells, although no proteolytic activity has been demonstrated (including against HA).[63] Although serum YKL-40 has been reported to be increased in patients with knee OA or hip OA in some[65,66] but not all[67] studies, its clinical utility in OA remains unclear because it does not correlate with radiologic damage[67] and progression.[68] YKL-40 may be a more interesting marker of disease progression in patients with RA[69] or cancer.[70-72]

More recently, YKL-39 or chitinase-3-like protein 2 has been identified.[64] It has been shown that YKL-39 (but not YKL-40) was overexpressed in cartilage from patients with OA compared to healthy cartilage.[73,74] Autoantibodies to YKL-39 have also been reported in a proportion of patients with OA (similar to that found in patients with RA), suggesting that humoral response to this molecule may be involved in the pathophysiology of these arthritic diseases.[75,76] Altogether, these preliminary data suggest that YKL-39 may be more specific for cartilage than YKL-40 and that it may prove to be a more sensitive biochemical marker of joint damage in OA—although data for synovial fluid and serum YKL-39 are still lacking.

## Marker of Synovium Turnover and Systemic Inflammation

### Marker of Systemic Inflammation

Investigation of synovial tissue metabolism in OA has received little attention. However, there is increasing evidence indicating alterations in synovial tissue metabolism in a non-negligible proportion of patients with OA,[77] as well as a correlation between the severity of synovitis and the progression of joint destruction.[78]

Thus, the development of biological markers specific to the synovial membrane is of particular interest.

Several markers have been proposed to assess synovitis and inflammation in OA. Increased systemic inflammation in OA can be detected by ultrasensitive assays for CRP, but some discrepant findings have been generated. Although most studies found an association between serum CRP levels with the degree of joint damage and/or progression of the disease in OA,[79,80] this relationship may be confounded by obesity (as recently shown in American populations).[81] In addition, CRP is not joint specific and can be affected by other chronic medical conditions—suggesting that it is unlikely to be a useful marker in OA.

### Marker of Synovial Tissue Activity

Activity of the synovial membrane can be more specifically evaluated by the measurement of serum levels of N-propeptide of type III procollagen, reflecting the synthesis of one of the most abundant collagens of synovial tissue: non-collagenous proteins such as YKL-40, HA, and the various enzymes secreted by the synoviocytes (including MMP-3).

HA can be measured by employing the specific binding of the G1 domain of aggrecan to HA.[82] HA is carried from the joint to the blood by lymph and is rapidly taken up by the liver, although a minor part may be removed by the kidney and thus its levels are markedly increased in patients with liver diseases.[83] Increased HA serum levels have been reported in patients with knee and hip OA—these levels correlating with the number of joints involved[84] and radiological progression.[68,85,86] Thus, serum HA appears as a potential prognostic marker of joint destruction in OA provided that hepatic function is not altered.

As discussed previously, proteases such as the collagenases MMP-1 and MMP-13 and stromelysin-1 (MMP-3) are considered to play an important role in joint damage associated with OA. When synovitis is present, these enzymes are secreted by synovial cells in increased amounts. In patients with OA, increased levels of MMP-3 in the synovial fluid were found.[87] More recently, higher serum levels of MMP-3 were reported to be associated with greater risk of radiologic progression in a subgroup of women with knee OA participating in a randomized trial of doxycycline. The association between increased baseline MMP-3 and higher progression was observed in the placebo group, but not in patients randomized to doxycycline.[88]

### New Synovial Tissue Marker

Not all of the biochemical markers previously discussed are specific to synovial tissue. We have characterized a glycosylated pyridinoline derivative, glucosyl-galactosyl-pyridinoline (Glc-Gal-PYD), which is found in large amounts in human synovium and in very low levels in the cartilage and other soft tissues[89] (Fig. 8.5). The specificity of Glc-Gal-PYD for synovial tissue has also been demonstrated in ex vivo models of human joint tissue degradation showing that this marker was released in the supernatant of synovial tissue, but not of cartilage and bone (Fig. 8.5). Urinary Glc-Gal-PYD has been found to be significantly increased in patients with knee OA,[67,90,91] especially in those presenting with knee swelling.[90] Increased levels were also found to be associated with decreased joint space width[67,91] and worse clinical symptoms.[67]

## New Marker Methodologies

The biochemical markers previously discussed have been measured using single immunoassay. In a study measuring 10 of these individual markers in patients with hip OA, we found that they can be grouped into five independent clusters derived from principal component analyses.[92] Interestingly, these independent groups of markers provided different and complementary information on joint metabolism, suggesting

that a combination of different biochemical markers may be useful to more accurately describe the complex physiopathologic processes of OA. New approaches have recently been applied for identifying and assaying OA biochemical markers, including genomics, proteomics, and metabolomics. These new methodologies coupled with sophisticated statistical methods allow the simultaneous analysis of multiple markers and are especially promising for early diagnosis of OA.

Using a genomic approach based on isolation of mRNA from circulating blood and subsequent reverse transcription polymerase chain reaction (PCR), Marshall et al.[93] identified six genes that were significantly downregulated in patients with mild OA (according to arthroscopy assessment) compared to healthy controls. Combination of these six genes in a multiple variable model was able to correctly identify 85% with mild OA and controls. Proteomic analysis generally involves separation of proteins by 2D electrophoresis, followed by their identification using mass spectroscopy.

Proteomic analysis has recently been successfully used to identify biochemical markers related to disease

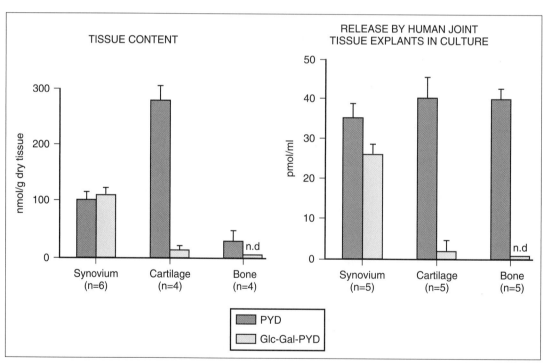

**Fig. 8.5** Glucosyl-galactosyl pyridinoline (Glc-Gal-PYD) as a specific biochemical marker of synovial tissue turnover. Samples of synovium, bone, and cartilage tissues were obtained at the time of surgery for total hip replacement from patients with OA. Left panel: the tissue concentration of pyridinoline (PYD) and Glc-Gal-PYD was determined by HPLC after acid and alkaline hydrolysis, respectively. Right panel: human joint tissues were cultured for 5 days in the presence of Il-1 beta (+ plasminogen for cartilage only). The concentrations of PYD and Glc-Gal-PYD in the supernatant were determined by HPLC. PYD is present at high concentration in synovium, cartilage, and bone tissues—whereas the glycosylated derivative Glc-Gal-PYD is present in large amount in synovium, very little in cartilage, and could not be detected (n.d.) in bone. Analysis of other soft tissues (including muscle and liver) also demonstrated little concentration of Glc-Gal-PYD. During degradation of joint tissues in culture, only synovium released a significant amount of Glc-Gal-PYD. (From Gineyts E, Garnero P, Delmas PD. Urinary excretion of glucosyl-galactosyl pyridinoline: A specific biochemical marker of synovium degradation. Rheumatology 2001;40:315–23, with permission.)

development and progression and to autoimmunity in OA. Applying 2D electrophoresis to human chondrocyte extracts followed by reaction with serum samples from 20 patients with OA, 20 patients with RA, and 20 healthy controls, Xiang et al.[94] identified 19 autoantigens specific to OA, 11 specific to RA, and 22 common to the two diseases. Triosephosphate isomerase (TPI) was subsequently identified by mass spectroscopy as one of the unique OA autoantigens. Indeed, immunoglobulin anti-TPI autoantibodies were detected in about 25% of OA serum and synovial fluid samples but in less than 6% of patients with RA or lupus.

The presence of anti-TPI autoantibodies in patients with OA was associated with lower radiographic grade. This study underscores the importance of autoimmunity (a well-recognized etiologic factor in RA) in the physiopathology of OA and to the potential of using autoantibodies as diagnostic biochemical markers of OA. Another new approach is metabolomic, which consists of the determination of a profile of metabolites specific to patients with OA. Using nuclear MR spectroscopy followed by principal component analysis, it has been reported that urinary hydroxybutyrate, pyruvate, creatine/creatinine, and glycerol were increased in 45 patients with knee or hip OA compared to healthy controls—suggesting altered energy utilization in OA.[95]

These technical developments will ultimately allow the identification of a panel of biochemical markers that could then be assessed simultaneously by microarray platforms. This strategy was recently used in a case-control study of the Baltimore Longitudinal Study of Aging to analyze 160 candidate blood proteins implicated in tissue matrix degradation, cellular activation, and inflammation. It was shown that a combination of a few of these proteins was already differently expressed in the 21 patients with no OA at the time of investigation who developed OA in the following 10 years compared to the 66 individuals who remained free of radiologic disease.[96] Because the outcome of the studies using these novel technologies is highly dependent on sample collection and data processing (for which standardization is still lacking), these findings obtained on a small number of patients will have to be independently replicated in larger samples.

## Potential Confounding Factors of Biochemical Markers of Osteoarthritis

Levels of biochemical markers measured in blood or urine (because assessment of synovial fluid is often not practical) provide information on systemic skeletal tissue turnover and are not necessarily specific to the alterations occurring in the signal joint. For example, it has been shown that degenerative disease of the knees, hips, hands, and lumbar discs contributed independently and additively to urinary CTX-II levels—clearly illustrating the total body contribution to systemic levels[97,98] (Fig. 8.6). The potential contribution of intervertebral discs is of particular relevance

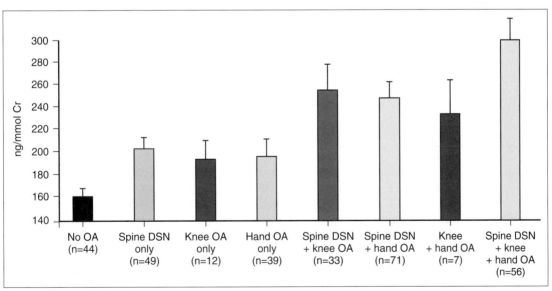

**Fig. 8.6** Urinary CTX-II reflects whole-body cartilage degradation in OA. Postmenopausal women were categorized according to presence or absence of radiologic lumbar spine disc narrowing (DSN) and/or radiologic knee OA and/or clinical hand OA. Bars represent the mean ($\pm$ SD) of urinary CTX-II levels in the different groups of women. In ANOVA (including spine DSN, knee and hand OA, age, and BMI), spine DNS ($p = 0.005$), knee OA ($p = 0.006$), and hand OA ($p = 0.006$) were significantly associated with urinary CTX-II levels. There was no significant interaction ($p = 0.84$) between spine DSN and knee-and-hand OA on urinary CTX-II levels, indicating independent and additive contribution of each joint to urinary CTX-II levels. (From Garnero P, Sornay-Rendu E, Arlot M, et al. Association between spine disc degeneration and type II collagen degradation in postmenopausal women: The OFELY study. Arthritis Rheum 2004;50:3137–44, with permission.)

because disc degeneration is common with aging. Adjusting systemic levels by a total body OA score based on radiographic damage and cartilage volume estimated by quantitative MRI may in part overcome this limitation.[99]

The clearance of the markers from the joint compartment to the bloodstream is complex, and potential excretions in the urine vary across individuals and can increase with inflammation after joint mobilization and exercise. A recent study of 20 patients with OA demonstrated that serum HA increased within the first hour after rising from bed and then remained stable.[100] Serum COMP was shown to increase significantly during running exercise[101] and after moderate walking activity, although changes were modest and transient.[102]

Serum and urinary levels of most biochemical markers also vary with sex, age, menopausal status, ethnicity, and OA risk factors such as body mass index (BMI). In a 6-week randomized controlled trial of patients with painful knee OA, it has been reported that ibuprofen (and the COX-2-specific inhibitor rofecoxib) prevented the significant elevation of CTX-II and Glc-Gal-PYD observed in patients receiving placebo.[90] Although it remains to be determined whether non-steroidal anti-inflammatory drugs have disease-modifying effects, these data underscore that commonly prescribed therapy in OA may be a confounding factor in biochemical marker clinical studies. Clearly, pre-analytical factors contribute to the intra- and inter-subject variability of biochemical marker levels and consequently need to be investigated under conditions as tightly controlled as possible.

## CLINICAL USES OF BIOLOGIC MARKERS FOR OSTEOARTHRITIS

The clinical researcher and the rheumatologist dream of a biochemical marker that can be used to diagnose the presence of the disease, preferably before radiologic evidence of joint damage, to identify patients at increased risk for disease progression and to monitor the efficacy of treatments (including DMOADs).

### Diagnosis

Several cross-sectional studies have found elevated or decreased levels of biologic markers in knee and hip OA, as compared to healthy sex- and age-matched controls.[27] Because the levels of most of these markers in both affected and unaffected individuals are influenced by sex, age, BMI, and hormone replacement therapy, it is important to adjust for these factors to judge the diagnostic value of markers. These studies clearly demonstrated, however, that there is a large overlap in marker levels between persons with and without OA (Fig. 8.7)—indicating that the measurements of one of the currently available markers are probably insufficiently sensitive to be useful for the diagnosis of OA.

An important limitation of most of these cross-sectional studies is the lack of radiologic assessment of the controls. Thus, it is likely that a significant proportion of controls have asymptomatic OA in one or a few joints that would lead to an underestimation of the true diagnostic accuracy of the markers. Another issue is that these studies included mainly patients with advanced disease, in that the selection was based on a

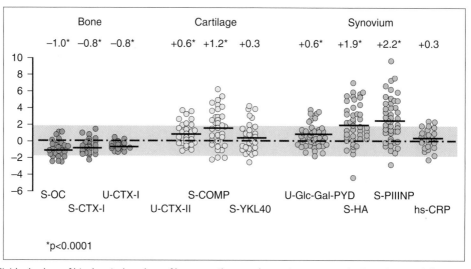

**Fig. 8.7** Individual values of biochemical markers of bone, cartilage, and synovium turnover in 67 patients with knee OA. Each value is expressed in Z-score (i.e., in number of standard deviations from the mean of 67 healthy age-matched controls). Note that p < 0.0001 versus 0. For abbreviations of the biochemical markers see Table 8.1. (From Garnero P, Piperno M, Gineyts E, et al. Cross sectional evaluation of biochemical markers of bone, cartilage and synovial tissue metabolism in patients with knee osteoarthritis: Relations with disease activity and joint damage. Ann Rheum Dis 2001;60:619–26, with permission.)

radiologic Kellgren–Lawrence (KL) score at or above 2.

Because biochemical markers reflect dynamic changes in tissue turnover, their levels are likely to be altered well before radiologic damage can be observed (as suggested by the proteomic analyses discussed previously). Consequently, for assessing the diagnostic utility of biochemical markers it may be more appropriate to include patients with early OA (who may be identified using sensitive imaging modalities such as MRI). We recently reported an association between urinary CTX-II and the severity of bone marrow abnormalities score by MRI,[103] which has been suggested to be an early feature of OA. In the near future, many more studies relating biochemical markers with the various MRI features of the joint will be undertaken and should bring valuable information for the biologic interpretation of both of these two new diagnostic modalities.

## Prediction of Progression

Progression in OA shows considerable variation across individuals, and the predictive capacity of clinical indices is poor. Because of the current inability to differentiate patients who will progress from nonprogressors, both groups of patients are included in clinical trials of DMOAD. This results in a limited sensitivity in measurement of disease progression and consequently adds to duration, number of patients, and cost of the study. Recruiting a more homogeneous population of OA progressors in clinical trials will be thus highly advantageous to faster drug development.

Recent longitudinal studies are in this respect encouraging because they suggest that some new biochemical markers may have a role in predicting disease progression. In a 4-year prospective study in postmenopausal women, urinary CTX-I and NTX-I were found to be higher in women with progressive knee OA compared to nonprogressive patients.[104] Although the definition for progressive disease may not be the most adequate because it included a decrease of joint space width (JSW) or an increase in osteophyte grade, these data suggest that increased bone resorption may be associated with progression.

In a large population-based cohort of 1,235 men and women, it was found that the baseline level of urinary CTX-II in the highest quartile was associated with a higher risk of radiologic progression of knee and hip OA in the subsequent 6.6 years[105] (Table 8.2). Increased baseline COMP levels were also shown to be associated with loss of JSW over 3 years in a small sample of patients with established knee OA.[106] Sharif et al.[30] followed a group of patients with early knee OA (40% with a KL score < 2) prospectively for 5 years. They showed that progression was not linear over this period and that serum COMP (measured every

**TABLE 8.2  INCREASED URINARY CTX-II AND THE RISK OF RADIOLOGIC PROGRESSION OF KNEE AND HIP OSTEOARTHRITIS: THE ROTTERDAM STUDY**[a]

| CTX-II at Baseline | Adjusted Odds Ratio of Progression[b] | |
|---|---|---|
| • Quartile | • Knee OA<br>• (JSN ≥2 mm)<br>• N = 26 | • Hip OA<br>• (JSN ≥1.5 mm)<br>• N = 24 |
| • First | • 1 | • 1 |
| • Second | • 4.1 (0.8–20.5) | • 3.9 (0.4–36.9) |
| • Third | • 4.5 (0.9–23.0) | • 8.3 (1.0–72.2) |
| • Fourth | • 6.0 (1.2–30.8) | • 8.4 (1.0–72.9) |
| • P for trend | • 0.064 | • 0.005 |
| • Change in risk per SD | • 1.6 (1.0–2.5) | • 1.9 (1.2–3.0) |

[a]The study consisted of 1,235 women and men ages ≥55 years from a population-based cohort. Among these individuals, 237 women and 123 men had radiologic evidence of knee and hip OA at baseline (Kellgren–Lawrence score ≥2 in one or both joints). Subjects were followed prospectively for an average 6.6 years and progression was assessed by joint space narrowing using weight-bearing anterioposterior radiographs. The table shows the risk of radiologic progression adjusted for age, sex, body mass index, lower limb disability index, baseline radiographic OA, and follow-up time for baseline levels of urinary CTX-II in quartiles or per SD (after log transformation).
[b]At a 95% confidence interval.
Source: Reijman M, Hazes JM, Bierna-Zeinstra SM, et al. A new marker for osteoarthritis: Cross-sectional and longitudinal approach. Arthritis Rheum 2004;50:2471–76, with permission.

6 months) was associated with this phasic pattern of progression.[107]

One could argue that assessment of progression in these studies is unreliable because it is based on the measurement of joint space narrowing (JSN) using conventional extended-knee standing anterior-posterior radiographs. This concern is especially relevant for short-term studies in knee OA but of less critical importance for the hip and long-term evaluation. Interestingly, higher levels of serum stromelysin have recently been reported to be associated with greater JSN measured over 30 months using a semi-flexed knee X-ray with fluoroscopic confirmation of joint position in women with knee OA participating in a randomized trial of doxycycline.[88]

### Combination of Markers to Improve Prediction of Disease Progression

Because of the complex involvement of bone, cartilage, and synovial tissue in joint damage in OA, it likely that only a combination of several biochemical markers will adequately predict disease progression. In a study including 12 patients with rapidly destructive hip OA and 28 patients with slowly progressive disease, we found that the combination of urinary CTX-II and

Helix-II (two biochemical markers of type II collagen breakdown) was more effective than one of these markers alone in identifying patients with rapidly progressive hip OA.[44]

In a prospective study of 52 patients with established knee OA, we found that low serum levels of PIIANP (as in late OA type II collagen synthesis decreases) or high urinary CTX-II excretion levels were associated with faster joint destruction as evaluated over a 1-year period by plain radiographs or by arthroscopy.[108] Combining these two biologic markers to obtain an index of uncoupling of type II collagen synthesis and breakdown based on the standardized difference between CTX-II and PII-IANP was more effective in predicting cartilage destruction than measurements of a single marker (Fig. 8.8).

Similar findings were reported in a community-based cohort of patients with knee OA in which the ratio between serum C2C and serum PIICP was associated with an increased risk of radiologic progression over the 18-month period, whereas individual markers were not predictive.[109] In a longitudinal 5-year study of 84 patients with early knee OA, we also recently reported that the combination of increased serum

PIIANP (as in early OA type II collagen synthesis increases) and increased urinary CTX-II allowed the identification of 92% of patients who showed radiologic progression—whereas one of these two markers when used alone could identify 40 to 70% of patients who progressed.[36]

In the evaluation of the **cho**ndromodulating effect of **dia**cerein in osteoarthritis of the **hip** (ECHODIAH) cohort of patients with hip OA followed over 3 years, we found that the combination of urinary CTX-II and HA that belonged to two of these independent groups of markers (cartilage degradation and synovitis, respectively) was more predictive than one of these markers alone.[68] Indeed, the patients with highest levels of CTX-II *or* HA had a risk of progression that was increased by 1.8- to 2.0-fold compared to the rest of the patients, whereas this risk was multiplied by 3.7 in the 13% of the patients who had *both* markers elevated.

## Monitoring Efficacy of Disease-modifying Osteoarthritis Treatment

One of the main issues that currently impair efficient development of structure-modifying therapies for OA

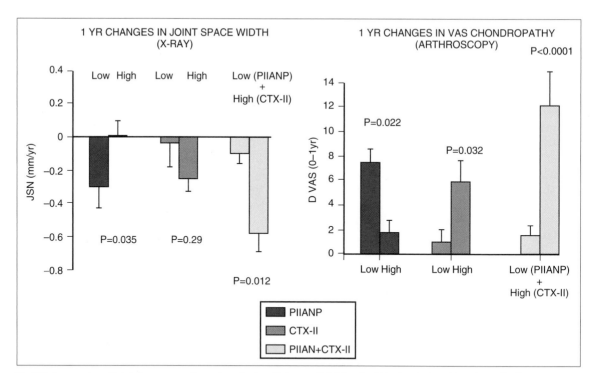

**Fig. 8.8** Progression of joint damage over 1 year in patients with low and high levels of biochemical markers of type II collagen synthesis, and degradation at baseline in 52 patients with established knee osteoarthritis. Low levels of serum N-propeptide of type IIA procollagen (PIIANP, marker of type IIA collagen synthesis) were those below the mean minus 1 standard deviation (SD) of healthy controls. High levels of urinary C-terminal cross-linking telopeptide of type II collagen (CTX-II, type II collagen degradation) were those that exceeded the mean plus 1 SD of healthy controls. The bars show the mean (+SD) of radiologic joint space narrowing (JSN, left-hand panel) or changes of a visual analogue scale (VAS) score of arthroscopic chondropathy over 1 year according to levels of biochemical markers at baseline. P values refer to the difference between the two groups of baseline levels of molecular markers. (From Garnero P, Ayral X, Rousseau J-C, et al. Uncoupling of type II collagen synthesis and degradation predicts progression of joint damage in patients with knee osteoarthritis. Arthritis Rheum 2002;46:2613–24, with permission.)

is the low sensitivity of radiographic methods, requiring long-term studies to show a significant difference between placebo- and active-drug-treated patients. Biologic markers may prove capable of providing earlier information compared to demonstration of slowing of joint space narrowing by X-ray. The paucity of data on the potential role of biologic markers for monitoring the treatment of OA is chiefly ascribed to the absence of medications with established chondroprotective activity.

In a randomized clinical trial of 137 subjects with knee pain, no significant effect of glucosamine sulfate could be demonstrated on the serum and urinary levels of the type II collagen neoepitopes C2C and C12C after 6 months of treatment.[110] Similar findings were reported in another 3-year placebo-controlled trial of glucosamine sulfate.[111] These negative findings can be explained either by the lack of sensitivity of the particular markers utilized in these studies to this particular treatment and/or the lack of efficacy of glucosamine sulfate to decrease cartilage damage (the disease-modifying activity of this compound is still debated).

However, in the second trial a significant effect of glucosamine sulfate on urinary CTX-II was observed in the subgroup of patients who had high pre-treatment CTX-II levels[111]—suggesting that patients with high cartilage turnover may have a greater therapeutic response to DMOADs. A small placebo-controlled study has shown increased cartilage tissue levels of epitope 846 in patients with knee OA following treatment with an oral MMP inhibitor,[112] but larger studies with serum measurements are waiting to draw conclusions on the potential use of this marker to monitor treatment efficacy.

## Anti-catabolic Bone Agents

Anti-catabolic bone agents currently used for the treatment of postmenopausal osteoporosis have been suggested to play a role as DMOADs mainly because of the importance of subchondral bone remodeling in OA initiation and/or progression. Animal models of OA have indeed shown that agents such as the bisphosphonates risedronate, alendronate, and zoledronate; calcitonin; estrogens; and selective estrogen-receptor modulators (SERMs) could partially prevent progression of joint damage.

A series of recent studies have investigated the effects of these treatments on urinary CTX-II using stored samples from randomized placebo-controlled clinical trials in postmenopausal women. They showed that bone-effective doses of oral and transdermal 17 beta estradiol,[113] the SERM levormeloxifene,[114] and the bisphosphonates alendronate and ibandronate[115] significantly decrease urinary CTX-II within 3 to 6 months. The decrease of CTX-II was dose dependent for the bisphosphonates and calcitonin, but not for estradiol and levormeloxifene. The magnitude of reduction of CTX-II was about 50% lower than that observed for the type I collagen biochemical markers of bone resorption urinary NTX-I and CTX-I, with the exception of levormeloxifene.

More recently, a dose-dependent effect of the bisphosphonate risedronate on urinary CTX-II was also found in patients with knee OA (Fig. 8.9).[116,117] The biologic and clinical interpretation of these findings requires further investigation. Indeed, the decrease of CTX-II could result from indirect effects of these drugs on subchondral bone turnover and/or a direct action on cartilage metabolism, which has been

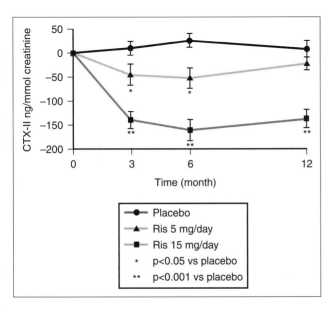

**Fig. 8.9** Effect of the bisphosphonate risedronate on urinary CTX-II in patients with knee OA. Two hundred & twenty-four patients with symptomatic and radiologic knee OA were randomized to oral risedronate 5 mg/day (n = 96), risedronate 15 mg/day (n = 90), or placebo (n = 98) for 1 year. The graph shows the mean (+SD) of changes in absolute values of urinary CTX-II after 3, 6, and 12 months compared to baseline. (From Spector TD, Conaghan PG, Buckland-Wright JC, et al. Effect of risedronate on joint structure and symptoms of knee osteoarthritis: Results of the brisk randomized, controlled trial. Arthritis Res Ther 2005;7:R625–33, with permission.)

suggested, for example, for calcitonin. Given the uncertainty regarding whether these therapies have disease-modifying activity in humans with OA, the clinical relevance of these changes to predict efficacy on joint damage also remains to be investigated.

RA may serve as a model for validating biochemical markers as surrogate markers of efficacy because efficient disease-modifying antirheumatic drugs (DMARDs) are available. In a randomized study of the combined sulfasalazine-methotrexate-prednisone therapy in early RA, we showed that the magnitude of CTX-II decrease at 3 months was associated with the changes in radiologic scores after 5 years independent of the changes in disease activity and inflammation.[118] These data suggest that early changes of biochemical markers of cartilage turnover may predict long-term structural efficacy of treatment in RA and potentially in OA—a hypothesis that will be possible to validate once effective DMOADs are available.

# REFERENCES

1. Gehron-Robey P. Bone matrix proteoglycans and glycoproteins. In JP Bilezikian, LG Raisz, GA Rodan (ed.), *Principles of Bone Biology*. San Diego: Academic Press 2002, 225–37.
2. Garnero P, Delmas PD. Investigation of bone: Bone turnover. In MC Hochberg, AJ Silman, JS Smolen, ME Weinblatt, MH Weisman (ed.), *Rheumatology*, Third Edition. London: Harcourt Health Sciences 2003, 2043–57.
3. Debri E, Reinholt FP, Heinegard D, Mengarelliholm S, Norgard M, Svensson O. Bone sialoprotein and osteopontin distribution at the osteocartilaginous interface. Clin Orthop 1996;330:251.
4. Sandell LJ, Heinegard D, Hering TM. Cell biology, biochemistry and molecular biology of articular cartilage in osteoarthritis. In Moskowitz RW, Altman RD, Hochberg MC, Goldberg VM (ed.). *Osteoarthritis: Diagnosis and Medical/Surgical Management*, Fourth Edition. Philadelphia: Wolters Kluwer/Lippincott Williams & Wilkins 2006, 73–106.
5. Aigner T, Zhu Y, Chansky HH, Matsen FA III, Maloney WJ, Sandell LJ. Re-expression of type II A procollagen by adult articular chondrocytes in osteoarthritic cartilage. Arthritis Rheum 1999;42:1443.
6. Mudget JS, Hutchinson NI, Chatrain NA, Forsyth AJ, Mc Donnell J, Singer II, et al. Susceptibility of stromelysin 1-deficient mice to collagen-induced arthritis and cartilage destruction. Arthritis Rheum 1998;41:110–21.
7. Billinghurst RC, Dahlberg L, Ionescu M, Reiner A, Bourne R, Rorabeck C, et al. Enhanced cleavage of type II collagen by collagenase in osteoarthritic articular cartilage. J Clin Invest 1997;99:1534.
8. Burrage PS, Mix KS, Brinckerhoff CE. Matrix metalloproteinases: Role in arthritis. Front Biosci 2006;11:529.
9. Yasuda Y, Kaleta J, Brömme D. The role of cathepsins in osteoporosis and arthritis: Rationale for the design of new therapies. Adv Drug Delivery Reviews 2005;57:973.
10. Garnero P, Borel O, Byrjalsen I, Ferreras M, Drake FH, McQueney S, et al. The collagenolytic activity of cathepsin K is unique among mammalian proteinases. J Biol Chem 1998;273:323–47.
11. Kafienah W, Bromme D, Buttle DJ, Croucher LJ, Hollander AP. Human cathepsin K cleaves native type I and II collagens at the N-terminal end of the triple helix. Biochem J 1998;331:727.
12. Konttinen YT, Mandelin J, Li TF, Salo J, Lassus J, Lijestrom M, et al. Acidic cysteine endoproteinase cathepsin K in the degeneration of the superficial articular hyaline cartilage in osteoarthritis. Arthritis Rheum 2002;46:953–60.
13. Morko JP, Soderstrom M, Saamanen AM, Salminen HJ, Vuorio EI. Up-regulation of cathepsin K expression in articular chondrocytes in a transgenic mouse model for osteoarthritis. Ann Rheum Dis 2004;63:649–55.
14. Hou WS, Li Z, Buttner FH, Bartnik E, Bromme D. Cleavage site specificity of cathepsin K toward cartilage proteoglycans and protease complex formation. Biol Chem 2003;384(6):891.
15. Watanabe H, Yamada Y, Kimata K. Roles of aggrecan, a large chondroitin sulfate proteoglycan, in cartilage structure and function. J Biochem 1998;124:667.
16. Glasson S, Askew R, Sheppard N, Carito B, Blanchet T, Ma HI, et al. Deletion of active ADMATS5 prevents cartilage degradation in a murine model of osteoarthritis. Nature 2005;434:644.
17. Caterson B, Flannery CR, Hughes CE, Little CB. Mechanisms involved in cartilage proteoglycan catabolism. Matrix Biology 2000;19:333.
18. Dudhia J, Davidson CM, Wells TM, Vynios DH, Hardingham TE, Bayliss MT. Age-related changes in the content of the C-terminal region of aggrecan in human articular cartilage. Biochem J 1996;313:933.
19. Edwards JC. The nature and origin of synovium: Experimental approaches to the study of synoviocyte differentiation. J Anat 1994;184:493.
20. Linck G, Stocker S, Grimaud JA, Porte A. Distribution of immunoreactive fibronectin and collagen (type I, III, IV) in mouse joints. Histochemistry 1983;77:117.
21. Stevens CR, Blacke DR, Merry P, Revell PA, Levick IR. A comparative study by morphometry of the microvasculature in normal and rheumatoid synovium. Arthrirtis Rheum 1991;34:150.
22. Swann DA, Radin EL. The molecular basis of articular lubrication. I. Purification and properties of a lubricating fraction from bovine synovial fluid. J Biol Chem 1972;40:414.
23. Jay GD, Britt DE, Cha CJ. Lubricin is a gene product of megakaryocyte stimulating factor gene expression by human synovial fibroblasts. J Rheumatol 2000;27:594.
24. Schumacher BL, Block JA, Schmid TM, Aydelotte MB, Kuettner KE. A novel protein glycan synthesized and secreted by chondrocytes of the superficial zone of articular cartilage. Arch Biochem Biophys 1994;311:144.
25. Marcelino J, Carpten JD, Suwairi WM, Gutierrez OM, Schwartz S, Robbins C, et al. CACP: Encoding a secreted proteoglycan, is mutated in camptodactyly-arthropathy-coxa vara-pericarditis syndrome. Nat Genet 1999;23:319.
26. Brown TJ, Laurent UBG, Fraser JRE. Turnover of hyaluronan in synovial joints. Exp Physiol 1991;76:125.
27. Garnero P, Rousseau JC, Delmas PD. Molecular basis and clinical use of biochemical markers of bone, cartilage, and synovium in joint diseases. Arthritis Rheum 2000;43:953.
28. Caterson B, Christner JE, Baker JR, Couchman JR. Production and characterization of monoclonal antibodies directed against connective tissue proteoglycans. Fed Proc 1985;44:386.
29. Visco DM, Johnstone B, Jolly Ga, Caterson B. Immunohistochemical analysis of 3B3 (-) and 7D4 epitope expression in canine osteoarthritis. Arthritis Rheum 1993;36:1718.
30. Rizkalla G, Reiner A, Bogoch E, Poole AR. Studies of the articular cartilage proteoglycan aggrecan in health and osteoarthritis: Evidence for molecular heterogeneity and extensive molecular changes in disease. J Clin Invest 1992;30:2268.
31. Glant TT, Mikecz K, Roughley PJ, Buzaz E, Poole AR. Age-related changes in protein-related epitopes of human articular cartilage proteoglycans. Biochem J 1986;236:71.
32. Slater RR, Bayliss MT, Lachiewicz PF, Visco DM, Caterson B. Monoclonal antibodies that detect biochemical markers of arthritis in humans. Arthritis Rheum 1995;5:665.
33. Antoniou J, Steffen T, Nelson F, Winterbottom N, Hollander AP, Poole AR. The human intervertebral disc: Evidence for changes in the biosynthesis and denaturation of the extracellular matrix with growth maturation, aging and degeneration. J Clin Invest 1996;98:996.
34. Poole AR, Webber A, Reiner A, Roughley PJ. Studies of a monoclonal antibody to skeletal keratan sulfate: Importance of antibody valency. Biochem J 1989;260:846.
35. Sharif M, Osborne DJ, Meadows K, Woodhouse SM, Colvin EM, Shepstone L, et al. The relevance of chondroitin and keratan sulfate markers in normal and arthritic synovial fluid. Brit J Rheumatol 1996;35:951.

36. Sharif M, Kirwan J, Charni N, Sandell LJ, Whittles C, Garnero P. A 5 year longitudinal study of type IIA collagen synthesis and total type II collagen degradation in patients with knee osteoarthritis: Association with disease progression. Rheumatology (in press).

37. Rousseau JC, Sandell LJ, Delmas PD, Garnero P. Development and clinical application in arthritis of a new immunoassay for serum type IIA procollagen NH2 propeptide. Human Reproduction, Methods Mol Med 2004;101:25.

38. Lippiello L, Hall D, Mankin HJ. Collagen synthesis in normal and osteoarthritic human cartilage. J Clin Invest 1997;59:593.

39. Chu Q, Lopez M, Hayashi K, et al. Elevation of collagenase generated type II collagen neoepitope and proteoglycan epitopes in synovial fluid following induction of joint instability in the dog. Osteoarthritis Cartilage 2002;10:662.

40. Cibere J, Thorne A, Kopec JA, Singer J, et al. Glucosamine sulfate and cartilage type II collagen degradation in patients with knee osteoarthritis: Randomized discontinuation trial employing biomarkers. J Rheumatol 2005;32:896.

41. Charni N, Juillet F, Garnero P. Urinary type II collagen helical peptide (Helix II) as a new biochemical marker of cartilage degradation in patients with osteoarthritis and rheumatoid arthritis. Arthritis Rheum 2005;52:1081.

42. Christgau S, Garnero P, Fledelius C, Moniz C, Ensig M, Gineyts E, et al. Collagen type II C-telopeptide fragments as an index of cartilage degradation. Bone 2001;29:209.

43. Garnero P, Desmarais S, Charni N, Percival MD. The type II collagen fragments HELIX-II and CTX-II reveal distinct enzymatic pathways of cartilage collagen degradation: Diagnostic and therapeutic implications in rheumatoid arthritis and osteoarthritis. Arthritis Rheum 2005;44:S56.

44. Garnero P, Charni N, Juillet F, Conrozier T, Vignon E. Increased urinary type II collagen helical and C telopeptide levels are independently associated with a rapidly destructive hip osteoarthritis. Ann Rheum Dis. 2006;65(12):1639.

45. Deberg M, Labasse A, Christgau S, et al. New serum biochemical markers (Coll 2-1 and Coll 2-1 NO2) for studying oxidative-related type II collagen network degradation in patients with osteoarthritis and rheumatoid arthritis. 2005;13(3):258.

46. Deberg M, Labasse AH, Collette J, et al. One year increase of Coll 2-1, a new marker of type II collagen is highly predictive of radiological OA progression. Osteoarthritis Cart 2005;13:258.

47. Verzijl N, Banlk RA, Tekoppele JM, DeGroot J. Ageing and osteoarthritis: A different perspective. Curr Opin Rheumatol 2003;15:616.

48. Senolt L, Braun M, Olejarova M, Forejtova S, Gatterova J, Pavelka K. Increased pentosidine, an advanced glycation end product, in serum and synovial fluid from patients with knee osteoarthritis and its relation with cartilage oligomeric matrix protein. Ann Rheum Dis 2005;64:886.

49. Hunter DJ, LaValley MP, Li J, Nevitt M, DeGroot J, Felson DT. Pentosidine does not predict cartilage loss among subjects with knee OA: The BOKS study. Osteoarthritis Cart 2005;13(A):S36.

50. Hedhom E, Antonsson P, Hjerpe A, Aeschlimann D, Paulsaon M, Rosa-Pimentel E, et al. Cartilage matrix proteins: An acidic oligomeric protein (COMP) detected only in cartilage. J Biol Chem 1992;267:6132.

51. Morgelin M, Heinegard D, Engel J, Paulsson M. Electron microscopy of native cartilage oligomeric matrix protein purified from the Swarm rat chondrosarcoma revealed a five-armed structure. J Biol Chem 1992;267:6137.

52. Oldberg A, Antonsson P, Lindblom K, Heinegard D. COMP (cartilage oligomeric matrix protein) is structurally related to the thrombospondins. J Biol Chem 1992;267:22346.

53. Briggs MD, Hoffman SM, King LM, Olsen AS, Mohrenweiser H, Leroy JG, et al. Pseudoachondroplasia and multiple epiphyseal dysplasia due to mutations in the cartilage oligomeric matrix protein gene. Nat Genet 1995;10:330.

54. Hecht JT, Nelsaon LD, Crowder E, Wang Y, Elder FFB, Harrison WR, et al. Mutations in exon 17B of cartilage oligomeric matrix protein (COMP) cause pseudoachondroplasia. Nat Genet 1995;10:325.

55. Posey KL, Hayes E, Haynes R, Hecht JT. Role of TSP-5/COMP in pseudoachondroplasia. Int J Cell Biol 2004;36:1005.

56. Svensson L, Aszodi A, Heinegard D, Hunziker EB, Reinholt FP, Fässler R, et al. Cartilage oligomeric matrix protein-deficient mice have normal skeletal development. Mol Cell Biol 2002;22:4366.

57. Muller G, Michel A, Altenburg E. COMP (cartilage oligomeric matrix protein) is synthesized in ligament, tendon, meniscus, and articular cartilage. Connect Tissue Res 1998;39:233.

58. Di Cesare PE, Carlson CSN, Stolerman ES, Hauser N, Tulli H, Paulsson M. Increased degradation and altered tissue distribution of cartilage oligomeric matrix protein in human rheumatoid and osteoarthritic cartilage. J Orthop Res 1996;14:946.

59. Dickinson SSC, Vankemmelbeke MN, Buttle DJ, Rosenberg K, Heinegard D, Hollander AP. Cleavage of cartilage oligomeric matrix protein (thrombospondin-5) by matrix-metalloproteinases and a disintegrin and metalloproteinase with thrombospondin motifs. Matrix Biology 2003;22:267.

60. Saxne T, Heinegard D. Cartilage oligomeric matrix protein: A novel marker turnover detectable in synovial fluid and blood. Brit J Rheumatol 1992;31:583.

61. Vilim V, Voburka Z, Vytasek R, et al. Monoclonal antibodies to human cartilage oligomeric matrix protein: Epitope mapping and characterization of sandwich ELISA. Clin Chim Acta 2003;328:59.

62. Henrissat B, Bairoch A. New families in the classification of glycosyl hydrolases based on amino-acid sequences similarities. Biochem J 1993;293:781.

63. Hakala BE, White C, Recklies AD. Human cartilage gp-39, a major secretory product of articular chondrocytes and synovial cells, is a mammalian member of a chitinase protein family. J Biol Chem 1993;293:781.

64. Hu B, Trinh K, Figueira WF, Price PA. Isolation and sequence of a novel human chondrocyte protein related to mammalian members of the chitinase protein family. J Biol Chem 1996;271:19415.

65. Johansen JS, Hvolris J, Hansen M, Backer V, Lorenszen I, Price PA. Serum YKL-40 levels in healthy children and adults: Comparison with serum and synovial fluid levels of YKL-40 in patients with osteoarthritis or trauma of the knee joint. Brit J Rheumatol 1996;35:553.

66. Conrozier T, Carlier MC, Mathieu P, Colson F, Debard AL, Richard S, et al. Serum levels of YKL-40 and C reactive protein in patients with hip osteoarthritis and healthy subjects: A cross sectional study. Ann Rheum Dis 2000;59(10):828.

67. Garnero P, Piperno M, Gineyts E, et al. Cross-sectional evaluation of biochemical markers of bone, cartilage and synovial tissue metabolism in patients with knee osteoarthritis: Relations with disease activity and joint damage. Ann Rheum Dis 2001;60:619.

68. Mazieres B, Garnero P, Gueguen A, et al. Molecular markers of cartilage breakdown and synovitis are strong independent predictors of structural progression of hip osteoarthritis: The ECHODIAH cohort. Ann Rheum Dis 2006;65:354.

69. Johansen JS, Stoltenberg M, Hansen M, Florescu A, Horslev-Petersen L, Price P. Serum YKL-40 concentrations in patients with rheumatoid arthritis: Relation to disease activity. Rheumatology (Oxford) 1999;38:618.

70. Johansen JS, Cintin C, Jorgensen M, et al. Serum YKL-40: A new potential marker of prognosis and location of metastases of patients with recurrent breast cancer. Eur J Cancer 1995;31A:1437.

71. Johansen JS, Drivsholm L, Price PA, Christensen IJ. High serum YKL-40 level in patients with small cell lung cancer is related to early death. Lung Cancer 2004;46(3):333.

72. Brasso K, Christensen IJ, Johansen JS, Teisner B, Garnero P, Price PA, et al. Prognostic value of PINP, bone alkaline phosphatase, CTX-I, and YKL-40 in patients with metastatic prostate carcinoma. Prostate (in press).

73. Steck E, Breit SD, Breusch SJ, Axt M, Ritcher W. Enhanced expression of the human chitinase 3-like 2 gene (YKL-39) but not chitinase 3-like 1 gene (YKL-40) in osteoarthritic cartilage. Biochem Biophys Res Commun 2002;299:109.

74. Knorr T, Obermayr F, Bartnick E, Zien A, Aighner T. YKL-39 (chitinase 3-like protein 2), but not YKL-40 (chitinase 3-like protein 1) is up regulated in osteoarthritic chondrocytes. Ann Rheum Dis 2003;62:995.

75. Tsuruha J, Masuko-Hongo K, Kato T, Sakata M, Nakamura H, Sekine T, et al. Autoimmunity against YKL-39, a human cartilage derived protein, in patients with osteoarthritis. J Rheumatol 2002;29:1459.

76. Du H, Masuko-Hongo K, Nakamura H, Xiang Y, Bao CD, Wang XD, et al. The prevalence of autoantibodies against cartilage intermediate layer protein, YKL-39, osteopontin and cyclic citrullinated pain patients with early-stage knee osteoarthritis: Evidence of a variety of autoimmune processes. Rheumatol Int 2005;26(1):35.

77. Pelletier JP, Martel-Pelletier J, Abramson SB. Osteoarthritis, an inflammatory disease. Arthritis Rheum 2001;44:1237.

78. Ayral X, Pickering EH, Woodworth TG, Mackillop N, Dougados M. Synovitis: A potential predictive factor of structural progression of medial tibiofemoral knee osteoarthritis. Results of a 1 year

longitudinal arthroscopic study in 422 patients. Osteoarthritis Cartilage 2005;13(5):361.

79. Spector TD, Hart DJ, Nandra D, Doyle DV, Mackillop N, Gallimore JR, et al. Low-level increases in serum C-reactive protein are present in early osteoarthritis of the knee and predict progressive disease. Arthritis Rheum 1997;40:723.

80. Sharif M, Shepstone L, Elson CJ, Dieppe PA, Kirwan JR. Increased serum C reactive protein may reflect events that precede radiographic progression in osteoarthritis of the knee. Ann Rheum Dis 2000;59(1):71.

81. Sowers M, Jannausch M, Stein E, et al. C-reactive protein as a biomarker of emergent osteoarthritis. Osteoarthritis Cartilage 2002;10:595.

82. Golderg R. Enzyme-linked immunosorbent assay for hyaluronate using cartilage proteoglycan and an antibody for keratan sulfate. Anal Biochem 1998;174:448.

83. Laurent TC, Larent UBG, Fraser RE. Serum hyaluronan as a disease marker. Ann Med 1996;28:241.

84. Elliot AL, Kraus VB, Luta G, et al. Serum hyaluronan levels and radiographic knee and hip osteoarthritis in African Americans and Caucasians in the Johnston County Osteoarthritis Project. Arthritis Rheum 2005;52:105.

85. Sharif M, George L, Shepstone J, Knudson W, Thonar EJ-MA, Cushnagan J, et al. Serum hyaluronic acid level as a predictor of disease progression in osteoarthritis of the knee. Arthritis Rheum 1995;38:760.

86. Pavelka K, Forejtova S, Olejarova M, Gatterova J, Senolt L, Spacek P, et al. Hyaluronic acid levels may have predictive value for the progresson of knee osteoarthritis. Osteoarthritis Cart 2004;12:277.

87. Lohmander LS, Hoerrner LA, Lark MW. Metalloproteinase-tissue-inhibitor and proteoglycan fragments in knee synovial fluid in human osteoarthritis. Arthritis Rheum 1993;36:181.

88. Lohmander LS, Brandt KD, Mazzuca SA, et al. Use of plasma stromelysin (matrix metalloproteinase 3) concentration to predict joint space narrowing in knee osteoarthritis. Arthritis Rheum 2005;52:3160.

89. Gineyts E, Garnero P, Delmas PD. Urinary excretion of glucosyl-galactosyl pyridinoline: A specific biochemical marker of synovium degradation. Rheumatology 2001;40:315.

90. Gineyts E, Mo JA, Ko A, Henriksen DB, et al. Effects of ibuprofen on molecular markers of cartilage and synovium turnover in patients with knee osteoarthritis. Ann Rheum Dis 2004;63:857.

91. Jordan KM, Syddall HE, Garnero P, Gineyts E, Dennison EM, Sayer AA, et al. Urinary CTX-II and glucosyl-galactosyl-pyridinoline are associated with presence and severity of radiographic knee osteoarthritis in men. (Submitted to Ann Rheum Dis 2006;65:871.)

92. Garnero P, Mazières B, Guéguen A, Abbal M, Berdah L, Lequesne M, et al. Cross-sectional association of ten molecular markers of bone, cartilage and synovium with disease activity and radiological joint damage in hip osteoarthritis patients: The ECHODIAH Cohort. J Rheum 2005;32:697.

93. Marshall KW, Zhang H, Yager TD, et al. Blood-based biomarkers for detecting mild osteoarthritis. Osteoarthritis Cart 2005;13:861.

94. Xiang Y, Sekine T, Nakamura H, et al. Proteomic surveillance of autoimmunity in osteoarthritis: Identification of triosephosphate isomerase as an autoantigen in patients with osteoarthritis. Arthritis Rheum 2004;50:1511.

95. Lamers RJAN, van Nessselrooij JHJ, Kraus VB, et al. Identification of a urinary profile associated with osteoarthritis. Osteoarthritis Cart 2005;13:762.

96. Ling QM, Patel D, Zhan M, et al. Changes in selected proteins associated with osteoarthritis development in the Baltimore Longitudinal study of aging (BSLA). Arthritis Rheum 2005;52:S256.

97. Garnero P, Sornay-Rendu E, Arlot M, et al. Association between spine disc degeneration and type II collagen degradation in postmenopausal women: The OFELY study. Arthritis Rheum 2004;50:3137.

98. Meulenbelt I, Kloppenburg M, Kroon HM, et al. Urinary CTX-II levels are associated with radiographic subtypes of osteoarthritis (OA) in hip, knee, and facet joints in subjects with familial OA at multiple sites: The GARP study. Ann Rheum Dis 3 August 2005 [e-pub ahead of print].

99. Moscowitz RW, Holderbaum D, Hooper MM. Total quantitative osteoarthritis load (TQOL) assessment tool: A proposed methodology for biomarker correlations. Arthritis Rheum 2005;52:S71.

100. Crisione LG, Elliot AL, Stabler T, et al. Variation of serum hyaluronan with activity in individual with knee osteoarthritis. Osteoarthritis Cart 2005;13:837.

101. Kerstin UG, Studbendorff JJ, Schmidt MC, Bruggemann GP. Changes in knee cartilage volume and serum COMP concentration after running exercise. Osteoarthritis Cart 2005;13:925.

102. Mundermann A, Dyrby CO, Andriacchi TP, et al. Serum concentration of oligomeric matrix protein (COMP) is sensitive to physiological cyclic loading in healthy adults. Osteoarthrtis Cart 2005;13:34.

103. Garnero P, Peterfy C, Zaim S, Schoenharting M. Bone marrow abnormality on magnetic resonance imaging is associated with type II collagen degradation in knee osteoarthritis: A three-month longitudinal study. Arthritis Rheum 2005;52:2822.

104. Bettica P, Cline G, Hart DJ, et al. Evidence for increased bone resorption in patients with progressive knee osteoarthritis: Longitudinal results from the Chingford study. Arthritis Rheum 2002;46:3178.

105. Reijman M, Hazes JM, Bierna-Zeinstra SM, et al. A new marker for osteoarthritis: Cross-sectional and longitudinal approach. Arthritis Rheum 2004;50:2471.

106. Vilim V, Olejarova M, Machacek S, et al. Serum levels of cartilage oligomeric matrix protein (COMP) correlate with radiographic progression of knee osteoarthritis. Osteoarthritis Cartilage 2002;10:707.

107. Sharif M, Kirwan JR, Elson CJ, et al. Suggestion of nonlinear or phasic progression of knee osteoarthritis based on measurements of serum cartilage oligomeric matrix protein levels over five years. Arthritis Rheum 2004;50:2479.

108. Garnero P, Ayral X, Rousseau J-C, et al. Uncoupling of type II collagen synthesis and degradation predicts progression of joint damage in patients with knee osteoarthritis. Arthritis Rheum 2002;46:2613.

109. Sharma L, Dunlop D, Ionescu M, et al. The ratio of collagen breakdown to collagen synthesis and its relationships with progression of knee osteoarthritis. Arthritis Rheum 2005; 50(1):S282.

110. Cibere J, Thorne A, Kopec JA, Singer J, et al. Glucosamine sulfate and cartilage type II collagen degradation in patients with knee osteoarthritis: Randomized discontinuation trial employing biomarkers. J Rheumatol 2005;32:896.

111. Christgau S, Henrotin Y, Tanko LB, et al. Osteoarthritis patients with high cartilage turnover show increased responsiveness to the cartilage protecting effect of glucosamine sulphate. Clin Exp Rheumatol 2004;22:36.

112. Leff RL, Elias I, Ionescu A, Poole R. Molecular changes in human osteoarthritis cartilage after 8 weeks of oral administration of BAY 12-9566, a matrix metalloproteinase inhibitor. J Rheumatol 2003;30:544.

113. Ravn P, Warning L, Christgau S, Christiansen C. The effect on cartilage of different forms of application of postmenopausal estrogen therapy: Comparison of oral and transdermal therapy. Bone 2004;35:1216.

114. Christgau S, Tanko LB, Cloos PAC, et al. Suppression of elevated cartilage turnover in postmenopausal women and in ovariectomized rats by estrogen and a selective estrogen-receptor modular (SERM). Menopause 2004;11:508.

115. Lehmann HJ, Mouritzen U, Christgau S, et al. Effect of bisphosphonates on cartilage turnover assessed with a newly developed assay for collagen type II degradation products. Ann Rheum Dis 2002;61:530.

116. Spector TD, Conaghan PG, Buckland-Wright JC, et al. Effect of risedronate on joint structure and symptoms of knee osteoarthritis: Results of the brisk randomized, controlled trial. Arthritis Res Ther 2005;7:R625–33.

117. Bingham CO, Buckland-Wright JC, Garnero P, et al. Risedronate decreases biochemical markers of cartilage degradation but does not decrease symptoms or slow radiographic progression in patients with medial compartment osteoarthritis of the knee: Results of the two-year multinational knee osteoarthritis structural arthritis study. Arthritis Rheum 2006, 54:3494.

118. Landewé R, Geusens P, Maarten B, et al. Markers for type II collagen breakdown predict the effect of disease modifying treatment on long-term radiographic progression in patients with rheumatoid arthritis: The Cobra study. Arthritis Rheum 2004;50:1390.

# 9 Radiographic Imaging in Osteoarthritis of the Hip and Knee

Eric Vignon and Marie-Pierre Hellio Le Graverand

## INTRODUCTION

Conventional radiography is the simplest and least expensive method of imaging joints in osteoarthritis (OA). Radiographs clearly visualize bony features (including marginal osteophytes, subchondral sclerosis, and subchondral cysts) associated with OA but provide only an estimate of cartilage thickness by the interbone distance or joint space width (JSW). Radiography is used in clinical practice in OA patients to establish the diagnosis and to monitor the progression of the disease. The radiographic definition of OA mainly relies on the evaluation of both osteophytes and joint space narrowing (JSN).

Because osteophytes are considered specific for OA, develop at an earlier stage than JSN, and are more correlated with knee pain and are easier to ascertain than other radiographic features, they represent a widely applied criterion for defining the presence of OA.[1,2] However, various radiographic definitions of OA have been proposed[1-4] (representing subtle differences in the identification of early OA among specialists). Assessment of OA severity mainly relies on JSN and subchondral bone lesions. Progression of JSN is the most commonly used criterion for the assessment of OA progression, and the complete loss of JSW characterized by bone-on-bone contact is a factor considered in the decision for joint replacement.

Radiographs are a 2D projection of a 3D joint and are subject to problems with variability (in joint repositioning in particular). Radiographs have for some time been known to perform poorly in the detection of early OA and to be relatively insensitive in the determination of disease progression. These limitations have been confirmed by the concurrent investigation of joints using more sophisticated imaging methods, including contrast arthrography, arthroscopy, computed tomography (CT) scan, and magnetic resonance imaging (MRI). Awareness of these limitations has not lessened the use of conventional radiography in

clinical practice, perhaps because of its history spanning decades and because X-rays are easily interpreted.

The growing number of publications on radiographic assessment of OA over recent years highlights a renewed interest in improving the performance of radiographic approaches. This interest was likely stimulated by the awareness that OA is a major widespread chronic health problem that leads to joint pain and disability and that its prevalence is expected to increase significantly over the upcoming decades as the population ages. In the past, longitudinal studies generally used standard plain radiographs (i.e., an anteroposterior [AP] view of the pelvis for the hip and standing AP view of the femorotibial joint for the knee).

Over the past few years, the validity of these radiographs for the accurate detection of early OA and the sensitive measurement of disease progression has been questioned. In addition, the demonstration of chondro-protection in disease-modifying OA drug (DMOAD) randomized controlled clinical trials (RCT) has been very difficult using conventional radiography. These issues have led to the considerable efforts and significant progress summarized in the following pages.

## ASSESSMENT OF OSTEOARTHRITIS ON RADIOGRAPHS

The severity of the individual radiographic lesions of OA can be estimated using semi-quantitative scoring systems. Published atlases (e.g., OARSI atlas) provide images that represent specific grades.[5,6] Several grading scales incorporating combinations of features have also been developed, including the most widely employed Kellgren–Lawrence scale. The Kellgren–Lawrence system suffers from limitations based on the invalid assumptions that changes in radiographic features (e.g., osteophytes, JSN) are linear over the course of the disease and that the relationship between these features is constant. Given the lower sensitivity to

131

change of OA qualitative scoring systems, they have been applied not in smaller and relatively short-term DMOAD clinical trials but predominantly in large longitudinal epidemiologic studies.

Among the various radiographic features of OA, JSW is considered the surrogate for articular cartilage thickness. In addition, according to guidance documents from regulatory agencies at present the only acceptable surrogate for a clinical endpoint (i.e., arthroplasty) is the measurement of JSW in serial radiographs in order to assess structural progression of OA.

Methods of measurement of JSW can be either manual (using calipers or a simple graduated rule and a micrometric eyepiece) or semiautomated using computer software.[7-16] Both manual and semiautomated measurement methods quantify the minimum JSW (i.e., interbone distance at the narrowest point of the joint compartment), whereas only computer software allows for the determination of a mean JSW in either a constant area or a region of interest. Minimum JSW was found more reproducible and more sensitive to change than mean JSW or a joint space area.[17,18] Although in some reports mean JSW has been suggested to perform better, minimum JSW remains the generally recommended and accepted outcome measurement.[13,14,20]

It is unclear whether the manual or semiautomated method of measurement of minimum JSW is superior. High reliability in the remeasurement of minimum JSW in the same radiograph (short-term reproducibility) has been reported for both manual and semiautomated methods.[7-16] Comparative evaluations (i.e., true head-to-head comparisons) of various measurement methods are rare and have yielded conflicting results. For example, for the hip joint both manual and semiautomated methods were suggested to have equivalent reliability and sensitivity in one study[12] but superiority of a computerized method was found in another study.[17]

The semiautomated measurement was also found superior to the manual method in a knee OA study,[13] but the converse finding was observed in another study.[21] However, superiority of the manual measurement method in the latter report was attributed to the correction of magnification inherent to that knee radiographic view. Interpretation of these study results is complicated by several factors, including the reliability of the observer related to his/her degree of expertise in identifying the location of minimum JSW and the performance of the semiautomated method used. A clear conclusion requires a head-to-head comparison of observers as well as computer software available in the field, which has not as yet been done.

Independently of the measurement method used, literature reports appear to describe JSW measurement as a simple task. This is probably true when measuring normal joints or joints with early OA in high-quality radiographs. However, when the quality of the radiograph and/or the progression of OA bony changes obscure the delineation of the original bone edges that form the articular surface the accurate measurement of minimum JSW may not be straightforward (Fig. 9.1). For example, poor tibial plateau alignment (i.e., inadequate superimposition of the anterior and posterior tibial rims) has been suggested to alter the reliability of the measurement of minimum JSW.[16]

In addition, the determination of the location of minimum JSW is observer dependent and can vary between observers in difficult radiographs. In one report, statistically significant differences in minimum JSW were observed between manual and semiautomated methods (as well as between two computerized methods) in both hip and knee OA joints.[18] In this study, large differences in minimum JSW (up to 1 mm) between measurement methods were reported— suggesting that these differences were likely related to divergence in the choice of the location of minimum JSW by the observers/computers rather than failure of the measurement methods themselves.

In the ECHODIAH study, the determination of the superolateral, concentric, or superomedial location of minimum JSW differed between two experts in nearly 20% of hips.[18] Notably, when the location of minimum JSW was not clearly superolateral agreement between the two experts was only 60%. The problem of the determination of the location of minimum JSW is not specific to the hip joint. In the femorotibial joint, the location of minimum JSW can substantially vary with minimal change in the delineation of bone edges and can be complicated by osteophytes.

Thus, the accurate determination of the location of minimum JSW is a difficult task and requires either an expert reader or the selection of indisputable radiographs. It is also important to note that the smallest standard deviation (SD) of the difference between test-retest measurements of minimum JSW hardly reaches 0.1 mm in the most reproducible methods.[15,16,22] This indicates a smallest detectable difference (SDD) of at least 0.2 mm, which remains relatively large considering the 0.10- to 0.15-mm expected average annual JSN of OA hip and knee joints.

## ACCURACY OF RADIOGRAPHS IN IMAGING OSTEOARTHRITIS JOINT LESIONS

Although standard AP radiographs of the hip and knee joints have been commonly used to score JSN for staging the severity of OA and to measure minimum JSW for assessing the progression of OA, it is now

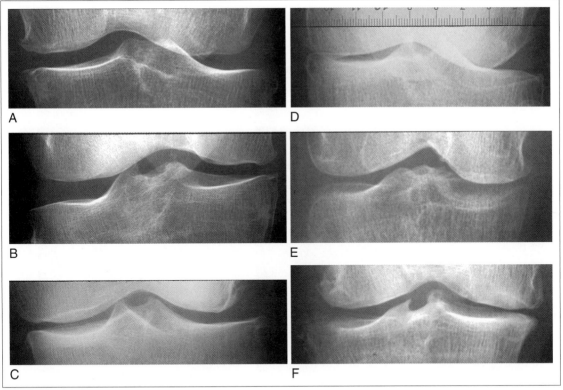

**Fig. 9.1** Illustration of the difficulty in the measurement of medial femorotibial minimum JSW in radiographs. (A) Proper alignment of the medial joint space, clear delineation of femoral and tibial bone edges, and projection of osteophytes out of the joint space facilitate the identification of the location of minimum JSW and its measurement. (B) Depending on one's estimate of the contour of the medial femoral condyle osteophyte, the selection of the site for minimum medial JSW measurement could vary substantially. (C) Duplicate edges of the medial femoral condyle and poorly individualized contour of the medial femoral osteophyte obscure the location of minimum medial JSW. (D) Poor alignment of the medial tibial plateau and projection of the medial femoral condyle in the joint space complicate the measurement of minimum JSW. (E) Dramatic lack of alignment of the medial tibial plateau obscures the delineation of the edge of the medial tibial plateau. (F) Delineation of the medial tibial plateau is vanishing in the medial part of the joint, making measurement of minimum JSW problematic.

well recognized that standard AP radiographs present major limitations. Consequently, in recent years additional acquisition protocols and radiographic views of the hip and knee joints have been developed and evaluated.

## Hip Joint Radiographs

In clinical practice, the acquisition of hip radiographs relies on the AP pelvis view in the weight-bearing position. Other hip radiograph protocols include the AP radiograph centered on one hip and the hip profile of Lequesne.[23] The latter requires complex patient positioning, but clearly identifies the joint space—which in non-OA subjects increases progressively from the inferoposterior region of the femoral head to the superoanterior part of the joint (Fig. 9.2).

In two studies, the comparison of the AP pelvis view with the hip profile of Lequesne clearly indicated that the former view misrepresented both the location and magnitude of minimum JSW in about 30% of the patients—in particular when the migration of the femoral head was not superolateral.[24,25] However, the AP pelvis view performed better than the hip profile in a number of other hip OA joints. These results suggest the benefit of acquiring both views for a complete and accurate assessment of JSN in the hip joint. Alternatively, these results suggest that at least in theory the AP pelvis radiograph alone may provide acceptable precision for longitudinal JSN measurement in those with a superolateral or concentric minimum JSW location.

## Knee Joint Radiographs

The standing AP radiograph of the knees in extension in the weight-bearing position has typically been the most commonly used radiographic view in knee OA studies, and continues to be the usual approach in clinical X-ray units. The standing AP radiograph exhibits

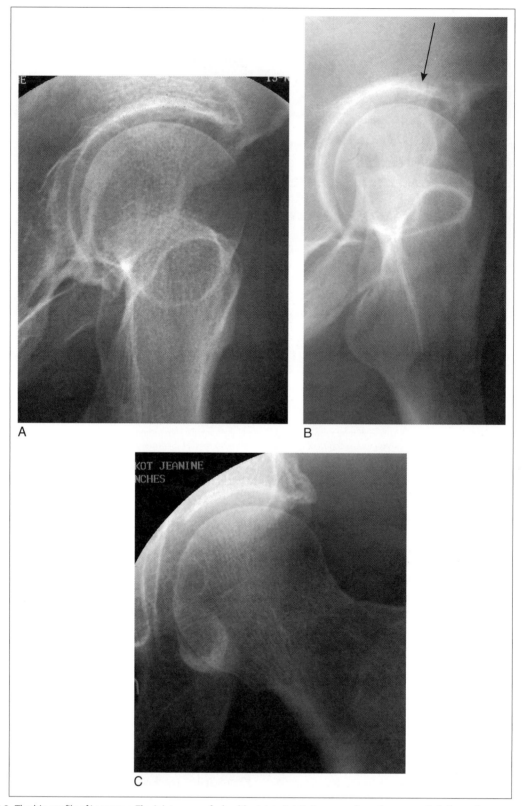

**Fig. 9.2** The hip profile of Lequesne. The joint space of a healthy joint slightly increases from the posteroinferior to the superoanterior part of the joint (A). The hip profile facilitates the identification of minute JSN located in the anterosuperior part of the joint (arrow). JSN is scored 1 (possible) in the pelvis radiograph (C) and scored 2 (definite) in the profile radiograph (B) of the same hip. Conversely, osteophytes of the superior and inferior region of the acetabulum are better identified in the pelvis view than in the profile view.

only the femorotibial joint and provides no information about the patellofemoral joint. Imaging of the latter requires a lateral or skyline view of the knee. Both lateral and skyline radiographic views have been recently reevaluated.[26,27] Both views appear similar for both the diagnosis and severity assessment of OA of the patellofemoral joint. However, the skyline view would appear more suitable for the measurement of patellofemoral JSW. JSN in patellofemoral OA is well known to vary greatly with conditions, including quadriceps contraction and the degree of knee flexion—suggesting that in this case the accurate measurement of JSN is unlikely to be straightforward.

It has also been known for some time that X-raying the knee in flexion improves detection of JSN. Several radiographic protocols that image the knee in flexion have been developed, including the Lyon-schuss and tunnel views. Current flexed-knee protocols differ by AP or PA positioning of the knee relative to the X-ray beam source, degree of knee flexion, inclination of the X-ray beam, and use of fluoroscopy to provide alignment of the anterior and posterior medial tibial rims.[28-38] These current protocols of the knee in flexion include the semiflexed AP view, the PA Lyon-schuss view, the PA fixed-flexion (FF) view, and the semiflexed PA metatarsophalangeal (MTP) view.[8,15,22,34]

The Lyon-schuss (PA) view positions the patient's patella, thigh, pelvis, and thorax flush with the table and co-planar with the tip of the great toe—resulting in a fixed flexion of the knee of approximately 20 degrees.[34] A quantitative comparison between the conventional extended AP and Lyon-schuss views indicated that the latter performed significantly better in detecting minimum JSW.[34] In knees with medial compartment OA, the average medial JSN score and the average minimum medial JSW were 1.5 ± 1.2 and 3.5 ± 1.5 (respectively) in the conventional AP compared to 2.5 ± 1.2 and 2.8 ± 1.8 mm (respectively) in the Lyon-schuss view.

In knees with lateral compartment OA, the average lateral JSN score and the average minimum lateral JSW were 2.2 ± 1.2 and 3.7 ± 1.7 (respectively) in the standing AP compared to 3.8 ± 0.9 and 1.2 ± 1.2 mm (respectively) in the Lyon-schuss view. Better exposure of the greater cartilage loss that occurs in the posterior area of the femoral condyles has been proposed to explain the greater sensitivity of radiographs of the knee in flexion than extended knee X-rays. It has also been reported that differences in JSW between the standing extended and flexed radiographs existed in normal knee joints, suggesting that changes observed in the flexed knee were related to anatomic factors (i.e., to a generally thinner JSW in the posterior part of the femorotibial joint).[39] In contrast, in another report in normal knees

JSW of the medial femorotibial joint was found similar in both standing extended and flexed radiographs—whereas lateral compartment JSW alone was significantly larger in the Lyon-schuss view compared to the standing AP view (5.3 ± 0.7 mm and 3.7 ± 1.4 mm, respectively).[34]

Importantly, it has also been demonstrated that the sensitivity of the conventional extended knee AP view for the identification of early femorotibial OA was poor. In 52% of patients with unilateral knee OA, contralateral knees considered normal on conventional AP radiographs exhibited femorotibial OA on semiflexed AP radiographs.[40] More dramatically, the standing AP view was shown to be potentially misleading with regard to the determination of the location of minimum JSW in the medial or lateral femorotibial compartments. Although this finding was mainly observed in patients with osteophytes but no obvious JSN, it is of importance when considering that those patients are common candidates for longitudinal studies (in particular, for DMOAD clinical trials).

In 73 patients with medial knee OA recruited into a DMOAD RCT on the basis of a possible medial JSN (score 1) in standing AP radiographs, the medial location of minimum JSW was confirmed in only about 7% of the knees—whereas 40% of the knees showed a definite JSN (score > 1) in the lateral compartment in Lyon-schuss radiographs.[41] A statistically significant inverse correlation between medial JSW and lateral JSW was observed in a cross-sectional study of OA knees presenting various stages of medial or lateral JSN.[41]

This finding suggests that the compartment contralateral to the narrowed one progressively enlarges during the narrowing of the affected compartment and outlines the importance of the appropriate identification of medial or lateral JSN in knees with early OA at baseline for an accurate evaluation of JSN in follow-up images. In summary, the standing AP radiograph of the pelvis appears to be an acceptable view for imaging hip OA—whereas the standing AP radiograph of the knee in extension shows deceiving performance in accurately imaging the location of maximum cartilage loss in femorotibial OA.

## MEASUREMENT OF OSTEOARTHRITIS PROGRESSION

The reliability in remeasuring JSW in one radiograph is greater than the reliability in measuring the progression of JSN in serial radiographs of the same joint. Evaluation of hip or knee JSN in serial radiographs has clearly emerged as a difficult task.[18] The main issues that have been identified include the acquisition of high-quality clinically relevant joint images and the reacquisition of the same joint image in serial radiographs.

The difficulty of the task appears to differ for hip and knee OA joints.

## Measurement of Hip Osteoarthritis Progression

Progression of JSN in hip OA has been commonly measured using the AP pelvis radiograph in the weight-bearing position.[42-46] The distribution of weight borne by each limb can be expected to vary with the degree of joint pain. Although minimum JSW was not substantially different, between radiographs taken in the supine and weight-bearing positions in OA hips in general[47,48] minimum JSW was significantly less in weight-bearing than supine positions in hips with a minimum JSW less than 2.5 mm.[48] Studies reporting the reproducibility of the hip joint image in serial films using the AP pelvis radiograph protocol are scarce.

Minimum JSW did not vary significantly between two pelvis radiographs of the same OA hip joints taken on the same day, even when foot rotation was modified.[49] However, significant variability in minimum JSW was reported in pelvis radiographs when the X-ray beam was centered on the umbilicus.[49] The SDD in this study was 0.46 mm. In another study, minimum JSW was measured in 100 normal hips of patients without OA—radiographed twice at different centers and at various intervals.[18] In agreement with the previous study, the SD of the difference between the two radiographs was 0.25 mm. The potential for measurement error in minimum JSW in serial radiographs is clearly larger than that in the same radiograph, suggesting that the precision error in the measurement of JSN is predominantly related to the variability in the reacquisition.

The sensitivity to change in JSW measurement in the pelvic AP radiograph can be estimated by analyzing JSN in the placebo group of reported DMOAD RCTs.[44-46] Data from three randomized clinical trials are illustrated in Table 9.1. Large differences in JSN between trials were observed. However, the SD of the mean JSN was regularly smaller than the mean JSN—indicating that erroneous JSW enlargement was uncommon and that the standardized response mean was acceptable.

The identification of the location of minimum JSW in serial radiographs is an important issue in longitudinal measurement. Measurements are usually made by an observer blinded to the sequence of serial films from the same subject. JSW measurement approaches vary between observers. For example, Lequesne selects the location of minimum JSW in the radiograph showing the greatest JSN and then consistently measures JSW at that particular location in the other films.[50] Often, investigators do not specify their measurement approach. It is reasonable to assume that computerized JSW measurements compute minimum JSW in each film regardless of its location. Differences in these measurement approaches may affect the sensitivity to change in JSN. The optimal or most clinically relevant methodology remains unknown.

In the ECHODIAH study, OA progression was analyzed by comparing the number of JSN progressors in each treatment group—which may be a more clinically relevant and interpretable outcome than the difference between two JSN means. A cutoff value of 0.5 mm was selected to identify patients in whom JSN was not the result of measurement error. This cutoff value was established by the blind remeasurement of 50 pairs of radiographs and represents twice the SD of test-retest differences.

In this study, the choice of analyzing the number of progressors was legitimate considering that the average JSN (and in this case JSN in the majority of the patients) was larger than the 0.5-mm SDD cutoff value over the 3-year period. It is important to note that the analysis of progressors as a dichotomous outcome measure is only usable when the cutoff value is smaller than the expected average JSN of the study. In other words, analyzing the number of progressors in a study with a 0.5-mm SDD cutoff value and a 0.2- to 0.3-mm expected average JSN could be misleading because it would represent the selection of patients with an abnormally high JSN.

Most importantly, measurement of hip OA JSN in the AP pelvis radiograph has been shown to be a clinically relevant outcome measure. In a retrospective analysis, the delay between onset of symptoms and total hip replacement in patients with hip OA was

| TABLE 9.1 JSN IN THE PLACEBO GROUP OF DMOAD CLINICAL TRIALS USING PELVIS AP RADIOGRAPHS | | | | |
|---|---|---|---|---|
| Reference | No. of Hips | Duration (Years) | JSN ± SD | SRM |
| Pavelka et al. 2000 | 66 | 5 | 0.22 ± 0.08 | 2.75 |
| Dougados et al. 2001 | 252 | 3 | 0.69 ± 0.67 | 1.02 |
| Lequesne et al. 2002 | 53 | 2 | 0.86 ± 0.62 | 1.39 |

shown to be inversely related to the annual rate of JSN.[42] This was confirmed prospectively in the ECHODIAH study, in which on the basis of a predicted need for future total hip replacement a JSN of 0.2 mm over 1 year and 0.4 mm over 2 years was found clinically relevant.[51] In the same study, a change of at least 0.4 mm in JSW over 3 years has also been suggested to be clinically relevant.[52] In addition, in this study progression of JSN in patients with hip OA has been correlated with elevated levels of some biomarkers at baseline.[53,54]

The reliability of JSW measurement in the AP radiograph centered on one hip and the hip profile has recently been compared to JSW from the AP pelvis radiograph. Sensitivity to change in JSN after 3 years was also evaluated.[55] Results suggested that the AP pelvis radiograph performed better than either of the two other views. This finding is likely related to the difficulty in acquiring reproducible hip joint images in serial radiographs using these other radiographic protocols.

In summary, reproducibility of the hip joint image in serial radiographs using the AP pelvis radiographic protocol is acceptable—and the measurement of JSN is a clinically relevant outcome measure, which is reasonable for longitudinal studies including DMOAD clinical trials.[56] However, the marginal sensitivity of radiographic measurement of hip OA progression justifies clinical trials of at least 3 years in length. Ensuring proper radiographic imaging of JSW by quality-control review and selection of patients with superolateral or concentric JSN could potentially reduce this time frame.

## Measurement of Knee Osteoarthritis Progression

The measurement of OA progression is more complex in the knee than in the hip. To date, the clinical relevance of knee OA radiographs has not been unequivocally demonstrated—in that the literature reports conflicting results. In a recent report of 70 patients with knee OA and Kellgren–Lawrence grade 1 and 2 radiographs, painful knees were found to be more frequently related to meniscal lesions (approximately 71% of cases) than to early OA (approximately 7.5% of cases).[57] Probably due to a slower progression of the disease in the knee than in the hip joint, the relationships among the first radiograph of a symptomatic knee OA joint, the rate of radiographic progression, and the necessity for a subsequent joint replacement have not been well established.[58]

JSW was shown to reliably measure cartilage thickness in the medial but not the lateral compartment in a study comparing JSW from weight-bearing plain films and cartilage thicknesses measured from double-contrast macroarthrograms of the same regions of the same knees.[60] In a prospective controlled study of patients with medial meniscal lesions, the comparison of JSW before and immediately after meniscectomy did not show a significant difference in JSW in standing AP or flexed-knee radiographs.[61]

In recent reports of MRI longitudinal studies, early radiographic OA was found to be associated with substantial changes in cartilage volume.[62,63] However, no statistical correlation between loss of cartilage volume on MRI and JSN on radiographs over 2 years was found.[59] In the doxycycline randomized controlled clinical trial, medial femorotibial JSN over 30 months was found to correlate with deterioration in pain and function.[64] In addition, in a recent report of an 8-year prospective longitudinal study the magnitude of JSN of the medial femorotibial joint over a 3-year period predicted subsequent joint replacement.[65]

Another reason for the complexity associated with knee radiography hinges on the fact that most reported studies used the conventional standing AP radiograph of the knee in extension, which is now recognized as a poor radiographic view for accurately measuring femorotibial minimum JSW and for detecting changes in JSN in serial films.[66-68] The measurement of JSW in the medial femorotibial compartment of healthy and OA knees has been reported to vary significantly with changes in a number of parameters, including foot rotation,[9] X-ray beam inclination,[9] degree of knee flexion,[9,34] degree of weight bearing,[34] intensity of knee pain,[69] and alignment of the medial tibial plateau.[40,70-72]

Changes in each of these parameters have been related to relatively large differences in JSW measurements (0.2 to 0.4 mm), which represent 2 to 3 years of JSN in knee OA (Table 9.2). Strikingly, in our own experience changes in knee positioning in serial conventional AP radiographs can induce change in JSW as large as 1 mm or even several millimeters. The requirement for an exact repositioning of the knee joint has been advocated for some time. However, no study has demonstrated that this improves the performance of the conventional standing AP radiograph.

As a result of this variability, the sensitivity to change in JSN in conventional standing AP radiographs in longitudinal cohorts or in the placebo group of reported DMOAD clinical trials[67,74-78] is relatively small. Table 9.3 outlines mean JSN and standardized response mean (SRM) for recently completed knee OA studies. The magnitude of the SD of the change in JSN suggests that erroneous measurement of JSW enlargement, often greater than 0.5 mm, was probably not uncommon. The rather small SD found in some studies is surprising and might be the result of a highly standardized radiographic procedure. In 336 pairs of knee conventional standing AP radiographs from a

| TABLE 9.2  JSN IN LONGITUDINAL OA COHORTS AND IN THE PLACEBO GROUP OF DMOAD CLINICAL TRIALS USING KNEE STANDING AP RADIOGRAPHS | | | |
|---|---|---|---|
| Reference | Duration (Years) | JSN ± SD | SRM |
| Mazzuca et al. 2002 | 2.6 | 0.37 ± 1.25 | 0.29 |
| Dieppe et al. 1997 | 3 | 0.30 ± 0.99 | 0.30 |
| Reginster et al. 2002 | 3 | 0.31 ± 0.90 | 0.34 |
| Pavelka et al. 2002 | 3 | 0.19 ± 0.50 | 0.38 |
| Pham et al. 2004 | 2 | 0.12 + 0.32 | 0.37 |
| Pham et al. 2004 | 1 | 0.09 ± 0.50 | 0.18 |

1-year ongoing trial, we found a mean JSN of 0.13 ± 1.13 mm (with a range as large as −4.7 to 5 mm). Thus, the precision error in the measurement of JSN in serial standing AP radiographs of the knee appears to be considerably larger than the progression of JSN—indicating that the conventional standing AP view of the knee performs poorly as a tool for measuring knee OA progression (Figs. 9.3 and 9.4).

To improve the performance of knee radiographs, four standardized radiograph protocols have been developed and characterized in recent years—including the semiflexed AP view, the Lyon-schuss view, the fixed-flexion view, and the semiflexed MTP view.[8,15,22,79-86] All of these radiograph protocols are schuss or tunnel views.

Among these four radiographic protocols, two are fluoroscopy guided (semiflexed AP and Lyon-schuss views). The semiflexed AP protocol alone uses an anteroposterior orientation of the X-ray beam. Although the AP semiflexed view has been shown to perform better than the conventional standing AP view, its performance can be affected by the requirement for magnification correction inherent in the method (as demonstrated by Mazzuca et al.).[21] In contrast, posteroanterior views of the knee in flexion do not require magnification correction and thus appear to be simpler and preferable. In the AP semiflexed view, the degree of knee flexion varies between 0 and 35 degrees in relation to the variable anatomic angle of the medial tibial plateau with horizontality.[81]

Although the positioning of the knee is identical in both the Lyon-schuss and FF views, the major differences between these two radiographic protocols being the use of fluoroscopy to individually adjust the inclination of the X-ray beam for an optimal alignment of the medial tibial plateau in the former and the use of a Plexiglas positioning device to optimally standardize knee flexion and foot positioning in the latter. In the semiflexed MTP protocol, the degree of knee flexion is not standardized and is smaller than that in the FF and Lyon-schuss views proportionally to the length of the big toe (in that the base of the toe is co-planar with the film in the former and the tip of the toe is in contact with the table in the others).

A head-to-head comparison of the various radiographic protocols of the knee in flexion has not been reported. Measurement characteristics of these radiographic protocols are summarized in Table 9.4. In the Lyon-schuss view, knee flexion was shown to improve sensitivity to change in comparison to the conventional standing AP view (potentially by imaging more precisely the location of cartilage maximum loss).[80] However, the optimal degree of knee flexion remains unknown. Standardization of knee positioning in the FF and Lyon-schuss views is very likely to improve the reproducibility of the knee flexion angle.

| TABLE 9.3  MAIN CHARACTERISTICS OF RADIOGRAPH PROTOCOLS OF THE KNEE IN FLEXION | | | | | | |
|---|---|---|---|---|---|---|
| Radiographic View | AP/PA | Degree of Knee Flexion | Standardization of Degree of Knee Flexion | Fluoroscopy | Alignment of the Medial Tibial Plateau | Reproducible Knee Rotation |
| Semiflexed AP | AP | Variable | No | Yes | Yes | ++ |
| Lyon-schuss | PA | 20–30° | Yes | Yes | Yes | + |
| Fixed-flexion | PA | 20–30° | Yes | No | Variable | ++ |
| MTP | PA | 7–10° | No | No | Variable | + |

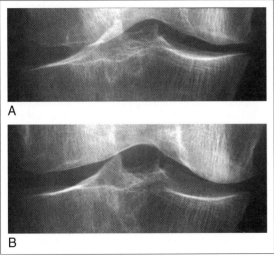

A

B

**Fig. 9.3** Variability in minimum JSW with alignment of the medial tibial plateau. Two radiographs of the same knee taken on the same day. Proper alignment of medial plateau with the X-ray beam in A and poor alignment in B. Minimum JSW is 0.51 mm larger in B than in A.

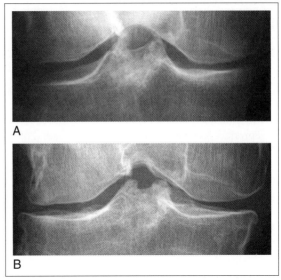

A

B

**Fig. 9.4** Dramatic variability in minimum JSW in relation to alteration in knee positioning. Two radiographs of the same knee taken on the same day. Minimum JSW is 2.2 mm larger in B than in A. The difference is related to alterations in both medial tibial plateau alignment (poor in A and acceptable in B) and in the degree of knee flexion as assessed by the depth of the femoral notch.

Knee flexion was indeed shown to be greater in the FF than in the MTP semiflexed and semiflexed AP views.[73] Although reproducibility of the degree of knee rotation can be expected with all four radiograph protocols of the knee in flexion (given the use of foot maps, positioning device, or fluoroscopy), knee rotation was shown to be better reproduced in semi-flexed AP radiographs than in FF radiographs.[73]

High performance in the reacquisition of the same knee image (short-term reproducibility of knee positioning) has been reported for the AP semiflexed, the FF, and the MTP semiflexed views.[79,82-86] However, long-term reproducibility of knee positioning—assessed by the variability in the inter-margin distance (IMD), the distance between the anterior and posterior rims of the medial tibial plateau in serial radiographs—was shown to be significantly less satisfactory in MTP semiflexed and FF radiographs compared to semiflexed AP radiographs.[73,87] Similar to the semiflexed AP view, the Lyon-schuss view showed reproducible alignment of the medial tibial

plateau in nearly 90% of knees in a single-center study[81] and in 70% of knees in a multicenter setting.[80]

Another critical parameter that differentiates the four radiograph protocols of the knee in flexion is the inclination of the X-ray beam, which is constant in the FF and MTP semiflexed views and fluoroscopy-adjusted in the semiflexed AP and Lyon-schuss views. Because the anatomic inclination of the medial tibial plateau varies significantly between individuals, the use of a constant X-ray beam angle implies that the medial tibial plateau will not be aligned with the X-ray beam in a large number of knees. In a recent study comparing the performance of the AP semiflexed, FF, and MTP semiflexed views, satisfactory alignment of the medial tibial plateau (defined by an IMD <1.4 mm) was achieved significantly more frequently with the fluoroscopically guided positioning used in the semiflexed

**TABLE 9.4 JSN IN LONGITUDINAL OA COHORTS AND IN THE PLACEBO GROUP OF DMOAD CLINICAL TRIALS USING RADIOGRAPH PROTOCOLS OF THE KNEE IN FLEXION**

| Reference | Fluoroscopy | Radiographic View | Follow-up (Years) | JSN ± SD | SRM |
|---|---|---|---|---|---|
| Brandt et al. 2003 | + | AP semiflexed | 2.5 | 0.45 ± 0.70 | 0.64 |
| Vignon et al. 2003 | + | Lyon-schuss | 2 | 0.24 ± 0.50 | 0.48 |
| Michel et al. 2005 | − | PA semiflexed | 2 | 0.14 ± 0.57 | 0.24 |
| Buckland-Wright et al. 2003 | + | AP semiflexed | 1 | 0.12 ± 0.41 | 0.29 |

AP protocol than with either the non-fluoroscopic FF or MTP protocols.[73]

The benefit of fluoroscopy to reproducibly align the medial tibial plateau has been shown in knees positioned according to the Lyon-schuss protocol.[81] Thus, non-fluoroscopic protocols propose to reproduce a constant degree of inclination of the tibial plateau within patients—whereas fluoroscopic protocols aim to reproduce a constant alignment of the medial tibial plateau within and between patients. Reproducibility of the alignment of the medial tibial plateau, assessed by the IMD, has been shown to be a critical factor for measuring reliably changes in JSW in serial radiographs and therefore to provide greater sensitivity to change in JSN.[70,73,80] Notably, only paired radiographs with satisfactory alignment of the medial tibial plateau have been shown to repeatedly exhibit a mean rate of JSN that was more rapid and less variable than that measured in all knees.[70,73,80] In the Lyon-schuss view, an IMD smaller than 1.2 mm was identified as the cutoff value for medial tibial plateau alignment that provides the greatest sensitivity to change for JSN.[72]

Recent reports of JSN in longitudinal OA studies using radiographs of the knee in flexion are presented in Table 9.4. In studies of at least 2 years, the sensitivity to change in JSN (assessed by the SRM) was significantly improved compared to that reported using the conventional standing AP radiograph protocol.[64,80] The SRM was greater in studies using a fluoroscopy protocol of at least 2 years in duration. The SRM did not reach the level observed in hip OA. However, the difference might be related to a slower progression of

the disease in the knee compared to the hip. Nevertheless, the magnitude of the reported SDs clearly indicates a significant improvement in the performance of radiographic protocols of the knee in flexion for the evaluation of knee OA progression.

In summary, imaging the progression of OA using radiographs is a more complex task for the knee than for the hip joint. The conventional standing AP radiograph of the knee is not a sensitive technique. The greater performance of some radiographic protocols of the knee in flexion can be expected to provide (1) a more precise determination of the location of maximum cartilage loss, improving patient selection for longitudinal studies, and (2) more reproducible joint positioning enhancing sensitivity to change in JSN. The most suitable radiographic view of the knee in flexion in large multicenter studies with regard to the sensitivity to change in JSN remains to be determined.

## SUMMARY

Given the great difficulty in obtaining high-quality reproducible radiographs of hip and knee OA joints, the precision of JSW measurement in serial radiographs remains marginal considering the expected average annual JSN of OA joints. Therefore, structure-modifying OA drug trials of long duration remain necessary. Efforts aimed at further improving the acquisition of clinically relevant high-quality joint images will continue to increase the performance of the radiographic assessment of OA progression in the hip and knee joints.

## REFERENCES

1. Altman R, Asch E, Bloch D, et al. Development of criteria for the classification and reporting of osteoarthritis. Arthritis Rheum 1986;29:1039–49.
2. Altman R, Alarcon D, Appelrouth D, American College of Rheumatology Subcommittee on Criteria for Osteoarthritis. The American College of Rheumatology criteria for the classification and reporting of osteoarthritis of the hip. Arthritis Rheum 1991;34:505–11.
3. Spector TD, Hart DJ, Byrne J, et al. Definition of osteoarthritis of the knee for epidemiological studies. Ann Rheum Dis 1993;52:790–94.
4. Reijman M, Hazes JM, Koes BW, et al. Validity, reliability, and applicability of seven definitions of hip osteoarthritis used in epidemiological studies: A systematic appraisal. Ann Rheum Dis 2004;63:226–32.
5. Altman R, Hochberg M, Murphy W, et al. Atlas of individual radiographic features in osteoarthritis. Osteoarthritis Cart 1995;3(A):3–70.
6. Scott WW Jr., Lethbridge-Cejku M, Reichle R, et al. Reliability of grading scales for individual radiographic features of osteoarthritis of the knee: The Baltimore longitudinal study of aging atlas of knee osteoarthritis. Invest Radiol 1993;28:497–501.
7. Dacre JE, Scott DL, Da Silva JAP, et al. Joint space in radiologically normal knees. Br J Rheumatol 1991;30:426–28.
8. Buckland-Wright JC, MacFarlane DG, Jasani MK, et al. Quantitative microfocal radiographic assessment of osteoarthritis of the knee

from weight bearing tunnel and semi-flexed standing views. J Rheum 1994;21:1734–41.
9. Ravaud P, Auleley GR, Chastang C, et al. Knee joint space width measurement: An experimental study of the influence of radiographic procedure and joint positioning. Br J Rheum 1996;35:761–66.
10. Gordon CL, Wu C, Peterfy CG, et al. Automated measurement of radiographic hip joint-space width. Med Phys 2001;28:267–77.
11. Hilliquin P, Pessis E, Coste J, et al. Quantitative assessment of joint space width with an electronic calliper. Osteoarthritis Cartilage 2002;10:542–46.
12. Maillefert JF, Sharp JT, Aho LS, et al. Comparison of a computer based method and the classical manual method for radiographic joint space width assessment in hip osteoarthritis. J Rheum 2002;29:2592–96.
13. Bruyere O, Henrotin YE, Honore A, et al. Impact of the joint space width measurement method on the design of knee osteoarthritis studies. Aging Clin Exp Res 2003;15:136–41.
14. Duryea J, Zaim S, Genant HK. New radiographic-based surrogate outcome measures for osteoarthritis of the knee. Osteoarthritis Cartilage 2003;11:102–10.
15. Peterfy C, Li J, Zaim S, et al. Comparison of fixed-flexed positioning with fluoroscopic semiflexed positioning for quantifying radiographic joint space width in the knee: Test-retest reproducibility. Skeletal Radiol 2003;32:128–32.

16. Conrozier T, Favret H, Mathieu P, et al. Influence of the quality of tibial plateau alignment on the reproducibility of computer joint space measurement from Lyon-schuss radiographic views of the knee in patients with knee osteoarthritis. Osteoarthritis Cartilage 2004;12:765–70.

17. Conrozier T, Lequesne M, Favret H, et al. Measurement of the radiological hip joint space width: An evaluation of various methods of measurement. Osteoarthritis Cartilage 2001; 9:281–86.

18. Vignon E. Radiographic issues in imaging the progression of hip and knee osteoarthritis. J Rheumatol Suppl 2004;70:36–44.

19. Michel BA, Stucki G, Frey D, et al. Chondroitins 4 and 6 sulfate in osteoarthritis of the knee: A randomized, controlled trial. Arthritis Rheum 2005;52:779–86.

20. Ravaud P, Chastang C, Auleley GR, et al. Assessment of joint space width in patients with osteoarthritis of the knee: A comparison of 4 measuring instruments. J Rheum 1996;23:1749–55.

21. Mazzuca SM, Brandt KD, Buckwalter KA, et al. Pitfalls in the accurate measurement of joint space narrowing in semiflexed anteroposterior radiographic image of the knee. Arthritis Rheum 2004;50:2508–15.

22. Buckland-Wright JC, Ward RJ, Peterfy C, et al. Reproducibility of the semiflexed (metatarsophalangeal) radiographic knee position and automated measurements of medial tibiofemoral joint space width in a multicenter clinical trial of knee osteoarthritis. J Rheum 2004;31:1588–97.

23. Lequesne M. The false profile view of the hip: Role, interest, economic considerations. Joint Bone Spine 2002;69:109–13.

24. Lequesne MG, Laredo JD. The faux profil (oblique view) of the hip in the standing position: Contribution to the evaluation of osteoarthritis of the adult hip. Ann Rheum Dis 1998;57:676–81.

25. Conrozier T, Bochu M, Gratacos J, et al. Evaluation of the "Lequesne's false profile" of the hip in patients with hip osteoarthritis. Osteoarthritis Cartilage 1999;7:295–300.

26. Chaisson CE, Gale DR, Gale E, et al. Detecting radiographic knee osteoarthritis: What combination of views is optimal? Rheumatology 2000;39:1218–21.

27. Elias DA, White LM. Imaging of patellofemoral disorders. Clin Radiol 2004;59:543–57.

28. Ahlback S. Osteoarthritis of the knee: A radiographic investigation. Acta Radiol Suppl (Stockh) 1968;277:1–71.

29. Leach RE, Gregg T, Siber FJ. Weight-bearing radiography in osteoarthritis of the knee. Radiology 1970;97:265–68.

30. Marklund T, Myrnerts R. Radiographic determination of cartilage height in the knee joint. Acta Orthop Scand 1974;45:752–55.

31. Resnick D, Vint V. The tunnel view in assessment of cartilage loss in osteoarthritis of the knee. Radiology 1980;137:547–48.

32. Railhac JJ, Fournie A, Gay R, et al. Exploration radiologique du genou de face en légère flexion et en charge. J Radiol 1981; 62:157–66.

33. Messieh SS, Fowler PJ, Munro T. Anteroposterior radiographs of the osteoarthritic knee. J Bone Joint Surg (Br) 1990;72B:639–40.

34. Piperno M, Hellio MP, Conrozier T, et al. Quantitative evaluation of joint space width in femorotibial osteoarthritis: Comparison of three radiographic views. Osteoarthritis and Cartilage 1998;6:252–59.

35. Rosenberg TD, Lonnie EP, Richard DP, et al. The forty-five-degree posteroanterior flexion weight-bearing radiograph of the knee. J Bone Joint Surg 1988;70A:1479–83.

36. Dervin GF, Feibel RJ, Rody K, et al. 3-foot standing AP versus 45 degrees PA radiograph for osteoarthritis of the knee. Clin J Sport Med 2001;11:10–16.

37. Inoue S, Nagamine R, Miura H, et al. Anteroposterior weight-bearing radiography of the knee with both knees in semiflexion, using new equipment. J Orthop Sci 2001;6:475–80.

38. Ritchie JF, Al-Sarawan M, Worth R, et al. A parallel approach: The impact of schuss radiography of the degenerate knee on clinical management. Knee 2004;11:283–37.

39. Deep K, Norris M, Smart C, et al. Radiographic measurement of joint space height in non-osteoarthritic tibiofemoral joints: A comparison of weight-bearing extension and 30 degrees flexion views. J Bone Joint Surg Br 2003;85:980–82.

40. Mazzuca SM, Brandt KD, German NC, et al. Development of radiographic changes of osteoarthritis in the Chingford knee reflects progression of disease or non-standardised positioning

of the joint rather than incident disease. Ann Rheum Dis 2003; 62:1061–65.

41. Merle-Vincent F, Piperno M, Favret H, et al. Tentative definition of medial and lateral femorotibial osteoarthritis. Arthritis Rheum 2004;50:250.

42. Conrozier T, Jousseaume CA, Mathieu P, et al. Quantitative measurement of joint space narrowing progression in hip osteoarthritis: A longitudinal retrospective study of patients treated by total hip arthroplasty. Br J Rheum 1998;37:961–68.

43. Goker B, Doughan AM, Schnitzer TJ, et al. Quantitation of progressive joint space narrowing in osteoarthritis of the hip: Longitudinal analysis of the contralateral hip after total hip arthroplasty. Arthritis Rheum 2000;43:988–94.

44. Pavelka K, Gatterova J, Gallerova V, et al. A 5-year randomized controlled double-blind study of glycosaminoglycan polysulfuric acid complex (Rumalon) as a structure-modifying therapy in osteoarthritis of the hip and knee. Osteoarthritis Cart 2000; 8:335–42.

45. Dougados M, Nguyen M, Berdah L, et al. ECHODIAH investigators study group. Evaluation of the structure-modifying effects of diacerein in hip osteoarthritis: ECHODIAH, a three-year, placebo controlled trial. Arthritis Rheum 2001;44:2539–47.

46. Lequesne M, Maheu E, Cadet C, et al. Structural effect of avocado/soybean unsaponifiables on joint space loss in osteoarthritis of the hip. Arthritis Rheum 2002;47:50–8.

47. Auleley GR, Rousselin B, Ayral X, et al. Osteoarthritis of the hip: Agreement between joint space width measurements on standing and supine conventional radiographs. Ann Rheum Dis 1998;57:519–23.

48. Conrozier T, Lequesne M, Tron AM, et al. The effect of position on the radiographic joint space width in osteoarthritis of the hip. Osteoarthritis Cartilage 1997;5:17–22.

49. Auleley GR, Duche A, Drape JL, et al. Measurement of joint space width in hip osteoarthritis: Influence of joint positioning and radiographic procedure. Rheumatology 2001;40:414–19.

50. Lequesne M. Chondrometry: Quantitative evaluation of joint space width and rate of joint space loss in osteoarthritis of the hip. Rev Rhum Engl Ed 1995;62:155–58.

51. Maillefert JF, Gueguen A, Nguyen M, et al. Relevant change in radiological progression in patients with hip osteoarthritis. I. Determination using predictive validity for total hip arthroplasty. Rheumatology 2002;41:142–47.

52. Maillefert JF, Gueguen A, Nguyen M, et al. Relevant change in radiological progression in patients with hip osteoarthritis. II. Determination using an expert opinion approach. Rheumatology 2002;41:148–52.

53. Garnero P, Mazieres B, Gueguen A, et al. Cross-sectional association of 10 molecular markers of bone, cartilage, and synovium with disease activity and radiological joint damage in patients with hip osteoarthritis: The ECHODIAH Cohort. J Rheum 2005;32:697–703.

54. Garnero P, Conrozier T, Christgau S, et al. Urinary type II collagen C-telopeptide levels are increased in patients with rapidly destructive hip osteoarthritis. Ann Rheum Dis 2003;62:939–43.

55. Maheu E, Cadet C, Marty M, et al. Reproducibility and sensitivity to change of various methods of joint space width measurements in osteoarthritis of the hip: A double reading of three different radiographs taken within a 3 year time interval. Arthritis Research and Therapy. Arthritis-research.com/content/7/6/R1375.

56. Altman RD, Bloch DA, Dougados M, et al. Measurement of structural progression in osteoarthritis of the hip: The Barcelona consensus group. Osteoarthritis Cartilage 2004;12:515–24.

57. Karachalios T, Zibis A, Papanagiotou P, et al. MR imaging findings in early osteoarthritis of the knee. Eur J Radiol 2004;50:225–30.

58. Bruyere O, Honore A, Rovati LC, et al. Radiologic features poorly predict clinical outcomes in knee osteoarthritis. Scand J Rheum 2002;31:13–16.

59. Raynauld JP, Martel-Pelletier J, Berthiaume MJ, et al. Quantitative magnetic resonance imaging evaluation of knee osteoarthritis progression over two years and correlation with clinical symptoms and radiologic changes. Arthritis Rheum 2004;50:476–87.

60. Buckland-Wright JC, MacFarlane DG, Lynch JA, et al. Joint space width measures cartilage thickness in osteoarthritis of the knee: High resolution plain film and double contrast macroradiographic investigation. Ann Rheum Dis 1995;54:263–68.

61. Ayral X, Bonvarlet JP, Simonnet J, et al. Influence of medial meniscectomy on tibiofemoral joint space width. Osteoarthritis Cartilage 2003;11:285–89.

62. Jones G, Ding C, Scott F, et al. Early radiographic osteoarthritis is associated with substantial changes in cartilage volume and tibial bone surface area in both males and females. Osteoarthritis Cartilage 2004;12:169–74.

63. Cicuttini FM, Wluka AE, Forbes A, et al. Comparison of tibial cartilage volume and radiologic grade of the tibiofemoral joint. Arthritis Rheum 2003;48:682–88.

64. Brandt KD, Mazzuca SA, Katz BP, et al. Effects of doxycycline on progression of osteoarthritis: Results of a randomized, placebo-controlled, double-blind trial. Arthritis Rheum 2005;52:2015–25.

65. Bruyere O, Richy F, Reginster JY. Three-year joint space narrowing predicts long-term incidence of knee surgery in patients with osteoarthritis: An 8-year prospective follow-up study. Ann Rheum Dis online 20 April 2005; doi:10.1136/ard.2005.037309.

66. Fife RS, Brandt KD, Braustein EM, et al. Relationship between arthroscopic evidence of cartilage damage and radiographic evidence of joint space narrowing in early osteoarthritis of the knee. Arthritis Rheum 1991;34:377–82.

67. Brandt KD, Mazzuca SA, Conrozier T, et al. Which is the best radiographic protocol for a clinical trial of a structure-modifying drug in patients with knee osteoarthritis? J Rheum 2002; 29:1308–20.

68. Mazzuca SA, Brandt KD. Is knee radiography useful for studying the efficacy of a disease-modifying osteoarthritis drug in humans? Rheum Dis Clin North Am 2003;29:819–30.

69. Mazzuca SA, Brandt KD, Lane KA, et al. Knee pain reduces joint space width in conventional standing anteroposterior radiographs of osteoarthritic knees. Arthritis Rheum 2002; 46:1223–27.

70. Mazzuca SA, Brandt KD, Dieppe PA, et al. Effect of alignment of the medial tibial plateau and X-ray beam on apparent progression of osteoarthritis in the standing anteroposterior knee radiograph. Arthritis Rheum 2001;44:1786–94.

71. Mazzuca SA, Brandt KD, Buckwalter KA, et al. Field test of the reproducibility of the semiflexed metatarsophalangeal view in repeated radiographic examinations of subjects with osteoarthritis of the knee. Arthritis Rheum 2002;46:109–13.

72. Conrozier T, Mathieu P, Piperno M, et al. Selection of knee radiographs for trials of structure-modifying drugs in patients with knee osteoarthritis: A prospective, longitudinal study of Lyon Schuss knee radiographs with the definition of adequate alignment of the medial tibial plateau. Arthritis Rheum 2005; 52:1411–17.

73. Hellio le Graverand MP, Mazzuca S, Lassere M, et al. Assessment of the radio-anatomic positioning of the osteoarthritic knee in serial radiographs: Comparison of three acquisition techniques. Radiography Working Group of the OARSI-OMERACT Imaging Workshop. Osteoarthritis Cartilage (in press).

74. Dieppe PA, Cushnaghan J, Shepstone L. The Bristol "OA500" study: Progression of oseoarthritis over 3 years and the relationship between clinical and radiographic changes at the knee joint. Osteoarthritis Cartilage 1997;5:87–97.

75. Reginster JY, Deroisy R, Rovati LC, et al. Long-term effects of glucosamine sulphate on osteoarthritis progression: A randomised, placebo-controlled clinical trial. Lancet 2001;357:251–56.

76. Pavelka K, Gatterova J, Olejarova M, et al. Glucosamine sulfate use and delay of progression of knee osteoarthritis: A 3-year, randomized, placebo-controlled, double-blind study. Arch Intern Med 2002;162:2113–23.

77. Pham T, Le Henanff A, Ravaud P, et al. Evaluation of the symptomatic and structural efficacy of a new hyaluronic acid compound, NRD101, in comparison with diacerein and placebo in a 1 year randomised controlled study in symptomatic knee osteoarthritis. Ann Rheum Dis 2004;63:1611–17.

78. Pham T, Maillefert JF, Hudry C, et al. Laterally elevated wedged insoles in the treatment of medial knee osteoarthritis: A two-year prospective randomized controlled study. Osteoarthritis Cartilage 2004;12:46–55.

79. Buckland-Wright JC, Bird CF, Ritter-Hrncirik CA, et al. X-ray technologist's reproducibility from automated measurements of the medial tibiofemoral joint space width in knee osteoarthritis for a multicenter, multinational clinical trial. J Rheum 2003;30:329–38.

80. Vignon E, Piperno M, Le Graverand MP, et al. Measurement of radiographic joint space width in the tibiofemoral compartment of the osteoarthritic knee: Comparison of standing anteroposterior and Lyon-schuss views. Arthritis Rheum 2003;48:378–84.

81. Conrozier T, Mathieu P, Piperno M, et al. Lyon-schuss radiographic view of the knee: Utility of fluoroscopy for the quality of tibial plateau alignment. J Rheum 2004;31:584–90.

82. Buckland-Wright JC, Wolfe F, Ward RJ, et al. Substantial superiority of semiflexed (MTP) views in knee osteoarthritis: A comparative radiographic study, without fluoroscopy, of standing extended, semiflexed (MTP), and schuss views. J Rheum 1999; 26:2664–74.

83. Dupuis DE, Beynnon BD, Richard MJ, et al. Precision and accuracy of joint space width measurements of the medial compartment of the knee using standardized MTP semi-flexed radiographs. Osteoarthritis Cartilage 2003;11:716–24.

84. Wolfe F, Lane NE, Buckland-Wright C. Radiographic methods in knee osteoarthritis: A further comparison of semiflexed (MTP), schuss-tunnel, and weight-bearing anteroposterior views for joint space narrowing and osteophytes. J Rheum 2002; 29:2597–2601.

85. Duddy J, Kirwan JR, Szebenyi B, et al. A comparison of the semiflexed (MTP) view with the standing extended view (SEV) in the radiographic assessment of knee osteoarthritis in a busy routine X-ray department. Rheumatology 2005;44:349–51.

86. Kothari M, Guermazi A, von Ingersleben G, et al. Fixed-flexion radiography of the knee provides reproducible joint space width measurements in osteoarthritis. Eur Radiol 2004; 14:1568–73.

87. Mazzuca SA, Brandt KD, Buckwalter KA. Detection of radiographic joint space narrowing in subjects with knee osteoarthritis: Longitudinal comparison of the metatarsophalangeal and semiflexed anteroposterior views. Arthritis Rheum 2003;48:385–90.

88. Buckland-Wright JC, Cline G, Meyer J. Structural progression in knee osteoarthritis over 12 months. Arthritis Rheum 2003;30(2):329–38.

# 10 Magnetic Resonance Imaging in Osteoarthritis

Timothy Mosher

## INTRODUCTION

With the recent development of disease-modifying interventions for osteoarthritis (OA), there is a need for objective markers of disease activity—particularly for the identification and monitoring of cartilage damage. Historically, radiography has been the primary imaging tool for diagnosis of OA. However, it is insensitive to soft tissue damage of the joint, and provides only an indirect 2D evaluation of articular cartilage loss. A unique property of magnetic resonance (MR) imaging (MRI) is the capacity to noninvasively image articular cartilage, bone marrow, and important articular soft tissues related to the pathogenesis of OA. Currently, MRI techniques are used in clinical practice to evaluate cartilage morphology—primarily in the diagnosis of focal lesions.

Quantitative MRI techniques for measuring cartilage morphology such as volume, thickness, and surface area have been developed and validated for clinical research applications. More recently, research MRI techniques have been developed that demonstrate sensitivity to biochemical and structural changes in the extracellular cartilage matrix that precede visible changes in the tissue. In the future, these techniques may serve as useful image markers for studying human cartilage physiology and for providing an objective assessment of chondro-protective therapies. The purpose of this chapter is to provide an overview of MRI physics and techniques used in the evaluation of OA, with particular emphasis on evaluation of articular cartilage. The first half of the chapter provides a brief overview of MRI physics and acquisition techniques used in musculoskeletal imaging. The second half of the chapter deals specifically with clinical and emerging research applications of MRI in cartilage imaging and OA.

Although MRI has substantial potential to provide new information on the pathogenesis of OA and response to therapy, clinical and research applications in OA have been surprisingly limited. Historically, clinical indications for musculoskeletal MRI studies have primarily been for diagnosis of surgically correctable lesions such as meniscal or ligamentous injuries in younger patients. Until recently, identification of cartilage pathology has been a secondary objective—and this has been primarily focused on detection of focal cartilage lesions, which can mimic the clinical presentation of surgical lesions such as meniscal tears. Few studies have validated MRI in the diagnosis of more extensive cartilage damage seen in patients with OA.

The limited research application of MRI in OA has been a result of several factors. Although the diversity of MRI techniques allows evaluation of many important properties of cartilage, the complexity involved has served to limit validation of specific techniques. Compared to radiographs, MRI provides a vast array of potential image markers for study. There is no clear consensus on which markers should be evaluated. Rapid progress in the development of MRI technology and new methods of signal acquisition make it difficult to perform the necessary standardized longitudinal studies on diagnostic efficacy. Standardization of techniques is further complicated by differences in instrumentation and image acquisition techniques among manufacturers.

The volume of data produced by MRI is a substantial limitation in applying this technology to clinical trials. Sophisticated automated or semiautomated image analysis tools are needed to efficiently reduce the MRI data set into useful endpoints that can be analyzed. Finally, the expense of MRI technology has limited both clinical and research development. Although newer techniques have made the MRI examination shorter, this examination method still requires substantially greater time to perform compared to higher-energy X-ray-based techniques. In addition, it is unlikely that the cost of MRI can be significantly reduced through economies of scale. To justify the use of MRI in the clinical or research assessment of OA, the value of information obtained must outweigh the expense.

## OVERVIEW OF MRI PHYSICS

### The MRI Signal

The science of MRI is based on the technique of nuclear magnetic induction (i.e., nuclear magnetic resonance [NMR]), discovered in 1945 in the laboratories of Felix Bloch[1] and Edward Purcell.[2] Using the NMR signal to generate an image is a more recent development, pioneered by Paul Lauterbur[3] and Peter Mansfield[4] in the early 1970s.

The source of the MRI signal is the hydrogen nucleus (i.e., proton) found in the water and fatty acid molecules of tissue. Specifically, the source is the weak magnetic field generated by the spin of the positively charged proton (termed the *nuclear magnetic moment*). The nuclear magnetic moment of the proton can occupy one of two energy levels. In the absence of an applied magnetic field, these levels have the same energy. Because the energy levels are equivalent, transitions between the energy levels would not result in a net release or absorption of energy and therefore would not yield a detectable signal. However, when placed into a large magnet interaction of the nuclear magnetic moment with the external magnetic field causes these levels to have different energy.

As a proton transitions from the high-energy level to the low-energy level it releases a small amount of radiofrequency (RF) energy. The transition of a proton from the low- to the high-energy state absorbs energy. The signal used to generate the MR image is produced by the net difference between energy released and energy absorbed by the proton as it makes transitions between energy levels. Compared to other imaging techniques—such as computed tomography (CT) or nuclear medicine—this energy is extremely small. The weak signal is a fundamental limitation of MRI and contributes to the long imaging times and significant expense of MRI equipment.

The amount of RF energy released or absorbed by the proton as it moves between energy levels is directly proportional to the strength of the external magnetic field. This relationship is defined by the Larmor equation (Equation 10.1).

$$\omega_0 = \gamma \bar{B}_0 \qquad (10.1)$$

Here, the Larmor frequency ($\omega_0$) is the frequency of the RF energy in megahertz (MHz), $B_0$ is the strength of the applied magnetic field in Tesla (T), and $\gamma$ is a proportionality constant (termed the *gyromagnetic ratio*, which is 42.6 MHz/T for the proton). The energy of the MRI signal is directly related to the resonance (Larmor frequency). The higher energy available from a higher $\omega_0$ increases the strength of the MRI signal. As can be seen from the Larmor equation, one way to increase the strength of the MRI signal is to use larger magnets.

The strength of most clinical MRI magnets is in the range of 0.3 to 3.0 T. For comparison, the strength of the earth's magnetic field is 0.5 gauss (0.00005 T). At 1.5 T, $\omega_0$ is approximately 63.9 MHz—increasing to 127.9 MHz at 3.0 T. The need for additional MRI signal is what drives the move to higher field strengths for clinical MRI magnets. The greater energy obtained at higher field strength provides a higher signal to noise ratio (SNR)—a key factor for high-resolution images needed for visualization of small structures such as articular cartilage.

High-field MRI scanners use cylindrical superconducting magnets to generate a magnetic field stronger than 1 T. Claustrophobia can be an issue with these systems. Newer high-field magnets are shorter in length, with flared openings to reduce the sensation of enclosure. Scanners of lower magnetic field strength (such as that provided by "open MRI" platforms) allow greater flexibility in magnet shape and are less confining. However, image acquisition times are longer in terms of obtaining signal strength comparable to that of a high-field scanner. The weaker MRI signal of low-field scanners can be problematic when imaging requires high spatial resolution or short imaging times, but are less of a problem in the evaluation of large joints such as knees and shoulders.

Because of the low energy of the MRI signal, accurate models of MRI physics can be described using a model based on classical mechanics. In this model, the nuclear magnetic moment of the proton can be described as a small bar magnet or dipole. In the absence of a magnetic field, the orientation of the magnetic dipole is random. In an external magnetic field, the dipole will be oriented either parallel or anti-parallel to the direction of the applied magnetic field—which by convention corresponds to the Z axis.

Because the proton dipoles are spinning, they undergo a complex motion about the Z axis called precession. This motion is similar to the motion of a top as it begins to lose rotational energy and begins to wobble in response to the force of gravity. If we consider a large number of protons, such as would be contained in a person, the number of dipoles aligned parallel to the external magnetic field is slightly greater than the number aligned anti-parallel to the magnetic field. As a result, the net nuclear magnetic moment of the protons within tissue can be represented by a small magnetic vector aligned parallel with the direction of the external magnetic field (Fig. 10.1).

This orientation of spins needed to generate the magnetic vector does not occur instantaneously. A few

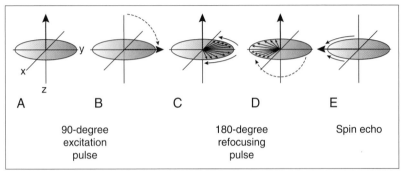

A           B           C           D           E

90-degree
excitation
pulse

180-degree
refocusing
pulse

Spin echo

**Fig. 10.1** The spin echo. (A) At equilibrium the net sum of the magnetic dipoles produced by the protons results in a small magnetic vector aligned along the direction of the applied magnetic field (Z axis). (B) A 90-degree excitation pulse generated by the RF transmitter rotates the magnetization into the XY plane. (C) Over time, small fluctuations in the magnetic field cause the individuals to diphase in the transverse plane. (D) A 180-degree refocusing pulse flips the transverse magnetization. (E) The differences in magnetic field that caused the spins to diphase now refocus the magnetization. The transient increase in the transverse magnetization that occurs following the 180-degree refocusing pulse is called a spin echo. In contrast to spin echo or FSE techniques, gradient echo sequences do not use a 180-degree refocusing pulse to refocus the transverse magnetization. Instead, refocusing is achieved by a transient reversal of the magnetic field gradients.

seconds after the patient is placed in the magnet, the orientations of the proton magnetic dipoles reach an equilibrium in which the vector is aligned along the Z axis and there is no net magnetization in the transverse (XY) plane. Once the spins are at equilibrium there is no net transfer of energy, and therefore no signal for generating an MR image. To generate an MRI signal, the protons must be perturbed from equilibrium by applying an external RF magnetic field. The RF magnetic field is applied perpendicular to the static magnetic field. The RF field is also called the B1 field, to differentiate it from the static B0 field generated by the large magnet.

The B1 field is generated by the RF transmit coil, which in most current clinical MRI systems is a large-body transmit coil that surrounds the patient. When the frequency of the B1 field is at the Larmor frequency $(\omega_0)$, the magnetic dipoles generated by the protons precess around B1 rather than B0. As a result, the magnetic vector rotates from the equilibrium position along the Z axis toward the XY plane. A B1 pulse sufficient to tip the magnetization 90 degrees from the Z axis into the XY plane is referred to as a 90-degree excitation pulse. To acquire an MR image, this process of tipping the magnetization into the transverse plane is repeated many times—depending on the specific MRI sequence used and the desired spatial resolution of the image. The interval between sequential 90-degree pulses is known as the time to repetition (TR), which can range from approximately 10 milliseconds (ms) to 10 seconds. As will be discussed later, selecting the appropriate TR is an important parameter affecting image contrast.

At the conclusion of the 90-degree pulse, the B1 field is turned off and the magnetic vector now located in

the XY plane will again precess around the Z axis as it slowly resumes its equilibrium orientation along the Z axis. The rotating component of the magnetic vector in the XY plane can induce a small current in a receiver coil, which is the signal used to generate the MR image. Because the precessing magnetic field is very weak, the receiver coil must be placed in close proximity to the region of interest.

For musculoskeletal MRI examinations, specialized receiver coils are optimized for different joints. Newer MRI platforms frequently use an array of small receiver coils, termed a *phased array coil*, to efficiently collect the signal. The shape and size of the receiver coil will vary with the joint imaged. For examinations of extremities such as the knee or wrist, the receiver coil is generally cylindrical in shape—whereas flat or flexible coil geometries are used in the imaging of the hips and shoulders.

After several milliseconds, the orientations of magnetic dipoles in the XY plane begin to lose phase coherence as the spins begin to fan out and lose a preferential orientation. The dephasing of the magnetic vectors causes the net magnetic vector to decrease in magnitude. This dephasing of the spins is a result of many factors, such as microscopic differences in the magnetic fields experienced by different protons and the exchange of energy between protons. The loss in magnetization caused by differences in the magnetic field can be partially recovered by applying a 180-degree B1 pulse to refocus the magnetization. The resultant increase in magnetization following the refocusing B1 pulse is termed a *spin echo*, which forms the basis for spin echo MRI techniques used in clinical imaging.

The process of obtaining a spin echo signal is illustrated in Fig. 10.1. The interval between the 90-degree pulse and the center of the spin echo is the time to echo (TE time). Along with TR, TE is the second important image acquisition parameter affecting image contrast. In the case of imaging via fast-spin echo (FSE, also called turbo-spin echo), a series of refocusing pulses is rapidly applied—resulting in a train of spin echoes. Another frequently used family of MRI techniques is gradient echo imaging. In the case of gradient echo imaging, a rapid reversal of magnetic field gradients rather than an RF pulse is used to refocus the transverse magnetization.

## Generating the MR Image

An MR image represents the 3D spatial localization of the MRI signal within the body. This is accomplished using three magnetic field gradients that generate a linear spatial variation in the static magnetic field along the three orthogonal planes. It is the process of turning the gradients on and off that generates the loud knocking sound experienced by the patient during the MRI exam. As can be seen from the Larmor equation (Equation 10.1), the resonant frequency of the proton is a function of the magnetic field.

A linear magnetic field across the body produces a spatial dependency of the Larmor frequency of the protons. For example, a linear gradient applied in the head-to-foot direction will cause protons in the feet to resonate at a different frequency from protons located in the head. When the linear gradient is applied, the resultant Larmor frequency of the proton can be used to determine the precise location of that proton along the direction of the gradient. To achieve 3D localization, it is necessary to use three magnetic field gradients. The order in which and method by which these gradients are applied determine the orientation of the acquired image.

Standard imaging planes are transverse, sagittal, and coronal planes. By convention, the transverse plane is displayed as if the viewer were positioned at the patient's feet with the patient in the supine position. The perspective of the sagittal plane is from the patient's left side, and the coronal is presented as if viewing the patient from the front. Although conventional views are acquired in these anatomic orientations, using a combination of gradients it is possible to acquire images in any arbitrary plane. By varying the way the slice selection gradient is applied, it is possible to acquire the images as a series of 2D parallel sections or as a 3D volume. Because of the long time needed to acquire the image data for a 3D volume, 3D acquisitions are generally limited to gradient echo techniques. Spin echo and FSE techniques are generally acquired using 2D acquisitions.

An important parameter of the MR image is resolution. Spatial resolution is determined by the size of the individual volume elements (voxels) that comprise the 3D tissue section represented in the 2D image displayed in the image. The voxel resolution is a function of the section thickness and the cross-sectional area. For 2D sequences used in the imaging of most joints, section thickness is typically in the range of 3 to 5 mm. Greater section thickness decreases spatial resolution and may make it more difficult to visualize small structures. When the voxel includes the interface between tissues (such as at the articular surface), the signal from the two tissues is averaged (making it difficult to resolve the surface). This artifact (termed *volume averaging*) is more severe for thicker sections. Thinner sections (such as in the range of 1 to 3 mm) are possible using 3D acquisitions.

The cross-sectional area of the voxel (pixel resolution) is a function of the size of the area imaged—termed the *field of view* (FOV)—and the number of voxels within that area (termed the *image matrix*). The in-plane resolution for most clinical musculoskeletal examination is in the range of 300 to 800 microns per pixel. Although higher spatial resolution is desirable, there are factors that limit spatial resolution. Decreasing voxel size reduces the MRI signal generated by each individual voxel, making the image appear grainy (similar to poor television reception). The reduced SNR can be recovered through signal averaging, but this is at the cost of increased imaging time. Although spatial resolution impacts image quality, the critical parameter influencing diagnostic interpretation of the images is the ability to clearly differentiate tissue types. This property is described by contrast resolution and is a function of both spatial resolution and image contrast.

## MRI Pulse Sequences

Adjusting the application and timing of the magnetic field gradients and RF pulses used to acquire the signal provides a large array of MRI techniques with quite different appearances. These variations in MRI acquisition techniques are referred to as pulse sequences. Clinical MRI pulse sequences can be clustered into three families: conventional spin echo techniques, FSE (turbo spin) techniques, and gradient echo techniques. Current clinical MRI evaluations of joints use all three pulse sequences.

### Conventional Spin Echo Techniques

Spin echo imaging techniques were developed in the late 1970s and remain an important tool in musculoskeletal imaging. The hallmark of the conventional spin echo sequence is the 180-degree refocusing pulse used to reestablish phase coherence of the transverse magnetization—resulting in a spin echo. This refocusing pulse corrects for differences in magnetic field that may be produced by the different chemical environments of fat and water (chemical shift) or by inhomogeneity of the magnetic field that occurs around metallic hardware or at air/tissue interfaces.

The primary advantage of spin echo MRI is the excellent soft tissue contrast, particularly for evaluation of connective tissues with high collagen content (such as menisci, tendons, and ligaments). Because these techniques have been available since the early 1980s, there is substantial experience and published literature using them for musculoskeletal MRI. Compared with other MRI techniques (such as FSE), there are fewer differences among manufacturers with regard to implementing the conventional spin echo technique. As a result, it is easier to standardize this technique across platforms. The major disadvantage of spin echo MRI is its inefficient collection of imaging data, which leads to long image acquisition times and/or to images of lower spatial resolution.

### Fast-spin (Turbo-spin) Echo Techniques

FSE imaging techniques were developed to improve the efficiency of signal collection regarded as a limitation of conventional spin echo imaging. The terms *fast* and *turbo* reflect differences among manufacturer nomenclature. However, all technologies for FSE are based on the "rapid acquisition with relaxation enhancement" (RARE) technique originally described by Henning et al. in 1984.[5,6] In RARE techniques, the initial 90-degree excitation pulse is followed by a train of 180-degree refocusing pulses and intervening phase encoding gradients that generate a series of spin echoes with differing spatial encoding.

The RARE techniques are more efficient than conventional spin echo techniques because multiple lines of spatial information are obtained following each 90-degree pulse. The increase in efficiency is directly related to the number of echoes collected (echo train length). For musculoskeletal MRI, echo train lengths generally range from 3 for T1-weighted or proton-density-weighted images to 10 or more for T2-weighted images. Thus, compared to conventional spin echo RARE images can be obtained 3 to 10 times faster. Although the improved efficiency in data collection can be used to decrease imaging time, it is also possible to use this efficiency to acquire images with higher spatial resolution.

As illustrated in Fig. 10.2, the major disadvantages of RARE imaging are image blurring and RF heating—which can be problematic in high-field systems.[7,8] In addition, the train of 180-degree refocusing pulses increases the amount of magnetization transfer between large macromolecules such as proteins and nearby water molecules. This provides an additional mechanism of contrast that is important in collagen-rich connective tissues such as menisci, tendons, ligaments, and articular cartilage.

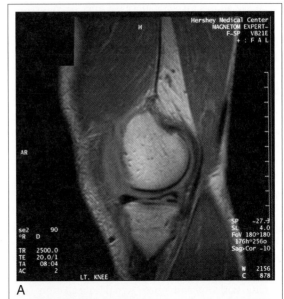

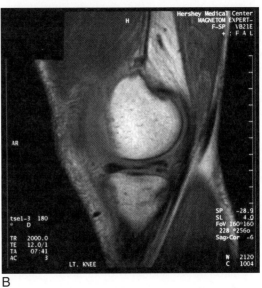

**Fig. 10.2** Conventional spin echo versus FSE in visualization of meniscal tear: (A) a conventional spin echo (TR/TE: 2,500 ms/20 ms) and (B) an FSE [TR/TE (eff): 2,000 ms/12 ms] with an echo train length of 3. Both images were obtained at 1.0 T. Although the FSE image is obtained at slightly higher spatial resolution, the margins of the horizontal cleavage tear of the posterior horn of the medial meniscus are indistinct compared to the conventional spin echo. The blurring on the FSE is an artifact produced by T2 modulation of the acquired spin echoes and can decrease sensitivity for detection of subtle meniscal tears.

### Gradient Echo Techniques

In contrast to spin echo techniques, gradient echo techniques do not use a 180-degree refocusing pulse to refocus the transverse magnetization. Instead, this is accomplished using a pair of inverted gradient pulses to generate a gradient echo. The absence of a 180-degree

RF pulse allows for very short TR and TE values and substantially reduces the amount of magnetization transfer. Because of the short TR, it is possible to perform 3D gradient echo acquisitions that can provide high spatial resolution images of an entire tissue volume. The gradient echo also differs from a spin echo in that the lack of a 180-degree refocusing pulse does not recover signal lost due to differences in chemical shift or to inhomogeneity of the magnetic field. This can be both beneficial and problematic.

The sensitivity of the gradient echo technique to the chemical environment of the proton makes it possible to determine the relative fat and water content within a voxel—a technique referred to as chemical shift imaging. In musculoskeletal imaging, this technique has been used to characterize bone marrow—aiding in the differentiation of benign from pathologic marrow-replacement processes.[9-11] However, for voxels containing both fat and water signal cancellation from differences in chemical shift produces spurious signal loss at the interface between fat and water within tissue. Because gradient echo techniques are sensitive to magnetic field inhomogeneity, they are sensitive to blood degradation products and can be used for lesion characterization—such as identifying hemosiderin deposition in synovium in the setting of pigmented villonodular synovitis.

Major disadvantages of gradient echo techniques are their relatively poor image contrast in terms of the evaluation of connective tissues and their production of artifacts from magnetic field inhomogeneity near air/tissue interfaces and around orthopedic hardware. Finally, the 3D techniques suffer from long image acquisition times—ranging from 5 to 10 minutes in length. Recent modifications (such as the use of water excitation and application of parallel imaging technology) have helped shorten examinations employing 3D techniques.

Terminology for gradient echo imaging varies widely among manufacturers. There are two basic forms of gradient echo imaging, distinguished based on whether the residual transverse magnetization is spoiled or refocused following collection of the gradient echo signal. Spoiled gradient echo images are used in T1-weighted techniques. Common acronyms for these techniques include spoiled-GRASS, FLASH, and RF-FAST. As illustrated in Fig. 10.3, these techniques are useful in obtaining high-resolution anatomic images for small joints such as the wrist and ankle[12,13] or in tailoring the technique to visualize small structures such as articular cartilage.[14,15]

In steady-state techniques, the transverse magnetization is refocused—increasing the relative contribution of the T2*-weighted signal. T2* contrast is generated by gradient echo images, in contrast to T2 contrast,

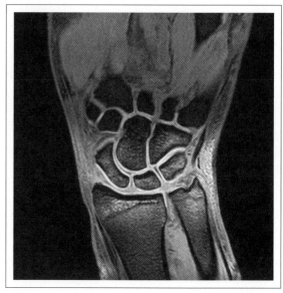

**Fig. 10.3** 1.5-T gradient echo image of wrist cartilage. A 3D water-excited T1-weighted gradient echo image of the wrist provides excellent visualization of the thin cartilage of the carpal bones. The 3D acquisition possible with the gradient echo technique provides high spatial resolution (section thickness: 1.5 mm, pixel resolution: 250 microns per pixel). A drawback of the gradient echo sequence is the relatively poor contrast for evaluation of other articular tissues and long image acquisition times.

which is generated by SE techniques. Common acronyms for these techniques include GRASS, FISP, and SSFP (steady-state free precession). More recent modifications of these techniques—such as balanced fast-field echo (balanced FFE) and true FISP techniques—demonstrate potential for improved visualization of articular cartilage.[16,17]

## Image Contrast

In viewing an MR image, the striking feature is the ability to visualize and differentiate soft tissues. This characteristic is a function of image contrast. In X-ray techniques, image contrast is primarily a function of tissue density—which determines the number of photons that strike the radiographic film or detector. In MRI, many different physical properties can be exploited to generate image contrast, and more continue to be developed into MRI techniques. Common sources of MR image contrast include density of mobile protons and the tissue relaxation times T1 and T2. Motion can also be used to generate contrast. For example, differences between moving and stationary protons can be exploited to generate MR angiographic images.

On a smaller scale, differences in microscopic translational motions that occur as a result of diffusion of protons can be used to generate contrast—and have been particularly useful in the clinical evaluation of cerebral ischemia. In addition to methods that use the intrinsic properties of tissue to generate image contrast, methods that make use of agents of exogenous contrast are available. Using a combination of pulse sequences optimized to enhance different contrast mechanisms, it is possible to characterize tissues and to develop clinical images that are sensitive to particular pathologies.

## Proton Density

Although all protons generate an MRI signal, only those protons located on molecules with sufficient mobility contribute to the signal detected by the MRI receiver (which is converted into an image). Protons located on large macromolecules (such as proteins or nucleic acids) have limited motion and lose signal before they can be detected. However, these molecules can contribute significantly to image contrast through interactions with nearby mobile protons (discussed further later in the chapter). The density of mobile protons in a voxel is a primary source of contrast in the MR image. Tissues with a high concentration of mobile protons (such as synovial fluid) can generate a strong MRI signal, whereas tissues with a low mobile-proton concentration (such as cortical bone and fibrous tissue) generate a weak signal and appear dark on images obtained with standard clinical MRI techniques.

## Relaxation Times T1 and T2

The RF pulses applied to tissue to generate the MR image introduce energy into the body, perturbing the magnetization of the protons from the equilibrium condition. The process by which the protons release this energy and return to thermal equilibrium is known as relaxation, which can be described using two relaxation times: T1 and T2. The relaxation time constant T1 is the spin lattice relaxation time, which describes the rate at which energy is transferred from the protons to the surrounding environment (lattice).

Using the classical model of a magnetic vector, the T1 relaxation time describes the rate at which magnetization is restored along the Z axis following the initial excitation pulse—and is thus occasionally referred to as the longitudinal relaxation time. The second relaxation time (T2) is the spin-spin relaxation time constant, which describes the rate at which transverse magnetization in the XY plane decays back to zero after the initial excitation pulse. For this reason, it is frequently called the transverse relaxation time.

## T1 Relaxation

Pulse sequences optimized to enhance differences in tissue T1 values are T1 weighted. For spin echo or FSE

images, this is accomplished using short TR and TE values. For gradient echo images, it is accomplished using short TR and TE values, a large flip angle on the excitation pulse, and spoilage of the transverse magnetization. Most tissues have T1 values in the range of 500 ms to 3 seconds. When the TR is less than the tissue T1, there is less time for the longitudinal magnetization to recover following the excitation pulse.

After applying a few excitation pulses, the spins reach a new equilibrium in which the saturation of spins from the repeated RF pulse is balanced with recovery of the longitudinal magnetization during the TR period. Tissues with short T1 values, such as fat, recover longitudinal magnetization faster and will contribute more signal to the resultant image. Tissue such as synovial fluid, which has a long T1, recovers less magnetization during the TR period and thus will appear dark on a T1-weighted image.

For T1 relaxation to occur, energy must be transferred from the proton to the surrounding lattice. After applying the RF pulses, the protons in the tissue contain slightly more energy than was present at the initial equilibrium condition. Because of the extremely small difference in energy between the two spin states, protons do not spontaneously release this energy. It is estimated that in a T1 field it would take $10^{19}$ seconds for an excited proton to spontaneously reverse its magnetic moment, a time longer than the estimated age of the universe. The transfer of energy from the proton to the surrounding lattice occurs through stimulated emission. For protons in biologic systems, the major mechanism for T1 relaxation is through interaction of the proton with small random fluctuating magnetic fields generated by the motion of nearby charged particles such as proteins.

When the frequency of the fluctuating magnetic field of these macromolecules is at the Larmor frequency, it stimulates the proton to release energy and return to the equilibrium state. Only those molecules tumbling at a rate sufficient to generate a magnetic field that is at the Larmor frequency can produce T1 relaxation. In biologic systems, it is primarily large macromolecules such as proteins that facilitate T1 relaxation of nearby water protons—thereby shortening the T1 relaxation time of the tissue. The T1 of tissue increases with increased magnetic field strength. This is because there are fewer macromolecules tumbling at the necessary rate to produce magnetic field fluctuations at the Larmor frequency.

Exogenous MRI contrast agents can be administered to facilitate T1 relaxation. Metal ions such as gadolinium contain unpaired electrons and will generate a magnetic field that is much larger than the small magnetic field generated by a nucleus. As a result, these compounds are very efficient in causing T1 relaxation of protons over a larger area. Gadolinium chelates are the primary class of MRI contrast agents. The free gadolinium ion is not used as a contrast agent. Not only is it toxic but its rotational and translational motions are too fast to cause efficient $T_1$ relaxation. Binding the gadolinium ion to a macromolecular chelate slows the motion into the proper range for $T_1$ relaxation to occur. It also decreases toxicity.

The biodistribution of gadolinium chelates is similar to that of iodinated contrast agents used in CT and radiography. Using rapid acquisitions, it is possible to acquire dynamic enhanced images with the contrast agent in the intravascular space. Such techniques form the basis of dynamic contrast enhanced MR angiography. Within several minutes, the contrast agent distributes in proportion to extracellular fluid volume and thus enhances areas of edema or inflammation. Gadolinium contrast agents are well tolerated, with low incidences of allergic reactions and nephrotoxicity. They are cleared by renal excretion.

## T2 Relaxation

The spin-spin (transverse) relaxation time constant $T_2$ describes the rate at which protons lose coherent magnetization in the transverse plane. For spin echo techniques, $T_2$ weighting is achieved by increasing TE and thereby allowing tissues with short $T_2$ to decay prior to acquiring the MRI signal. Tissues with long $T_2$ times, such as fluid, will retain coherent magnetization and therefore contribute a relatively larger component of the acquired signal—making them appear bright on $T_2$-weighted images.

Pathologic processes that increase water content of tissue such as edema will lengthen the $T_2$ relaxation time. In addition to the long TE, it is necessary to use a long TR value to minimize $T_1$ weighting of the signal. With FSE, the displayed image is a composite of spin echoes acquired with different TE values and thus different degrees of $T_2$ weighting. For this reason, these techniques are termed *effective TEs*—describing the TE value that contributes the majority of signal used to achieve the desired contrast.

The interaction of magnetic fields that produces $T_1$ relaxation also causes $T_2$ relaxation. In addition, processes that lead to randomization of spins in the transverse plane will contribute to $T_2$ relaxation. This includes the exchange of protons between water and exchangeable protons on macromolecules, diffusion of protons through small magnetic field gradients occurring in tissue, and residual quadrupolar interactions in highly anisotropic tissues such as tendons, ligaments, and cartilage. As a result, for all biologic tissues the $T_2$ relaxation time is shorter than $T_1$—ranging from 250 microseconds for highly organized tissues such as tendons and ligaments to 400 ms for synovial fluid.

## Magnetization Transfer

The MRI signal detected is comprised of three pools of protons based on their relative mobility and $T_2$ relaxation times.[18] Highly mobile protons have long $T_2$ values measured in milliseconds and give rise to the signal used to derive the anatomic image. Protons located on large macromolecules make up a second pool. Because these protons have a very short $T_2$, on the order of several microseconds, the signal decays rapidly and is not detected with standard MRI techniques.

The third population is the hydration layer, consisting of protons that are interacting with protons on the macromolecules through hydrogen bonding and are exchanging with the mobile proton pool. As the name implies, magnetization transfer is a process whereby the magnetization from a proton in the macromolecule pool is transferred to the mobile proton pool.[19] As a result of magnetization transfer, it is possible to indirectly obtain information from the macromolecules in tissue that do not contribute directly to the MR image.

In connective tissues rich in collagen, the transfer of magnetization from protons located on proteins such as collagen to mobile protons surrounding these proteins is an important source of image contrast. This is particularly true for techniques (such as multi-slice FSE techniques) that use a large number of RF pulses. In multi-slice FSE techniques, there is rapid application of off-resonance RF energy that quickly saturates the bound proton pool but does not saturate the mobile pool.[20] This saturated magnetization is then transferred either through chemical exchange or exchange of magnetization to nearby water protons in the mobile pool, thereby decreasing signal intensity on the MR image.[21,22]

As a result of magnetization transfer, tissue containing significant hydrophilic protein will have lower signal intensity.[20] Types I and II collagen demonstrate substantial magnetization transfer with FSE techniques.[23,24] For cartilage, incidental magnetization transfer reduces signal intensity by 15 to 20% as the number of slices (and thus the amount of off-resonance irradiation) increases.[25] Because gradient echo techniques use significantly fewer RF pulses, there is less incidental magnetization transfer with gradient echo techniques compared to spin echo and FSE techniques.

Magnetization transfer can have both beneficial and deleterious effects on image contrast. In the case of meniscal tears, magnetization transfer from fibrillated margins of the meniscal tear decreases signal intensity of fluid located within the tear. Because the meniscus is dark on MRI, decreasing the signal intensity of fluid within the tear decreases the contrast with the dark meniscus and can make it more difficult to identify meniscal tears.

On FSE sequences, the high degree of magnetization transfer leads to regional differences in signal intensity on T2-weighted images of articular cartilage. At sites of fibrillation with exposed collagen fibers, magnetization transfer between surface collagen and adjacent fluid increases contrast between cartilage and synovial fluid on T2 sequences—thereby improving sensitivity as applied to the detection of focal lesions.[26,27]

### Tissue Anisotropy

In connective tissues such as tendons, ligaments, and articular cartilage, the highly ordered arrangement of collagen fibers produces residual quadrupolar coupling—an efficient mechanism for T2 relaxation. For these tissues with a highly preferred or anisotropic organization of collagen fibrils, T2 is dependent on the relative orientation of the collagen fibers with Bo.[28,29] Tissues containing fibers oriented parallel or perpendicular to Bo have efficient T2 relaxation. The short T2 value decreases signal intensity. However, when fibers are oriented 54 degrees relative to Bo there is averaging of the residual quadrupolar coupling—which minimizes this contribution to T2 relaxation and leads to an increase in signal intensity. Because of this effect, 54 degrees is termed the *magic angle*.[30]

In tendons, the orientational dependence of T2 varies from 250 microseconds (when the tendon is aligned parallel to Bo) to 20 ms (when the tendon is oriented at the magic angle[28])—leading to an increase in signal intensity that may be mistaken for degenerative change.[31,32] Similar orientation dependence occurs in the radial zone of articular cartilage as a result of the anisotropic architecture of the type II collagen matrix.[33]

## Fat Suppression

In T1-weighted images, and in most FSE images, subcutaneous fat and fat within bone marrow have the brightest signal and set the dynamic range of the image. To identify subtle lesions within fat-containing tissues (as with inflammation or bone marrow abnormalities) it is necessary to suppress the dominating signal produced by fat. This can be accomplished using selective chemical shift fat-suppression techniques or using short tau inversion recovery (STIR)—a non chemical-shift-dependent method of fat suppression.

Chemical-shift-selective techniques selectively irradiate protons located on fat immediately prior to applying the excitation pulse. As a result, protons from fat are saturated—and only protons on water remain to contribute signal to the MR image. In general, fat-suppression techniques work well at high magnetic field strengths—where the resonant frequency of fat and water are far enough apart to allow selective suppression. These techniques are used following administration of MRI contrast to identify areas of tissue enhancement.

Chemical-shift fat suppression is less effective where the magnetic field uniformity is distorted, such as by tissue surrounding orthopedic hardware or by air/tissue interfaces. The STIR technique relies on a difference in the T1 relaxation rate of fat versus water to achieve fat suppression. It is not chemically selective. The STIR sequence is less sensitive to magnetic field inhomogeneity and therefore is a useful form of fat suppression for large areas of coverage, for areas with complex curved anatomy (such as the foot and ankle), and for areas near metallic hardware.

## Image Artifacts

The weak signal of MRI makes it particularly susceptible to a variety of image artifacts that can degrade image quality and interfere with diagnosis. Common artifacts encountered in MRI of joints include motion artifacts, chemical shift artifacts, truncation artifacts, and artifacts resulting from differences in magnetic susceptibility of tissues and/or implanted metallic materials.

### Motion Artifacts

Long image acquisition times in MRI make it particularly sensitive to image artifact from motion. This can be a result of physiologic motion (such as breathing or blood flow) or of movement of the patient during the scan. Artifacts from motion will appear as blurring or ghosting of the image along the phase-encoding direction of the image. For MRI images of the extremities, motion artifact can be reduced by restraining the limb in a comfortable position. Young pediatric patients and patients who are in discomfort, are claustrophobic, or are suffering from dementia are particularly prone to motion artifact.

These individuals may require sedation or adequate pain control to obtain a diagnostic examination. Periodic motion from breathing can produce artifact in MRI studies of the shoulder, particularly in patients with respiratory problems. Swapping the phase and frequency axes and using motion suppression techniques may reduce artifact in these examinations. In MRI examinations of the knee, pulsatile blood flow in the popliteal artery can produce ghost artifacts that may mimic pathology in the patellar cartilage in images acquired with an anterior/posterior phase-encoding axis. Swapping the phase and frequency axes will reduce the diagnostic impact of this artifact.

### Chemical Shift Artifacts

In MRI of articular cartilage, the close proximity of fat in bone marrow and peri-articular soft tissues poses problems with chemical shift artifact. Differences in the local magnetic field experienced by protons located on fat and water cause them to resonate at different frequencies. As a result, signal from fat can be misregistered and potentially obscure nearby tissues (such as articular cartilage). Chemical shift artifact always occurs along the frequency-encoding direction. Changing the orientation of the frequency-encoding direction so that it runs parallel to the bone cartilage interface prevents the fat signal from obscuring the articular cartilage.

Although this approach works for relatively flat articular surfaces such as the patella, it has limited utility for round surfaces such as the femoral head or condyle—for which changing the frequency-encoding direction simply transposes the artifact from one region of the joint to another. Fat-suppression techniques can be used to minimize chemical shift artifact. It is important to remember that the magnitude of the artifact is dependent on the strength of the magnetic field. Non fat-suppressed images obtained on 3.0-T systems must use higher receiver bandwidths to prevent significant chemical shift artifact.

### Truncation Artifacts

Truncation artifacts are a result of post-processing of MRI data. To reduce the image acquisition time, a limited quantity of MRI data is collected, filtered, and transformed into an MR image using a Fourier transform algorithm. Truncation of data at the edge of the data set produces artifactual bright and dark bands within the image. These are most conspicuous near the interfaces of tissues with large differences in signal intensity. In cartilage MRI, this frequently occurs in fat-suppressed gradient echo images when there is a narrow transition zone between the bright cartilage and the dark bone. The truncation artifact has been shown to be at least partially responsible for the banded appearance of cartilage when imaged with these techniques.[34,35]

### Magnetic Susceptibility Artifacts

Magnetic susceptibility is a measure of the propensity of a material to become magnetized when placed in a magnetic field. When placed in the MRI magnet, most body tissues generate a small but extremely weak magnetic field in a direction opposite that of the applied magnetic field. These tissues are termed *diamagnetic.* Materials such as stainless-steel orthopedic implants generate a small magnetic field in the same direction as the applied magnetic field and are called *paramagnetic.* Materials that generate a large magnetic field (such as iron) are *ferromagnetic.* Ferromagnetic materials are strongly attracted to the MRI magnet, and may cause injury to the patient if they are accidentally brought within the stray field of the magnet.

Differences in magnetic susceptibilities of tissues or implanted metallic devices distort the homogeneity of the magnetic field and produce a variety of image artifacts. The size of the induced magnetic field distortion is dependent on the relative difference in magnetic susceptibility of the two materials, on the geometry and orientation of the material to the magnetic field, and on the strength of the magnetic field. Stainless steel (e.g., implants) generates greater field distortion than titanium, which has a magnetic susceptibility closer to that of tissue. Cylindrical metallic devices concentrate the magnetic flux along the long axis of the device, causing larger field distortion at the ends of the cylinder than adjacent to the shaft of the cylinder. As with chemical shift artifact, the artifact produced by differences in magnetic susceptibility increases with increasing magnetic field strength—and thus will be more severe at 3.0 T compared to 1.5 T.

Magnetic susceptibility artifacts can be subdivided into two groups based on the size of the magnetic field distortion. Large differences in magnetic susceptibility, such as around stainless-steel orthopedic implants, generate large distortions in the linearity of the magnetic field gradient used to spatially encode the MRI data. This results in geometric distortion of the voxel dimensions, resulting in bright and dark bands around the object. The artifacts will be present on both gradient echo and spin echo images.

Smaller field distortion results in loss of the MRI signal due to rapid dephasing of the transverse magnetization. This artifact will result in a signal-void (black) area within the image, and will be most severe on gradient echo images. It can be minimized using spin echo or FSE techniques with short TE values to reduce signal loss from diffusion. Small differences in the magnetic susceptibility of trabecular bone and hyaline cartilage produce macroscopic magnetic field gradients in the tidemark zone of cartilage. These field distortions lead to loss of signal in the deeper layers of cartilage, particularly on images acquired with gradient echo techniques. This artifact may cause the cartilage to appear artificially thin, which can result in an underestimation of cartilage thickness and volume.[36]

## CLINICAL MRI EVALUATION IN OSTEOARTHRITIS

Early studies in experimental models of OA indicated MRI had a high sensitivity in the identification of cartilage pathology.[37] Subsequent studies have confirmed a high level of sensitivity for MRI. A major advantage of MRI is that it provides the ability to visualize in their entirety the soft tissues that contribute to the multifactorial disease process[38,39] and that are associated with symptoms of OA.[40] In addition to those associated with articular cartilage, MRI identifies pathologies of the meniscus, synovium, joint fluid, subchondral bone marrow, and soft tissues that help to maintain joint stability (including the joint capsule, ligaments, muscles, and tendons).[39,41]

The ability to concurrently evaluate intra-articular and extra-articular pathology provides a means of evaluating changes in OA in terms of how they affect the whole organ of the joint, as well as a means of monitoring these changes over time.[42,43] To address the total joint involvement in OA, scoring systems such as the Whole Organ Magnetic Resonance Imaging Score (WORMS) have been developed to provide a semiquantitative evaluation.[43] In future studies, this ability should shed new light on the important roles played by subchondral bone, joint stability, and altered joint biomechanics in regard to disease progression.

## MRI of Articular Cartilage

### Technical Considerations

Currently, the primary MRI pulse sequences used in evaluating articular cartilage are 3D fat-suppressed T1-weighted spoiled gradient echo and 2D proton-density-weighted FSE techniques. Each has relative advantages and disadvantages with respect to contrast resolution and the visualization of articular cartilage.

The major advantage of the 3D T1-weighted gradient echo techniques is high spatial resolution. As shown in Fig. 10.3, this is particularly important in the evaluation of small joints and of curved articular cartilage surfaces such as the femoral head (where thin sections are needed to clearly delineate cartilage interfaces and minimize volume averaging). Using this technique at 1.5 T, it is possible to obtain images with a 1.0- to 2.0-mm section thickness and in-plane resolution of 200 to 350 microns per pixel. For comparison, 2D FSE techniques are generally limited to 3- to 4-mm section thickness and 300- to 500-micron in-plane resolution.

Several disadvantages limit routine clinical application of this technique. The gradient echo technique is relatively inefficient for generating contrast resolution, resulting in long image acquisition times—ranging, for example, from 6 to 10 minutes to acquire a 3D volume of the knee cartilage in the sagittal plane. The lack of substantial magnetization transfer reduces sensitivity for detection of superficial cartilage lesions and degeneration of the collagen matrix in deeper layers of the tissue. Although the technique produces high-contrast images of cartilage, it is relatively poor for the evaluation of other internal derangements (such as tears of menisci, ligaments, and tendons) and is relatively insensitive to bone marrow pathology.

More recent clinical evaluation of articular cartilage, particularly in the knee, has relied heavily on proton-density-weighted FSE images either with or without fat suppression.[44,45] The primary advantage of this technique is excellent soft tissue contrast with relatively modest image acquisition times of 3 to 4 minutes. The technique also provides clinically useful information regarding other articular tissues (such as menisci and bone marrow), making it particularly useful in the clinical setting where it is necessary to evaluate the entire joint. The primary disadvantage of the technique is lower spatial resolution. This is less of a limitation at 3.0 T, where higher signal compared to noise can permit higher spatial resolution. Although clinical experience with 3.0 T in cartilage is limited, preliminary results suggest that the higher field strength provides greater diagnostic accuracy in the detection of focal defects.[46,47]

New techniques based on the steady-state free precession sequence[16,17] and multi-echo T2* sequences[48] have been proposed for cartilage imaging. These techniques provide high-resolution images of cartilage with image contrast similar to that obtained with FSE techniques. Although preliminary results are promising, these techniques are not widely available and have undergone limited validation for routine clinical use.

### Focal Cartilage Lesions

Current MRI grading systems of articular cartilage damage are based on modifications of the Outerbridge classification originally described for surgical grading of patellar lesions.[49] As represented in Table 10.1, the original Outerbridge classification is based on size of surface fragmentation and fissuring. The MRI modification of the Outerbridge classification incorporates the depth of the lesion from the articular surface.

### Grade 0: Normal Cartilage

By definition, grade 0 cartilage has both normal morphology and signal intensity. However, signal intensity of normal cartilage varies with location in the joint, and with the particular pulse sequence used to acquire the image. This is primarily a function of regional and zonal differences in the type II collagen matrix, which has a strong influence on the T2 relaxation of cartilage.[50] In cartilage subjected to repetitive compressive strain, type II collagen demonstrates a highly organized zonal architecture.[51] Regional differences in local biomechanics have also been shown to alter chondrocyte density and morphology and produce variation in properties of the extracellular matrix, depending on location within the knee joint.[52] As seen in Fig. 10.4, these zonal differences in the extracellular matrix vary the signal intensity on fat-suppressed proton-density-weighted MR images.

With polarized light microscopy, the radial zone near bone is characterized by dense condensations of collagen fibrils oriented perpendicular to bone.[51]

**TABLE 10.1 ORIGINAL OUTERBRIDGE CLASSIFICATION (SURGICAL)[49] AND MODIFIED OUTERBRIDGE CLASSIFICATION (MRI) OF FOCAL ARTICULAR CARTILAGE LESIONS**

| Grade | Outerbridge (Surgical) | Modified Outerbridge (MRI) |
|---|---|---|
| 0 | Normal | Normal |
| I | Softening and swelling | Hyperintense T2-weighted signal with smooth surface |
| II | Fragmentation and fissuring <1/2-inch diameter | Fragmentation and fissuring <50% of cartilage thickness |
| III | Fragmentation and fissuring >1/2-inch diameter | Fragmentation and fissuring >50% of cartilage thickness |
| IV | Erosion of cartilage down to bone | Full-thickness cartilage defect |

The high content and anisotropic orientation of collagen provides efficient T2 relaxation, leading to low signal intensity on proton density or T2-weighted images.[53-55] With very high-resolution images, the darker radial zone has a striated appearance—with alternating fine bands of high and low signal intensity radiating from the bone cartilage interface.[56-58]

These dark bands correlate closely with areas of condensed collagen fibers[59] and freeze fracture patterns in cartilage.[57,58] Closer to the articular surface, the lower anisotropy and oblique orientation of the collagen matrix lead to a gradual increase in T2 relaxation time—leading to a gradual increase in signal intensity. Collagen fibers are oriented parallel to the articular surface. This layer, which is approximately 200 microns thick and is too thin to resolve on most clinical MR images, has been termed the *lamina splendens*.[51] The layers of signal intensity described previously are most conspicuous in the patella and tibial plateau.[34] In thin cartilage (such as the femoral condyle, ankle, and hip) there is generally insufficient spatial resolution to resolve zonal differences in cartilage T2.

Recognizing the heterogeneous MRI appearance of cartilage is important in avoiding erroneously interpreting nonuniform signal as disease.[60] In addition to differences in cartilage T2 with respect to depth from the articular surface, there are differences in cartilage T2 with respect to location in the joint and relative orientation of the cartilage to the applied magnetic field. As illustrated in Fig. 10.5, near the periphery of the tibial plateau the oblique orientation of the collagen matrix results in higher signal intensity on fat-suppressed proton-density-weighted FSE images.[56,61] Regional differences in cartilage T2 are most pronounced in the femoral condyle.[62]

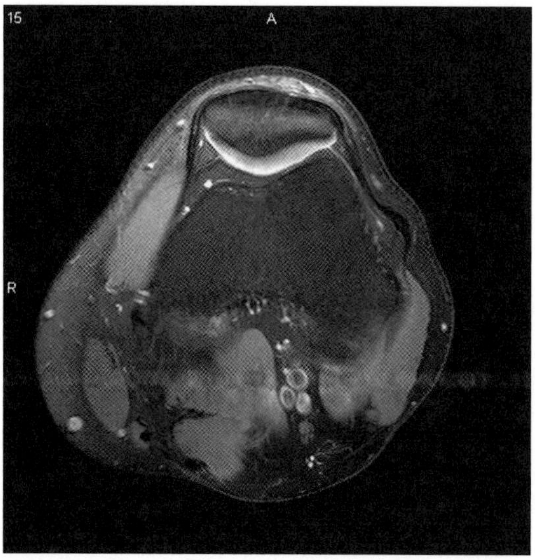

Fig. 10.4 Normal cartilage demonstrating regional variation in signal intensity. Axial 3.0-T fat-suppressed proton-density-weighted image demonstrates lower signal intensity in the radial zone of articular cartilage produced by the relatively high concentration of type II collagen and the highly anisotropic arrangement of the extracellular cartilage matrix. Signal intensity increases toward the articular surface in the transitional zone, where there is less anisotropy and higher water content.

This is a result of two processes. First, there are substantial differences in the organization of extracellular matrix and chondrocytes between the central femoral surface and posterior femoral condyles.[52] Although the type II collagen in the central femoral condyle has a high degree of anisotropy, results from electron microscopy and X-ray diffraction indicate that the collagen matrix in the posterior femoral condyle has less anisotropy and has a fine fibrillar organization.[63,64] This region of cartilage lacks the regular bands of condensed collagen seen in the central femoral condyle. Second, the oblique orientation of collagen in this region with respect to the direction of Bo is close to the magic angle of 54 degrees.[62]

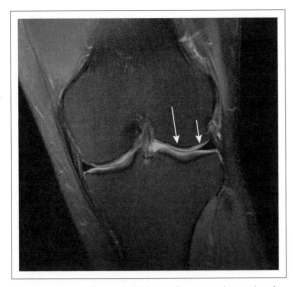

**Fig. 10.5** Coronal femoral tibial joint demonstrating regional variation in tibial cartilage. Regional differences in the extracellular cartilage matrix produce differences in cartilage T2-weighted signal intensity. In the central femoral cartilage (arrow), the anisotropic arrangement of collagen fibrils produces low signal intensity in the radial zone near the bone cartilage interface. Near the periphery of the femoral cartilage, fibers have a more oblique orientation—producing more uniform high-signal intensity in cartilage (arrowhead). Similar regional variation is seen in tibial cartilage.

As a result of differences in organization and orientation of the type II collagen matrix, cartilage in the posterior femoral condyle demonstrates uniformly high signal intensity compared to the layered pattern of signal intensity observed in the central femoral condyle. This regional variation in cartilage signal intensity highlights the high sensitivity of cartilage T2 to the organization and content of the type II collagen matrix.[65]

### Grade I Lesions

In the Outerbridge classification, grade I lesions are identified by a subjective assessment of cartilage softening with an intact articular surface. Because there is no direct MRI finding that corresponds to cartilage softening, this has been modified to reflect MRI signal changes without morphologic changes of the cartilage surface. Early studies found poor correlation between grade I MRI lesions and arthroscopy,[66,67] as well as low sensitivity in MRI detection of patellar cartilage softening found at arthroscopy.[68]

More recent studies suggest that the poor correlation reflects differences in the properties of cartilage evaluated with the two techniques. In studies on enzymatically treated cartilage specimens, degradation of the type II collagen matrix was strongly correlated with elevation in cartilage T2—whereas removal of proteoglycans using either trypsin or IL-2 had minimal effect.[69] Similarly, it has been shown that although removal of proteoglycan significantly decreases cartilage stiffness elevation of T2 with degradation of the collagen matrix correlated poorly with Young's modulus.[70,71] Based on results of ex vivo studies, it is likely that focal elevation in T2-weighted signal intensity reflects structural changes of the collagen matrix that do not substantially alter compressibility of cartilage.

Remote areas of T2 hyperintensity are frequently found in patients with more advanced areas of focal cartilage loss. Although the clinical significance of this finding is unknown, small longitudinal studies suggest that grade I lesions are common and progress to sites of morphologic damage.[72] The pattern of T2 elevation can reflect the underlying mechanism of cartilage injury. Linear T2 elevation at the bone/cartilage interface can be a result of cartilage delamination, which occurs when high shear strain cleaves the collagen fibrils traversing the tidemark zone.[73,74] As illustrated in Fig. 10.6, a more diffuse heterogeneous pattern of high T2-weighted signal can be observed following acute trauma—frequently in association with hyperintensity in the adjacent subchondral bone marrow.

Isolated areas of T2 hyperintensity are infrequently identified in cartilage of patients with no reported history of trauma. This is most often seen in thicker patellar cartilage, where the cartilage is sufficiently thick to

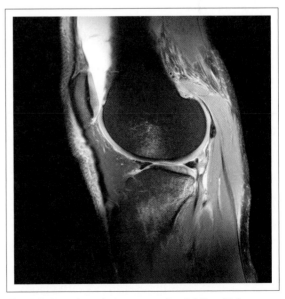

**Fig. 10.6** Acute bone marrow contusion. 3.0-T sagittal fat-suppressed proton density images in patient with acute ACL tear demonstrates high signal in lateral femoral condyle and posterior lateral tibial plateau consistent with a pivot shift mechanism of injury.

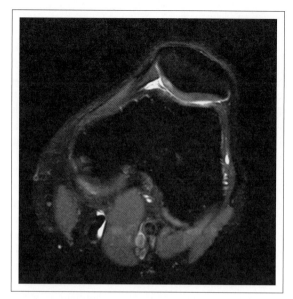

**Fig. 10.7** Cartilage blister, grade I lesion. 1.5-T axial fat-suppressed proton density image of the patella from a 37-year-old male with a 1-year history of aching retropatellar pain demonstrates focally increased T2 signal intensity and smooth contour bulge of the articular surface.

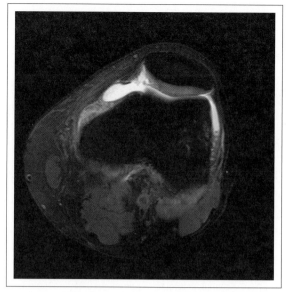

**Fig. 10.8** Cartilage flap tear, grade II lesion. 3.0-T axial fat-suppressed proton density image of the patella from a 41-year-old male with ACL tear and focal flap tear of the medial patellar facet. The linear area of fluid signal intensity involves the superficial 50% of articular cartilage consistent with a grade II lesion.

resolve the deep layer of cartilage. As shown in Fig. 10.7, this can be associated with a focal blister or smooth contour abnormality of the overlying articular surface. Similar findings of focal swelling and alterations in the fibril density in the superficial zone of patellar cartilage have been reported in the electron microscopy literature,[75,76] supporting the hypothesis that these lesions represent structural reorganization/degeneration of the collagen matrix. In contrast to focal elevation in T2 seen with type I lesions, a diffuse increase in the T2 of cartilage occurs with aging.[77] This begins near the articular surface in the mid forties, extending to the deeper layers of cartilage with increasing age.[78]

### Grade II Lesions

Grade II lesions represent fissures, erosion, ulceration, or fibrillation involving the superficial 50% of cartilage thickness. There is no general consensus in the MRI literature regarding the terminology used to report cartilage lesions. Fissures represent linear clefts of the articular surface. They are most frequently observed following joint trauma, particularly in patellar cartilage. As shown in Fig. 10.8, obliquely oriented fissures or flap tears can be seen following patellar dislocation—most frequently near the median ridge. Ulceration of superficial cartilage blisters results in a small and irregular focal crater (Fig. 10.9). Erosion refers to a smoothly marginated area of thinned cartilage frequently seen in older patients.

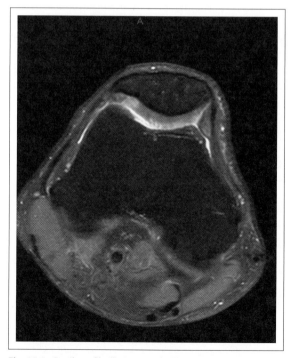

**Fig. 10.9** Cartilage fibrillation, grade II lesion. Axial 1.5-T fat-suppressed proton density image of the patella with diffuse surface irregularity of the patellar surface consistent with fibrillation.

Cartilage erosion is often identified in the posterior tibial plateau and femoral condyle, particularly in patients with chronic tears of the anterior cruciate ligament. Fibrillation or fraying of the articular surface appears visually as a fine velvety surface and is a common finding in subjects with OA. MRI has insufficient spatial resolution to resolve the individual fibrillations,[79] which generally appear as an indistinct articular margin.

MRI has relatively poor sensitivity and accuracy in identifying grade II lesions when using arthroscopy as the gold standard. This is in part due to limited spatial resolution of MRI,[80] and in part to the subjective nature in estimating lesion depth with arthroscopy. Because of greater contrast between the bright signal intensity of synovial fluid and intermediate signal intensity of cartilage, T2-weighted images have greater sensitivity in identifying superficial fibrillation.[81] Magnetization transfer enhances the surface contrast resolution and can improve conspicuity of these lesions. Despite higher spatial resolution, on T1-weighted gradient echo images the low signal intensity of fluid and resulting poor contrast make it difficult to identify sites of superficial fibrillation.[81]

### Grade III Lesions

As illustrated in Fig. 10.10, lesions that extend to more than 50% of the depth of the articular cartilage but do not result in exposure of the underlying bone are classified as grade III lesions. In correlation with arthroscopy or surgical grading, both T1-weighted fat-suppressed spoiled gradient echo and proton-density FSE MRI have high diagnostic accuracy in the identification of grade III lesions.[44,45,82,83]

### Grade IV Lesions

Full-thickness lesions with exposure of the underlying subchondral bone are classified as grade IV lesions. The margin of the lesion can suggest the mechanism of cartilage injury. Sharply marginated borders, such as those seen in Fig. 10.11, are characteristic of traumatic cartilage injuries—whereas shallow or irregular margins are features more characteristic of chronic degeneration. Abnormal signal from the underlying bone marrow and central osteophytes is frequently associated with grade IV lesions. MRI has demonstrated high specificity and sensitivity for the detection of grade IV defects.

## Associated Findings in Osteoarthritis
### Subchondral Marrow Abnormalities

Abnormal signal from the subchondral bone marrow is a frequent finding in acute traumatic cartilage injury and in the setting of OA.[84-86] Similar MRI findings

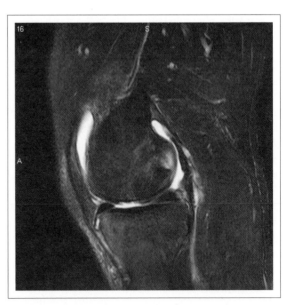

**Fig. 10.11** Grade IV lesion with sharply marginated shoulders. 1.5-T fat-suppressed T2-weighted images (TR/TE: 3,400 ms/60 ms) of a 28-year-old female with a clinically diagnosed ACL tear. Fluid intensity signal extends to the bone surface consistent with a grade IV lesion. The relative preservation of adjacent cartilage and the sharp margins of the chondral lesion are consistent with a traumatic injury. The long TE increases T2 weighting, making the sequence sensitive to marrow contusion (see posterior femoral condyle). However, articular cartilage is hypointense—making it difficult to assess cartilage thickness and internal signal abnormality.

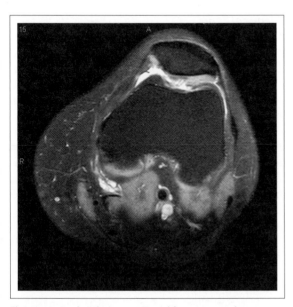

**Fig. 10.10** Grade III lesion. 3.0-T axial fat-suppressed proton density image of the patella demonstrates a large area of cartilage erosion and fibrillation involving the medial patellar facet and median ridge. Although cartilage thickness of the more peripheral lateral facet is preserved, the diffusely increased signal intensity is consistent with degenerative change in the collagen matrix. (See Color Plate 5.)

are observed following high-intensity exercise or with altered joint biomechanics.[87] It is a nonspecific MRI finding but can be associated with pain[85] and with internal derangement in the knee.[88,89]

The signal abnormality typically follows the characteristics of water, which is dark on short TE sequences and bright on fluid-sensitive sequences such as fat-suppressed proton-density or T2-weighted SE or FSE sequences or on STIR images.[90] Because the abnormal signal closely follows water, this finding has been erroneously termed *bone marrow edema*.[91] Correlation studies with histology indicate that a mixture of tissue types contributes to the abnormal marrow signal. In the setting of acute trauma, areas of fluid-like signal were associated with regions of trabecular microfracture, hemorrhage, necrosis, and edema.[92]

In this setting, the marrow findings represent a bone marrow contusion. Follow-up studies have shown that the abnormal marrow signal can persist for several months following resolution of symptoms. In the presence of OA, the region of abnormal marrow signal has a heterogeneous histology consisting of necrosis, fibrosis, subchondral cysts, edema, hemorrhage, and granulation tissue.[91,93,94]

One study has shown that the presence of abnormal marrow signal involving greater than 33% of the subchondral surface within a knee compartment was closely correlated with pain.[95] However, this correlation has not been observed in other studies.[96] The pattern of abnormal T2 signal appears to be prognostic. Patients demonstrating lesions with ill-defined margins are more likely to have resolution of symptoms compared to lesions with marginated serpentine borders suggestive of osteonecrosis.[97] Altered biomechanics with increased loading of the subchondral bone is a well-known cause of abnormal marrow signal and thus may reflect joint mal-alignment or increased loading that places the overlying cartilage at risk for further degeneration. Mal-alignment has been shown to be a prognostic indicator of OA progression.[98] Similarly, marrow edema in the medial compartment is associated with genu varus and is prognostic of further radiographic progression.[99]

Although more common in the hip,[100] transient bone marrow edema in the absence of trauma has been observed in the knee. For the hip, this condition is most frequently observed in middle-aged males.[101,102] Similar findings are seen in association with subchondral insufficiency fractures of the medial femoral condyle in middle-aged and elderly females, often in association with meniscal tears.[103] Although this lesion has been referred to as a spontaneous osteonecrosis of the knee (SONK), more recent studies suggest that this entity is likely a result of increased loading forces on the subchondral bone.[89,104]

The risk of fracture and development of stress-related marrow abnormality in the subchondral marrow is likely influenced by osteoporosis. In a study of more than 800 postmenopausal women, there was a significantly lower prevalence of subchondral bone marrow edema-like lesions in women receiving alendronate and estrogen compared to women not receiving antiresorptive therapy.[105]

## Osteophytes

Osteophytes are a radiographic hallmark of OA.[88,106-108] Because of high signal from bone marrow, osteophytes are best demonstrated on T1-weighted or non fat-suppressed proton-density-weighted images with high sensitivity.[38,109,110] In the setting of fat-suppressed images, thickening of ligament or capsular images can simulate osteophytes. Two types of osteophytes occur in the setting of OA. Central osteophytes occur centrally in the articular surface in association with full-thickness loss of articular cartilage and meniscal tear.[111]

Marginal osteophytes occur at the periphery by new bone formation in response to the traction of capsular attachments. Recent studies demonstrate an association between marginal osteophytes and an increase in tibial surface area.[112,113] Marginal osteophytes are also associated with cartilage defects seen on MRI in the femorotibial[114,115] and the patellofemoral joint.[116] Recent studies indicate good inter-reader agreement using MRI in the assessment of marginal osteophytes.[117,118]

## Meniscal Tears

Since the pioneering work of Fairbanks in 1948, there has been growing recognition of the important role of the meniscus in preserving articular cartilage and maintaining healthy joint biomechanics.[119] As a result, a primary goal of meniscal repair is maintaining meniscal tissue and function.[120] The meniscus serves a variety of biomechanical and physiologic functions, including absorbing and redistributing compressive load across the joint surface.[121,122] Meniscal dysfunction, particularly in the setting of the ACL-deficient knee, is a significant risk factor for development of knee OA in clinic-based studies.[72,123-126]

Meniscal tears are a frequent finding in patients with articular cartilage defects.[127,128] In patients with meniscal tears, cartilage lesions located centrally in the medial femoral tibial compartment progressed to a greater degree than those located in the anterior or posterior regions of the medial compartment or within the lateral compartment.[72] Although tears are relatively prevalent in an elderly asymptomatic population,[88,129,130] the incidence is higher in subjects with pain and with greater severity of radiographic knee OA.[131]

Radial displacement or extrusion of the meniscus, sometimes referred to as the Fairbank's sign, is frequently seen in association with OA.[132-135] Meniscal extrusion is also a common finding in radial tears[136] involving the posterior insertional ligaments. These tears are particularly damaging to normal meniscal function because they transect the hoop fibers that help to constrain the meniscus within the joint space and redistribute the compressive load by converting it into tensile hoop strain.

Detection of meniscal tear continues to be the primary diagnostic indication for clinical knee MRI. The diagnosis of meniscal tear with MRI relies on detection of linear increased signal intensity extending to an articular surface,[137,138] identification of displaced meniscal fragments,[139] or morphologic change in the meniscal contour such as truncation of the free edge seen with longitudinal bucket handle tears.[140,141] MRI has been a valuable clinical diagnostic tool for the evaluation of patients with suspected meniscal pathology. In a summary of results from prospective studies containing more than 200 cases with surgical correlation, the sensitivity of MRI for diagnosis of meniscal tear was 87% for conventional spin echo techniques, 83% for FSE techniques, and 87% for gradient echo techniques. Specificity for MRI was similar for all three techniques, ranging from 92% for FSE to 95% for gradient echo.[142]

The lower sensitivity of FSE techniques has been attributed to image blurring resulting from T2 modulation of the MRI signal, and has led to recommendations by some authors for abandoning FSE techniques for meniscal evaluation.[143,144] Sensitivity for detection of tears involving the posterior horn of the lateral meniscus has consistently been lower than that for the medial meniscus.[145-147] This is partly interpretative error,[148] but also reflects the complex anatomy of the posterior insertional ligament of the lateral meniscus—which runs obliquely through all three standard anatomic planes, making it prone to artifact from volume averaging and increased signal intensity due to the magic angle effect.[149] Lower sensitivity is also observed in the diagnosis of meniscal tears in knees with multi-trauma[150] radial tears involving the posterior horn of the medial meniscus[151] and in the detection of longitudinal bucket handle tears.[152]

False positive MRI studies are more common in the elderly, where there is increased internal signal intensity in the meniscus attributed to degenerative changes of the fibrocartilage matrix.[130,153-155] Less frequently transient elevated signal intensity in the setting of trauma, or meniscal contusion, has been described as a potential false positive finding.[156] High false positive rates have also been reported in the anterior horn of the meniscus.[157,158]

# CLINICAL RESEARCH APPLICATIONS OF MRI IN OSTEOARTHRITIS

The need to develop sensitive and reliable markers of cartilage damage has been a growing area of OA research. The ability of MRI to noninvasively provide high-resolution images of articular cartilage makes it a valuable tool for both basic science and clinical research. Clinical research applications have focused on methods that will allow quantitative cartilage morphometry to evaluate anatomic changes of tissue, and more recently parametric mapping techniques that will provide evaluation of biochemical changes in the extracellular matrix associated with cartilage degradation.

## Anatomic Techniques: Quantitative Cartilage Morphometry

### Techniques

Historically, imaging markers in clinical OA research have relied on radiographic measures of disease severity such as joint space narrowing (JSN) and osteophyte formation.[159] Because these findings are an indirect measure of cartilage loss, radiography is insensitive and nonspecific for early tissue damage in OA. A primary research application of MRI in OA has been the development and validation of techniques for deriving direct quantitative measures of cartilage morphology.[160] Methods and applications of this quantitative cartilage morphometry have been recently reviewed.[161] Although there is no clear consensus on the specific image marker to be analyzed with these techniques, most studies have evaluated cartilage volume, mean cartilage thickness, and surface area.

Nearly all studies using quantitative MRI in the evaluation of OA have been directed toward the knee. Although this in part is driven by the high prevalence of knee OA, it is also a function of the ability to provide particularly high-resolution MR images of knee articular cartilage that are more difficult to obtain in other joints. The cylindrical shape of the leg and relatively superficial location of the knee joint allow high-sensitivity phased array coils to be placed in close proximity to the joint. These geometric considerations are not as optimal in joints with thinner cartilage or that are located deeper in the body.

Gradient echo imaging techniques are used to acquire the data used in the morphometric analysis of cartilage.[16,161] Because the thin cartilage layer of the knee has complex curved geometry, it is necessary to obtain images with high spatial resolution. Established protocols for quantitative assessment of cartilage morphology use volumetric 3D T1-weighted fat-suppressed or water-excited gradient echo acquisitions with a section thickness of <2 mm and in-plane resolution of <300 microns per pixel.[161-164]

The use of thin-section 3D acquisition reduces errors from volume averaging that occur when cartilage interfaces are oriented obliquely to the imaging plane.[80,163,165,166] However, recent studies have questioned the need for thin-section acquisition.[167,168] The use of a short TE (<10 ms) is necessary to capture signal from the deep radial zone of cartilage that has short TE values in the range of 10 to 30 ms.[36,169] In addition, high bandwidths are necessary for the minimization of chemical shift artifact from subchondral fatty marrow that may obscure the bone/cartilage interface.

Because both artifacts are more severe at higher field strength and because these artifacts may lead to underestimation of cartilage thickness, particular caution should be taken when using 3.0-T systems. Although initial validation of quantitative cartilage MRI was performed at 1.5 T, recent preliminary results indicate that measured cartilage thickness is similar between 3.0 and 1.5 T.[47]

### Validation and Reproducibility

Before applying a technique to longitudinal studies, it is necessary to first demonstrate that the result is valid (a true representation of the underlying disease process), reliable (provides a reproducible result), and responsive to clinically significant changes in the disease status. Quantitative MRI protocols have undergone several technical validation studies comparing cartilage volume measurements derived from MRI with anatomic reference methods using cadaver or surgical knee specimens[161,170-175] and in vivo validation of cartilage thickness with high-resolution CT arthrography.[176]

In a recent review of published MRI validation studies, systematic differences for MRI determination of cartilage volume and thickness compared with reference methods range from 5 to 10%.[161] It should be noted that compared to radiography (which has received only limited validation for evaluation of the medial femoral tibial compartment[177]) MRI has demonstrated high accuracy in the evaluation of all three compartments of the knee. Although validation studies of normal joints are applicable to normative studies or to the early stages of OA (when there is minimal tissue loss), they may not be representative of advanced OA in which thinning of cartilage introduces greater error from artifact and limited resolution.

Similar validations have been performed in the setting of severe OA.[178,179] Comparative studies have shown that smaller tibial[180,181] and patellar[182] cartilage volumes are correlated with radiographic findings of OA. In patients with severe knee OA, MRI underestimated tibial cartilage volume by 13% compared to water displacement of excised cartilage. However, precision remained high, with a coefficient of variation ranging from 3.8% in the lateral compartment to 5.5% medially.[178]

Several studies have evaluated the reliability of quantitative cartilage morphometry. Errors due to low reproducibility or precision of the MRI determination of morphometry are relatively small compared to the annual rate of change in the image marker, with a pooled coefficient of variation (CV%) generally less than 5% for determination of cartilage volume.[161] Because cartilage volume is smaller in the setting of OA, the CV% is higher for OA subjects compared to healthy controls. However, it is still in the range of 5%. Because of errors from volume averaging, which is related to the shape and orientation of cartilage relative to the acquisition planes, precision varies with joint compartment and orientation of the imaging plane.[161]

The highest reproducibility is obtained using axial images of patellar cartilage with a pooled coefficient of variation of 1%,[183,184] and from the central regions of the tibial femoral joint.[185] Lower precision is obtained in assessment of thinner femoral and tibial cartilage evaluated in the sagittal plane, with reported reproducibility ranging from 2[186] to 9%.[163] Precision in assessment of femoral cartilage volume appears to be better using coronal acquisition.[179] This may be due to in-plane volume averaging of femoral cartilage that occurs near the inter-condylar notch with sagittal acquisitions. Coronal acquisition has also been shown to provide greater precision in the evaluation of tibial cartilage volume and thickness.[187]

Because there is less curvature in tibial cartilage, reproducibility is higher than that of femoral cartilage. One study indicates that for both normal individuals and individuals with radiographic findings of OA there is a strong correlation between femoral and tibial cartilage volumes.[180] As a result, it may be possible to use compartmental measures of tibial cartilage as an indicator of femoral tibial disease severity. However, others have shown significant individual variation in cartilage morphometry between different articular surfaces within the joint.[188]

The precision in determining mean cartilage thickness and cartilage surface area is similar to that of cartilage volume.[161] There is limited experience applying quantitative MRI techniques to multi-center trials in which differences in MRI instrumentation and experience may lead to greater variation due to contribution of systematic bias between sites. Preliminary findings from a small multi-center trial found no substantial systematic differences between sites in determination of cartilage volume.[189]

### Research Applications of MRI Cartilage Morphometry

Quantitative assessment of cartilage morphometry has been applied to several cross-sectional human studies to identify factors that influence cartilage morphology.

The primary focus of these studies has been the association of age, gender, body habitus, level of activity, and joint biomechanics on cartilage volume, thickness, and surface area.

Several studies have demonstrated an inverse correlation of knee cartilage thickness with age,[190-193] although the association of age with cartilage volume is variable.[191] With increasing age there is a higher prevalence of focal cartilage lesions,[191] which has been shown to be prognostic for loss of cartilage volume.[194]

MRI results demonstrate significant gender effects in cartilage volumes, with young males having 16 to 31% greater volume than young females.[195] Similarly, greater tibial and patellar cartilage volumes have been demonstrated in male adults.[196-198] This difference in volume is primarily a result of gender differences in cartilage surface area rather than cartilage thickness.[199,200] For children and adolescents, the gender difference was partially explained by differences in physical activity.[195] This differs from results in older adults, for whom there is no significant association with level of activity.[201] Other studies in male adults report an inverse association of BMI and physical activity with total and medial cartilage volumes.[192,202]

Other studies suggest that the observed gender differences in cartilage volume are driven primarily by body size, independent of gender.[203] Hormonal influences may also contribute to gender differences in cartilage volume. There is a positive correlation between serum testosterone and medial tibial cartilage volume measured with MRI.[202] Results with estrogen replacement therapy (ERT) are less clear. Women on long-term ERT have been shown to have 10% more knee cartilage than age-matched women not on ERT,[204] whereas no significant effect on patella cartilage volume was observed in women on ERT.[205]

Body habitus has been shown to influence cartilage morphology. An inverse association of patellar cartilage volume and BMI has been established in an obese population.[206] Along with increased biomechanical force from elevated BMI, increased compartmental loading from knee mal-alignment has been associated with progressive loss of cartilage volume.[207] In contrast to BMI, increased muscle mass has been correlated with larger cartilage volumes[208] and is associated with a reduction in the rate of tibial cartilage loss.[209] Several studies have looked for correlations among cartilage morphometric parameters of volume, mean thickness, and surface area using anthropomorphic measures such as height and weight.

Knee cartilage volume and surface area were closely correlated with height. However, there was no correlation with cartilage thickness.[188] Within subjects, the difference in cartilage volume, mean thickness, and surface area between the right and left knee were 5.0, 3.8,

and 3.4%, respectively—substantially less than the corresponding inter-subject variability (respectively) of 24.8, 14.4, and 14.1%.[210] In this study, differences within subjects were associated with differences in muscle cross-sectional area—suggesting that biomechanical forces contribute to the observed differences in cartilage morphology between joints.

As has been previously observed with radiographic features of OA, there is a poor association between cartilage morphometry measured with MRI and clinical findings. Hunter et al. demonstrated an inverse association between patellar cartilage volume and (collectively) pain, function, and global Western Ontario MacMaster Osteoarthritis Index (WOMAC) score[211]—with no association between symptoms and cartilage volume measurements derived from other compartments. A weak association between medial tibial cartilage volume and pain has recently been demonstrated.[212] Link et al. found no significant association between MRI findings and symptoms.[213]

A critical feature of an image marker for monitoring disease progression is responsiveness to change. There have been few technical validation studies of MRI responsiveness. Phantom validation studies have used tissue samples to subjectively evaluate incremental thinning.[214] Studies in humans indicate that MRI is more sensitive than radiographs in detecting and monitoring loss of articular cartilage, and that MRI is responsive to changes in cartilage morphometry that occur over a period of 1 to 2 years. A longitudinal study of 28 subjects with knee OA comparing medial compartment joint space width measured from standing radiographs and MRI cartilage volume found no significant correlation in longitudinal change of these measures over a 2-year period.[215]

In this study, cartilage volume was found to be a better predictor of knee replacement. Substantial reduction in cartilage volume and increase in bone surface area have been demonstrated in subjects with mild radiographic OA (KL score 1), suggesting that MRI is more sensitive than radiographs in the detection of early cartilage loss.[112] In a study of 32 subjects with symptomatic knee OA, Raynauld et al. demonstrated a global cartilage loss of 6.1% after 2 years.[216] A 2-year longitudinal cohort study of 123 subjects with radiographic OA have shown an annual loss in tibial cartilage volume of 5.3% and suggested that baseline cartilage volume was a primary determinant in rate of cartilage loss.[217]

A similar study evaluating 28 healthy men over a 2-year period observed a decrease in tibial cartilage volume of 2.8% per year.[218] Similar responsiveness to cartilage loss has been demonstrated in the patellofemoral joint. In a 2-year longitudinal study of patellofemoral OA, patellar cartilage was shown to decrease at a rate of

4.5% per year and was not correlated with loss of tibial cartilage volume—suggesting that the pathogenesis between the two compartments is different.[219]

Quantitative MRI has been useful in following cartilage loss in populations at risk for developing OA. A 2-year longitudinal study in eight subjects with normal radiographs and partial meniscectomy has shown a significant loss of knee cartilage volume compared to non-surgical controls.[220] Quantitative MRI has been used to follow cartilage thinning following acute spinal cord injury, with a decrease in mean thickness ranging from 9% in the patella to 13% in the lateral tibia and a total reduction in cartilage volume of 10%.[221]

Some studies indicate that cartilage volume is an insensitive marker of disease progression. Longitudinal studies in patients with radiographically established knee OA[222] and rheumatoid arthritis[223] failed to demonstrate a change in cartilage volume, raising concern over the responsiveness of this endpoint for monitoring structural changes. A limitation of cartilage volume as a quantitative endpoint is the lack of regional sensitivity to focal sites of cartilage damage. There is the potential to improve sensitivity by evaluating regional changes in cartilage thinning through regional thickness maps.

This necessitates methodology for spatially co-registering images obtained at different sessions. Waterton et al. have used this approach to evaluate diurnal variation in articular cartilage.[224] Analysis of variance demonstrated no significant change in cartilage volume between scans obtained in the early morning and those obtained in the late afternoon. However, a decrease in cartilage thickness of up to 0.6 mm was identified in sites under primarily compressive load. Other regions demonstrated an increase in cartilage thickness, suggesting that there is a diurnal redistribution of cartilage water reflecting regional differences in biomechanical load.

Applications of quantitative MRI for cartilage morphometry are less well established in joints other than the knee. Quantitative MRI morphometry has been applied to the hip,[225] elbow,[226] and shoulder.[227] The high spatial resolution available with the 3D acquisition makes the gradient echo technique useful in the evaluation of the small joints, such as the wrist and hand, and in small animal models of OA.[165]

Validation studies have shown that MRI provides a reliable and reproducible assessment of cartilage volume of the metacarpophalangeal joints.[228] There has been limited validation of the techniques in the interphalangeal or wrist joints. There has been limited validation of the 3D fat-suppressed T1-weighted spoiled gradient echo technique in the evaluation of cartilage thickness of the ankle,[229-231] with several studies suggesting lower accuracy of MRI compared to CT arthrography.[232,233]

## Biochemical Techniques: Parametric Mapping

Knowledge gained from animal studies indicates that anatomic changes of cartilage damage such as surface fibrillation and erosion represent relatively late manifestations of the disease and are preceded by biochemical and structural changes in tissue. The sensitivity of the MRI signal to the macromolecular environment of tissue provides the potential to use measurements of MRI relaxation parameters to detect and monitor these early changes in cartilage in the intact human joint. Potential MRI parameters that have been proposed for the study of cartilage are summarized in Table 10.2.

Initial results from these studies indicate that MRI parametric mapping techniques are sensitive to (and in some cases specific for) a broad range of properties in the cartilage matrix that are relevant to the study of early OA. In many cases these techniques have been limited to proof-of-concept studies in excised osteochondral specimens. Other techniques, such as delayed gadolinium enhanced MRI of cartilage (dGEMRIC) and cartilage T2 mapping, have been validated and applied to several cross-sectional human studies.

### Proteoglycan-sensitive Techniques

The depletion of proteoglycan from cartilage is an early finding in OA, and is strongly correlated with changes in biomechanical properties of the tissue. MRI methods of measuring regional proteoglycan concentration consist of sodium MRI, T1rho imaging, and dGEMRIC.

#### Sodium MRI

Although all clinical MRI is derived from the signal generated by the proton, any nucleus with an odd number of protons and/or neutrons possesses a nuclear magnetic moment and is capable of generating an MRI signal. The $^{23}Na$ nucleus is one such nucleus that can generate an MRI signal. However, the signal generated by the $^{23}Na$ nucleus has less than half the energy of the signal generated by the proton. In addition, the relatively low concentration of sodium in cartilage (approximately 320 $\mu M$) compared to water (and the very short T2 time of the sodium signal) make in vivo $^{23}Na$ MRI challenging.

Sodium imaging requires the use of specific transmit and receive coils that are not readily available for clinical systems. With the introduction of ultra-high-field human 7.0-T MRI systems, sodium imaging with spatial resolution similar to that currently observed with proton MRI may be possible in the future. In cartilage,

**TABLE 10.2  POTENTIAL MRI PARAMETERS FOR EVALUATION OF ARTICULAR CARTILAGE**

| Cartilage Property | MRI Parameter | References |
|---|---|---|
| Water content | Proton density | (234) |
| | T1 | (235, 236) |
| | T2 | (237) |
| Proteoglycan content | Sodium MRI | (238, 239) |
| | T1rho | (240, 241) |
| | DGEMRIC | (242–245) |
| Collagen content | MT | (23, 246, 247) |
| | T2 | (69, 248, 249) |
| Collagen orientation | T2 | (55, 249–252) |
| | Diffusion tensor imaging | (253) |
| Water mobility | Diffusion | (254–257) |
| | T2 | (58, 249) |
| Regional cartilage compressibility | MRI tagging | (258) |
| | MR elastography | (259) |
| | T2 Mapping | (260, 261) |

sodium ions are associated with the negatively charged keratan sulfate and chondroitin sulfate side chains of the glycosaminoglycans (GAGs), and are the primary component of the fixed-charged density (FCD) in the extracellular matrix.[262,263]

Preliminary studies in excised tissue samples have shown that sodium MRI is sensitive to small changes in sodium concentration with enzymatic depletion of GAG.[238,264-267] Techniques have been proposed for obtaining quantitative measures of sodium concentration in cartilage,[239,268] and for selectively obtaining the signal from sodium bound to macromolecules in the extracellular matrix.[269,270] Although in vivo human images have been demonstrated,[238,270] clinical research application of sodium MRI has been limited to proof-of-concept studies.

## T1rho Imaging

Although differences in T1 relaxation between tissues is a primary source of image contrast in clinical MRI, T1rho contrast has received limited attention. To review, the relaxation constant T1 refers to the spin lattice relaxation time constant in the presence of a static magnetic field. The relaxation time constant T1rho refers to spin lattice relaxation in the rotating frame (relaxation in the presence of the RF magnetic field). T1rho has been shown to be sensitive to the molecular interactions of water with large rotating macromolecules.

In the case of early cartilage degeneration, T1rho appears to be sensitive to the interaction of water protons with proteoglycans.[271] However, with further GAG depletion there also appears to be contribution from collagen water interaction similar to that seen with magnetization transfer and T2 relaxation maps.[272-274] Regatte and co-workers have demonstrated a strong correlation between T1rho in tissue and spectrophotometric assays of cartilage proteoglycan content.[275,276]

In isolated tissue specimens, T1rho increases with proteoglycan depletion (using trypsin digestion[240,277,278]) but not with collagenase treatment. A recent study using IL-1 depletion of proteoglycan in a rabbit model demonstrated promise for using T1rho in vivo to monitor changes in proteoglycan content.[241] There is a strong correlation between T1rho and fixed-charge density as assessed using sodium MRI.[279]

Initial application of T1rho in humans was limited to single-slice acquisition,[280] although more recently multi-slice[281] and 3D acquisitions[282-284] have been developed. A potential limitation of the T1rho technique is the relatively large amount of RF power applied, which can result in tissue heating. However, newer versions of the technique suggest this is not a significant limitation at current clinical field strengths. These initial feasibility studies have demonstrated elevated T1rho in subjects with symptomatic OA. However, there has been limited clinical experience with this technique. There have been no published studies evaluating the reproducibility and responsiveness of this technique in humans.

### Delayed Gadolinium Enhanced MRI of Cartilage

Unlike sodium MRI, which measures the FCD directly, the dGEMRIC technique uses a negatively charged contrast agent to indirectly measure regional GAG content.[285,286] Following intravenous injection, the MRI contrast agent Gd(DTPA)-2 (which goes by the trade name Magnevist) slowly diffuses into synovial fluid (and over time will equilibrate with articular cartilage). Because of steric hindrance and electrostatic repulsion of Gd(DTPA)-2, the partitioning of the contrast agent within cartilage is inversely proportional to the distribution of GAG.[287] Areas of low GAG will contain a higher content of contrast agent, which results in more rapid $T_1$ relaxation of adjacent water protons. After obtaining a series of $T_1$-weighted images, a $T_1$ map can be calculated that provides a regional assessment of relative Gd(DTPA)-2 concentration inversely proportional to regional GAG content.[288]

Technical issues related to optimization of the dGEMRIC technique for human clinical applications have been reviewed.[242] The compound Gd(DTPA)-2 has been approved for clinical use as an MRI contrast agent. However, the dGEMRIC technique represents an off-label application. The standard clinical dose is 0.1 mM/kg body weight. However, a dose up to 0.3 mM/kg has been used in neuroimaging applications. There is a dose-dependent response of $T_1$ relaxation in cartilage over the range of 0.1 to 0.3 mM/kg body weight.[289]

Reproducibility of the technique using a test-retest paradigm was slightly better using a double dose of Gd(DTPA)-2 and was in the range of +/-15% for regional $T_1$ measurements.[242] Some authors have advocated using a triple dose to improve sensitivity to small changes in GAG.[289] To increase uptake in synovial fluid, it is recommended that subjects exercise the joint for 10 minutes after intravenous injection. It is necessary to wait 2 hours before obtaining $T_1$ maps to allow penetration into thicker patellar cartilage.[289] For thinner cartilage (such as the hip), the interval after injection can be reduced to 90 minutes.[242]

A limitation of the dGEMRIC technique is the delay period between injection and imaging, and the long imaging time needed to acquire the series of $T_1$-weighted images used to calculate the $T_1$ maps. Using standard spin echo imaging techniques, total imaging time approaches 1 hour and has limited spatial coverage. The long imaging interval makes it necessary to correct for patient motion that may occur between acquisitions. More recently, techniques have been developed for rapid $T_1$ mapping of tissue that can reduce acquisition times to several minutes with improved spatial coverage. These newer pulse sequences are currently undergoing validation.

Several validation studies have shown a strong correlation between GAG content determined using the dGEMRIC technique and biochemical or histologic measures.[243,287,288,290-292] In isolated cartilage samples, the correlation between GAG content determined using dGEMRIC and histologic measurement of GAG is better in superficial cartilage than in deeper layers (where MRI can overestimate GAG).[270] Differences between observers in the selection and calculation of regional $T_1$ have been shown not to be a significant source of variation.[293]

Several groups are exploring clinical research applications of dGEMRIC in evaluation of OA. In a cohort of 15 subjects with pre-radiographic knee OA, increased uptake of Gd(DTPA)-2 was observed in compartments with fibrillation and softening identified arthroscopically.[294] Greater uptake of Gd (DTPA) has been seen in subjects with acetabular dysplasia, which correlated well with both pain and degree of dysplasia.[244] dGEMRIC has been used to monitor serial changes in GAG following osteochondral allograft.[295] However, more recent studies suggest that baseline differences in cartilage $T_1$ make it necessary to measure $T_1$ both before and after contrast administration in order to accurately assess GAG content.

Several studies have used dGEMRIC to evaluate cartilage in the setting of acute or chronic soft tissue derangements of the knee. Areas of increased contrast uptake have been associated with sites of meniscal or ligamentous injuries.[245] In patients with acute (less than 3 weeks) ACL tears, increased uptake of contrast was observed in cartilage of the medial compartment and in the lateral compartment adjacent to sites of subchondral marrow contusion.[296] The $T_1$ value of cartilage correlated well with GAG content measured in synovial fluid at the time of arthroscopy.

Results of dGEMRIC have demonstrated a high level of responsiveness to changes in cartilage GAG. The dGEMRIC technique has been used to monitor GAG repletion following interleukin-1-induced depletion.[297] Several studies have shown that changes observed with dGEMRIC are closely associated with the biomechanical properties of cartilage. Increased uptake of Gd(DTPA)-2 indicative of low GAG content is associated with increased cartilage compressibility.[70,71,298] Preliminary findings in osteochondral allografts demonstrate a similar association between indentation stiffness and low GAG as determined using dGEMRIC.[299]

A recent study of 37 subjects suggests that dGEMRIC may be useful in monitoring the adaptive response of cartilage to exercise.[300] Using the dGEMRIC technique, baseline $T_1$ values correlated strongly with level of physical activity—with the longest $T_1$ values (high GAG) observed in elite runners and lowest $T_1$ values in sedentary individuals. This study supports previous work in animals, suggesting that load-bearing exercise can increase GAG content in cartilage.[301] These intriguing results point toward future translational research opportunities in understanding the important role of joint biomechanics in cartilage physiology and the role of exercise in the development of OA.

## Collagen-sensitive Techniques

Along with the large aggregating proteoglycan aggrecan, type II collagen is the other major macromolecule present in the extracellular cartilage matrix. It is the confining properties of collagen in response to the swelling properties of aggrecan that provide cartilage with the high interstitial pressure and ability to restrain water movement needed to achieve the normal response to physiologic stress.[302,303] In addition, the collagen fibrils are an essential component of normal cartilage response to shear stress.[304,305]

As discussed earlier in the chapter, routine clinical FSE imaging is remarkably sensitive to regional variation in the organization and content of the type II collagen matrix of cartilage.[51] Two MRI parameters, in particular magnetization transfer and T2 of cartilage, have demonstrated sensitivity to changes in cartilage collagen. Although both techniques are sensitive to the collagen content in cartilage, T2 is also sensitive to orientation of collagen fibrils in the extracellular matrix.

### Magnetization Transfer

The potential for magnetization transfer is present in any multi-slice MRI technique. It is particularly prominent in FSE techniques because of the rapid application of multiple off-resonance RF pulses. For standard clinical imaging, substantial incidental magnetization transfer leading to lower signal intensity from cartilage can occur with multi-slice FSE sequences.[20,25,306] Because gradient echo techniques do not have a 180-degree refocusing RF pulse and use less energy for the excitation RF pulse, there is substantially less magnetization transfer in gradient echo images. By applying an off-resonance RF pre-pulse immediately before the gradient echo sequence, it is possible to impart magnetization transfer contrast to the image. By subtracting images with magnetization transfer preparation from control images obtained without the pre-pulse, it is possible to isolate the contribution from magnetization transfer.[307]

Variability from multiple factors such as RF power, pulse profile, and offset frequency limit quantification of magnetization transfer—making it difficult to implement as a parametric mapping technique.[308,309] Because calculation of MT is derived from a subtraction of two image sets, the resulting signal compared to noise is very poor and is prone to artifact from any motion occurring between the two acquisitions. Furthermore, for human studies the additional RF power needed for magnetization transfer is limited by safety guidelines for specific absorption rate in place to limit RF heating. As a result, most magnetization transfer applications have been non-quantitative.

There have been few demonstrations of quantitative magnetization transfer techniques in humans.[27,310,311] The primary application of magnetization transfer in the evaluation of articular cartilage has been to improve contrast resolution between cartilage and the overlying synovial fluid,[26,312] which has been shown to increase the accuracy of focal cartilage lesion detection.[170,313] Substantial magnetization transfer has been demonstrated in articular cartilage.[24,314] Studies in excised tissue samples,[23,27,315-317] bioengineered cartilage tissue,[318] and animal models[246,319] have shown that collagen water interaction is the major contributor to this effect—with little variation in magnetization transfer occurring with the removal of proteoglycan. A few studies have questioned whether proteoglycan depletion contributes to increased magnetization transfer.[247,320]

### Cartilage T2 Mapping

The spin-spin (transverse) relaxation time is an MRI time constant sensitive to the slow molecular motions of protons as they move through the macromolecular environment. Early in the development of biologic NMR it was recognized that changes in tissue T2 provide a sensitive marker of disease.[321] In cartilage, T2 is sensitive to changes in water content,[234,237,322-324] collagen content,[69,248,273,274,325,326] and orientation of the highly organized anisotropic arrangement of collagen fibrils in the extracellular cartilage matrix.[24,33,50,55,56,250-252,327-331]

The orientational dependence of T2 is a result of residual quadrupolar relaxation mechanisms present in cartilage as a result of the anisotropic arrangement of collagen fibrils[33,273,332-334] and is most pronounced in the radial zone of cartilage, where there is a preferential orientation of fibers perpendicular to bone.[327,328,331] Correlation studies in tissue samples have demonstrated a strong inverse correlation between cartilage T2 and optical methods of assessing collagen fiber anisotropy.[54,55,65,250,335] Most studies have observed a negligible effect on T2 following enzymatic depletion of proteoglycan from cartilage,[272,275,336,337] as well as poor regional correlation between T2 and histologic staining for proteoglycan.[248]

A few studies suggest that proteoglycan depletion may lead to an increase in cartilage T2.[338-340] A study on cartilage with genetic mutation leading to lack of aggrecan in the extracellular matrix suggests that depletion of the large aggregating proteoglycan does not substantially change the mean T2 value but substantially increases the range of distribution of T2, likely due to increased availability of additional water binding sites (thereby increasing the heterogeneity of the macro-molecular environment).[341]

Sensitivity to structural changes in the cartilage collagen matrix and the concurrent changes that occur with respect to changes in water content make cartilage T2 mapping a useful probe for the study of early OA.[249] Changes in collagen fibril organization are observed during the process of cartilage development,[325,342-345] aging,[346-349] and early OA.[350-354] Weakening of the collagen fibril mesh decreases the constraining forces on the hydrated proteoglycan, leading to an increase in water content and an increase in the permeability of cartilage.[355,356] Compressibility and permeability of cartilage are highly correlated with water content. As water content increases the matrix of the tissue becomes more compressible,[303] and a greater portion of the load is carried by the solid components of the extracellular matrix.[357] This subsequently leads to increased stress, structural fatigue and fragmentation of the solid extracellular matrix, and ultimately to visible changes such as cartilage fibrillation and ulceration.

Several studies have demonstrated a strong association with T2 and histologic measures of OA in tissue sample[70,272,358] and animal models of OA.[235,359,360] Using MRI microscopy, cartilage T2 mapping has been used to follow chondral repair in a rat model.[326,361] Although elevated T2 is most frequently associated with cartilage damage, areas of low T2-weighted signal intensity are not infrequently observed in adjacent cartilage. Low T2 values can be associated with focal areas of increased collagen deposition[235] and chondrocalcinosis.[318,362]

Although most validation studies have been performed using high-field MRI microscopy scanners on excised tissue, in vivo human cartilage T2 maps have been obtained from the patellofemoral joint,[363] the adult[62,364,365] and pediatric femoral tibial joint,[366] and the proximal interphalangeal joint of the hand.[367] Quantitative T2 maps are derived from multi-echo imaging sequences by fitting the signal intensity of each pixel to a single exponential decay, with image acquisition times ranging from 5 to 10 minutes. Recently, preliminary results of a rapid T2 mapping sequence have been presented.[365] Technical considerations for human cartilage T2 mapping have also been recently reviewed.[249,254]

As illustrated in Fig. 10.12, high-resolution T2-mapping studies in humans have demonstrated a spatial variation in T2 similar to that observed with MR microscopy of tissue samples.[56] Shorter T2 values in the range of 30 to 40 ms are observed in subchondral bone, increasing to 50 ms near the articular surface. Based on correlation studies in tissue samples, this spatial dependency is a result of regional differences in the

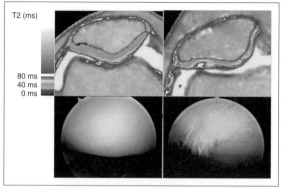

**Fig. 10.12** Cartilage T2 maps. Representative cartilage T2 maps and corresponding arthroscopy images are presented for a 29-year-old female with normal cartilage (left) and a 67-year-old female with grade III ulceration of the lateral patellar facet (right) confirmed at arthroscopy. Normal cartilage demonstrates spatial variation in cartilage T2, with short T2 values observed near bone (blue: 30 to 40 ms). Because of lower anisotropy of collagen fibers in the transitional zone of cartilage, T2 values increase near the articular surface (yellow: 50 to 60 ms). Focal degeneration of the collagen matrix elevates cartilage T2—in this example to values greater than 80 ms. (See Color Plate 5.)

organization of the collagen matrix. Age appears to alter the magnitude of this spatial dependency.

Preliminary results in a pediatric population demonstrate a spatial variation in T2 similar to that observed in young adults.[368] However, beginning about age 45 there is a statistically significant increase in T2 of the superficial layer of cartilage compared to individuals younger than 45 years.[77,78] For individuals older than 65 years, statistically significant elevation in T2 is observed throughout the entire thickness of cartilage.[78] This pattern differs from the multi-focal T2 elevation described in symptomatic individuals.[77] The results support the hypothesis that aging is associated with degeneration or reorganization of the collagen matrix beginning at the articular surface and progressing to deeper layers with age. In contrast to age, gender does not appear to have a significant influence on cartilage T2.[369]

Although subjective interpretation of changes in T2 contrast is a standard tool in clinical evaluation of cartilage damage, there has been limited application of quantitative T2 mapping in evaluating arthritis. In a study of young females with juvenile rheumatoid arthritis, there was a diffuse elevation in cartilage T2 compared to healthy age-matched controls. However, the spatial dependency of T2 was similar between the two groups.[370] Two studies have applied quantitative T2 mapping in subjects with OA. A recent study has demonstrated a strong association between the serum biomarker Col 2-3/4–long mono (a collagenase-derived neoepitope of type II collagen) and knee cartilage T2.[371]

This same study found an association between serum cartilage oligomeric matrix protein (COMP) and cartilage volume. This study illustrates the potential for using serum biomarkers in combination with selective image markers to identify specific degenerative pathways in cartilage. Dunn et al. have shown elevation in cartilage T2 in patients with mild radiographic knee OA. However, there was no significant difference between groups with mild and moderate OA.[372] It appears that cartilage T2 has a nonlinear response to collagen degeneration.

It is possible that early degenerative change in organization of the collagen matrix produces elevation in T2. However, further degeneration does not lead to further elevation in T2. In the future, longitudinal studies are needed to determine the significance of isolated T2 changes. It is unknown if changes associated with T2 elevation are irreversible, if they invariably progress to morphologic sites of damage, or if they can be modified through intervention.

## Functional Cartilage Imaging

A relatively new research application of MRI is the study of cartilage biomechanics. Several studies have used quantitative MRI to measure changes in cartilage thickness in response to compressive loading. Initial studies with osteochondral plugs used MRI to monitor real-time change in cartilage thickness during compression creep experiments performed with an MRI-compatible compression device.[373,374] These ex vivo applications have been extended to studies in intact human joints.[375] Slight differences in the degree of patellar cartilage change were observed between static loading (squatting) and dynamic loading (deep knee bends) of the patellofemoral joint.[184]

Patellar cartilage volume was observed to decrease 6% in young males immediately after performing 50 deep knee bends.[376] The degree of deformation was less (3%) in an elderly cohort.[200] Differences in patellar cartilage deformation have been observed with different exercise. The greatest change occurs after performing deep knee bends (−5.9%), whereas the least occurs after walking (−2.8%).[377] Patellar cartilage deformation following deep knee bends was similar for elite weight lifters, runners, and sedentary controls—suggesting that prior training did not significantly alter patellar cartilage response to compressive load.

Although bulk properties of cartilage biomechanics have been well evaluated with standard biomaterial testing techniques, specialized techniques using confocal microscopy have shown significant differences in the biomechanical properties of cartilage in relation to depth from the articular surface.[378,379] When compressed, the superficial layer of cartilage develops large compressive and tensile strain—resulting in significant tissue consolidation and high fluid flow. Little compressive strain occurs in the deep radial zone. Tensile strain develops at the surfaces of cartilage. Understanding the heterogeneous response of cartilage to physiologic loads will likely improve understanding of the role of biomechanics in OA.

A potential application of MRI in the evaluation of cartilage biomechanics is the ability to nondestructively evaluate regional properties of cartilage in intact tissue specimens.[260,380] Using double quantum-filtered deuterium NMR of cartilage plugs, Shinar et al. were able to demonstrate a loss of collagen fiber anisotropy of the deep radial zone in cartilage placed under static compression.[333] Loss of anisotropy occurs when cartilage is cleaved from bone, indicating that fibers anchored in the tidemark zone are essential to the maintenance of normal fibril orientation and suggesting that an intact bone cartilage interface is essential to the evaluation of cartilage biomechanics.[334]

Recently, regional changes in cartilage biomechanics have been explored using MRI tagging techniques to place MRI-visible fiducial markers ("tags") within the cartilage that can be tracked with MRI microscopy techniques.[258,381] Similar regional biomechanics have been explored using MR elastography to visualize propagation of pressure waves through cartilage,[259] and with diffusion tensor imaging to visualize changes in collagen fibril orientation in response to static compressive load.[253]

Another approach is to use changes in signal intensity to monitor changes in cartilage during compression.[382] An early study by Rubenstein demonstrated a decrease in cartilage signal intensity when osteochondral plugs were placed under compressive load. This signal change was attributed to the extrusion of cartilage water and to alteration in the orientation of collagen fibers, leading to a decrease in cartilage T2. The important role of fiber anisotropy in evaluating regional biomechanical response was confirmed by a strong association between changes in collagen fiber orientation and T2 when cartilage plugs were placed under a static compressive load.[260]

Interestingly, alteration in collagen fiber orientation appears to be different between static and cyclic loading conditions.[383] Greater deformation of collagen fibers with static loading is observed in deeper layers of cartilage, whereas fiber deformation in cyclic loading is limited to the superficial region. In initial feasibility studies, a decrease in cartilage T2 of the femoral tibial joint was measured when static compression was applied to the leg within the magnet[384] and in patellar cartilage following deep knee bends.[324] More recently, using quantitative T2 mapping of cartilage plugs zone-specific changes in cartilage T2 were observed during compressive loading.[385]

These observations indicate that changes in T2 anisotropy may be a potential method for obtaining regional information on cartilage deformation. In an initial study using quantitative T2 mapping in humans, localized decreases in cartilage T2 were observed in the superficial 30% of femoral cartilage immediately after 30 minutes of running exercise.[386] These in vivo results in humans are consistent with prior studies in excised samples, indicating greater compressibility of superficial cartilage[379] and changes in superficial collagen orientation with cyclical loading.[383] The ability to study human cartilage response to physiologic loads provides an opportunity for new translational research toward understanding the role of cartilage biomechanics in cartilage physiology and the pathogenesis of OA.

## REFERENCES

1. Bloch F, Hansen W, Packard M. Nuclear induction. Phys Rev 1946;69:127.
2. Purcell E, Torrey H, Pound R. Resonance absorption by nuclear magnetic moments in a solid. Phys Rev 1946;69:3738.
3. Lauterbur PC. Image formation by induced local interactions: Examples employing nuclear magnetic resonance. Nature 1973;242(5394):190–91.
4. Mansfield P, Maudsley AA. Medical imaging by NMR. Br J Radiol 1977;50(591):188–94.
5. Hennig J, Nauerth A, Friedburg H, Ratzel D. New rapid imaging procedure for nuclear spin tomography. Radiologe 1984;24(12):579–80.
6. Hennig J, Nauerth A, Friedburg H. RARE imaging: A fast imaging method for clinical MR. Magn Reson Med 1986;3(6):823–33.
7. Jaramillo D, Laor T, Mulkern RV. Comparison between fast spin-echo and conventional spin-echo imaging of normal and abnormal musculoskeletal structures in children and young adults. Invest Radiol 1994;29(9):803–11.
8. Fellner C, Geissler A, Held P, Strotzer M, Treibel W, Fellner F. Signal, contrast, and resolution in optimized PD- and T2-weighted turbo SE images of the knee. J Comput Assist Tomogr 1995;19(1):96–105.
9. Zampa V, Cosottini M, Michelassi C, Ortori S, Bruschini L, Bartolozzi C. Value of opposed-phase gradient-echo technique in distinguishing between benign and malignant vertebral lesions. Eur Radiol 2002;12(7):1811–18.
10. Vande Berg BC, Malghem J, Lecouvet FE, Maldague B. Classification and detection of bone marrow lesions with magnetic resonance imaging. Skeletal Radiol 1998;27(10):529–45.
11. Disler DG, McCauley TR, Ratner LM, Kesack CD, Cooper JA. In-phase and out-of-phase MR imaging of bone marrow: Prediction of neoplasia based on the detection of coexistent fat and water. AJR 1997;169(5):1439–47.
12. Potter HG, Asnis-Ernberg L, Weiland AJ, Hotchkiss RN, Peterson MG, McCormack RR Jr. The utility of high-resolution magnetic resonance imaging in the evaluation of the triangular fibrocartilage complex of the wrist. J Bone Joint Surg Am 1997;79(11):1675–84.
13. Totterman SM, Miller RJ, McCance SE, Meyers SP. Lesions of the triangular fibrocartilage complex: MR findings with a three-dimensional gradient-recalled-echo sequence. Radiology 1996;199(1):227–32.
14. Disler DG, McCauley TR, Kelman CG, Fuchs MD, Ratner LM, Wirth CR, et al. Fat-suppressed three-dimensional spoiled gradient-echo MR imaging of hyaline cartilage defects in the knee: Comparison with standard MR imaging and arthroscopy. AJR 1996;167(1):127–32.
15. Disler DG, Peters TL, Muscoreil SJ, Ratner LM, Wagle WA, Cousins JP, et al. Fat-suppressed spoiled GRASS imaging of knee hyaline cartilage: Technique optimization and comparison with conventional MR imaging. AJR 1994;163(4):887–92.
16. Hargreaves BA, Gold GE, Beaulieu CF, Vasanawala SS, Nishimura DG, Pauly JM. Comparison of new sequences for high-resolution cartilage imaging. Magn Reson Med 2003;49(4):700–09.
17. Gold GE, Fuller SE, Hargreaves BA, Stevens KJ, Beaulieu CF. Driven equilibrium magnetic resonance imaging of articular cartilage: Initial clinical experience. J Magn Reson Imaging 2005;21(4):476–81.
18. Harrison R, Bronskill MJ, Henkelman RM. Magnetization transfer and T2 relaxation components in tissue. Magn Reson Med 1995;33(4):490–96.
19. Morris GA, Freemont AJ. Direct observation of the magnetization exchange dynamics responsible for magnetization transfer contrast in human cartilage in vitro. Magn Reson Med 1992;28(1):97–104.
20. Dixon WT, Engels H, Castillo M, Sardashti M. Incidental magnetization transfer contrast in standard multislice imaging. Magn Reson Imaging 1990;8(4):417–22.
21. Wolff SD, Balaban RS. Magnetization transfer contrast (MTC) and tissue water proton relaxation in vivo. Magn Reson Med 1989;10(1):135–44.
22. Constable RT, Anderson AW, Zhong J, Gore JC. Factors influencing contrast in fast spin-echo MR imaging. Magn Reson Imaging 1992;10(4):497–511.
23. Kim DK, Ceckler TL, Hascall VC, Calabro A, Balaban RS. Analysis of water-macromolecule proton magnetization transfer in articular cartilage. Magn Reson Med 1993;29(2):211–15.
24. Henkelman RM, Stanisz GJ, Kim JK, Bronskill MJ. Anisotropy of NMR properties of tissues. Magn Reson Med 1994;32(5):592–601.
25. Yao L, Gentili A, Thomas A. Incidental magnetization transfer contrast in fast spin-echo imaging of cartilage. J Magn Reson Imaging 1996;6(1):180–84.
26. Wolff SD, Chesnick S, Frank JA, Lim KO, Balaban RS. Magnetization transfer contrast: MR imaging of the knee. Radiology 1991;179(3):623–38.
27. Vahlensieck M, Dombrowski F, Leutner C, Wagner U, Reiser M. Magnetization transfer contrast (MTC) and MTC-subtraction: Enhancement of cartilage lesions and intracartilaginous degeneration in vitro. Skeletal Radiol 1994;23(7):535–39.
28. Fullerton GD, Cameron IL, Ord VA. Orientation of tendons in the magnetic field and its effect on T2 relaxation times. Radiology 1985;155(2):433–35.
29. Peto S, Gillis P. Fiber-to-field angle dependence of proton nuclear magnetic relaxation in collagen. Magn Reson Imaging 1990;8(6):705–12.
30. Erickson SJ, Prost RW, Timins ME. The "magic angle" effect: Background physics and clinical relevance. Radiology 1993;188(1):23–5.
31. Hayes CW, Parellada JA. The magic angle effect in musculoskeletal MR imaging. Top Magn Reson Imaging 1996;8(1):51–6.
32. Timins ME, Erickson SJ, Estkowski LD, Carrera GF, Komorowski RA. Increased signal in the normal supraspinatus tendon on MR imaging: Diagnostic pitfall caused by the magic-angle effect. AJR 1995;165(1):109–14.
33. Xia Y. Magic-angle effect in magnetic resonance imaging of articular cartilage: A review. Invest Radiol 2000;35(10):602–21.
34. Waldschmidt JG, Rilling RJ, Kajdacsy-Balla AA, Boynton MD, Erickson SJ. In vitro and in vivo MR imaging of hyaline cartilage: Zonal anatomy, imaging pitfalls, and pathologic conditions. Radiographics 1997;17(6):1387–1402.

35. Frank LR, Brossmann J, Buxton RB, Resnick D. MR imaging truncation artifacts can create a false laminar appearance in cartilage. AJR 1997;168(2):547–54.

36. Freeman DM, Bergman G, Glover G. Short TE MR microscopy: Accurate measurement and zonal differentiation of normal hyaline cartilage. Magn Reson Med 1997;38(1):72–81.

37. Sabiston CP, Adams ME, Li DK. Magnetic resonance imaging of osteoarthritis: Correlation with gross pathology using an experimental model. J Orthop Res 1987;5(2):164–72.

38. Fernandez-Madrid F, Karvonen RL, Teitge RA, Miller PR, Negendank WG. MR features of osteoarthritis of the knee. Magn Reson Imaging 1994;12(5):703–09.

39. Karachalios T, Zibis A, Papanagiotou P, Karantanas AH, Malizos KN, Roidis N. MR imaging findings in early osteoarthritis of the knee. Eur J Radiol 2004;50(3):225–30.

40. Hill CL, Gale DG, Chaisson CE, Skinner K, Kazis L, Gale ME, et al. Knee effusions, popliteal cysts, and synovial thickening: Association with knee pain in osteoarthritis. J Rheumatol 2001; 28(6):1330–37.

41. Guermazi A, Zaim S, Taouli B, Miaux Y, Peterfy CG, Genant HG. MR findings in knee osteoarthritis. Eur Radiol 2003;13(6): 1370–86.

42. Peterfy CG. Imaging of the disease process. Curr Opin Rheumatol 2002;14(5):590–96.

43. Peterfy CG, Guermazi A, Zaim S, Tirman PF, Miaux Y, White D, et al. Whole-Organ Magnetic Resonance Imaging Score (WORMS) of the knee in osteoarthritis. Osteoarthritis Cartilage 2004; 12(3):177–90.

44. Potter HG, Linklater JM, Allen AA, Hannafin JA, Haas SB. Magnetic resonance imaging of articular cartilage in the knee: An evaluation with use of fast-spin-echo imaging. J Bone Joint Surg Am 1998;80(9):1276–84.

45. Bredella MA, Tirman PF, Peterfy CG, Zarlingo M, Feller JF, Bost FW, et al. Accuracy of T2-weighted fast spin-echo MR imaging with fat saturation in detecting cartilage defects in the knee: Comparison with arthroscopy in 130 patients. AJR 1999;172(4): 1073–80.

46. Fischbach F, Bruhn H, Unterhauser F, Ricke J, Wieners G, Felix R, et al. Magnetic resonance imaging of hyaline cartilage defects at 1.5T and 3.0T: Comparison of medium T2-weighted fast spin echo, T1-weighted two-dimensional and three-dimensional gradient echo pulse sequences. Acta Radiol 2005;46(1):67–73.

47. Kornaat PR, Reeder SB, Koo S, Brittain JH, Yu H, Andriacchi TP, et al. MR imaging of articular cartilage at 1.5T and 3.0T: Comparison of SPGR and SSFP sequences. Osteoarthritis Cartilage 2005;13(4):338–44.

48. Schmid MR, Pfirrmann CW, Koch P, Zanetti M, Kuehn B, Hodler J. Imaging of patellar cartilage with a 2D multiple-echo data image combination sequence. AJR 2005;184(6):1744–48.

49. Outerbridge RE. The etiology of chondromalacia patellae. J Bone Joint Surg Br 1961;43-B:752–57.

50. Rubenstein JD, Kim JK, Morova-Protzner I, Stanchev PL, Henkelman RM. Effects of collagen orientation on MR imaging characteristics of bovine articular cartilage. Radiology 1993;188(1):219–26.

51. Jeffery AK, Blunn GW, Archer CW, Bentley G. Three-dimensional collagen architecture in bovine articular cartilage. J Bone Joint Surg Br 1991;73(5):795–801.

52. Quinn TM, Hunziker EB, Hauselmann HJ. Variation of cell and matrix morphologies in articular cartilage among locations in the adult human knee. Osteoarthritis Cartilage 2005;13(8): 672–78.

53. Xia Y, Moody JB, Alhadlaq H, Hu J. Imaging the physical and morphological properties of a multi-zone young articular cartilage at microscopic resolution. J Magn Reson Imaging 2003;17(3): 365–74.

54. Xia Y, Moody JB, Burton-Wurster N, Lust G. Quantitative in situ correlation between microscopic MRI and polarized light microscopy studies of articular cartilage. Osteoarthritis Cartilage 2001;9(5):393–406.

55. Nieminen MT, Rieppo J, Toyras J, Hakumaki JM, Silvennoinen J, Hyttinen MM, et al. T2 relaxation reveals spatial collagen architecture in articular cartilage: A comparative quantitative MRI and polarized light microscopic study. Magn Reson Med 2001;46(3):487–93.

56. Goodwin DW, Wadghiri YZ, Zhu H, Vinton CJ, Smith ED, Dunn JF. Macroscopic structure of articular cartilage of the tibial plateau: Influence of a characteristic matrix architecture on MRI appearance. AJR 2004;182(2):311–18.

57. Goodwin DW, Dunn JF. High-resolution magnetic resonance imaging of articular cartilage: Correlation with histology and pathology. Top Magn Reson Imaging 1998;9(6):337–47.

58. Goodwin DW, Zhu H, Dunn JF. In vitro MR imaging of hyaline cartilage: Correlation with scanning electron microscopy. AJR 2000;174(2):405–09.

59. Foster JE, Maciewicz RA, Taberner J, Dieppe PA, Freemont AJ, Keen MC, et al. Structural periodicity in human articular cartilage: Comparison between magnetic resonance imaging and histological findings [see comments]. Osteoarthritis Cartilage 1999;7(5):480–85.

60. Yoshioka H, Stevens K, Genovese M, Dillingham MF, Lang P. Articular cartilage of knee: Normal patterns at MR imaging that mimic disease in healthy subjects and patients with osteoarthritis. Radiology 2004;231(1):31–8.

61. Goodwin DW. Visualization of the macroscopic structure of hyaline cartilage with MR imaging. Semin Musculoskelet Radiol 2001;5(4):305–12.

62. Smith HE, Mosher TJ, Dardzinski BJ, Collins BG, Collins CM, Yang QX, et al. Spatial variation in cartilage T2 of the knee. J Magn Reson Imaging 2001;14(1):50–5.

63. Gomez S, Toffanin R, Bernstorff S, Romanello M, Amenitsch H, Rappolt M, et al. Collagen fibrils are differently organized in weight-bearing and not-weight-bearing regions of pig articular cartilage. J Exp Zool 2000;287(5):346–52.

64. Xia Y, Moody JB, Alhadlaq H, Burton-Wurster N, Lust G. Characteristics of topographical heterogeneity of articular cartilage over the joint surface of a humeral head. Osteoarthritis Cartilage 2002;10(5):370–80.

65. Alhadlaq HA, Xia Y, Moody JB, Matyas JR. Detecting structural changes in early experimental osteoarthritis of tibial cartilage by microscopic magnetic resonance imaging and polarised light microscopy. Ann Rheum Dis 2004;63(6):709–17.

66. Gagliardi JA, Chung EM, Chandnani VP, Kesling KL, Christensen KP, Null RN, et al. Detection and staging of chondromalacia patellae: relative efficacies of conventional MR imaging, MR arthrography, and CT arthrography. AJR Am J Roentgenol 1994; 163(3):629–36.

67. van Leersum M, Schweitzer ME, Gannon F, Finkel G, Vinitski S, Mitchell DG. Chondromalacia patellae: An in vitro study: Comparison of MR criteria with histologic and macroscopic findings. Skeletal Radiol 1996;25(8):727–32.

68. De Smet AA, Monu JU, Fisher DR, Keene JS, Graf BK. Signs of patellar chondromalacia on sagittal T2-weighted magnetic resonance imaging. Skeletal Radiol 1992;21(2):103–05.

69. Nieminen MT, Toyras J, Rieppo J, Hakumaki JM, Silvennoinen J, Helminen HJ, et al. Quantitative MR microscopy of enzymatically degraded articular cartilage. Magn Reson Med 2000;43(5): 676–81.

70. Nissi MJ, Toyras J, Laasanen MS, Rieppo J, Saarakkala S, Lappalainen R, et al. Proteoglycan and collagen sensitive MRI evaluation of normal and degenerated articular cartilage. J Orthop Res 2004;22(3):557–64.

71. Kurkijarvi JE, Nissi MJ, Kiviranta I, Jurvelin JS, Nieminen MT. Delayed gadolinium-enhanced MRI of cartilage (dGEMRIC) and T2 characteristics of human knee articular cartilage: Topographical variation and relationships to mechanical properties. Magn Reson Med 2004;52(1):41–6.

72. Biswal S, Hastie T, Andriacchi TP, Bergman GA, Dillingham MF, Lang P. Risk factors for progressive cartilage loss in the knee: A longitudinal magnetic resonance imaging study in forty-three patients. Arthritis Rheum 2002;46(11):2884–92.

73. Levy AS, Lohnes J, Sculley S, LeCroy M, Garrett W. Chondral delamination of the knee in soccer players. Am J Sports Med 1996;24(5):634–39.

74. Kendell SD, Helms CA, Rampton JW, Garrett WE, Higgins LD. MRI appearance of chondral delamination injuries of the knee. AJR 2005;184(5):1486–89.

75. Hwang WS, Li B, Jin LH, Ngo K, Schachar NS, Hughes GN. Collagen fibril structure of normal, aging, and osteoarthritic cartilage. J Pathol 1992;167(4):425–33.

76. Mori Y, Kubo M, Okumo H, Kuroki Y. A scanning electron microscopic study of the degenerative cartilage in patellar chondropathy. Arthroscopy 1993;9(3):247–64.

77. Mosher TJ, Dardzinski BJ, Smith MB. Human articular cartilage: Influence of aging and early symptomatic degeneration on the spatial variation of T2; preliminary findings at 3 T. Radiology 2000;214(1):259–66.

78. Mosher TJ, Liu Y, Yang QX, Yao J, Smith R, Dardzinski BJ, et al. Age dependency of cartilage magnetic resonance imaging T2 relaxation times in asymptomatic women. Arthritis Rheum 2004;50(9):2820.

79. Rubenstein JD, Li JG, Majumdar S, Henkelman RM. Image resolution and signal-to-noise ratio requirements for MR imaging of degenerative cartilage. AJR 1997;169(4):1089–96.

80. Link TM, Majumdar S, Peterfy C, Daldrup HE, Uffmann M, Dowling C, et al. High resolution MRI of small joints: Impact of spatial resolution on diagnostic performance and SNR. Magn Reson Imaging 1998;16(2):147–55.

81. Mosher TJ, Pruett SW. Magnetic resonance imaging of superficial cartilage lesions: Role of contrast in lesion detection. J Magn Reson Imaging 1999;10(2):178–82.

82. Disler DG, McCauley TR, Wirth CR, Fuchs MD. Detection of knee hyaline cartilage defects using fat-suppressed three-dimensional spoiled gradient-echo MR imaging: Comparison with standard MR imaging and correlation with arthroscopy. AJR 1995;165(2):377–82.

83. Macarini L, Perrone A, Murrone M, Marini S, Stefanelli M. Evaluation of patellar chondromalacia with MR: Comparison between T2-weighted FSE SPIR and GE MTC. Radiol Med (Torino) 2004;108(3):159–71.

84. Felson DT. An update on the pathogenesis and epidemiology of osteoarthritis. Radiol Clin North Am 2004;42(1):1–9, v.

85. Hofmann S, Kramer J, Vakil-Adli A, Aigner N, Breitenseher M. Painful bone marrow edema of the knee: differential diagnosis and therapeutic concepts. Orthop Clin North Am 2004;35(3):321–33, ix.

86. Mandalia V, Fogg AJ, Chari R, Murray J, Beale A, Henson JH. Bone bruising of the knee. Clin Radiol 2005;60(6):627–36.

87. Lazzarini KM, Troiano RN, Smith RC. Can running cause the appearance of marrow edema on MR images of the foot and ankle? Radiology 1997;202(2):540–42.

88. Zanetti M, Pfirrmann CW, Schmid MR, Romero J, Seifert B, Hodler J. Patients with suspected meniscal tears: Prevalence of abnormalities seen on MRI of 100 symptomatic and 100 contralateral asymptomatic knees. AJR 2003;181(3):635–41.

89. Yao L, Stanczak J, Boutin RD. Presumptive subarticular stress reactions of the knee: MRI detection and association with meniscal tear patterns. Skeletal Radiol 2004;33(5):260–64.

90. Arndt WF, 3rd, Truax AL, Barnett FM, Simmons GE, Brown DC. MR diagnosis of bone contusions of the knee: Comparison of coronal T2-weighted fast spin-echo with fat saturation and fast spin-echo STIR images with conventional STIR images. AJR 1996;166(1):119–24.

91. Zanetti M, Bruder E, Romero J, Hodler J. Bone marrow edema pattern in osteoarthritic knees: Correlation between MR imaging and histologic findings. Radiology 2000;215(3):835–40.

92. Rangger C, Kathrein A, Freund MC, Klestil T, Kreczy A. Bone bruise of the knee: Histology and cryosections in 5 cases. Acta Orthop Scand 1998;69(3):291–94.

93. Bergman AG, Willen HK, Lindstrand AL, Pettersson HT. Osteoarthritis of the knee: Correlation of subchondral MR signal abnormalities with histopathologic and radiographic features. Skeletal Radiol 1994;23(6):445–48.

94. Nolte-Ernsting CC, Adam G, Buhne M, Prescher A, Gunther RW. MRI of degenerative bone marrow lesions in experimental osteoarthritis of canine knee joints. Skeletal Radiol 1996;25(5):413–20.

95. Felson DT, Chaisson CE, Hill CL, Totterman SM, Gale ME, Skinner KM, et al. The association of bone marrow lesions with pain in knee osteoarthritis. Ann Intern Med 2001;134(7):541–49.

96. Sowers MF, Hayes C, Jamadar D, Capul D, Lachance L, Jannausch M, et al. Magnetic resonance-detected subchondral bone marrow and cartilage defect characteristics associated with pain and X-ray-defined knee osteoarthritis. Osteoarthritis Cartilage 2003;11(6):387–93.

97. Lotke PA, Ecker ML, Barth P, Lonner JH. Subchondral magnetic resonance imaging changes in early osteoarthrosis associated with tibial osteonecrosis. Arthroscopy 2000;16(1):76–81.

98. Sharma L, Song J, Felson DT, Cahue S, Shamiyeh E, Dunlop DD. The role of knee alignment in disease progression and functional decline in knee osteoarthritis. JAMA 2001;286(2):188–95.

99. Felson DT, McLaughlin S, Goggins J, LaValley MP, Gale ME, Totterman S, et al. Bone marrow edema and its relation to progression of knee osteoarthritis. Ann Intern Med 2003;139(5/1):330–36.

100. Watson RM, Roach NA, Dalinka MK. Avascular necrosis and bone marrow edema syndrome. Radiol Clin North Am 2004;42(1):207–19.

101. Moosikasuwan JB, Miller TT, Math K, Schultz E. Shifting bone marrow edema of the knee. Skeletal Radiol 2004;33(7):380–85.

102. Arjonilla A, Calvo E, Alvarez L, Fernandez Yruegas D. Transient bone marrow oedema of the knee. Knee 2005;12(4):267–69.

103. Uetani M, Hashmi R, Ito M, Okimoto T, Kawahara Y, Hayashi K, et al. Subchondral insufficiency fracture of the femoral head: Magnetic resonance imaging findings correlated with micro-computed tomography and histopathology. J Comput Assist Tomogr 2003;27(2):189–93.

104. Ramnath RR, Kattapuram SV. MR appearance of SONK-like subchondral abnormalities in the adult knee: SONK redefined. Skeletal Radiol 2004;33(10)575–81.

105. Carbone LD, Nevitt MC, Wildy K, Barrow KD, Harris F, Felson D, et al. The relationship of antiresorptive drug use to structural findings and symptoms of knee osteoarthritis. Arthritis Rheum 2004;50(11):3516–25.

106. Kellgren JLJ. Radiological assessment of osteoarthritis. Ann Rheum Dis 1957;16:494–501.

107. Ravaud P, Dougados M. Radiographic assessment in osteoarthritis. J Rheumatol 1997;24(4):786–91.

108. Felson DT, McAlindon TE, Anderson JJ, Naimark A, Weissman BW, Aliabadi P, et al. Defining radiographic osteoarthritis for the whole knee. Osteoarthritis Cartilage 1997;5(4):241–50.

109. Chan WP, Lang P, Stevens MP, Sack K, Majumdar S, Stoller DW, et al. Osteoarthritis of the knee: Comparison of radiography, CT, and MR imaging to assess extent and severity. AJR 1991;157(4):799–806.

110. Beattie KA, Boulos P, Pui M, O'Neill J, Inglis D, Webber CE, et al. Abnormalities identified in the knees of asymptomatic volunteers using peripheral magnetic resonance imaging. Osteoarthritis Cartilage 2005;13(3):181–86.

111. McCauley TR, Kornaat PR, Jee WH. Central osteophytes in the knee: Prevalence and association with cartilage defects on MR imaging. AJR 2001;176(2):359–64.

112. Jones G, Ding C, Scott F, Glisson M, Cicuttini F. Early radiographic osteoarthritis is associated with substantial changes in cartilage volume and tibial bone surface area in both males and females. Osteoarthritis Cartilage 2004;12(2):169–74.

113. Wluka AE, Wang Y, Davis SR, Cicuttini FM. Tibial plateau size is related to grade of joint space narrowing and osteophytes in healthy women and in women with osteoarthritis. Ann Rheum Dis 2005;64(7):1033–37.

114. Boegard T, Rudling O, Petersson IF, Jonsson K. Correlation between radiographically diagnosed osteophytes and magnetic resonance detected cartilage defects in the tibiofemoral joint. Ann Rheum Dis 1998;57(7):401–07.

115. Ding C, Garnero P, Cicuttini F, Scott F, Cooley H, Jones G. Knee cartilage defects: Association with early radiographic osteoarthritis, decreased cartilage volume, increased joint surface area and type II collagen breakdown. Osteoarthritis Cartilage 2005;13(3):198–205.

116. Boegard T, Rudling O, Petersson IF, Jonsson K. Correlation between radiographically diagnosed osteophytes and magnetic resonance detected cartilage defects in the patellofemoral joint. Ann Rheum Dis 1998;57(7):395–400.

117. Roemer FW, Guermazi A, Lynch JA, Peterfy CG, Nevitt MC, Webb N, et al. Short tau inversion recovery and proton density-weighted fat suppressed sequences for the evaluation of osteoarthritis of the knee with a 1.0 T dedicated extremity MRI: Development of a time-efficient sequence protocol. Eur Radiol 2005;15(5):978–87.

118. Kornaat PR, Ceulemans RY, Kroon HM, Riyazi N, Kloppenburg M, Carter WO, et al. MRI assessment of knee osteoarthritis: Knee

Osteoarthritis Scoring System (KOSS)-inter-observer and intra-observer reproducibility of a compartment-based scoring system. Skeletal Radiol 2005;34(2):95–102.

119. Wojtys EM, Chan DB. Meniscus structure and function. Instr Course Lect 2005;54:323–30.

120. Boyd KT, Myers PT. Meniscus preservation; rationale, repair techniques and results. Knee 2003;10(1):1–11.

121. Messner K, Gao J. The menisci of the knee joint: Anatomical and functional characteristics, and a rationale for clinical treatment. J Anat 1998;193(2):161–78.

122. Aagaard H, Verdonk R. Function of the normal meniscus and consequences of meniscal resection. Scand J Med Sci Sports 1999;9(3):134–40.

123. Burks RT, Metcalf MH, Metcalf RW. Fifteen-year follow-up of arthroscopic partial meniscectomy. Arthroscopy 1997;13(6):673–79.

124. Roos H, Lauren M, Adalberth T, Roos EM, Jonsson K, Lohmander LS. Knee osteoarthritis after meniscectomy: Prevalence of radiographic changes after twenty-one years, compared with matched controls. Arthritis Rheum 1998;41(4):687–93.

125. Englund M, Roos EM, Roos HP, Lohmander LS. Patient-relevant outcomes fourteen years after meniscectomy: Influence of type of meniscal tear and size of resection. Rheumatology (Oxford) 2001;40(6):631–39.

126. Wu WH, Hackett T, Richmond JC. Effects of meniscal and articular surface status on knee stability, function, and symptoms after anterior cruciate ligament reconstruction: A long-term prospective study. Am J Sports Med 2002;30(6):845–50.

127. Noble J, Hamblen DL. The pathology of the degenerate meniscus lesion. J Bone Joint Surg Br 1975;57(2):180–86.

128. Zamber RW, Teitz CC, McGuire DA, Frost JD, Hermanson BK. Articular cartilage lesions of the knee. Arthroscopy 1989;5(4):258–68.

129. LaPrade RF, Burnett QM II, Veenstra MA, Hodgman CG. The prevalence of abnormal magnetic resonance imaging findings in asymptomatic knees, with correlation of magnetic resonance imaging to arthroscopic findings in symptomatic knees. Am J Sports Med 1994;22(6):739–45.

130. Jerosch J, Castro WH, Assheuer J. Age-related magnetic resonance imaging morphology of the menisci in asymptomatic individuals. Arch Orthop Trauma Surg 1996;115(3-4):199–202.

131. Bhattacharyya T, Gale D, Dewire P, Totterman S, Gale ME, McLaughlin S, et al. The clinical importance of meniscal tears demonstrated by magnetic resonance imaging in osteoarthritis of the knee. J Bone Joint Surg Am 2003;85-A(1):4–9.

132. Kenny C. Radial displacement of the medial meniscus and Fairbank's signs. Clin Orthop 1997(339):163–73.

133. Miller TT, Staron RB, Feldman F, Cepel E. Meniscal position on routine MR imaging of the knee. Skeletal Radiol 1997;26(7):424–27.

134. Sugita T, Kawamata T, Ohnuma M, Yoshizumi Y, Sato K. Radial displacement of the medial meniscus in varus osteoarthritis of the knee. Clin Orthop Relat Res 2001(387):171–77.

135. Lerer DB, Umans HR, Hu MX, Jones MH. The role of meniscal root pathology and radial meniscal tear in medial meniscal extrusion. Skeletal Radiol 2004;33(10):569–74.

136. Tuckman GA, Miller WJ, Remo JW, Fritts HM, Rozansky MI. Radial tears of the menisci: MR findings. AJR 1994;163(2):395–400.

137. Kaplan PA, Nelson NL, Garvin KL, Brown DE. MR of the knee: The significance of high signal in the meniscus that does not clearly extend to the surface. AJR 1991;156(2):333–36.

138. De Smet AA, Norris MA, Yandow DR, Quintana FA, Graf BK, Keene JS. MR diagnosis of meniscal tears of the knee: Importance of high signal in the meniscus that extends to the surface. AJR 1993;161(1):101–07.

139. Vande Berg BC, Malghem J, Poilvache P, Maldague B, Lecouvet FE. Meniscal tears with fragments displaced in notch and recesses of knee: MR imaging with arthroscopic comparison. Radiology 2005;234(3):842–50.

140. Dorsay TA, Helms CA. Bucket-handle meniscal tears of the knee: Sensitivity and specificity of MRI signs. Skeletal Radiol 2003;32(5):266–72.

141. Aydingoz U, Firat AK, Atay OA, Doral MN. MR imaging of meniscal bucket-handle tears: A review of signs and their relation to arthroscopic classification. Eur Radiol 2003;13(3):618–25.

142. Rubin DA, Paletta GA Jr. Current concepts and controversies in meniscal imaging. Magn Reson Imaging Clin N Am 2000;8(2):243–70.

143. Blackmon GB, Major NM, Helms CA. Comparison of fast spin-echo versus conventional spin-echo MRI for evaluating meniscal tears. AJR 2005;184(6):1740–43.

144. Helms CA. The meniscus: Recent advances in MR imaging of the knee. AJR Am J Roentgenol 2002;179(5):1115–22.

145. Mesgarzadeh M, Moyer R, Leder DS, Revesz G, Russoniello A, Bonakdarpour A, et al. MR imaging of the knee: Expanded classification and pitfalls to interpretation of meniscal tears. Radiographics 1993;13(3):489–500.

146. Cheung LP, Li KC, Hollett MD, Bergman AG, Herfkens RJ. Meniscal tears of the knee: Accuracy of detection with fast spin-echo MR imaging and arthroscopic correlation in 293 patients. Radiology 1997;203(2):508–12.

147. Winters K, Tregonning R. Reliability of magnetic resonance imaging of the traumatic knee as determined by arthroscopy. N Z Med J 2005;118(1209):U1301.

148. Justice WW, Quinn SF. Error patterns in the MR imaging evaluation of menisci of the knee. Radiology 1995;196(3):617–21.

149. Peterfy CG, Janzen DL, Tirman PF, van Dijke CF, Pollack M, Genant HK. "Magic-angle" phenomenon: A cause of increased signal in the normal lateral meniscus on short-TE MR images of the knee. AJR Am J Roentgenol 1994;163(1):149–54.

150. De Smet AA, Graf BK. Meniscal tears missed on MR imaging: Relationship to meniscal tear patterns and anterior cruciate ligament tears. AJR 1994;162(4):905–11.

151. Bin SI, Kim JM, Shin SJ. Radial tears of the posterior horn of the medial meniscus. Arthroscopy 2004;20(4):373–78.

152. Helms CA, Laorr A, Cannon WD Jr. The absent bow tie sign in bucket-handle tears of the menisci in the knee. AJR 1998;170(1):57–61.

153. Hajek PC, Gylys-Morin VM, Baker LL, Sartoris DJ, Haghighi P, Resnick D. The high signal intensity meniscus of the knee: Magnetic resonance evaluation and in vivo correlation. Invest Radiol 1987;22(11):883–90.

154. Hodler J, Haghighi P, Pathria MN, Trudell D, Resnick D. Meniscal changes in the elderly: Correlation of MR imaging and histologic findings. Radiology 1992;184(1):221–25.

155. Guten GN, Kohn HS, Zoltan DJ. "False positive" MRI of the knee: A literature review study. WMJ 2002;101(1):35–8.

156. Cothran RL Jr., Major NM, Helms CA, Higgins LD. MR imaging of meniscal contusion in the knee. AJR 2001;177(5):1189–92.

157. Shankman S, Beltran J, Melamed E, Rosenberg ZS. Anterior horn of the lateral meniscus: Another potential pitfall in MR imaging of the knee. Radiology 1997;204(1):181–4.

158. Shepard MF, Hunter DM, Davies MR, Shapiro MS, Seeger LL. The clinical significance of anterior horn meniscal tears diagnosed on magnetic resonance images. Am J Sports Med 2002;30(2):189–92.

159. Kellgren J, Lawrence J. Radiologic assessment of osteoarthrosis. Ann Rheum Dis 1957;16:494–501.

160. Raynauld JP. Quantitative magnetic resonance imaging of articular cartilage in knee osteoarthritis. Curr Opin Rheumatol 2003;15(5):647–50.

161. Eckstein F, Glaser C. Measuring cartilage morphology with quantitative magnetic resonance imaging. Semin Musculoskelet Radiol 2004;8(4):329–53.

162. Marshall KW, Guthrie BT, Mikulis DJ. Quantitative cartilage imaging. Br J Rheumatol 1995;34(1):29–31.

163. Hardya PA, Newmark R, Liu YM, Meier D, Norris S, Piraino DW, et al. The influence of the resolution and contrast on measuring the articular cartilage volume in magnetic resonance images. Magn Reson Imaging 2000;18(8):965–72.

164. Kornaat PR, Doornbos J, van der Molen AJ, Kloppenburg M, Nelissen RG, Hogendoorn PC, et al. Magnetic resonance imaging of knee cartilage using a water selective balanced steady-state free precession sequence. J Magn Reson Imaging 2004;20(5):850–56.

165. Link TM, Lindner N, Haeussler M, Reimer P, Allkemper T, Jerosch J, et al. Artificially produced cartilage lesions in small joints: Detection with optimized MRI-sequences. Magn Reson Imaging 1997;15(8):949–56.

166. McGibbon CA, Bencardino J, Yeh ED, Palmer WE. Accuracy of cartilage and subchondral bone spatial thickness distribution from MRI. J Magn Reson Imaging 2003;17(6):703–15.

167. Cicuttini F, Morris KF, Glisson M, Wluka AE. Slice thickness in the assessment of medial and lateral tibial cartilage volume and accuracy for the measurement of change in a longitudinal study. J Rheumatol 2004;31(12):2444–48.

168. Zhai G, Ding C, Cicuttini F, Jones G. Optimal sampling of MRI slices for the assessment of knee cartilage volume for cross-sectional and longitudinal studies. BMC Musculoskelet Disord 2005;6(1):10.

169. Cova M, Toffanin R, Szomolanyi P, Vittur F, Pozzi-Mucelli RS, Jellus V, et al. Short-TE projection reconstruction MR microscopy in the evaluation of articular cartilage thickness. Eur Radiol 2000;10(8):1222–26.

170. Peterfy CG, van Dijke CF, Janzen DL, Gluer CC, Namba R, Majumdar S, et al. Quantification of articular cartilage in the knee with pulsed saturation transfer subtraction and fat-suppressed MR imaging: Optimization and validation. Radiology 1994;192(2):485–91.

171. Dupuy DE, Spillane RM, Rosol MS, Rosenthal DI, Palmer WE, Burke DW, et al. Quantification of articular cartilage in the knee with three-dimensional MR imaging. Acad Radiol 1996;3(11):919–24.

172. Kladny B, Bail H, Swoboda B, Schiwy-Bochat H, Beyer WF, Weseloh G. Cartilage thickness measurement in magnetic resonance imaging. Osteoarthritis Cartilage 1996;4(3):181–86.

173. Eckstein F, Schnier M, Haubner M, Priebsch J, Glaser C, Englmeier KH, et al. Accuracy of cartilage volume and thickness measurements with magnetic resonance imaging. Clin Orthop Relat Res 1998(352):137–48.

174. Graichen H, von Eisenhart-Rothe R, Vogl T, Englmeier KH, Eckstein F. Quantitative assessment of cartilage status in osteoarthritis by quantitative magnetic resonance imaging: Technical validation for use in analysis of cartilage volume and further morphologic parameters. Arthritis Rheum 2004;50(3):811–16.

175. Cohen ZA, McCarthy DM, Kwak SD, Legrand P, Fogarasi F, Ciaccio EJ, et al. Knee cartilage topography, thickness, and contact areas from MRI: In-vitro calibration and in-vivo measurements. Osteoarthritis Cartilage 1999;7(1):95–109.

176. Haubner M, Eckstein F, Schnier M, Losch A, Sittek H, Becker C, et al. A non-invasive technique for 3-dimensional assessment of articular cartilage thickness based on MRI. Part 2: Validation using CT arthrography. Magn Reson Imaging 1997;15(7):805–13.

177. Buckland-Wright JC, Macfarlane DG, Lynch JA, Jasani MK, Bradshaw CR. Joint space width measures cartilage thickness in osteoarthritis of the knee: High resolution plain film and double contrast macroradiographic investigation. Ann Rheum Dis 1995;54(4):263–68.

178. Burgkart R, Glaser C, Hyhlik-Durr A, Englmeier KH, Reiser M, Eckstein F. Magnetic resonance imaging-based assessment of cartilage loss in severe osteoarthritis: Accuracy, precision, and diagnostic value. Arthritis Rheum 2001;44(9):2072–77.

179. Glaser C, Burgkart R, Kutschera A, Englmeier KH, Reiser M, Eckstein F. Femoro-tibial cartilage metrics from coronal MR image data: Technique, test-retest reproducibility, and findings in osteoarthritis. Magn Reson Med 2003;50(6):1229–36.

180. Cicuttini FM, Wluka AE, Stuckey SL. Tibial and femoral cartilage changes in knee osteoarthritis. Ann Rheum Dis 2001;60(10):977–80.

181. Cicuttini FM, Wluka AE, Forbes A, Wolfe R. Comparison of tibial cartilage volume and radiologic grade of the tibiofemoral joint. Arthritis Rheum 2003;48(3):682–88.

182. Cicuttini FM, Wang YY, Forbes A, Wluka AE, Glisson M. Comparison between patella cartilage volume and radiological assessment of the patellofemoral joint. Clin Exp Rheumatol 2003;21(3):321–26.

183. Eckstein F, Westhoff J, Sittek H, Maag KP, Haubner M, Faber S, et al. In vivo reproducibility of three-dimensional cartilage volume and thickness measurements with MR imaging. AJR 1998;170(3):593–97.

184. Eckstein F, Lemberger B, Stammberger T, Englmeier KH, Reiser M. Patellar cartilage deformation in vivo after static versus dynamic loading. J Biomech 2000;33(7):819–25.

185. Koo S, Gold GE, Andriacchi TP. Considerations in measuring cartilage thickness using MRI: Factors influencing reproducibility and accuracy. Osteoarthritis Cartilage 2005;13(9):782–09.

186. Cicuttini F, Forbes A, Asbeutah A, Morris K, Stuckey S. Comparison and reproducibility of fast and conventional spoiled gradient-echo magnetic resonance sequences in the determination of knee cartilage volume. J Orthop Res 2000;18(4):580–84.

187. Hyhlik-Durr A, Faber S, Burgkart R, Stammberger T, Maag KP, Englmeier KH, et al. Precision of tibial cartilage morphometry with a coronal water-excitation MR sequence. Eur Radiol 2000;10(2):297–303.

188. Eckstein F, Winzheimer M, Hohe J, Englmeier KH, Reiser M. Interindividual variability and correlation among morphological parameters of knee joint cartilage plates: Analysis with three-dimensional MR imaging. Osteoarthritis Cartilage 2001;9(2):101–11.

189. Morgan SR, Waterton JC, Maciewicz RA, Leadbetter JE, Gandy SJ, Moots RJ, et al. Magnetic resonance imaging measurement of knee cartilage volume in a multicentre study. Rheumatology (Oxford) 2003;43(1):19-21.

190. Karvonen RL, Negendank WG, Teitge RA, Reed AH, Miller PR, Fernandez-Madrid F. Factors affecting articular cartilage thickness in osteoarthritis and aging. J Rheumatol 1994;21(7):1310–18.

191. Ding C, Cicuttini F, Scott F, Cooley H, Jones G. Association between age and knee structural change: A cross sectional MRI based study. Ann Rheum Dis 2005;64(4):549–55.

192. Dalla Palma L, Cova M, Pozzi-Mucelli RS. MRI appearance of the articular cartilage in the knee according to age. J Belge Radiol 1997;80(1):17–20.

193. Hudelmaier M, Glaser C, Hohe J, Englmeier KH, Reiser M, Putz R, et al. Age-related changes in the morphology and deformational behavior of knee joint cartilage. Arthritis Rheum 2001;44(11):2556–61.

194. Cicuttini F, Ding C, Wluka A, Davis S, Ebeling PR, Jones G. Association of cartilage defects with loss of knee cartilage in healthy, middle-age adults: A prospective study. Arthritis Rheum 2005;52(7):2033–39.

195. Jones G, Glisson M, Hynes K, Cicuttini F. Sex and site differences in cartilage development: A possible explanation for variations in knee osteoarthritis in later life. Arthritis Rheum 2000;43(11):2543–49.

196. Cicuttini F, Forbes A, Morris K, Darling S, Bailey M, Stuckey S. Gender differences in knee cartilage volume as measured by magnetic resonance imaging. Osteoarthritis Cartilage 1999;7(3):265–71.

197. Ding C, Cicuttini F, Scott F, Glisson M, Jones G. Sex differences in knee cartilage volume in adults: Role of body and bone size, age and physical activity. Rheumatology (Oxford) 2003;42(11):1317–23.

198. Eckstein F, Siedek V, Glaser C, Al-Ali D, Englmeier KH, Reiser M, et al. Correlation and sex differences between ankle and knee cartilage morphology determined by quantitative magnetic resonance imaging. Ann Rheum Dis 2004;63(11):1490–95.

199. Faber SC, Eckstein F, Lukasz S, Muhlbauer R, Hohe J, Englmeier KH, et al. Gender differences in knee joint cartilage thickness, volume and articular surface areas: Assessment with quantitative three-dimensional MR imaging. Skeletal Radiology 2001;30(3):144–150.

200. Eckstein F, Reiser M, Englmeier KH, Putz R. In vivo morphometry and functional analysis of human articular cartilage with quantitative magnetic resonance imaging: From image to data, from data to theory. Anat Embryol (Berl) 2001;203(3):147–73.

201. Muhlbauer R, Lukasz TS, Faber TS, Stammberger T, Eckstein F. Comparison of knee joint cartilage thickness in triathletes and physically inactive volunteers based on magnetic resonance imaging and three-dimensional analysis. Am J Sports Med 2000;28(4):541–46.

202. Cicuttini FM, Wluka A, Bailey M, O'Sullivan R, Poon C, Yeung S, et al. Factors affecting knee cartilage volume in healthy men. Rheumatology (Oxford) 2003;42(2):258–62.

203. Nishimura K, Tanabe T, Kimura M, Harasawa A, Karita K, Matsushita T. Measurement of articular cartilage volumes in the normal knee by magnetic resonance imaging: Can cartilage volumes be estimated from physical characteristics? J Orthop Sci 2005;10(3):246–52.

204. Wluka AE, Davis SR, Bailey M, Stuckey SL, Cicuttini FM. Users of oestrogen replacement therapy have more knee cartilage than non-users. Ann Rheum Dis 2001;60(4):332–36.

205. Cicuttini FM, Wluka AE, Wang Y, Stuckey SL, Davis SR. Effect of estrogen replacement therapy on patella cartilage in healthy women. Clin Exp Rheumatol 2003;21(1):79–82.

206. Ding C, Cicuttini F, Scott F, Cooley H, Jones G. Knee structural alteration and BMI: A cross-sectional study. Obes Res 2005;13(2):350–61.

207. Cicuttini F, Wluka A, Hankin J, Wang Y. Longitudinal study of the relationship between knee angle and tibiofemoral cartilage volume in subjects with knee osteoarthritis. Rheumatology (Oxford) 2004;43(3):321–24.

208. Hudelmaier M, Glaser C, Englmeier KH, Reiser M, Putz R, Eckstein F. Correlation of knee-joint cartilage morphology with muscle cross-sectional areas vs. anthropometric variables. Anat Rec 2003;270A(2):175–84.

209. Cicuttini FM, Teichtahl AJ, Wluka AE, Davis S, Strauss BJ, Ebeling PR. The relationship between body composition and knee cartilage volume in healthy, middle-aged subjects. Arthritis Rheum 2005;52(2):461–67.

210. Eckstein F, Muller S, Faber SC, Englmeier KH, Reiser M, Putz R. Side differences of knee joint cartilage volume, thickness, and surface area, and correlation with lower limb dominance—an MRI-based study. Osteoarthritis Cartilage 2002;10(12):914–21.

211. Hunter DJ, March L, Sambrook PN. The association of cartilage volume with knee pain. Osteoarthritis Cartilage 2003;11(10):725–29.

212. Wluka AE, Wolfe R, Stuckey S, Cicuttini FM. How does tibial cartilage volume relate to symptoms in subjects with knee osteoarthritis? Ann Rheum Dis 2004;63(3):264–68.

213. Link TM, Steinbach LS, Ghosh S, Ries M, Lu Y, Lane N, et al. Osteoarthritis: MR imaging findings in different stages of disease and correlation with clinical findings. Radiology 2003;226(2):373–81.

214. Tebben PJ, Pope TW, Hinson G, Batnitzky S, Wetzel LH, DePaolis DC, et al. Three-dimensional computerized reconstruction: Illustration of incremental articular cartilage thinning. Invest Radiol 1997;32(8):475–84.

215. Cicuttini F, Hankin J, Jones G, Wluka A. Comparison of conventional standing knee radiographs and magnetic resonance imaging in assessing progression of tibiofemoral joint osteoarthritis. Osteoarthritis Cartilage 2005;13(8):722–27.

216. Raynauld JP, Martel-Pelletier J, Berthiaume MJ, Labonte F, Beaudoin G, de Guise JA, et al. Quantitative magnetic resonance imaging evaluation of knee osteoarthritis progression over two years and correlation with clinical symptoms and radiologic changes. Arthritis Rheum 2004;50(2):476–87.

217. Wluka AE, Stuckey S, Snaddon J, Cicuttini FM. The determinants of change in tibial cartilage volume in osteoarthritic knees. Arthritis Rheum 2002;46(8):2065–72.

218. Hanna F, Ebeling PR, Wang Y, O'Sullivan R, Davis S, Wluka AE, et al. Factors influencing longitudinal change in knee cartilage volume measured from magnetic resonance imaging in healthy men. Ann Rheum Dis 2005;64(7):1038–42.

219. Cicuttini F, Wluka A, Wang Y, Stuckey S. The determinants of change in patella cartilage volume in osteoarthritic knees. J Rheumatol 2002;29(12):2615–19.

220. Cicuttini FM, Forbes A, Yuanyuan W, Rush G, Stuckey SL. Rate of knee cartilage loss after partial meniscectomy. J Rheumatol 2002;29(9):1954–56.

221. Vanwanseele B, Eckstein F, Knecht H, Spaepen A, Stussi E. Longitudinal analysis of cartilage atrophy in the knees of patients with spinal cord injury. Arthritis Rheum 2003;48(12):3377–81.

222. Gandy SJ, Dieppe PA, Keen MC, Maciewicz RA, Watt I, Waterton JC. No loss of cartilage volume over three years in patients with knee osteoarthritis as assessed by magnetic resonance imaging. Osteoarthritis Cartilage 2002;10(12):929–37.

223. Gandy SJ, Brett AD, Dieppe PA, Keen MC, Maciewicz RA, Taylor CJ, et al. Measurement of cartilage volumes in rheumatoid arthritis using MRI. Br J Radiol 2005;78(925):39–45.

224. Waterton JC, Solloway S, Foster JE, Keen MC, Gandy S, Middleton BJ, et al. Diurnal variation in the femoral articular cartilage of the knee in young adult humans. Magn Reson Med 2000;43(1):126–32.

225. Zhai G, Cicuttini F, Srikanth V, Cooley H, Ding C, Jones G. Factors associated with hip cartilage volume measured by magnetic resonance imaging: The Tasmanian Older Adult Cohort Study. Arthritis Rheum 2005;52(4):1069–76.

226. Graichen H, Springer V, Flaman T, Stammberger T, Glaser C, Englmeier KH, et al. Validation of high-resolution water-excitation magnetic resonance imaging for quantitative assessment of thin cartilage layers. Osteoarthritis Cartilage 2000;8(2):106–14.

227. Graichen H, Jakob J, von Eisenhart-Rothe R, Englmeier KH, Reiser M, Eckstein F. Validation of cartilage volume and thickness measurements in the human shoulder with quantitative magnetic resonance imaging. Osteoarthritis Cartilage 2003;11(7):475–82.

228. Peterfy CG, van Dijke CF, Lu Y, Nguyen A, Connick TJ, Kneeland JB, et al. Quantification of the volume of articular cartilage in the metacarpophalangeal joints of the hand: Accuracy and precision of three-dimensional MR imaging. AJR 1995;165(2):371–75.

229. Trattnig S, Breitenseher MJ, Huber M, Zettl R, Rottmann B, Haller J, et al. Determination of cartilage thickness in the ankle joint: an MRT (1.5)-anatomical comparative study. Rofo Fortschr Geb Rontgenstr Neuen Bildgeb Verfahr 1997;166(4):303–06.

230. Tan TC, Wilcox DM, Frank L, Shih C, Trudell DJ, Sartoris DJ, et al. MR imaging of articular cartilage in the ankle: Comparison of available imaging sequences and methods of measurement in cadavers. Skeletal Radiol 1996;25(8):749–55.

231. Al-Ali D, Graichen H, Faber S, Englmeier KH, Reiser M, Eckstein F. Quantitative cartilage imaging of the human hind foot: Precision and inter-subject variability. J Orthop Res 2002;20(2):249–56.

232. El-Khoury GY, Alliman KJ, Lundberg HJ, Rudert MJ, Brown TD, Saltzman CL. Cartilage thickness in cadaveric ankles: Measurement with double-contrast multi-detector row CT arthrography versus MR imaging. Radiology 2004;233(3):768–73.

233. Schmid MR, Pfirrmann CW, Hodler J, Vienne P, Zanetti M. Cartilage lesions in the ankle joint: comparison of MR arthrography and CT arthrography. Skeletal Radiol 2003;32(5):259–65.

234. Shapiro EM, Borthakur A, Kaufman JH, Leigh JS, Reddy R. Water distribution patterns inside bovine articular cartilage as visualized by 1H magnetic resonance imaging. Osteoarthritis Cartilage 2001;9(6):533–38.

235. Gahunia HK, Lemaire C, Babyn PS, Cross AR, Kessler MJ, Pritzker KP. Osteoarthritis in rhesus macaque knee joint: Quantitative magnetic resonance imaging tissue characterization of articular cartilage. J Rheumatol 1995;22(9):1747–56.

236. Potter K, Butler JJ, Horton WE, Spencer RG. Response of engineered cartilage tissue to biochemical agents as studied by proton magnetic resonance microscopy. Arthritis Rheum 2000;43(7):1580–90.

237. Lusse S, Claassen H, Gehrke T, Hassenpflug J, Schunke M, Heller M, et al. Evaluation of water content by spatially resolved transverse relaxation times of human articular cartilage. Magn Reson Imaging 2000;18(4):423–30.

238. Reddy R, Insko EK, Noyszewski EA, Dandora R, Kneeland JB, Leigh JS. Sodium MRI of human articular cartilage in vivo. Magn Reson Med 1998;39(5):697–701.

239. Shapiro EM, Borthakur A, Gougoutas A, Reddy R. 23Na MRI accurately measures fixed charge density in articular cartilage. Magn Reson Med 2002;47(2):284–91.

240. Duvvuri U, Kudchodkar S, Reddy R, Leigh JS. T(1rho) relaxation can assess longitudinal proteoglycan loss from articular cartilage in vitro. Osteoarthritis Cartilage 2002;10(11):838–44.

241. Wheaton AJ, Dodge GR, Borthakur A, Kneeland JB, Schumacher HR, Reddy R. Detection of changes in articular cartilage proteoglycan by T(1rho) magnetic resonance imaging. J Orthop Res 2005;23(1):102–08.

242. Burstein D, Velyvis J, Scott KT, Stock KW, Kim YJ, Jaramillo D, et al. Protocol issues for delayed Gd(DTPA)(2-)-enhanced MRI (dGEMRIC) for clinical evaluation of articular cartilage. Magn Reson Med 2001;45(1):36–41.

243. Bashir A, Gray ML, Burstein D. Gd-DTPA2 as a measure of cartilage degradation. Magn Reson Med 1996;36(5):665–73.

173

244. Kim YJ, Jaramillo D, Millis MB, Gray ML, Burstein D. Assessment of early osteoarthritis in hip dysplasia with delayed gadolinium-enhanced magnetic resonance imaging of cartilage. J Bone Joint Surg Am 2003;85-A(10):1987–92.

245. Williams A, Gillis A, McKenzie C, Po B, Sharma L, Micheli L, et al. Glycosaminoglycan distribution in cartilage as determined by delayed gadolinium-enhanced MRI of cartilage (dGEMRIC): Potential clinical applications. AJR 2004;182(1):167–72.

246. Laurent D, Wasvary J, O'Byrne E, Rudin M. In vivo qualitative assessments of articular cartilage in the rabbit knee with high-resolution MRI at 3 T. Magn Reson Med 2003;50(3):541–49.

247. Lattanzio PJ, Marshall KW, Damyanovich AZ, Peemoeller H. Macromolecule and water magnetization exchange modeling in articular cartilage. Magn Reson Med 2000;44(6):840–51.

248. Fragonas E, Mlynarik V, Jellus V, Micali F, Piras A, Toffanin R, et al. Correlation between biochemical composition and magnetic resonance appearance of articular cartilage. Osteoarthritis Cartilage 1998;6(1):24–32.

249. Mosher TJ, Dardzinski BJ. Cartilage MRI T2 relaxation time mapping: Overview and applications. Semin Musculoskelet Radiol 2004;8(4):355–68.

250. Grunder W, Wagner M, Werner A. MR-microscopic visualization of anisotropic internal cartilage structures using the magic angle technique. Magn Reson Med 1998;39(3):376–82.

251. Xia Y, Farquhar T, Burton-Wurster N, Lust G. Origin of cartilage laminae in MRI. J Magn Reson Imaging 1997;7(5):887–94.

252. Goodwin DW, Wadghiri YZ, Dunn JF. Micro-imaging of articular cartilage: T2, proton density, and the magic angle effect. Acad Radiol 1998;5(11):790–98.

253. Filidoro L, Dietrich O, Weber J, Rauch E, Oerther T, Wick M, et al. High-resolution diffusion tensor imaging of human patellar cartilage: Feasibility and preliminary findings. Magn Reson Med 2005;53(5):993–98.

254. Glaser C. New techniques for cartilage imaging: T2 relaxation time and diffusion-weighted MR imaging. Radiol Clin North Am 2005;43(4):641–53, vii.

255. Miller KL, Hargreaves BA, Gold GE, Pauly JM. Steady-state diffusion-weighted imaging of in vivo knee cartilage. Magn Reson Med 2004;51(2):3948.

256. Mlynarik V, Sulzbacher I, Bittsansky M, Fuiko R, Trattnig S. Investigation of apparent diffusion constant as an indicator of early degenerative disease in articular cartilage. J Magn Reson Imaging 2003;17(4):440–44.

257. Xia Y, Farquhar T, Burton-Wurster N, Vernier-Singer M, Lust G, Jelinski LW. Self-diffusion monitors degraded cartilage. Arch Biochem Biophys 1995;323(2):323–28.

258. Neu CP, Hull ML, Walton JH, Buonocore MH. MRI-based technique for determining nonuniform deformations throughout the volume of articular cartilage explants. Magn Reson Med 2005;53(2):321–28.

259. Hardy PA, Ridler AC, Chiarot CB, Plewes DB, Henkelman RM. Imaging articular cartilage under compression: Cartilage elastography. Magn Reson Med 2005;53(1):1065–73.

260. Grunder W, Kanowski M, Wagner M, Werner A. Visualization of pressure distribution within loaded joint cartilage by application of angle-sensitive NMR microscopy. Magn Reson Med 2000;43(6):884–91.

261. Mosher TJ, Smith HE, Collins C, Liu Y, Hancy J, Dardzinski BJ, et al. Change in knee cartilage T2 at MR imaging after running: A feasibility study. Radiology 2005;234(1):245–49.

262. Maroudas A, Muir H, Wingham J. The correlation of fixed negative charge with glycosaminoglycan content of human articular cartilage. Biochim Biophys Acta 1969;177(3):492–500.

263. Lesperance LM, Gray ML, Burstein D. Determination of fixed charge density in cartilage using nuclear magnetic resonance. J Orthop Res 1992;10(1):1–13.

264. Insko EK, Kaufman JH, Leigh JS, Reddy R. Sodium NMR evaluation of articular cartilage degradation. Magn Reson Med 1999;41(1):30–4.

265. Borthakur A, Shapiro EM, Beers J, Kudchodkar S, Kneeland JB, Reddy R. Sensitivity of MRI to proteoglycan depletion in cartilage: Comparison of sodium and proton MRI. Osteoarthritis Cartilage 2000;8(4):288–93.

266. Borthakur A, Shapiro EM, Beers J, Kudchodkar S, Kneeland JB, Reddy R. Effect of IL-1beta-induced macromolecular depletion on residual quadrupolar interaction in articular cartilage. J Magn Reson Imaging 2002;15(3):315–23.

267. Wheaton AJ, Borthakur A, Dodge GR, Kneeland JB, Schumacher HR, Reddy R. Sodium magnetic resonance imaging of proteoglycan depletion in an in vivo model of osteoarthritis. Acad Radiol 2004;11(1):21–8.

268. Shapiro EM, Borthakur A, Dandora R, Kriss A, Leigh JS, Reddy R. Sodium visibility and quantitation in intact bovine articular cartilage using high field (23)Na MRI and MRS. J Magn Reson 2000;142(1):24–31.

269. Duvvuri U, Kaufman JH, Patel SD, Bolinger L, Kneeland JB, Leigh JS, et al. Sodium multiple quantum spectroscopy of articular cartilage: Effects of mechanical compression. Magn Reson Med 1998;40(3):370–75.

270. Borthakur A, Hancu I, Boada FE, Shen GX, Shapiro EM, Reddy R. In vivo triple quantum filtered twisted projection sodium MRI of human articular cartilage. J Magn Reson 1999;141(2):286–90.

271. Duvvuri U, Goldberg AD, Kranz JK, Hoang L, Reddy R, Wehrli FW, et al. Water magnetic relaxation dispersion in biological systems: The contribution of proton exchange and implications for the noninvasive detection of cartilage degradation. Proc Natl Acad Sci USA 2001;98(22):12479–84.

272. Mlynarik V, Trattnig S, Huber M, Zembsch A, Imhof H. The role of relaxation times in monitoring proteoglycan depletion in articular cartilage. J Magn Reson Imaging 1999;10(4):497–502.

273. Mlynarik V, Szomolanyi P, Toffanin R, Vittur F, Trattnig S. Transverse relaxation mechanisms in articular cartilage. J Magn Reson 2004;169(2):300–07.

274. Menezes NM, Gray ML, Hartke JR, Burstein D. T2 and T1rho MRI in articular cartilage systems. Magn Reson Med 2004;51(3):503–09.

275. Regatte RR, Akella SV, Borthakur A, Kneeland JB, Reddy R. Proteoglycan depletion-induced changes in transverse relaxation maps of cartilage: Comparison of T2 and T1rho. Acad Radiol 2002;9(12):1388–94.

276. Regatte RR, Akella SV, Borthakur A, Reddy R. Proton spin-lock ratio imaging for quantitation of glycosaminoglycans in articular cartilage. J Magn Reson Imaging 2003;17(1):114–21.

277. Duvvuri U, Reddy R, Patel SD, Kaufman JH, Kneeland JB, Leigh JS. T1rho-relaxation in articular cartilage: Effects of enzymatic degradation. Magn Reson Med 1997;38(6):863–67.

278. Akella SV, Regatte RR, Gougoutas AJ, Borthakur A, Shapiro EM, Kneeland JB, et al. Proteoglycan-induced changes in T1rho-relaxation of articular cartilage at 4T. Magn Reson Med 2001;46(3):419–23.

279. Wheaton AJ, Casey FL, Gougoutas AJ, Dodge GR, Borthakur A, Lonner JH, et al. Correlation of T1rho with fixed charge density in cartilage. J Magn Reson Imaging 2004;20(3):519–25.

280. Akella SV, Regatte RR, Borthakur A, Kneeland JB, Leigh JS, Reddy R. T1rho MR imaging of the human wrist in vivo. Acad Radiol 2003;10(6):614–19.

281. Wheaton AJ, Borthakur A, Kneeland JB, Regatte RR, Akella SV, Reddy R. In vivo quantification of T1rho using a multislice spin-lock pulse sequence. Magn Reson Med 2004;52(6):1453–58.

282. Regatte RR, Akella SV, Borthakur A, Kneeland JB, Reddy R. In vivo proton MR three-dimensional T1rho mapping of human articular cartilage: Initial experience. Radiology 2003;229(1):269–74.

283. Borthakur A, Wheaton A, Charagundla SR, Shapiro EM, Regatte RR, Akella SV, et al. Three-dimensional T1rho-weighted MRI at 1.5 Tesla. J Magn Reson Imaging 2003;17(6):730–36.

284. Regatte RR, Akella SV, Wheaton AJ, Lech G, Borthakur A, Kneeland JB, et al. 3D-T1rho-relaxation mapping of articular cartilage: In vivo assessment of early degenerative changes in symptomatic osteoarthritic subjects. Acad Radiol 2004;11(7):741–49.

285. Gray ML, Burstein D, Xia Y. Biochemical (and functional) imaging of articular cartilage. Semin Musculoskelet Radiol 2001;5(4):329–43.

286. Gray ML, Burstein D. Molecular (and functional) imaging of articular cartilage. J Musculoskelet Neuronal Interact 2004;4(4):365–68.

287. Bashir A, Gray ML, Boutin RD, Burstein D. Glycosaminoglycan in articular cartilage: In vivo assessment with delayed Gd(DTPA)(2-)-enhanced MR imaging. Radiology 1997;205(2):551–58.

288. Bashir A, Gray ML, Hartke J, Burstein D. Nondestructive imaging of human cartilage glycosaminoglycan concentration by MRI. Magn Reson Med 1999;41(5):857–65.

289. Tiderius CJ, Olsson LE, de Verdier H, Leander P, Ekberg O, Dahlberg L. Gd-DTPA2)-enhanced MRI of femoral knee cartilage: A dose-response study in healthy volunteers. Magn Reson Med 2001;46(6):1067–71.

290. Gillis A, Gray M, Burstein D. Relaxivity and diffusion of gadolinium agents in cartilage. Magn Reson Med 2002;48(6):1068–71.

291. Trattnig S, Mlynarik V, Breitenseher M, Huber M, Zembsch A, Rand T, et al. MRI visualization of proteoglycan depletion in articular cartilage via intravenous administration of Gd-DTPA. Magn Reson Imaging 1999;17(4):577–83.

292. Nieminen MT, Rieppo J, Silvennoinen J, Toyras J, Hakumaki JM, Hyttinen MM, et al. Spatial assessment of articular cartilage proteoglycans with Gd-DTPA-enhanced T1 imaging. Magn Reson Med 2002;48(4):640–48.

293. Tiderius CJ, Tjornstrand J, Akeson P, Sodersten K, Dahlberg L, Leander P. Delayed gadolinium-enhanced MRI of cartilage (dGEMRIC): Intra- and interobserver variability in standardized drawing of regions of interest. Acta Radiol 2004;45(6):628–34.

294. Tiderius CJ, Olsson LE, Leander P, Ekberg O, Dahlberg L. Delayed gadolinium-enhanced MRI of cartilage (dGEMRIC) in early knee osteoarthritis. Magn Reson Med 2003;49(3):488–92.

295. Gillis A, Bashir A, McKeon B, Scheller A, Gray ML, Burstein D. Magnetic resonance imaging of relative glycosaminoglycan distribution in patients with autologous chondrocyte transplants. Invest Radiol 2001;36(12):743–48.

296. Tiderius CJ, Olsson LE, Nyquist F, Dahlberg L. Cartilage glycosaminoglycan loss in the acute phase after an anterior cruciate ligament injury: Delayed gadolinium-enhanced magnetic resonance imaging of cartilage and synovial fluid analysis. Arthritis Rheum 2005;52(1):120–27.

297. Williams A, Oppenheimer RA, Gray ML, Burstein D. Differential recovery of glycosaminoglycan after IL-1-induced degradation of bovine articular cartilage depends on degree of degradation. Arthritis Res Ther 2003;5(2):R97–105.

298. Samosky JT, Burstein D, Eric Grimson W, Howe R, Martin S, Gray ML. Spatially-localized correlation of dGEMRIC-measured GAG distribution and mechanical stiffness in the human tibial plateau. J Orthop Res 2005;23(1):93–101.

299. Vasara AI, Nieminen MT, Jurvelin JS, Peterson L, Lindahl A, Kiviranta I. Indentation stiffness of repair tissue after autologous chondrocyte transplantation. Clin Orthop Relat Res 2005(433):233–42.

300. Tiderius CJ, Svensson J, Leander P, Ola T, Dahlberg L. dGEMRIC (delayed gadolinium-enhanced MRI of cartilage) indicates adaptive capacity of human knee cartilage. Magn Reson Med 2004;51(2):286–90.

301. Arokoski JP, Jurvelin JS, Vaatainen U, Helminen HJ. Normal and pathological adaptations of articular cartilage to joint loading. Scand J Med Sci Sports 2000;10(4):186–98.

302. Maroudas A. Balance between swelling pressure and collagen tension in normal and degenerate cartilage. Nature 1976;260:808–09.

303. Armstrong CG, Mow VC. Variations in the intrinsic mechanical properties of human articular cartilage with age, degeneration, and water content. J Bone Joint Surg [Am] 1982;64(1):88–94.

304. Akizuki S, Mow VC, Muller F, Pita JC, Howell DS, Manicourt DH. Tensile properties of human knee joint cartilage: I. Influence of ionic conditions, weight bearing, and fibrillation on the tensile modulus. J Orthop Res 1986;4(4):379–92.

305. Guilak F, Ratcliffe A, Lane N, Rosenwasser MP, Mow VC. Mechanical and biochemical changes in the superficial zone of articular cartilage in canine experimental osteoarthritis. J Orthop Res 1994;12(4):474–84.

306. Santyr GE. Magnetization transfer effects in multislice MR imaging. Magn Reson Imaging 1993;11(4):521–32.

307. Schick F. Pulsed magnetization transfer contrast MRI by a sequence with water selective excitation. J Comput Assist Tomogr 1996;20(1):73–9.

308. Henkelman RM, Huang X, Xiang QS, Stanisz GJ, Swanson SD, Bronskill MJ. Quantitative interpretation of magnetization transfer. Magn Reson Med 1993;29(6):759–66.

309. Vahlensieck M, Traber F, Giesecke J, Schild H. Magnetization transfer contrast (MTC): Optimizing off-resonance and on-resonance frequency MTC methods at 0.5 and 1.5 T. Biomed Tech (Berl) 2001;46(1/2):10–17.

310. Peterfy CG vDC, Janzen DL, Gluer CC, Namba R, Majumdar S, Lang P, Genant HK. Quantification of articular cartilage in the knee with pulsed saturation transfer subtraction and fat-suppressed MR imaging: Optimization and validation. Radiology 1994;192:485–91.

311. Hohe J, Faber S, Stammberger T, Reiser M, Englmeier KH, Eckstein F. A technique for 3D in vivo quantification of proton density and magnetization transfer coefficients of knee joint cartilage. Osteoarthritis Cartilage 2000;8(6):426–33.

312. Niitsu M, Hirohata H, Yoshioka H, Anno I, Campeau NG, Itai Y. Magnetization transfer contrast on gradient echo MR imaging of the temporomandibular joint. Acta Radiol 1995;36(3):295–99.

313. Peterfy CG, Majumdar S, Lang P, van Dijke CF, Sack K, Genant HK. MR imaging of the arthritic knee: improved discrimination of cartilage, synovium, and effusion with pulsed saturation transfer and fat- suppressed T1-weighted sequences. Radiology 1994;191(2):413–19.

314. Koskinen SK, Komu ME. Low-field strength magnetization transfer contrast imaging of the patellar cartilage. Acta Radiol 1993;34(2):124–26.

315. Gray ML, Burstein D, Lesperance LM, Gehrke L. Magnetization transfer in cartilage and its constituent macromolecules. Magn Reson Med 1995;34(3):319–25.

316. Seo GS, Aoki J, Moriya H, Karakida O, Sone S, Hidaka H, et al. Hyaline cartilage: In vivo and in vitro assessment with magnetization transfer imaging. Radiology 1996;201(2):525–30.

317. Paajanen H, Komu M, Lehto I, Laato M, Haapasalo H. Magnetization transfer imaging of lumbar disc degeneration: Correlation of relaxation parameters with biochemistry. Spine 1994;19(24):2833–37.

318. Potter K, Leapman RD, Basser PJ, Landis WJ. Cartilage calcification studied by proton nuclear magnetic resonance microscopy. J Bone Miner Res 2002;17(4):652–60.

319. Laurent D, Wasvary J, Yin J, Rudin M, Pellas TC, O'Byrne E. Quantitative and qualitative assessment of articular cartilage in the goat knee with magnetization transfer imaging. Magn Reson Imaging 2001;19(10):1279–86.

320. Wachsmuth L, Juretschke HP, Raiss RX. Can magnetization transfer magnetic resonance imaging follow proteoglycan depletion in articular cartilage? Magma 1997;5(1):71–8.

321. Damadian R. Tumor detection by nuclear magnetic resonance. Science 1971;171(976):1151–53.

322. Lehner KB, Rechl HP, Gmeinwieser JK, Heuck AF, Lukas HP, Kohl HP. Structure, function, and degeneration of bovine hyaline cartilage: Assessment with MR imaging in vitro. Radiology 1989;170(2):495–99.

323. Lusse S, Knauss R, Werner A, Grunder W, Arnold K. Action of compression and cations on the proton and deuterium relaxation in cartilage. Magn Reson Med 1995;33(4):483–89.

324. Liess C, Lusse S, Karger N, Heller M, Gluer CC. Detection of changes in cartilage water content using MRI T(2)-mapping in vivo. Osteoarthritis Cartilage 2002;10(12):907–13.

325. Watrin A, Ruaud JP, Olivier PT, Guingamp NC, Gonord PD, Netter PA, et al. T2 mapping of rat patellar cartilage. Radiology 2001;219(2):395–402.

326. Watrin-Pinzano A, Ruaud JP, Cheli Y, Gonord P, Grossin L, Bettembourg-Brault I, et al. Evaluation of cartilage repair tissue after biomaterial implantation in rat patella by using T2 mapping. Magma 2004;17(3-6):219-28.

327. Xia Y, Farquhar T, Burton-Wurster N, Ray E, Jelinski LW. Diffusion and relaxation mapping of cartilage-bone plugs and excised disks using microscopic magnetic resonance imaging. Magn Reson Med 1994;31(3):273–82.

328. Xia Y. Relaxation anisotropy in cartilage by NMR microscopy (muMRI) at 14-microm resolution. Magn Reson Med 1998;39(6):941–49.

329. Mlynarik V, Degrassi A, Toffanin R, Vittur F, Cova M, Pozzi-Mucelli RS. Investigation of laminar appearance of articular cartilage by means of magnetic resonance microscopy. Magn Reson Imaging 1996;14(4):435–42.

330. Kim DJ, Suh JS, Jeong EK, Shin KH, Yang WI. Correlation of laminated MR appearance of articular cartilage with histology, ascertained by artificial landmarks on the cartilage. J Magn Reson Imaging 1999;10(1):57–64.

175

331. Xia Y, Moody JB, Alhadlaq H. Orientational dependence of T2 relaxation in articular cartilage: A microscopic MRI (microMRI) study. Magn Reson Med 2002;48(3):460–69.

332. Navon G, Shinar H, Eliav U, Seo Y. Multiquantum filters and order in tissues. NMR Biomed 2001;14(2):112–32.

333. Shinar H, Seo Y, Ikoma K, Kusaka Y, Eliav U, Navon G. Mapping the fiber orientation in articular cartilage at rest and under pressure studied by 2H double quantum filtered MRI. Magn Reson Med 2002;48(2):322–30.

334. Keinan-Adamsky K, Shinar H, Navon G. The effect of detachment of the articular cartilage from its calcified zone on the cartilage microstructure, assessed by 2H-spectroscopic double quantum filtered MRI. J Orthop Res 2005;23(1):109–17.

335. Xia Y, Elder K. Quantification of the graphical details of collagen fibrils in transmission electron micrographs. J Microsc 2001; 204(1):3–16.

336. Regatte RR, Kaufman JH, Noyszewski EA, Reddy R. Sodium and proton MR properties of cartilage during compression. J Magn Reson Imaging 1999;10(6):961–67.

337. Toffanin R, Mlynarik V, Russo S, Szomolanyi P, Piras A, Vittur F. Proteoglycan depletion and magnetic resonance parameters of articular cartilage. Arch Biochem Biophys 2001;390(2): 235–42.

338. Wayne JS, Kraft KA, Shields KJ, Yin C, Owen JR, Disler DG. MR imaging of normal and matrix-depleted cartilage: Correlation with biomechanical function and biochemical composition. Radiology 2003;228(2):493–99.

339. Watrin-Pinzano A, Ruaud JP, Olivier P, Grossin L, Gonord P, Blum A, et al. Effect of proteoglycan depletion on T2 mapping in rat patellar cartilage. Radiology 2004;234(1):162-70.

340. Watrin-Pinzano A, Ruaud JP, Olivier P, Grossin L, Gonord P, Blum A, et al. Effect of proteoglycan depletion on T2 mapping in rat patellar cartilage. Radiology 2005;234(1):162–70.

341. Mosher TJ, Chen Q, Smith MB. 1H magnetic resonance spectroscopy of nanomelic chicken cartilage: effect of aggrecan depletion on cartilage T2. Osteoarthritis Cartilage 2003;11(10):709–15.

342. Vogel HG. Influence of maturation and aging on mechanical and biochemical properties of connective tissue in rats. Mech Ageing Dev 1980;14(3-4):283–92.

343. Babyn PS, Kim HK, Lemaire C, Gahunia HK, Cross A, DeNanassy J, et al. High-resolution magnetic resonance imaging of normal porcine cartilaginous epiphyseal maturation. J Magn Reson Imaging 1996;6(1):172–79.

344. Aszodi A, Hunziker EB, Olsen BR, Fassler R. The role of collagen II and cartilage fibril-associated molecules in skeletal development. Osteoarthritis Cartilage 2001;9(A):S150–59.

345. Olivier P, Loeuille D, Watrin A, Walter F, Etienne S, Netter P, et al. Structural evaluation of articular cartilage: Potential contribution of magnetic resonance techniques used in clinical practice. Arthritis Rheum 2001;44(10):2285–95.

346. Bank RA, Bayliss MT, Lafeber FP, Maroudas A, Tekoppele JM. Ageing and zonal variation in post-translational modification of collagen in normal human articular cartilage: The age-related increase in non-enzymatic glycation affects biomechanical properties of cartilage. Biochem J 1998;330(1):345–51.

347. Hollander AP, Pidoux I, Reiner A, Rorabeck C, Bourne R, Poole AR. Damage to type II collagen in aging and osteoarthritis starts at the articular surface, originates around chondrocytes, and extends into the cartilage with progressive degeneration. J Clin Invest 1995;96(6):2859–69.

348. DeGroot J, Verzijl N, Budde M, Bijlsma JW, Lafeber FP, TeKoppele JM. Accumulation of advanced glycation end products decreases collagen turnover by bovine chondrocytes. Exp Cell Res 2001;266(2):303–10.

349. DeGroot J, Verzijl N, Wenting-van Wijk MJ, Jacobs KM, Van El B, Van Roermund PM, et al. Accumulation of advanced glycation end products as a molecular mechanism for aging as a risk factor in osteoarthritis. Arthritis Rheum 2004;50(4):1207–15.

350. Lanzer WL, Komenda G. Changes in articular cartilage after meniscectomy. Clin Orthop Relat Res 1990(252):41–8.

351. Pfander D, Rahmanzadeh R, Scheller EE. Presence and distribution of collagen II, collagen I, fibronectin, and tenascin in rabbit normal and osteoarthritic cartilage. J Rheumatol 1999;26(2): 386–94.

352. Freemont AJ, Byers RJ, Taiwo YO, Hoyland JA. In situ zymographic localisation of type II collagen degrading activity in osteoarthritic human articular cartilage. Ann Rheum Dis 1999;58(6):357–65.

353. Rogart JN, Barrach HJ, Chichester CO. Articular collagen degradation in the Hulth-Telhag model of osteoarthritis. Osteoarthritis Cartilage 1999;7(6):539–47.

354. Van De Lest CH, Brama PA, Van El B, DeGroot J, Van Weeren PR. Extracellular matrix changes in early osteochondrotic defects in foals: A key role for collagen? Biochim Biophys Acta 2004;1690(1):54–62.

355. Maroudas AI. Balance between swelling pressure and collagen tension in normal and degenerate cartilage. Nature 1976;260(5554):808–09.

356. Maroudas A, Venn M. Chemical composition and swelling of normal and osteoarthrotic femoral head cartilage. II. Swelling. Ann Rheum Dis 1977;36(5):399–406.

357. Mow VC, Holmes MH, Lai WM. Fluid transport and mechanical properties of articular cartilage: A review. J Biomech 1984;17(5): 377–94.

358. David-Vaudey E, Ghosh S, Ries M, Majumdar S. T2 relaxation time measurements in osteoarthritis. Magn Reson Imaging 2004;22(5):673–82.

359. Gahunia HK, Lemaire C, Cross AR, Babyn P, Kessler MJ, Pritzker KP. Osteoarthritis in rhesus macaques: Assessment of cartilage matrix quality by quantitative magnetic resonance imaging. Agents Actions Suppl 1993;39:255–59.

360. Spandonis Y, Heese FP, Hall LD. High resolution MRI relaxation measurements of water in the articular cartilage of the meniscectomized rat knee at 4.7 T. Magn Reson Imaging 2004;22(7):943–51.

361. Watrin-Pinzano A, Ruaud JP, Cheli Y, Gonord P, Grossin L, Gillet P, et al. T2 mapping: An efficient MR quantitative technique to evaluate spontaneous cartilage repair in rat patella. Osteoarthritis Cartilage 2004;12(3):191–200.

362. Beltran J, Marty-Delfaut E, Bencardino J, Rosenberg ZS, Steiner G, Aparisi F, et al. Chondrocalcinosis of the hyaline cartilage of the knee: MRI manifestations. Skeletal Radiol 1998;27(7): 369–74.

363. Dardzinski BJ, Mosher TJ, Li S, Van Slyke MA, Smith MB. Spatial variation of T2 in human articular cartilage. Radiology 1997;205(2):546–50.

364. Mosher TJ, Smith H, Dardzinski BJ, Schmithorst VJ, Smith MB. MR imaging and T2 mapping of femoral cartilage: In vivo determination of the magic angle effect. AJR 2001; 177(3):665–69.

365. Van Breuseghem I, Bosmans HT, Elst LV, Maes F, Pans SD, Brys PP, et al. T2 mapping of human femorotibial cartilage with turbo mixed MR imaging at 1.5 T: Feasibility. Radiology 2004;233(2):609–14.

366. Dardzinski BJ, Laor T, Schmithorst VJ, Klosterman L, Graham TB. Mapping T2 relaxation time in the pediatric knee: Feasibility with a clinical 1.5-T MR imaging system. Radiology 2002; 225(1):233–39.

367. Lazovic-Stojkovic J, Mosher TJ, Smith HE, Yang QX, Dardzinski BJ, Smith MB. Interphalangeal joint cartilage high-spatial-resolution in vivo MR T2 mapping: A feasibility study. Radiology 2004;233(1):292–96.

368. Dardzinski BJ, Laor T, Schmidthorst VJ, Klosterman L, Graham TB. Mapping T2 relaxation time in the pediatric knee: Feasibility with a clinical 1.5-T MR imaging system. Radiology 2002;225(1):233–39.

369. Mosher TJ, Collins CM, Smith HE, Moser LE, Sivarajah RT, Dardzinski BJ, et al. Effect of gender on in vivo cartilage magnetic resonance imaging T2 mapping. J Magn Reson Imaging 2004;19(3):323–28.

370. Kight AC, Dardzinski BJ, Laor T, Graham TB. Magnetic resonance imaging evaluation of the effects of juvenile rheumatoid arthritis on distal femoral weight-bearing cartilage. Arthritis Rheum 2004;50(3):901–05.

371. King KB, Lindsey CT, Dunn TC, Ries MD, Steinbach LS, Majumdar S. A study of the relationship between molecular biomarkers of joint degeneration and the magnetic resonance-measured characteristics of cartilage in 16 symptomatic knees. Magn Reson Imaging 2004;22(8):1117–23.

372. Dunn TC, Lu Y, Jin H, Ries MD, Majumdar S. T2 relaxation time of cartilage at MR imaging: Comparison with severity of knee osteoarthritis. Radiology 2004;232(2):592–98.

373. Kaufman JH, Regatte RR, Bolinger L, Kneeland JB, Reddy R, Leigh JS. A novel approach to observing articular cartilage deformation in vitro via magnetic resonance imaging. J Magn Reson Imaging 1999;9(5):653–62.

374. Neu CP, Hull ML. Toward an MRI-based method to measure non-uniform cartilage deformation: An MRI-cyclic loading apparatus system and steady-state cyclic displacement of articular cartilage under compressive loading. J Biomech Eng 2003;125(2):180–88.

375. Eckstein F, Adam C, Sittek H, Becker C, Milz S, Schulte E, et al. Non-invasive determination of cartilage thickness throughout joint surfaces using magnetic resonance imaging. J Biomech 1997;30(3):285–89.

376. Eckstein F, Tieschky M, Faber SC, Haubner M, Kolem H, Englmeier KH, et al. Effect of physical exercise on cartilage volume and thickness in vivo: MR imaging study. Radiology 1998;207(1):243–48.

377. Eckstein F, Lemberger B, Gratzke C, Hudelmaier M, Glaser C, Englmeier KH, et al. In vivo cartilage deformation after different types of activity and its dependence on physical training status. Ann Rheum Dis 2005;64(2):291–95.

378. Guilak F, Ratcliffe A, Mow VC. Chondrocyte deformation and local tissue strain in articular cartilage: A confocal microscopy study. J Orthop Res 1995;13(3):410–21.

379. Wong M, Carter DR. Articular cartilage functional histomorphology and mechanobiology: A research perspective. Bone 2003;33(1):1–13.

380. Herberhold C, Faber S, Stammberger T, Steinlechner M, Putz R, Englmeier KH, et al. In situ measurement of articular cartilage deformation in intact femoropatellar joints under static loading. J Biomech 1999;32(12):1287–95.

381. Neu CP, Hull ML, Walton JH. Heterogeneous three-dimensional strain fields during unconfined cyclic compression in bovine articular cartilage explants. J Orthop Res 2005;23(6):1390–08.

382. Stammberger T, Herberhold C, Faber S, Englmeier KH, Reiser M, Eckstein F. A method for quantifying time dependent changes in MR signal intensity of articular cartilage as a function of tissue deformation in intact joints. Med Eng Phys 1998;20(10):741–49.

383. Kaab MJ, Ito K, Clark JM, Notzli HP. Deformation of articular cartilage collagen structure under static and cyclic loading. J Orthop Res 1998;16(6):743–51.

384. Nag D, Liney GP, Gillespie P, Sherman KP. Quantification of T(2) relaxation changes in articular cartilage with in situ mechanical loading of the knee. J Magn Reson Imaging 2004;19(3):317–22.

385. Alhadlaq HA, Xia Y. The structural adaptations in compressed articular cartilage by microscopic MRI (microMRI) T(2) anisotropy. Osteoarthritis Cartilage 2004;12(11):887–94.

386. Mosher TJ, Smith HE, Collins C, Liu Y, Hancy J, Dardzinski BJ, et al. Change in knee cartilage T2 at MR imaging after running: A feasibility study. Radiology 2005;234(1):245–49.

# 11

# Nonsteroidal Anti-inflammatory Drugs for Osteoarthritis

Daniel H. Solomon and Nicola J. Goodson

## INTRODUCTION

The nonsteroidal anti-inflammatory drug (NSAID) class of medications includes nonselective agents (nsNSAIDs), selective cyclo-oxygenase-2 inhibitors (coxibs), and aspirin. All members of this class inhibit cyclo-oxygenase (COX)—the group of enzymes that initiate metabolism of arachidonic acid into various eicosanoids, including prostaglandin $E_2$, thromboxane $A_2$, prostacyclin, prostaglandin $D_2$, and prostaglandin $F_2$. These eicosanoids play critical tissue-specific functions in almost every system in the body. The ability of NSAIDs to inhibit pain, lower fever, and reduce inflammation makes them one of the most important classes of medications. However, their relatively narrow therapeutic index (modest benefit with substantial potential toxicity) has also guaranteed that concerns regarding adverse events will always surround this class.

The history of this class extends back hundreds of years. Aspirin was originally derived from willow bark (see Fig. 11.1), whose medicinal properties were recognized by Hippocrates. European chemists isolated salicin from willow in the 1800s. In 1899, Bayer first marketed acetyl salicylic acid as aspirin. Some claim that aspirin was the first major medicine in the world to be sold in pill form. The first non-aspirin NSAID developed was phenylbutazone, in 1949.[1] Since that time, more than 40 NSAIDs (nsNSAIDs and coxibs) have been developed and marketed, and approximately one quarter of these have been removed from the market because of toxicity (Fig. 11.2).

This chapter has several aims. First, we will review the pharmacology of these agents, including prostaglandin inhibition and their pharmacokinetic parameters. Second, their efficacy data for osteoarthritis (OA) will be assessed. Third, the side effect profiles of nsNSAIDs and coxibs will be examined. These sections focus on gastrointestinal and cardiovascular adverse events. Finally, the pharmaco-economic issues surrounding these agents will be discussed.

## MECHANISMS OF ACTION AND PHARMACOKINETICS

An understanding of the pharmacology of prostaglandins allows one to understand the diverse actions of nsNSAIDs and coxibs. This section explores the diverse functions of prostaglandins and their role in arthritis and in maintaining health. It also discusses the structure and pharmacokinetics of some commonly used nsNSAIDs and coxibs.

### Prostaglandin Metabolism

Prostaglandins were first isolated from human seminal fluid in the 1930s and were named prostaglandins, as initially it was thought they were derived from the prostate gland. It has since become apparent that prostaglandins can be generated by every cell in the body.

Prostanoids (along with leukotrienes and the epoxy-eicosatrienoic acids) are biologically active compounds collectively termed the *eicosanoids*. These substances participate in cell-to-cell communication and exert their actions on target cells at their site of synthesis. The common substrate for the generation of eicosanoids is arachidonic acid. This is a 20-carbon essential fatty acid that is esterified to the phospholipids of cell membranes. Arachidonic acid has to be released by the cell membrane to allow it to be metabolized into groups of biologically active eicosanoids.[2]

The prostanoids include prostaglandins, prostacyclin, and thromboxane—whose biosynthesis depends on three consecutive enzymatic steps[3] (see Fig. 11.3). First, phospholipases release arachidonic acid from the cell membrane phospholipids. Then arachidonic acid is transformed first into prostaglandin $G_2$ (PGG$_2$) and then into prostaglandin $H_2$ (PGH$_2$). The enzymes that carry out this step are called the prostaglandin H synthetases, which exist in two forms [cyclo-oxygenase (COX)-1 and COX-2]. The two isoforms of COX are strong determinants of the ultimate prostanoid. Cell- and tissue-specific isomerases metabolize the PGH$_2$

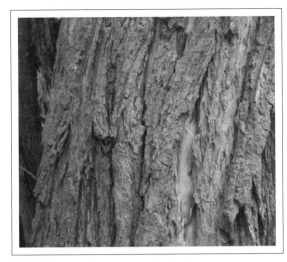

**Fig. 11.1** Willow bark.

into specific prostanoids. These specific prostanoids have different functions, depending on their sites of production.[4]

## Prostaglandins in Health and Disease

Classically, it has been described that the prostaglandins produced via the COX-1 pathway are involved in "housekeeping" functions in that they mediate physiologic responses. COX-2 is expressed by cells involved in inflammation and during disease states such as malignancy. It is primarily responsible for production of prostanoids involved in both acute and chronic inflammatory states.[5] This is probably an overstatement of differences in COX-1 and COX-2 in that they are both critical enzymes in health and disease. The physiologic and pharmacologic actions of COX-generated prostanoids are very heterogeneous and are summarized in Fig. 11.4.

### Inflammation and Arthritis

Both $PGE_2$ and prostacyclin ($PGI_2$) have been found in the synovial fluid of arthritis patients and appear to contribute to the development of inflammatory erythema and pain.[6] Both $PGE_2$ and $PGI_2$ can sensitize nociceptors on sensory nerve cell terminals to painful stimuli. Fever is caused by $PGE_2$ released by endothelial cells. Expression of both COX-1 and COX-2 are increased in inflamed joints. Medications that inhibit COX-2 will prevent the production of prostanoids and thus reduce inflammation, fever, and pain.

Prostanoids affect the immune system in a number of ways. $PGE_2$ inhibits IL-2 and interferon production by T lymphocytes and induces B-cell maturation from immature cells. It has been suggested that tumor cell production of $PGE_2$ causes depression of the immune system in malignancy. Therefore, the down-regulation of $PGE_2$ and immunosuppression by nsNSAIDs and coxibs may be factors involved in the proposed cancer-inhibiting actions of these agents.[7]

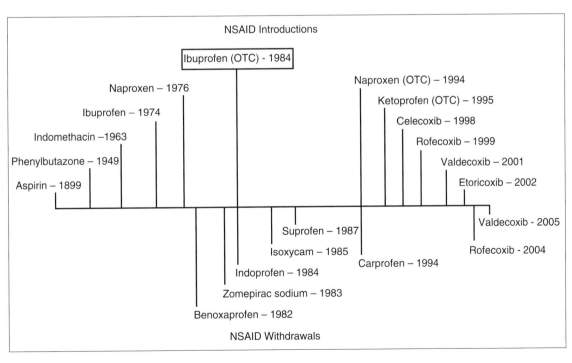

**Fig. 11.2** Timeline of NSAID development.

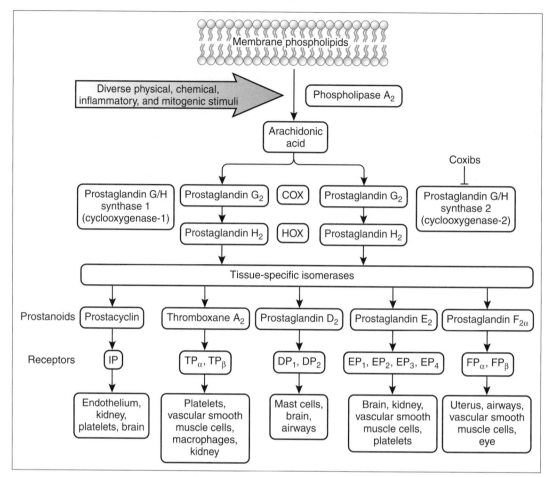

**Fig. 11.3** Prostaglandin metabolism.

## Gastrointestinal Tract

Prostanoids provide cytoprotection in the gastrointestinal tract by a number of mechanisms. $PGE_2$ and $PGI_2$ both reduce acid secretion and cause vasodilatation in blood vessels of the gastric mucosa. Both of these actions contribute to maintaining gastric mucosal integrity. In addition, $PGE_2$ stimulates the release of viscous mucus that coats the gastric mucosa but also allows a layer of secreted bicarbonate to form. This alkaline layer helps to neutralize the effects of the acidic stomach content on the gastric walls. Inhibiting COX-1 leads to reduced gastric $PGE_2$ synthesis and

**Fig. 11.4** Prostaglandins in various disease states and organs.

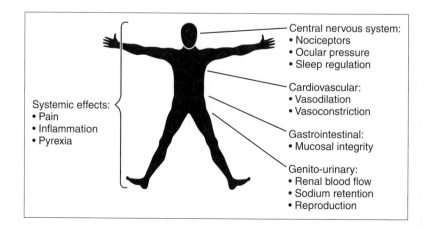

reduced gastric blood flow. However, studies in rats have shown that inhibition of both COX-1 and COX-2 are required to produce gastric mucosal ulceration.[8]

### Cardiovascular System

Endothelial cells contain prostacyclin synthase enzymes in high concentrations and secrete $PGI_2$. $PGI_2$ causes vascular smooth muscle relaxation, leading to increased blood flow. $PGE_2$ can also contribute to vascular dilatation responsible for the erythema observed with inflammation.[9]

Platelets only contain COX-1 that converts arachidonic acid to thromboxane $A_2$, an important regulator of vasoconstrictor and thrombosis. The balance of $PGI_2$ and thromboxane $A_2$ maintains normal vessel dilatation and hemostasis. After ingestion of aspirin, platelet thromboxane and vascular prostacyclin synthesis is inhibited. Platelets are unable to produce further COX, as they have no nucleus and thromboxane synthesis is prevented. Vascular cells are nucleated and are able to synthesize $PGI_2$ after a few hours.[10] Therefore, aspirin is a very effective treatment for thrombotic and occlusive vascular diseases.

Eicosanoids also seem to play a role in the atherosclerotic plaques, where high levels of COX-2 are expressed. However, the role of COX-2 in atherosclerosis is currently not well understood.[11] As well, it is important to note that prostanoids are required for maintaining a patent ductus arteriosus in utero and for its closure in the postnatal period. Not surprisingly, closure of the ductus is influenced by NSAIDs.

### Kidney

Normal kidneys produce $PGE_2$ and $PGI_2$, although the renal medulla predominantly produces $PGE_2$. These prostanoids act as vasodilators and are also natriuretic, inhibiting tubular reabsorption of sodium. The $PGI_2$ and $PGE_2$ produced in the renal cortex also control renin release. Therefore, renal prostanoids influence renal blood flow, glomerular filtration rate, and the release of renin. It seems that COX-1 inhibition leads to reduction in the glomerular filtration rate, whereas sodium retention is mediated by COX-2 inhibition. Patients with congestive heart failure, liver cirrhosis, or renal impairment are very dependent on vasodilator prostanoids to maintain kidney function. Blocking prostanoid synthesis by the use of nsNSAIDs or selective COX-2 inhibitors can lead to renal ischemia and impaired renal function.

### Other Organ Systems

The prostanoids have heterogeneous effects on bronchiolar tone, with $PGE_2$ and $PGI_2$ providing weak bronchodilatation and $PGF_2$-$\alpha$ and thromboxane $A_2$ providing bronchoconstriction. $PGD_2$, a potent vasoconstrictor, is released by mast cells and appears to play a key role in allergic asthma. Inflammatory stimuli cause differential release of prostanoids, and the true role of prostaglandins in asthma is unclear. Apart from the few individuals who have aspirin-sensitive asthma, the nsNSAIDS have little effect on airway function in most asthmatic patients. This is thought to be COX-1 mediated, and therefore specific COX-2 inhibitors may be safer in these patients.

$PGF_2$-$\alpha$ is produced by the endometrium and appears to be important for reproduction in that it influences ovulation and the menstrual cycle. $PGE_2$ is involved in ripening of the cervix prior to labor and can induce labor at any stage of pregnancy. Uterine contractions are stimulated by $PGF_2$-$\alpha$. Both of these prostaglandins are made by COX-1 and COX-2. Human seminal fluid contains high concentrations of prostanoids, including $PGE_2$, $PGE_1$, $PGE_3$, and $PGF_2$-$\alpha$. These prostaglandins may potentiate conception by stimulating contractions of the cervix, fallopian tubes, and uterus.

$PGE_2$ and $PGD_2$ are both synthesized in the brain. They have opposing actions on sleep, in that $PGE_2$ causes wakefulness and $PGD_2$ causes lowering of the body temperature and promotes sleep. COX-1 is found in abundance in the forebrain, and it is thought that prostaglandins are involved in sensory processing and in regulation of the autonomic nervous system.

## Chemical Structures and Pharmacokinetics of nsNSAIDs and Coxibs

Although all the nsNSAIDs cause COX inhibition, they have differing structures and different properties. Most NSAIDs are acidic agents, but there are a small number of non-acidic NSAIDs—including nabumetone (see Fig. 11.5).[12] NSAIDs can be classified according to their chemical structure. For example, diclofenac is classified as a phenyl acetic acid—and naproxen and ibuprofen are both propionic acids. More recent classification schemes are based on the degree of COX-2 selectivity.

Of the coxibs, both celecoxib and valdecoxib contain a sulfonamide group attached to the diarylheterocycles. Patients who are allergic to sulfonamides should avoid these particular preparations. Valdecoxib has currently been withdrawn from the market because of concerns over serious skin rashes, although it is not clear that such rashes were due to sulfonamide allergies. Rofecoxib and etoricoxib have phenylsulfone moieties attached and should be safer agents for those with sulfonamide hypersensitivity.[13]

Both of these agents are highly selective for COX-2 inhibition. Concerns over cardiovascular safety of rofecoxib have caused the withdrawal of this drug from the market. The most recently developed coxib is lumiracoxib. This drug appears to be different from the other

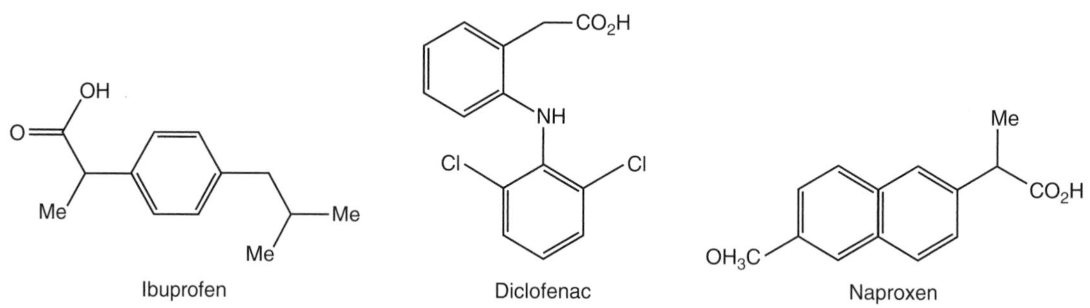

**Fig. 11.5** Structure of common nonselective NSAIDs (ibuprofen, naproxen, diclofenac).

selective coxibs in both its chemical structure and pharmacokinetics (see Table 11.1 and Fig. 11.6). It lacks a sulfur-containing moiety but has a carboxylic acid moiety. It is highly specific for COX-2 inhibition and has a relatively short half-life.

The pharmacokinetics of nsNSAIDs and coxibs have important similarities. After oral administration, there is rapid absorption of most nsNSAIDs and coxibs. They are both highly bound to plasma proteins, with less than 10% of the circulating drug remaining unbound and pharmacologically active. NSAID binding in plasma can be saturated if the concentration of drug exceeds that of albumin. The volume of distribution for most NSAIDs ranges between 0.1 and 0.3 L per kg. However, celecoxib appears to have a much higher volume of distribution and it is thought that this represents extensive tissue distribution.[14] It is interesting to note that the concentrations of NSAIDs are more sustained in synovial fluid than in plasma, perhaps explaining the prolonged effectiveness in the treatment of arthritic symptoms.[15]

With the exception of azapropazone, which is eliminated by the kidneys, most NSAIDs are metabolized by the liver and their metabolites are secreted into urine or bile. Hepatic NSAID elimination is dependent on the amount of unbound NSAID in the plasma and the enzyme activity of the liver. The plasma half-life of different NSAIDs varies from 0.25 to 70 hours. At therapeutic doses, there appears to be little difference in efficacy between drugs. However, the different half-lives and side effect profiles do influence the suitability of certain NSAIDs for different clinical situations.

In vitro assessment of the biochemical selectivity of NSAIDs for COX-1 and COX-2 inhibition is very dependent on drug concentrations. The inhibitory concentration ($IC_{50}$) is the amount of NSAID required to inhibit the activity of COX-1 and COX-2 by 50%.[16] This is often presented as an $IC_{50}$ ratio of a drug's COX-1 and COX-2 inhibitory concentrations. Larger values of $IC_{50}$ ratio represent more COX-2 selectivity (see Table 11.1).

| TABLE 11.1 PHARMACOKINETIC PROPERTIES AND TYPICAL DOSING OF SELECTED NSAIDs | | | |
|---|---|---|---|
| | Half-life (hours) | $IC_{50}$ ratio | Typical OA dosage |
| **NSAIDs** | | | |
| Diclofenac | 1–2 | 29 | 100–150 mg/day |
| Ibuprofen | 2–2.5 | 0.5 | 1,200 mg/day |
| Naproxen | 12–15 | 0.7 | 500–1,000 g/day |
| **Coxibs** | | | |
| Celecoxib | 11–16 | 30 | 200 mg/day |
| Etorixocib | 24 | 344 | 60 mg/day |
| Lumiracoxib | 3–6 | 700 | 400 mg/day |
| Rofecoxib | 16–18 | 272 | 12.5 mg/day |
| Valdecoxib | 8–11 | 61 | 10 mg/day |

$IC_{50}$ ratio refers to the ratio of $IC_{50}$ for COX-2 inhibition to COX-1 inhibition.

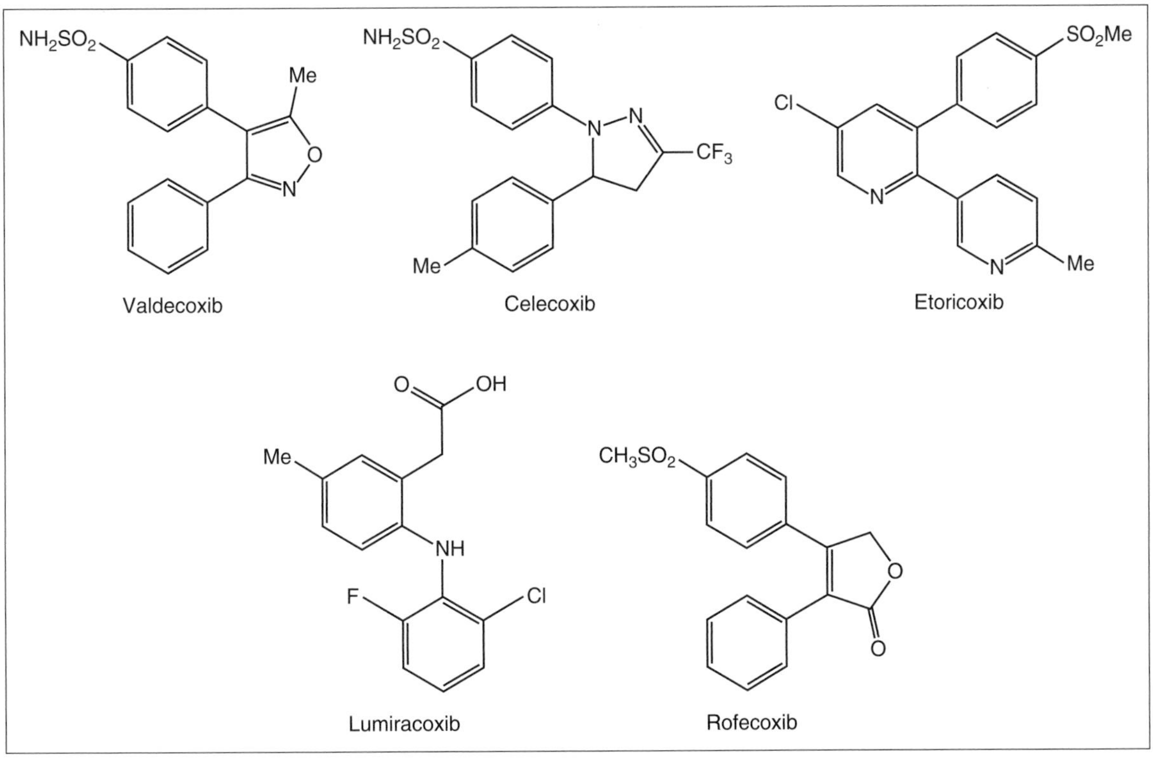

**Fig. 11.6** Structure of coxibs (celecoxib, etoricoxib, lumiracoxib, rofecoxib, valdecoxib).

# EFFICACY OF nsNSAIDS AND COXIBS IN OSTEOARTHRITIS: TREATMENT RECOMMENDATIONS

Almost all persons reading this chapter will have personally enjoyed the analgesic benefits of NSAIDs. Their efficacy in OA has been shown in numerous randomized controlled trials. This section does not address NSAIDs' efficacy in placebo-controlled trials. Instead, we focus on several areas more controversial: NSAIDs compared with acetaminophen, NSAIDs compared with opioids, and the use of topical NSAIDs. We do not focus on head-to-head comparisons between NSAIDs or coxibs because many of these trials are designed such that the comparisons are not of equal dosages, making interpretation problematic. The section ends with a summary of recommendations from the American College of Rheumatology and the European League Against Rheumatism for the use of NSAIDs in OA—noting recent quality indicators for their use.

## NSAIDs Compared with Acetaminophen for Osteoarthritis

Several trials have compared nsNSAIDs or coxibs with acetaminophen for OA of the hip and/or knee (see Table 11.2).[17-22] Although there are some data to support the efficacy of acetaminophen compared with nsNSAIDs and/or coxibs, most studies have found nsNSAIDs and/or coxibs to be superior to acetaminophen. Comparing the trials is somewhat problematic because of some important differences in design, patient populations, and outcomes measured. Subgroup analyses have suggested that perhaps more severe patients do better with nsNSAIDs or coxibs, but this finding has not been consistent.

Several "n-of-1" trials have compared acetaminophen with nsNSAIDs. These trials serially test two active comparators in a double-blind manner. In one of these n-of-1 studies, 20 patients with OA received diclofenac 100 mg/day or acetaminophen 2,000 mg/day.[23] Nineteen of the 20 patients found the trial useful for decision making. Eight patients found no difference between agents, five patients found the NSAID better, two found acetaminophen better, and five found neither agent acceptable.

## NSAIDs Compared with Opioids

There has been increasing interest in the role of opioids in patients with chronic nonmalignant pain. This interest partly stems from the recognition of cardiovascular side effects of the nsNSAIDs and coxibs. Several opioids have been compared with placebo on a background of nsNSAID use in OA (see Table 11.3).

**183**

**TABLE 11.2  SELECTED TRIALS COMPARING NSAIDs OR COXIBS WITH ACETAMINOPHEN**

| Author (year) | OA Site | Duration | NSAID or Coxib | Acetaminophen | Results* |
|---|---|---|---|---|---|
| Bradley (1991) | Knee | 4 weeks | N = 62, ibuprofen 1,200 mg/day | N = 61, 4,000 mg/day | No difference |
| | | | N = 61, ibuprofen 2,400 mg/day | … | No difference |
| Geba (2002) | Knee | 6 weeks | N = 96, rofecoxib 12.5 mg/day | N = 94, 4,000 mg/day | No difference |
| | | | N = 95, rofecoxib 25 mg/day | … | Better than acetaminophen |
| | | | N = 97, celecoxib 200 mg/day | … | No difference |
| Pincus (2001) | Hip or knee | 6 weeks | N = 112, diclofenac 150 mg/day | N = 112, 4,000 mg/day | Better than acetaminophen |
| Case (2003) | Knee | 12 weeks | N = 25, diclofenac 150 mg/day | N = 29, 4,000 mg/day | Better than acetaminophen |
| | | | N = 28, placebo | … | No difference |
| Boureau (2004) | Hip or knee | 2 weeks | N = 111, ibuprofen 1,200 mg/day | N = 111, 3,000 mg/day | Better than acetaminophen |
| Pincus (2004) | Hip or knee | 6 weeks | N = 121, celecoxib 200 mg/day | N = 114, 4,000 mg/day | Better than acetaminophen |

OA, osteoarthritis.
*Statistically significant difference in primary endpoint between NSAID (or coxib) comparator and acetaminophen.
The ellipse (…) refers to the same acetaminophen comparator dosage as the line above.

These trials use various designs, making comparison impossible.[24-27] As well, by using placebo as the comparator arm the opioids are assured of appearing superior.

The article from Schnitzer and colleagues[24] was the most rigorously conducted study. They used a 5-week open-label run-in phase, during which all patients were treated with naproxen to determine whether they would respond. Subjects were randomized in a stratified manner based on response to naproxen and then assigned to either placebo or tramadol. Among nonresponders to naproxen, tramadol was no better than placebo. However, among patients responding to

**TABLE 11.3  SELECTED TRIALS COMPARING TESTING OPIOIDS ON A BASELINE OF NSAIDs**

| Author (year) | OA Site | Duration | NSAID or Placebo | Opioid | Results* |
|---|---|---|---|---|---|
| Schnitzer (1999) | Knee | 8 weeks | N = 54,[†] placebo | N = 36, tramadol 200 mg/day | Better than placebo |
| | | | N = 68,[‡] placebo | N = 78, tramadol 200 mg/day | No difference |
| Caldwell (1999) | Back, neck, knee | 1 month | N = 36, placebo | N = 37, IR oxy/APAP | Better than placebo |
| | | | | N = 34, CR oxycodone | Better than placebo |
| Wilder-Smith (2001) | Knee, hip | 1 month | N = 30, any NSAID | N = 29, CR codeine 120 mg/day | Better than placebo |
| | | | | N = 28, tramadol 100 mg/day | Better than placebo |
| Emkey (2004) | Knee, hip | 3 months | N = 154, placebo | N = 153, tram/APAP 200–400 mg/day | Better than placebo |

OA, osteoarthritis; IR, immediate release; oxy, oxycodone; APAP, acetaminophen; CR, continuous release.
Statistically significant difference in primary endpoint between NSAID (or coxib) comparator and acetaminophen.
[†]This trial had two arms, naproxen responders and [‡]naproxen non-responders.
The ellipse (…) refers to the same acetaminophen comparator dosage as the line above.

naproxen tramadol was significantly better than placebo and allowed patients to reduce their dosage of naproxen. This finding is important in light of recent recommendations to use nsNSAIDs at the lowest possible effective dosage to reduce the risk of gastrointestinal and cardiovascular toxicity.

## Efficacy of Topical NSAIDs

Topical NSAIDs are an interesting option to consider for some patients. These preparations are not widely available in the United States but can be compounded by specialty pharmacies. They are marketed more widely in Europe and Asia. Diclofenac is one of the more commonly used topical NSAID preparations. A recent meta-analysis of these agents found that patients using topical NSAIDs were twice as likely to accrue benefit than those using placebo.[28] Numbers withdrawing from these trials due to an adverse event were equal across active topical agents and placebo. Because these agents do affect local musculoskeletal structures but have few systemic side effects, they are a good option for some patients and are part of standard recommendations (see material following).

## Recommendations for the Role of NSAIDs in Osteoarthritis

The American College of Rheumatology (ACR) and the European League Against Rheumatism (EULAR) include nsNSAIDs and coxibs as part of their recommendations for management of OA (see Table 11.4).[29,30] Both organizations consider acetaminophen first-line oral analgesia for OA. As well, the recommendations include risk stratification of patients based on known factors associated with nsNSAID-associated gastrointestinal toxicity. The similarities in the recommendations are more striking than the differences.

## Quality Indicators for Osteoarthritis

Recommendations have been further refined by the Arthritis Foundation's Quality Indicator Project into a set of "quality indicators" (see Table 11.5).[31] These quality indicators are based on the available evidence and allow recommendations to be operationalized as tools for measuring quality. Such indicators are used by a variety of consumer and employer groups when deciding on which health plan to use. The quality indicators go somewhat beyond the professional organizations' recommendations because they also recommend laboratory monitoring and methods for communicating risk.

## GASTROINTESTINAL ADVERSE EVENTS

The major source of NSAID-related adverse events is the gastrointestinal tract. As noted previously, prostaglandins are critical for maintaining the integrity of the mucosal layer within the stomach and duodenum. The major source of gastrointestinal toxicity related to NSAIDs is the upper tract lesions, from the common complaint of dyspepsia to the less common but not rare clinically evident ulcer. This chapter focuses on the upper gastrointestinal tract lesions associated with NSAIDs. First, we review the epidemiology of these lesions, including rates and risk factors. Second, we will examine some of the strategies for avoiding these lesions. Finally, the non upper-tract lesions, including liver and colon, are surveyed.

## Epidemiology of NSAID-associated Gastrointestinal Toxicity

The reported rate of gastrointestinal events in patients taking NSAIDs varies widely. This is mainly because of between-study differences in the definition

| TABLE 11.4  COMPARISON OF RECOMMENDATIONS FOR THE USE OF NSAIDs FOR OSTEOARTHRITIS* | |
|---|---|
| **American College of Rheumatology** | **European League Against Rheumatism** |
| Pharmacologic measures should be considered adjunctive to non-pharmacologic measures. | Optimal management of hip OA requires a combination of non-pharmacologic and pharmacologic treatments. |
| Acetaminophen is comparable to NSAIDs for many patients and an adequate trial should be attempted before use of an NSAID. | Because of its efficacy and safety, acetaminophen (paracetamol) up to 4 g/day is the oral analgesic of first choice for mild-moderate pain. It is the preferred long-term oral analgesic. |
| Before initiating treatment with NSAIDs, patient should be carefully screened for risk factors for NSAID-associated gastrointestinal toxicity. | NSAIDs at the lowest effective dose should be added or substituted in patients who respond inadequately to acetaminophen. |
| Options for patients with risk factors for NSAID-associated gastrointestinal toxicity include a coxib or an NSAID with misoprostol or a proton pump inhibitor. | In patients with increased gastrointestinal risk, non-selective NSAIDs plus a gastroprotective agent or a coxib should be used. |

The most recent recommendations from the European League Against Rheumatism concern hip osteoarthritis.

| TABLE 11.5 ARTHRITIS FOUNDATION QUALITY INDICATORS | |
|---|---|
| Informing patients about risk | 1. IF a patient is prescribed an NSAID (nonselective or selective), THEN the patient should be advised of the associated gastrointestinal bleeding risks and renal risks and the gastrointestinal risks should be documented. |
| | 2. IF a patient is prescribed low-dose (≤325 mg/day) aspirin, THEN the patient should be advised of the associated gastrointestinal bleeding risks. |
| | 3. IF a patient is prescribed acetaminophen AND the patient has risk factors for liver disease OR if the patient is treated with high-dose (≥4 gm/day) acetaminophen, THEN the patient should be advised of the associated risk of liver toxicity. |
| Gastrointestinal prophylaxis | 4. IF a patient is treated with a nonselective NSAID, AND the patient has risk factors for gastrointestinal bleeding,[†] THEN the patient should be treated concomitantly with either misoprostol or a PPI. |
| | 5. IF a patient is treated with a COX-2-selective NSAID AND the patient takes low-dose aspirin daily AND the patient has risk factors for gastrointestinal bleeding,[†] THEN the patient should be treated concomitantly with either misoprostol or a PPI. |
| | 6. IF a patient is treated with low-dose aspirin daily AND the patient has 2 or more risk factors for gastrointestinal bleeding,[†] THEN the patient should be treated concomitantly with either misoprostol or a PPI. |
| Selection of NSAID | 7. IF a patient who is NOT treated with low-dose aspirin has risk factors for gastrointestinal bleeding,[†] and is prescribed an NSAID, THEN the patient should receive EITHER a nonselective NSAID plus a gastroprotective agent (PPI or misoprostol) OR a COX-selective NSAID. |
| | 8. IF a patient who takes coumadin is prescribed an NSAID, THEN the NSAID should be either COX-2-selective or a nonacetylated salicylate. |
| Monitoring | 9. IF a patient is treated with daily NSAIDs (selective or nonselective) and has risk factors for gastrointestinal bleeding,[‡] THEN a CBC should be performed at baseline and during the first year after initiating therapy. |
| | 10. IF a patient is treated with daily NSAIDs (selective or nonselective) AND the patient has risk factors for developing renal insufficiency,[§] THEN a serum creatinine should be assessed at baseline and at least once in the first year following the initiation of therapy. |

NSAID = nonsteroidal antiinflammatory drug; COX = cyclooxygenase; PPI = proton pump inhibitor; CBC = complete blood count.
[†]Risk factors for gastrointestinal bleeding for indicators 4–7 defined as any of the following: age ≥75 years, peptic ulcer disease, gastrointestinal bleeding, or glucocorticoid use.
[‡]Risk factors for gastrointestinal bleeding for indicator 9 defined as any of the following: age ≥75 years, peptic ulcer disease, gastrointestinal bleeding, glucocorticoid use, or coumadin use.
[§]Risk factors for renal insufficiency defined as any of the following: age ≥75 years, diabetes mellitus, hypertension, angiotensin converting enzyme inhibitor use, or diuretic use.
Source: From Saag KG, Olivieri JJ, Patino F, Mikuls TR, Allison JJ, MacLean CH. Measuring quality in arthritis care: The Arthritis Foundation's quality indicator set for analgesics. Arthritis Rheum 2004;51:337–49.

of gastrointestinal events, the underlying risk for these events among the study populations, and the dosages of NSAIDs used. For example, the annual rate of upper gastrointestinal complications in the NSAID comparator arm of the original celecoxib new drug application was 0.5 versus 4.5% in the VIGOR trial.[32,33] The rate of gastrointestinal complications among short-term users (i.e., 1 to 2 weeks) of NSAIDs has not been carefully studied but is probably substantially lower.

Many epidemiologic studies have found an increased risk of gastrointestinal adverse events associated with nsNSAIDs. At least four meta-analyses have been published on the topic, and all find a greater than twofold increased risk for such events among users of

nsNSAIDs (range of odds ratios or relative risks from 2.7 to 5.4).[34-37] These gastrointestinal complications add up to substantial morbidity and mortality. The Arthritis, Rheumatism, and Aging Medical Information System (ARAMIS) investigators suggested that approximately 16,500 deaths and 107,000 hospitalizations annually appear related to nsNSAID-associated gastrointestinal toxicity.[38,39]

Although NSAID-associated gastrointestinal complications can affect anyone taking an nsNSAID or coxib, these events are somewhat predictable. A number of easily identified risk factors for nsNSAID-associated complications have been identified consistently across many studies (see Table 11.6).[40-45] These factors include

| Author, Year (ref.) | Study Design | GI Endpoints | Sample | Risk Factor | GI Risk OR or RR (95% CI) |
|---|---|---|---|---|---|
| Gabriel et al. 1991 (10) | Meta-analysis | Bleeds, perforations, or other GI events resulting in hospitalization or death | 8 studies pooled Not reported | Age ≥60 Concomitant corticosteroid use | 5.5 (4.6–6.6) 1.8 (1.2–2.8) |
| | | Subsequent or unspecified GI event | 10 studies pooled | History of GI AEs | 4.8 (4.1–5.6) |
| Hernandez-Diaz and Rodriguez 2000 (11) | Meta-analysis | Bleeds, perforations, or other GI events resulting in hospitalization or visit to a specialist | 7 studies pooled 12 studies pooled | Age >80 years History of ulcer | 9.2 (7.6–11.1) 5.9 (5.2–6.7) |
| Silverstein et al. 1995 (12) | Randomized, placebo-controlled trial | Perforations, gastric outlet obstructions, or bleeds | 8,843 RA patients | Age ≥75 years History of peptic ulcer History of GI bleeding | 2.5 (1.5–4.1) 2.3 (1.3–4.1) 2.6 (1.3–5.0) |
| Singh et al. 1996 (13) | Prospective cohort | Risk of hospitalization or death due to NSAID-induced GI events | 1,921 RA patients | Advancing age Previous NSAID GI side effect Prednisone use | 1.0 (1.0–1.1) 1.6 (1.0–2.4) 1.8 (1.2–2.7) |
| Shorr et al. 1993 (73) | Retrospective cohort | Hospitalization for hemorrhagic peptic ulcers | 2,203 person-years of oral anticoagulant (Medicaid enrollees) | Anticoagulant use | 12.7 (6.3–25.7) |
| Garcia Rodriguez and Jick 1994 (72) | Case control | Upper GI bleeds or perforations | 1,457 cases 10,000 controls | Anticoagulant use | 6.4 (2.8–14.6) |
| Piper et al. 1991 (88) | Case control | Hospitalization for gastric or duodenal ulcer | 1,415 cases, 7,063 controls (Medicaid enrollees) | Concomitant corticosteroid use | 4.4 (2.0–9.7) |
| Hernandez-Diaz and Rodriguez 2001 (89) | Case control | Upper GI complications | 2,105 cases 11,500 controls | Concomitant oral steroid use | 8.9 (5.0–15.8) |

Source: From Saag KG, Olivieri JJ, Patino F, Mikuls TR, Allison JJ, MacLean CH. Measuring quality in arthritis care: The Arthritis Foundation's quality indicator set for analgesics. Arthritis Rheum 2004;51:337–49.

older age, history of gastrointestinal bleeding or peptic ulcer, concomitant glucocorticoids, and concomitant anticoagulant use. Age is probably a continuous risk factor above age 60. Any one of these factors is associated with a significant increase in risk, and some have suggested that they can be combined into a predictive index.

## Strategies for Minimizing NSAID-associated Gastrointestinal Toxicity

By stratifying patients based on the previously cited risk factors, one can attempt to selectively prescribe nsNSAIDs to patients at lower risk of gastrointestinal toxicity. However, there are occasions when patients with OA have extremely good responses to nsNSAIDs but also have characteristics that put them at high risk of gastrointestinal toxicity. In these circumstances, several options exist, including topical NSAIDs (see previous material) and the addition of misoprostol or a proton pump inhibitor.

Before reviewing the data regarding misoprostol or proton pump inhibitors for nsNSAID-associated gastrointestinal complications, it is important to note two major limitations of these data. First, almost no studies have examined primary prevention of nsNSAID toxicity. Rather, studies have enrolled patients after an nsNSAID-associated bleeding episode and then examined healing or re-bleeding rates. Although these are interesting groups of patients and important endpoints, these results may not apply to the primary prevention of nsNSAID-associated toxicity. Second, very few studies have primarily examined clinical endpoints. Instead, they have relied on endoscopic data regarding ulcers. Endoscopic ulcers are related to actual clinical events but are far from an ideal surrogate endpoint.

Misoprostol is a prostaglandin analogue that has been shown to prevent clinically apparent nsNSAID-associated gastrointestinal bleeding.[46] The MUCOSA trial enrolled almost 9,000 patients with rheumatoid arthritis (RA) who were receiving continuous nsNSAID treatment for pain. Patients received misoprostol 200 mcg or placebo four times daily in a double-blind manner. At the end of the 6-month follow-up, 0.56% (25 of 4,404) of patients receiving misoprostol experienced a serious gastrointestinal complication.

This compared favorably with the 0.95% (42 of 4,439) of those taking placebo who reached the primary endpoint (p = 0.049). It is important to note that overall more adverse events were noted among subjects taking misoprostol than placebo. These included diarrhea (10%), abdominal pain (7%), dyspepsia (5%), nausea (5%), and flatulence (5%). However, this study demonstrates the effectiveness of misoprostol as co-therapy with nsNSAIDs. It also points out the relatively low rate of serious gastrointestinal complications, even among older patients (mean age = 68 years) with RA.

Although not as thoroughly tested as the dose of 200 mcg four times daily, many advocate lower-dose co-administration of misoprostol. A common dosage form of misoprostol combines 200 mcg with diclofenac 50 or 75 mg. This is generally given twice daily. It is also important to note that misoprostol is indicated by the Food and Drug Administration as an abortifascient. Thus, women of child-bearing age must have a negative pregnancy test before using it as co-therapy to reduce NSAID-associated gastrointestinal toxicity.

The second strategy shown to reduce actual clinical events is co-administration of a proton pump inhibitor.[47] Several endoscopic studies suggested that adding a proton pump inhibitor to an nsNSAID would reduce the risk of nsNSAID-associated gastrointestinal toxicity.[48,49] These studies compared omeprazole 20 or 40 mg per day to ranitidine or misoprostol in patients with nsNSAID-associated endoscopic ulcers. Both trials found improved endoscopic healing with omeprazole. As well, secondary endpoints that included clinical symptoms suggest that all strategies reduced symptoms—with omeprazole-treated patients reporting the least dyspepsia.

However, omeprazole has been shown in one randomized trial to produce rates of recurrent bleeding similar to those of celecoxib.[50] This trial enrolled nearly 300 patients with a known nsNSAID-associated gastrointestinal bleed. All patients were treated acutely. If patients were found to have *H. pylori*, this was eradicated. They were then randomized to celecoxib 200 mg twice daily versus diclofenac 75 mg twice daily plus omeprazole 20 mg daily. Over the 6 months of the study, recurrent ulcer bleeding defined as a clinical event with proven endoscopic ulcers were found in 4.9% of patients in the celecoxib arm and 6.4% in the diclofenac plus omeprazole arm. These rates were not statistically different. Based on these data, many recommend that an nsNSAID plus a proton pump inhibitor is equal in safety to a coxib.

## Clinical Management Algorithm

A strategy for initial management of symptomatic OA is outlined in Fig. 11.7. As noted previously, non-pharmacologic measures (exercise, weight loss, taping, bracing, or cane) should be tried in most patients. Acetaminophen, unless contraindicated, is first-line pharmacologic treatment for all patients. A 2-week trial of acetaminophen 1,000 mg tid-qid should be attempted. If this is not sufficient, a trial of low-dose nsNSAID may be warranted. Patients who will need nsNSAID treatment long term should be risk-stratified based on the factors listed in Fig. 11.7.

If they meet at least one of these factors, alternative strategies should be considered. These include topical NSAIDs and/or low-potency opioids in patients without contraindications. If the patient wants to pursue NSAID treatment and has a risk factor for nsNSAID-associated gastrointestinal toxicity, a coxib (or co-administration of misoprostol or a proton pump inhibitor) should be strongly considered. In addition, patients at high risk for future cardiovascular events may want to avoid coxibs and possibly nsNSAIDs (see material following).

## Miscellaneous Gastrointestinal Toxicity

Liver toxicity is a well-recognized but very rare adverse event related to nsNSAIDs and coxibs. Although it is a class warning across all nsNSAIDs and coxibs, it may occur more frequently with diclofenac. However, good estimates of hepatotoxicity by drug are not available.[51] The best estimates suggest that clinically important liver toxicity occurs in 1 per 10,000 patient courses of nsNSAIDs or coxibs.[52]

Many more patients will have slight elevations in liver enzymes. In fact, in one large trial comparing ibuprofen or diclofenac to celecoxib the rates of liver enzyme abnormalities were 2.3% (93 of 3,981) for the nsNSAIDs and 0.6% (24 of 3,987) for celecoxib.[53] The risk factors for drug-induced liver toxicity have not been well studied but probably include concomitant use of hepatotoxins (drugs, alcohol) and underlying liver disease (hepatitis B or C). The mechanisms underlying

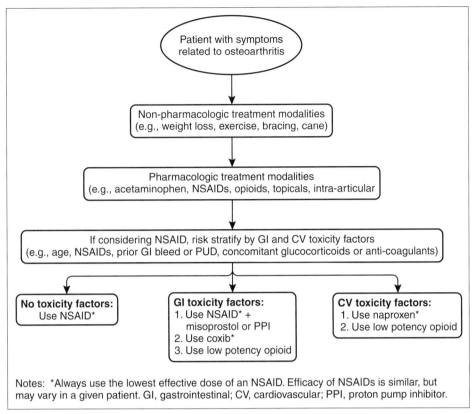

**Fig. 11.7** Recommendations to minimize gastrointestinal toxicity in NSAID users.

the hepatoxicity are immunologic and may vary by agent and person. The clinical presentations can include blood test abnormalities, mild cholestasis, and severe hepatocellular injury.

In addition to the well-recognized liver and upper gastrointestinal tract toxicities, nsNSAIDs and coxibs have been associated with lower tract adverse events. Ulcers can occur anywhere from the mouth to the anus, and nsNSAIDs are recognized as a common cause of large intestinal ulcers.[54] Colitis has been reported as a result of NSAID use, and at times the lesions can be confused with those of Crohn's disease.[55] The mechanisms of NSAID-induced lower tract toxicity are not clear. Although systemic prostaglandin inhibition probably plays a role, there may also be some direct effect of these agents within the large intestine.

## CARDIOVASCULAR ADVERSE EVENTS

The cardiovascular potential of NSAIDs was recognized long ago with the development of aspirin as an anti-thrombotic agent. However, the effect of these agents in the cardiovascular system has taken prominence as recent data have raised substantial concerns regarding the coxibs and nsNSAIDs. Many potential

mechanisms linking these agents to adverse events in the cardiovascular system have been suggested and reviewed.[56] This section reviews the proposed mechanisms for this link, examines the data from randomized controlled trials and observational epidemiology, and explores a possible interaction between some agents and aspirin.

## Mechanisms

Coxibs had initially been marketed for their analgesic and anti-inflammatory benefits without the bleeding risk from COX-1 inhibition. This claim was based on the understanding that platelet-derived COX-1 is the major source of thromboxane. However, the origins of circulating prostacyclin (the other important vasoactive eicosanoid) were not as clear. Prostacyclin plays a critical role in fibronolysis and vasodilatation, counterbalancing the effects of thromboxane on platelet aggregation and vasoconstriction.

Studies of healthy volunteers revealed that urinary levels of a prostacyclin metabolite were lowered in subjects taking rofecoxib, suggesting that endovascular production of prostacyclin may be COX-2 mediated.[57] These data suggest that COX-2 may play a role in vascular health. Furthermore, its inhibition may create an imbalance between thromboxane and prostacyclin, favoring thrombosis and vasoconstriction. The potential risk of thrombosis based on these mechanisms was articulated in an early review of coxibs.[58] A series of elegant knockout mice studies suggest that the imbalance between prostacyclin and thromboxane may account for some of the cardiovascular risk associated with these agents.[59,60] It is unclear whether this imbalance may also link nsNSAIDs with cardiovascular outcomes. Even the nsNSAIDs are differentially selective for COX-1 and COX-2,[61] and these agents may be associated with cardiovascular harm.

The vasoreactive potential of coxibs was further demonstrated in several human studies that measured flow-mediated dilatation and found that both celecoxib and rofecoxib had effects on endovascular function.[62-65] Other possible mechanisms linking certain nsNSAIDs and/or coxibs to long-term cardiovascular outcomes include changes in blood pressure and possible oxidative modification of biologic lipids.[66] The hypertensive potential of nsNSAIDs was recognized over a decade ago, with some suggestion that certain agents had greater effects on blood pressure than others.[67,68] A heterogeneous effect on blood pressure has been noted between celecoxib and rofecoxib.[69]

No one mechanism linking coxibs (or nsNSAIDs) to cardiovascular events has been proven. Several compelling possibilities have been described: thrombosis and vasoconstriction associated with an imbalance between thromboxane and prostacyclin, hypertension from inhibition of prostaglandin-dependent counter-regulatory mechanisms, and COX-independent oxidative stress. These potential mechanisms could explain both short-term and long-term risks, similar to those suggested by the clinical trial and observational data.

## Randomized Controlled Trials

Rofecoxib was withdrawn from the market by its manufacturer in late 2004 after determining that 25 mg daily was associated with a doubling of the risk for thrombotic cardiovascular events with long-term use. However, the potential for an elevated thrombotic risk with rofecoxib was widely appreciated in 2000 with publication of the VIGOR trial.[70] This trial compared 50 mg daily of rofecoxib versus 500 mg twice daily of naproxen in 8,076 patients with RA (see Table 11.7). Aspirin users were excluded from this trial. Although the patients in the rofecoxib arm experienced fewer gastrointestinal outcomes, they suffered five times more heart attacks and the relative risk for severe thrombotic cardiovascular events was doubled. The event curves diverged after approximately 6 weeks.

The APPROVe (Adenomatous Polyp Prevention on Vioxx) trial tested rofecoxib 25 mg daily against placebo among 2,586 patients with a prior adenomatous polyp

(see Table 11.7).[71] Aspirin use was reported by 17% at entry. Patients in the rofecoxib arm experienced a four- to fivefold increase in the risk of congestive heart failure. Severe thrombotic cardiovascular events were approximately twice as frequent in the rofecoxib arm than in the placebo arm. Divergence in these curves became apparent after 18 months of follow-up. Until the APPROVe trial, several other trials with rofecoxib 25 mg had not demonstrated an increased cardiovascular risk—although these were generally of shorter duration.[72]

### Celecoxib

The CLASS trial compared celecoxib 400 mg twice daily with ibuprofen 800 mg three times daily or diclofenac 75 mg twice daily (see Table 11.7).[73] Patients with OA and RA were enrolled, and regular aspirin use was reported at the trial's initiation by 22% of patients. Rates of cardiovascular events did not differ significantly between the celecoxib users and the combined nsNSAID user group.

The Adenoma Prevention with Celecoxib (APC) trial demonstrated that high-dose long-term celecoxib use is associated with an increase in the risk of thrombotic cardiovascular events (see Table 11.7).[74] This trial randomized 2,035 patients with prior adenomatous polyps to receive celecoxib 200 mg twice daily, celecoxib 400 mg twice daily, or placebo. At the trial outset, 30% of patients reported aspirin use. Thirty-three months after its initiation, the trial was halted because of an increase in the risk of cardiovascular events observed in both celecoxib arms (see Table 11.7). There appeared to be a dose-response effect, with the higher dosage of celecoxib associated with more frequent cardiovascular events.

A second adenomatous polyp prevention trial, the Prevention of Spontaneous Adenomatous Polyps (PreSAP), also tested celecoxib versus placebo (see Table 11.7).[75] This trial randomized 1,561 subjects to once-daily (not twice) dosing of celecoxib at 400 mg or placebo. After 33 months of follow-up, there was no increase in cardiovascular events observed in the celecoxib arm versus the placebo arm.

### Valdecoxib

There have been several short-term studies of valdecoxib in patients with arthritis who have not had adequate numbers of events to deem the medication safe or unsafe. However, the results of two trials in patients undergoing coronary artery bypass grafting, the CABG I[76] and CABG II,[77] have found an increased risk of cardiovascular events in patients using valdecoxib and its intravenous formulation parecoxib (see Table 11.7). These trials were designed to determine whether valdecoxib might have a role in postoperative pain management.

TABLE 11.7  CARDIOVASCULAR EVENTS OBSERVED IN LONG-TERM TRIALS OF COXIBS AND NSAIDs

| Trial (Reference) | Patient Population | Follow-up (Months)[a] | Aspirin (%) | Coxib Arm Dosage | N | Events | Rate[b] | Comparator Arm Dosage | N | Events | Rate[b] | Relative Risk (95% CI) |
|---|---|---|---|---|---|---|---|---|---|---|---|---|
| **Rofecoxib Trials** | | | | | | | | | | | | |
| Bombardier (2000) | RA | 9 | 0 | Rofecoxib 50 mg qd | 4,047 | 45 | 1.67 | Naproxen 500 mg bid | 4,029 | 19 | 0.70 | 2.38 (1.39–4.00) |
| Bresalier (2005) | Adenomatous polyp | 30 | 16 | Rofecoxib 25 mg qd | 1,287 | 46 | 1.50 | Placebo | 1,299 | 26 | 0.78 | 1.92 (1.19–3.11) |
| **Celecoxib Trials** | | | | | | | | | | | | |
| Silverstein (2000) | OA and RA | 9 | 22 | Celecoxib 400 mg bid | 3,987 | 34 | 1.5 | Ibuprofen 800 mg tid | 1,985 | 20 | 1.8 | 0.83[‡] |
| | | | | | | | | Diclofenac 75 mg bid | 1,996 | 15 | 1.4 | 1.07[‡] |
| Solomon (2005) | Adenomatous polyp | ≥33 | 30 | Celecoxib 200 mg bid | 685 | 16 | 0.78 | Placebo | 679 | 7 | 0.34 | 2.3 (0.9–5.5) |
| | | | | Celecoxib 400 mg bid | 671 | 23 | 1.14 | … | … | … | … | 3.4 (1.4–2.8) |
| PreSAP (2005) | Adenomatous polyp | ≥33 | 16 | Celecoxib 400 mg qd | 933 | 20 | 0.72 | Placebo | 628 | 12 | 0.64 | 1.1 (0.6–2.3) |

OA, osteoarthritis; RA, rheumatoid arthritis; AD, Alzheimer's disease; CABG, coronary artery bypass graft; NA, not available. The ellipse (…) signifies that the data are the same as the row above. Some of the cardiovascular events were not adjudicated in the references noted.
[a]Median duration of follow-up, unless noted.
[b]Rate refers to cardiovascular events per 100 person-years. The definition of event differed by study (see text for definitions).

*Continued*

## TABLE 11.7 CARDIOVASCULAR EVENTS OBSERVED IN LONG-TERM TRIALS OF COXIBS AND NSAIDs—cont'd

| Trial (Reference) | Patient Population | Follow-up (Months)[a] | Aspirin (%) | Coxib Arm | | | | Comparator Arm | | | | Relative Risk (95% CI) |
|---|---|---|---|---|---|---|---|---|---|---|---|---|
| | | | | N | Dosage | Events | Rate[b] | N | Dosage | Events | Rate[b] | |
| **Valdecoxib Trials** | | | | | | | | | | | | |
| Ott (2003) | Post CABG | 44 days | 100 | 311 | Parecoxib/valdecoxib 20 mg bid[d] | 24 | NA | 151 | Placebo/placebo | 4 | NA | 2.91[c] |
| Nussmeier (2005) | Post CABG | 40 days | 100 | 555 | Parecoxib/valdecoxib 20 mg bid[d] | 11 | NA | 560 | Placebo/placebo | 3 | NA | 2.0 (0.5–8.1) |
| | | | | 556 | Placebo/valdecoxib 20 mg bid | 6 | NA | … | … | … | … | 3.7 (1.0–13.5) |
| **Lumiracoxib Trial** | | | | | | | | | | | | |
| Farkouh (2004) | OA | 12 | 22 | 4,376 | Lumiracoxib 40 mg | 19 | 0.59 | 4,397 | Ibuprofen 800 mg tid | 23 | 0.74 | 0.76 (0.41–1.40) |
| | | | 25 | 4,741 | Lumiracoxib 40 mg | 40 | 1.10 | 4,730 | Naproxen 500 mg bid | 27 | 0.76 | 1.46 (0.89–2.37) |

[a]When not available, the relative risks were calculated as the crude event rate in coxib users divided by the crude event rate in the comparator group.
[d]In CABG I and CABG II, medications were administered by intravenous route (parecoxib) for the first 3 days and then by mouth for 11 more days in CABG I and for 7 more days in CABG II.
Source: Solomon D. Selective cyclooxygenase 2 inhibitors and cardiovascular events. Arthritis Rheum 2005;52(7):1968–78.

The risk ratio for confirmed cardiovascular events was significantly elevated in both trials.

### Lumiracoxib

Lumiracoxib has a structure different from other agents. It has a very short half-life but can be dosed once daily because of its lipophilic nature. It was approved for use by the European Medicines Agency for patients with OA, RA, or acute gouty arthritis. The TARGET trial compared 1 year of therapy with lumiracoxib 400 mg once daily to naproxen 500 mg twice daily or ibuprofen 800 mg three times daily.[78] Patients with OA aged 50 and older were randomized stratified on age and low-dose aspirin use. The rates for the primary cardiovascular endpoint were similar among lumiracoxib and NSAID users (see Table 11.7). The comparisons between lumiracoxib and each nsNSAID (ibuprofen and naproxen) individually suggested some possible differences, but none was statistically significant.

## Observational Epidemiology

Several pharmacoepidemiologic analyses have been published on coxibs and cardiovascular disease (see Table 11.8). Ray and colleagues examined celecoxib and rofecoxib use among Medicaid beneficiaries in Tennessee.[79] Subjects were required to be new users of these agents and comparisons were made with nonusers. Adjusted models used Poisson regression, which assumes a constant risk of outcomes over the full length of follow-up. This study found no increased risk with celecoxib, no increased risk with 25 mg or less daily of rofecoxib, but a doubling of the risk with rofecoxib above 25 mg daily.

Solomon and colleagues published a similar analysis using data from low-income Medicare beneficiaries who also have a drug benefit from Pennsylvania or New Jersey.[80] They drew from a source population of approximately 500,000 persons. The primary analysis used information from 1999 to 2000. All analyses were pre-specified, with the endpoint being heart attack. Users of coxibs were compared with non-users, as well as to each other and to nsNSAID users. Multivariable models included information on potential confounders that preceded use of the agents of interest.

The primary analysis found an increased risk of heart attack for rofecoxib users compared with non-users and to celecoxib users (see Table 11.8). The risk with rofecoxib tended toward an increase compared with nsNSAIDs but did not reach statistical significance. Pre-specified dosage analyses revealed a dose-response relationship between rofecoxib and heart attack with all comparators. In addition, secondary analysis among new users revealed that the first 90 days were the period of highest risk for rofecoxib use (odds ratio = 1.39) compared with later than 90 days (odds ratio = 0.96).

Celecoxib was not associated with an increased risk of acute myocardial infarction (AMI) in any of these analyses. Although the potential effect of confounders was deemed minimal by examining an external data set,[81] these analyses are limited by lack of information on some cardiovascular risk factors.

An FDA-sponsored epidemiologic analysis examined beneficiaries of a large health maintenance organization.[82] This analysis compared current use of coxibs and nsNSAIDs to remote use (>60 days prior) of these agents. The primary analysis found a statistically significant increase in cardiovascular risk with rofecoxib dosages above 25 mg daily (see Table 11.8). At dosages of 25 mg or less daily, the risk was elevated but did not reach statistical significance. Celecoxib was not associated with an increase in cardiovascular risk. Naproxen use was associated with a slight increase in risk. An important strength of this study was the use of patient surveys to augment cardiovascular risk factor data.

Kimmel and colleagues conducted a non-claims-based epidemiologic analysis in 36 hospitals located in five counties.[83] These investigators selected cases of heart attack from hospital discharge information. They then attempted to enroll these patients and controls from the same county. The response rate was 50 to 55% for each group. Drug exposure information was gathered as part of a detailed telephone survey conducted by trained interviewers. Modest response rates and potential recall bias limit this study, but the detailed collection of cardiovascular risk factor data and aspirin information is an important strength. The results of this study are in line with other analyses (see Table 11.8).

Two observational epidemiologic studies, from Ontario and Maryland, have found no increased risk with any coxib (see Table 11.8).[84,85] Each of these studies had potential limitations. The Canadian study restricted the analysis to persons who filled multiple prescriptions and thus may have missed events that occur with a first and only prescription. As well, these analyses may have over-controlled for potential mediators of the coxibs' effects on the cardiovascular system because they included hypertension, congestive heart failure, and angina diagnosed after the initiation of medications as adjusters in multivariable models. The methods used by the Maryland investigators are complex, but a key question is whether use of coxibs and/or nsNSAIDs was required to overlap with the event dates. If drug exposure was not confirmed on the event date, it is impossible to say anything meaningful about the potential association between coxibs and cardiovascular events.

## Possible Interactions with Aspirin

Clinical pharmacology studies have also raised the possibility that some nsNSAIDs may block the benefits

TABLE 11.8  RELATIVE RISK OF CARDIOVASCULAR EVENTS OBSERVED IN EPIDEMIOLOGIC STUDIES OF COXIBS

| Study (Reference) | Patient Population | Coxib | | | Comparator* | | | Relative Risk (95% CI) |
|---|---|---|---|---|---|---|---|---|
| | | Agent | N | Events | Group | N | Events[†] | |
| Ray (2002) | Medicaid, mean | Rofecoxib ≤25 mg | 20,245 | 55 | Non-use[‡] | 202,916 | 3,085 | 1.01 (0.77–1.33) |
| | age = 62 | Rofecoxib >25 mg | 3887 | 13 | … | … | … | 1.70 (0.98–2.95) |
| | | Celecoxib, any dose | 22,337 | 74 | … | … | … | 0.96 (0.76–1.21) |
| Mamdani (2003) | Ontario, | Rofecoxib, any dose | 12,156 | 58 | Non-use | 100,000 | 418 | 1.0 (0.8–1.4) |
| | mean age = 76 | Celecoxib, any dose | 15,271 | 75 | … | … | … | 0.9 (0.7–1.2) |
| Solomon (2004) | Medicare, | Rofecoxib ≤25 mg | 876 | 202 | Non-use | 49,044 | 9,793 | 1.21 (1.01–1.44) |
| | mean age = 79 | Rofecoxib >25 mg | 65 | 23 | … | … | … | 1.70 (1.07–2.71) |
| | | Celecoxib ≤200 mg | 1,767 | 341 | … | … | … | 0.92 (0.83–1.03) |
| | | Celecoxib >200 mg | 373 | 74 | … | … | … | 0.94 (0.74–1.19) |
| Graham (2005) | HMO, | Rofecoxib ≤25 mg | 246 | 58 | Remote use | 23,378 | 4,658 | 1.23 (0.89–1.71) |
| | mean age = 68 | Rofecoxib >25 mg | 18 | 10 | … | … | … | 3.00 (1.09–8.31) |
| | | Celecoxib, any dose | 617 | 126 | … | … | … | 0.84 (0.67–1.04) |
| Kimmel (2005) | Community, | Rofecoxib, any dose | 105 | 27 | Non-use | 5,845 | 1,354 | 1.16 (0.70–1.93) |
| | mean age = 55 | Celecoxib, any dose | 105 | 18 | … | … | … | 0.43 (0.23–0.79) |
| Shaya (2005) | Medicaid, | Rofecoxib, any dose | 497 | NA | Other NSAIDs | 5,245 | NA | 0.99 (0.76–1.30) |
| | mean age = NA | Celecoxib, any dose | 507 | NA | … | … | … | 1.19 (0.93–1.51) |

CI, confidence interval; HMO, health maintenance organization.
The ellipse (…) represents repeated rows of data.
Some of the studies included multiple comparator groups. To simplify comparisons across studies, the number of comparators has been limited.
[†]See text for study-specific definitions of cardiovascular events.
[‡]Non-use refers to no NSAID or coxib use.
Source: Solomon D. Selective cyclooxygenase 2 inhibitors and cardiovascular events. Arthritis Rheum 2005;52(7):1968–78.

of aspirin.[86] In one study, ibuprofen was shown to block aspirin's ability to inhibit platelet function. This may occur because of competitive inhibition by ibuprofen at the acetylation site in the platelet COX-1 enzyme. Without access to this site, aspirin is unable to irreversibly inhibit thromboxane $A_2$ production in the platelet. Some clinical studies of this issue have found an increased risk of cardiovascular events in patients taking aspirin and concomitant ibuprofen, but not all (see Table 11.9).[87-92] These authors have recommended limiting use of ibuprofen in patients requiring cardioprotective aspirin.[93]

## OTHER ADVERSE EVENTS

The gastrointestinal and cardiovascular toxicities of the NSAIDs are widely recognized. However, these agents also have notable side effects involving the renal, dermatologic, and central nervous systems (see Table 11.10).

### Renal Adverse Events

The nephrotoxicity of NSAIDs and coxibs is well recognized and has several different clinical manifestations. These include sodium retention, hyporeninemic hypoaldosteronism, pre-renal azotemia (acute tubular necrosis if untreated), acute interstitial nephritis, and nephrotic syndrome. Pre-renal azotemia is quite common in persons with already reduced renal blood flow and appears due to inhibition of the prostaglandin-mediated counter-regulatory mechanisms of the kidney. Edema, hypertension, and acute renal failure are several manifestations of pre-renal azotemia. As well, hyporeninemic hypoaldosteronism is not uncommon in diabetics using NSAIDs and manifests with hyperkalemia and a mild metabolic acidosis.

Acute renal function has been noted to be reduced in many studies with most agents, including nsNSAIDs and coxibs.[94-98] In addition, many of the nsNSAIDs have been implicated as causing chronic renal failure. Relative risks range from 2 to 8 in two well-done epidemiologic studies.[99,100] However, the existence of a chronic NSAID nephropathy has been debated by some.

### Cutaneous

Almost every type of cutaneous drug reaction has been described with NSAIDs. This includes morbilliform eruptions, fixed drug eruptions, erythema multiforme (Stevens–Johnson syndrome or toxic epidermal necrolysis), pseudoporphyria, and photosensitivity. The epidemiology of these reactions has not been extensively studied, but one estimate is that 27% of all adverse drug eruptions are from NSAIDs.[101] Although most of these reactions are mild, Stevens–Johnson syndrome

has been described in a relatively large number of patients taking valdecoxib and is one of the reasons the FDA requested that its manufacturer remove it from the market.[102]

## Central Nervous System Side Effects

Aseptic meningitis is well recognized among persons taking almost all NSAIDs. Many of the reported cases are with ibuprofen in patients with autoimmune diseases. However, normal hosts taking NSAIDs other than ibuprofen have developed well-documented cases of aseptic meningitis.

## PHARMACO-ECONOMICS

The advent of the coxibs created great controversy over the appropriate use of NSAIDs. The coxibs were developed to improve the gastrointestinal toxicity profile of NSAIDs but were then marketed widely and used beyond the high-risk gastrointestinal patients. Although much of the marketing frenzy quieted down when the potential cardiovascular toxicities of coxibs were revealed, the controversy regarding which patients should get which agents and the implications for health care costs provides an important pharmaco-economic lesson.

### NSAID Utilization

NSAIDs are very popular medications. Investigators from the Nurses Health Study found that among women 52 to 77 years of age 10.8% report using NSAIDs 6+ days per week, and 26.7% at least 1 day per week.[103] The recognition of how large a public health problem NSAID-associated gastrointestinal toxicity had become and the advent of coxibs have focused attention on NSAID utilization patterns.

Investigators using several different data sources have observed that many coxib users did not have clear indications for these drugs.[104,105] Much of the use of coxibs appears to have been driven by physician preferences and specialty, which may have been influenced by nonclinical factors.[106,107] One study found that patients who received concomitant aspirin were more likely to receive an nsNSAID.[108] It is also interesting to note that many patients receiving nsNSAIDs have risk factors for NSAID-associated gastrointestinal toxicity.[109,110] Thus, there appears to be both an overuse of coxibs and an underuse of strategies to reduce NSAID-associated gastrointestinal toxicity.

### Pharmaco-economics of Coxibs

Several different groups have investigated the economics of coxib use. These agents can cost from 5 to 10 times more than a generic NSAID and do not confer greater benefit to patients. In selected groups at high risk for

**TABLE 11.9 EPIDEMIOLOGIC STUDIES OF THE INTERACTION BETWEEN IBUPROFEN AND ASPIRIN**

| Author (Reference) | Study Population | Study Design | Source of Drug Information | Outcome of Interest | Exposure of Interest | N | Events N | Results Adjusted[a] |
|---|---|---|---|---|---|---|---|---|
| **Studies Demonstrating a Possible Increased Risk of CVD Events with Ibuprofen[b] and Aspirin Combinations** | | | | | | | | |
| MacDonald (2003) | Tayside general practice | Cohort | Medicines monitoring unit-prescription dispensing | CVD mortality | | | | HR (95% CI) |
| | | | | | ASA (Reference) | 6,285 | 1,350 | |
| | | | | | ASA and ibuprofen | 187 | 39 | 1.73 (1.05, 2.84) |
| | | | | | ASA and diclofenac | 206 | 44 | 0.80 (0.49, 1.31) |
| Kimmel (2004) | Hospital discharge after MI and community controls | Case control | Retrospective survey including OTC meds | First hospitalized non-fatal MI | | | | OR (95% CI) |
| | | | | | ASA (Reference) | 1,059 | 288 | |
| | | | | | ASA and NSAID users | 366 | 74 | 0.83 (0.58, 1.17) |
| | | | | | ASA and frequent ibuprofen[c] | NA | NA | 2.03 (0.60, 6.84) |
| Kurth (2003) | Male primary prevention (Physicians Health Study) | Randomized controlled trial | Prospective survey via mailed questionnaire every 6–12 months | First MI | | | | HR (95% CI) |
| | | | | | ASA (Reference) | 10,780 | 107 | |
| | | | | | ASA and NSAID[d] (1–59 days) | 195 | 26 | 1.19 (0.77, 1.85) |
| | | | | | ASA and NSAID[d] (≥60 days) | 25 | 6 | 2.84(1.24, 6.52) |

**Studies Demonstrating No Increased Risk of CVD Events with Ibuprofen* and Aspirin Combinations**

| Study | Population | Study design | Data source | Outcome | Exposure | | | |
|---|---|---|---|---|---|---|---|---|
| Curtis (2003) | Medicare patients post–MI (Cooperative Cardiovascular Project) | Cohort | Hospital discharge medications | 1-year mortality | ASA (Reference) | 66,739 | 11,546 | HR (95% CI) |
| | | | | | ASA and NSAIDs | 2,733 | 432 | 0.96 (0.86, 1.06) |
| | | | | | ASA and ibuprofen | 844 | 118 | 0.84 (0.70, 1.01) |
| Patel (2003) | Veterans Affairs patients | Cohort | Pharmacy records | MI | ASA (Reference) | 10,239 | 684 | RR (95% CI) |
| | | | | | ASA and ibuprofen | 3,859 | 138 | 0.61 (0.50, 0.73) |
| Garcia-Rodriguez (2004) | Primary care (GPRD) | Nested case control | Primary care prescriptions | MI and CVD mortality | ASA (Reference) | 3,515 | 1,119 | OR (95% CI) |
| | | | | | ASA and NSAID | 466 | 163 | 1.10 (0.89, 1.37) |
| | | | | | ASA and ibuprofen | 132 | 46 | 1.08 (0.74, 1.58) |

ASA, aspirin; HR, hazard ratio; CI, confidence interval; MI, myocardial infarction; RR, relative risk; NA, not available; OR, odds ratio; GPRD, general practice research database.
[a] Adjusted for demographics and measures of CVD risk in all but the Patel study.
[b] Some studies did not examine ibuprofen separately.
[c] Frequent ibuprofen use was defined as use ≥4 times/week.
[d] Type of NSAID not known. Duration of NSAID use was estimated for each year of the study from the frequency of use in the preceding month.
Source: Solomon DH, Goodson NJ. The cardiovascular system in rheumatic disease: The next "extra-articular" manifestation? J Rheumatol 2005;32:1415–18.

| TABLE 11.10 SELECTED OTHER NSAID- AND COXIB-RELATED TOXICITIES | |
|---|---|
| **Organ** | **Manifestation** |
| **Renal** | |
| | Pre-renal azotemia (acute tubular necrosis) |
| | Hyporeninemic hypoaldosteronism |
| | Acute interstitial nephritis |
| | Nephrotic syndrome |
| | Sodium retention |
| **Cutaneous** | |
| | Stevens–Johnson syndrome (erythema multiforme or toxic epidermal necrolysis) |
| | Photosensitivity |
| | Fixed drug eruption |
| | Morbilliform eruption |
| | Pseudoporphyria |
| **CNS** | |
| | Aseptic meningitis |
| | Hearing loss |

gastrointestinal toxicity, they may be a good deal from an economic standpoint. Analyses by two groups suggested that using coxibs in patients with at least one risk factor for an NSAID-associated gastrointestinal adverse event was economically reasonable.[111,112] However, coxib use in young patients without risk factors was associated with cost-effectiveness ratios much higher than accepted limits.

## Improving NSAID Utilization

Two large-scale interventions have attempted to improve the use of analgesics in the elderly living in nursing homes and the community.[113,114] Both interventions used educational programs to improve patient selection for nsNSAIDs and acetaminophen and attempted to reduce days of nsNSAID exposure. The nursing home intervention produced significant improvements in analgesia use, whereas the effects of the community-based intervention were much more modest.

## SUMMARY

As pain is one of the most prominent complaints in OA, NSAIDs will remain an important option for treatment. However, their relatively narrow therapeutic index will ensure that their use remains controversial. Choosing an NSAID for treatment requires balancing the potential risks and benefits for an individual patient. Pharmacologic research is concentrated on making safer NSAIDs, and epidemiologists are working on determining who are appropriate candidates for which medications.

## ACKNOWLEDGMENT

James Rossi provided excellent technical assistance in compiling figures, tables, and references.

## REFERENCES

1. Moreland LW, Russell AS, Paulus HE. Management of rheumatoid arthritis: The historical context. J Rheumatol 2001;50:1431–52.
2. Simmons DL, Botting RM, Hla T. Cyclooxygenase isozymes: The biology of prostaglandin synthesis and inhibition. Pharmacological Reviews 2004;56(3):387–437.
3. FitzGerald GA, Patrono C. The coxibs, selective inhibitors of cyclooxygenase-2. N Engl J Med 2001;345(6):433–42.
4. Simmons DL, Botting RM, Hla T. Cyclooxygenase isozymes: The biology of prostaglandin synthesis and inhibition. Pharmacological Reviews 2004;56(3):387–437.
5. Brune K, Hinz B. Selective cyclooxygenase-2 inhibitors: Similarities and differences. Scand J Rheumatol 2004;33(1):1–6.
6. Bombardieri S, Cattani P, Ciabattoni G, Di Munno O, Pasero G, Patrono C, et al. The synovial prostaglandin system in chronic inflammatory arthritis: Differential effects of steroidal and nonsteroidal anti-inflammatory drugs. Br J Pharmacol 1981;73(4):893–901.
7. Simmons DL, Botting RM, Hla T. Cyclooxygenase isozymes: the biology of prostaglandin synthesis and inhibition. Pharmacological Reviews 2004;56(3):387–437.
8. Wallace JR, McKnight W, Reuter BK, Vergnolle N. NSAID induced gastric damage in rats: Requirements for inhibition of both cyclooxygenase 1 and 2. Gastroenterology 2000;119:706–14.
9. Solomon LM, Juhlin L. Prostaglandins on cutaneous vasculature. J Invest Dermatol 1968;51:280–82.
10. Jaffe EA, Weksler B. Recovery of endothelial cell prostacyclin production after inhibition by low doses of aspirin. J Clin Invest 1979;63:532–35.
11. Simmons DL, Botting RM, Hla T. Cyclooxygenase isozymes: The biology of prostaglandin synthesis and inhibition. Pharmacological Reviews 2004;56(3):387–437.
12. Peplow PV. Properties and actions of non-steroidal anti-inflammatory drugs, including their effects on prostaglandin and macromolecular biosynthesis. Prostaglandins Leukotrienes & Essential Fatty Acids 1988;33(3):239–52.
13. Patrignani P, Sciulli MG. Pharmaceutical exploitation: Cyclooxygenase and lipooxygenase inhibitors. In: P Curtis-Prior (ed.), The Eicosenoids. Cambridge: John Wiley & Sons 2004: 599–612.
14. Davies NM, Skjodt N. Choosing the right NSAID. Clin Pharmacokin 2000;38(5):377–92.
15. Day RO, Mclachlan AJ, Graham GG, Williams KM. Pharmacokinetics of nonsteroidal anti-inflammatory drugs in synovial fluid. Clin Pharmacokinet 1999;36(3):191.
16. FitzGerald GA, Patrono C. The coxibs, selective inhibitors of cyclooxygenase-2. N Engl J Med 2001;345(6):433–42.

17. Bradley JD, Brandt KD, Katz BP, Kalasinski LA, Ryan SI. Comparison of an anti-inflammatory dose of ibuprofen, an analgesic dose of ibuprofen, and acetaminophen in the treatment of patients with osteoarthritis of the knee. N Engl J Med 1991;11;325:87–91.

18. Pincus T, Koch GG, Sokka T. A randomized, double-blind, crossover clinical trial of diclofenac plus misoprostol versus acetaminophen in patients with osteoarthritis of the hip or knee. Arthritis Rheum 2001;44:1587–98.

19. Geba GP, Weaver AL, Polis AB, Dixon ME, Schnitzer TJ. Efficacy of rofecoxib, celecoxib, and acetaminophen in osteoarthritis of the knee: A randomized trial. JAMA 2002;287:64–71.

20. Case JP, Baliunas AJ. Block JA. Lack of efficacy of acetaminophen in treating symptomatic knee osteoarthritis: A randomized, double-blind, placebo-controlled comparison trial with diclofenac sodium. Arch Intern Med 2003;163:169–78.

21. Boureau F, Schneid H, Zeghari N, Wall R, Bourgeois P. The IPSO study: Ibuprofen, paracetamol study in osteoarthritis. A randomised comparative clinical study comparing the efficacy and safety of ibuprofen and paracetamol analgesic treatment of osteoarthritis of the knee or hip. Ann Rheum Dis 2004;63: 1028–34.

22. Pincus T, Koch G, Lei H, Mangal B, Sokka T, Moskowitz R, et al. Patient preference for placebo, acetaminophen (paracetamol) or celecoxib efficacy studies (PACES): Two randomised, double blind, placebo controlled, crossover clinical trials in patients with knee or hip osteoarthritis. Ann Rheum Dis 2004;63:931–39.

23. March L, Irwig L, Schwarz J, Simpson J, Chock C, Brooks P. N of 1 trials comparing a non-steroidal anti-inflammatory drug with paracetamol in osteoarthritis. BMJ 1994;309:1041–45.

24. Schnitzer TJ, Kamin M, Olson WH. Tramadol allows reduction of naproxen dose among patients with naproxen-responsive osteoarthritis pain: A randomized, double-blind, placebo-controlled study. Arthritis Rheum 1999;42:1370–77.

25. Caldwell JR, Hale ME, Boyd RE, Hague JM, Iwan T, Shi M, et al. Treatment of osteoarthritis pain with controlled release oxycodone or fixed combination oxycodone plus acetaminophen added to nonsteroidal antiinflammatory drugs: A double blind, randomized, multicenter, placebo controlled trial. J Rheumatol 1999;26:862–69.

26. Wilder-Smith CH, Hill L, Spargo K, Kalla A. Treatment of severe pain from osteoarthritis with slow-release tramadol or dihydrocodeine in combination with NSAIDs: A randomised study comparing analgesia, antinociception and gastrointestinal effects. Pain 2001;91:23–31.

27. Emkey R, Rosenthal N, Wu SC, Jordan D, Kamin M. CAPSS-114 Study Group. Efficacy and safety of tramadol/acetaminophen tablets (ultracet) as add-on therapy for osteoarthritis pain in subjects receiving a COX-2 nonsteroidal antiinflammatory drug: A multicenter, randomized, double-blind, placebo-controlled trial. J Rheumatol 2004;31:150–56.

28. Mason L, Moore RA, Edwards JE, Derry S, McQuay HJ. Topical NSAIDs for chronic musculoskeletal pain: Systematic review and meta-analysis. BMC Musculoskeletal Disorders 2004;5:28.

29. American College of Rheumatology Subcommittee on Osteoarthritis Guidelines. Recommendations for the medical management of osteoarthritis of the hip and knee. Arthritis Rheum 2000;43:1905–15.

30. Zhang W, Doherty M, Arden N, Bannwarth B, Bijlsma J, Gunther KP, et al. EULAR evidence based recommendations for the management of hip osteoarthritis: Report of a task force of the EULAR Standing Committee for International Clinical Studies Including Therapeutics (ESCISIT). Ann Rheum Dis 2005;64: 669–81.

31. Saag KG, Olivieri JJ, Patino F, Mikuls TR, Allison JJ, MacLean CH. Measuring quality in arthritis care: The Arthritis Foundation's quality indicator set for analgesics. Arthritis Rheum 2004;51: 337–49.

32. http://www.fda.gov/medwatch/SAFETY/2004/jan_PI/Celebrex_PI.pdf. Accessed 22 July 2005.

33. Bombardier C, Laine L, Reicin A, Shapiro D, Burgos-Vargas R, Davis B, et al. Comparison of upper gastrointestinal toxicity of rofecoxib and naproxen in patients with rheumatoid arthritis: VIGOR Study Group. N Engl J Med 2000;343:1520–28.

34. Ofman JJ, MacLean CH, Straus WL, Morton SC, Berger ML, Roth EA, et al. A metaanalysis of severe upper gastrointestinal complications of nonsteroidal antiinflammatory drugs. J Rheumatol 2002;29:804–12.

35. Bollini P, Garcia Rodriguez LA, Perez Gutthann S, Walker AM. The impact of research quality and study design on epidemiologic estimates of the effect of nonsteroidal anti-inflammatory drugs on upper gastrointestinal tract disease. Arch Intern Med 1992;152:1289–95.

36. Gabriel SE, Jaakkimainen L, Bombardier C. Risk for serious gastrointestinal complications related to use of nonsteroidal anti-inflammatory drugs: A meta-analysis. Ann Intern Med 1991;115:787–96.

37. Hernandez-Diaz S, Rodriguez LA. Association between nonsteroidal anti-inflammatory drugs and upper gastrointestinal tract bleeding/perforation: An overview of epidemiologic studies published in the 1990s. Arch Intern Med 2000;160:2093.

38. Fries JF, Murtagh KF, Bennett M, Zatarain E, Lingala B, Bruce B. The rise and decline in nonsteroidal anti-inflammatory drug-associated gastropathy in rheumatoid arthritis. Arthritis Rheum 2004;50:2433–40.

39. Singh G, Ramey DR. NSAID-induced gastrointestinal complications: The ARAMIS perspective, 1997. J Rheumatol 1998;25(51): 8–16.

40. Hernandez-Diaz S, Rodriguez LA. Association between nonsteroidal anti-inflammatory drugs and upper gastrointestinal tract bleeding/perforation: An overview of epidemiologic studies published in the 1990s. Arch Intern Med 2000;160:2093.

41. Silverstein FE, Graham DY, Senior JR, Davies HW, Struthers BJ, Bittman RM, et al. Misoprostol reduces serious gastrointestinal complications in patients with rheumatoid arthritis receiving nonsteroidal anti-inflammatory drugs: A randomized, double-blind, placebo-controlled trial. Ann Intern Med 1995;123: 241–49.

42. Shorr RI, Ray WA, Daugherty JR, Griffin MR. Concurrent use of nonsteroidal anti-inflammatory drugs and oral anticoagulants places elderly persons at high risk for hemorrhagic peptic ulcer disease. Arch Intern Med 1993;153:1665–70.

43. Garcia Rodriguez LA, Jick H. Risk of upper gastrointestinal bleeding and perforation associated with individual non-steroidal anti-inflammatory drugs. Lancet 1994;343:769–72.

44. Piper JM, Ray WA, Daugherty JR, Griffin MR. Corticosteroid use and peptic ulcer disease: Role of nonsteroidal anti-inflammatory drugs. Ann Intern Med 1991;114:735–40.

45. Hernandez-Diaz S, Rodriguez LA. Steroids and risk of upper gastrointestinal complications. Am J Epidemiol 2001;153:1089–93.

46. Silverstein FE, Graham DY, Senior JR, Davies HW, Struthers BJ, Bittman RM, et al. Misoprostol reduces serious gastrointestinal complications in patients with rheumatoid arthritis receiving nonsteroidal anti-inflammatory drugs: A randomized, double-blind, placebo-controlled trial. Ann Intern Med 1995; 123:241–49.

47. Chan FK, Hung LC, Suen BY, Wu JC, Lee KC, Leung VK, et al. Celecoxib versus diclofenac and omeprazole in reducing the risk of recurrent ulcer bleeding in patients with arthritis. N Engl J Med 2002;347:2104–10.

48. Hawkey CJ, Karrasch JA, Szczepanski L, Walker DG, Barkun A, Swannell AJ, et al. Omeprazole compared with misoprostol for ulcers associated with nonsteroidal antiinflammatory drugs: Omeprazole versus Misoprostol for NSAID-induced Ulcer Management (OMNIUM) Study Group. N Engl J Med 1998;338: 727–34.

49. Yeomans ND, Tulassay Z, Juhasz L, Racz I, Howard JM, van Rensburg CJ, et al. A comparison of omeprazole with ranitidine for ulcers associated with nonsteroidal antiinflammatory drugs: Acid Suppression Trial: Ranitidine versus Omeprazole for NSAID-associated Ulcer Treatment (ASTRONAUT) Study Group. N Engl J Med 1998;338:719–26.

50. Chan FK, Hung LC, Suen BY, Wu JC, Lee KC, Leung VK, et al. Celecoxib versus diclofenac and omeprazole in reducing the risk of recurrent ulcer bleeding in patients with arthritis. N Engl J Med 2002;347:2104–10.

51. Bjorkman D. Nonsteroidal anti-inflammatory drug-associated toxicity of the liver, lower gastrointestinal tract, and esophagus. Am J Med 1998;105(5A)17S–21S.

52. Teoh NC, Farrell GC. Hepatotoxicity associated with non-steroidal anti-inflammatory drugs. Clinics Liver Disease 2003;7:401–13.

53. Silverstein FE, Faich G, Goldstein JL, Simon LS, Pincus T, Whelton A, et al. Gastrointestinal toxicity with celecoxib vs nonsteroidal anti-inflammatory drugs for osteoarthritis and rheumatoid arthritis: The CLASS study, a randomized controlled trial. JAMA 2000;284:1247–55.

54. Davies NM. Toxicity of nonsteroidal anti-inflammatory drugs in the large intestine. Dis Colon Rectum 1995;38:1311–21.

55. Gibson GR, Whitacre EB, Ricotti CA. Colitis induced by non-steroidal anti-inflammatory drugs: Report of four cases and review of the literature. Arch Intern Med 1992;152:625–32.

56. Solomon DH. Selective COX-2 inhibitors and cardiovascular outcomes. Arthritis Rheum 2005;52:1968–78.

57. McAdam BF, Catella-Lawson F, Mardini IA, Kapoor S, Lawson JA, Fitzgerald GA. Systemic biosynthesis of prostacyclin by cyclooxygenase (COX)-2: The human pharmacology of a selective inhibitor of COX-2. Proc Natl Acad Sci USA 1999;96:272–77.

58. FitzGerald GA, Patrono C. The coxibs, selective inhibitors of cyclooxygenase-2. N Engl J Med 2001;345:433–42.

59. Cheng Y, Austin SC, Rocca B, Koller BH, Coffman TM, Grosser T, et al. Role of prostacyclin in the cardiovascular response to thromboxane A2. Science 2002;296:539–41.

60. Egan KM, Lawson JA, Fries S, Koller B, Rader DJ, Smyth EM, et al. COX-2-derived prostacyclin confers atheroprotection on female mice. Science 2004;306:1954–57.

61. Fitzgerald G. http://www.fda.gov/ohrms/dockets/ac/05/slides/2005-4090S1_03_FDA-Fitzgerald.ppt. Accessed 12 March 2005.

62. Chenevard R, Hurlimann D, Bechir M, et al. Selective COX-2 inhibition improves endothelial function in coronary artery disease. Circulation 2003;107:405–09.

63. Widlansky ME, Price DT, Noyan G, et al. Short- and long-term COX-2 inhibition reverses endothelial dysfunction in patients with hypertension. Hypertension 2003;42:310–15.

64. Title LM, Giddens K, McInerney MM, McQuenn MJ, Nassar BA. Effective of cyclooxygease-2 inhibition with rofecoxib on endothelial dysfunction and inflammatory markers in patients with coronary artery disease. J Am Coll Cardiol 2003;42:1747–53.

65. Bogaty P, Brophy JM, Noel M, Boyer L, Simard S, Bertrand F, et al. Impact of prolonged cyclooxygenase-2 inhibition on inflammatory markers and endothelial function in patients with ischemic heart disease and raised C-reactive protein. Circulation 2004;110:934–39.

66. Walter MF, Jacob RF, Day CA, Dahlborg R, Weng Y, Mason RP. Sulfone COX-2 inhibitors increase susceptibility of human LDL and plasma to oxidative modification: Comparison to sulfonamide COX-2 inhibitors and NSAIDs. Atherosclerosis 2004;177:235–43.

67. Gurwitz JH, Avorn J, Bohn RL, Glynn RJ, Monane M, Mogun H. Initiation of antihypertensive treatment during nonsteroidal anti-inflammatory drug therapy. JAMA 1994;272:781–86.

68. Pope JE, Anderson JJ, Felson DT. A meta-analysis of the effects of nonsteroidal anti-inflammatory drugs on blood pressure. Arch Intern Med 1993;153:477–84.

69. Aw TJ, Haas SJ, Liew D, Krum H. Meta-analysis of cyclooxygenase-2 inhibitors and their effects on blood pressure. Arch Intern Med 2005;165:1–7.

70. Bombardier C, Laine L, Reicin A, Shapiro D, Burgos-Vargas R, Davis B, et al. VIGOR Study Group: Comparison of upper gastrointestinal toxicity of rofecoxib and naproxen in patients with rheumatoid arthritis. N Engl J Med 2000;343:1520–28.

71. Bresalier RS, Sandler RS, Quan H, et al. Cardiovascular events associated with rofecoxib in a colorectal adenoma chemoprevention trial. N Engl J Med 2005;352:1092–1102.

72. Weir MR, Sperling RS, Reicin A, Gertz BJ. Selective COX-2 inhibition and cardiovascular effects: A review of the rofecoxib development program. Am Heart J 2003;146:591–604.

73. Silverstein FE, Faich G, Goldstein JL, Simon LS, Pincus T, Whelton A, et al. Gastrointestinal toxicity with celecoxib vs nonsteroidal anti-inflammatory drugs for osteoarthritis and rheumatoid arthritis: The CLASS study, a randomized controlled trial. JAMA 2000;284:1247–55.

74. Solomon SD, McMurray JV, Pfeffer MA, et al. Cardiovascular risk associated with celecoxib in a clinical trial for colorectal adenoma prevention. N Engl J Med 2005;352(11):1071–80.

75. http://www.fda.gov/ohrms/dockets/ac/05/briefing/2005-4090B1_03_Pfizer-Celebrex-Bextra.pdf. Accessed 10 March 2005.

76. Ott E, Nussmeier NA, Duke PC, et al. Efficacy and safety of the cyclooxygenase 2 inhibitors parecoxib and valdecoxib in patients undergoing coronary artery bypass surgery. J Thoracic Cardiovasc Surg 2003;125:1481–90.

77. Nussmeier NA, Whelton AA, Brown MT, et al. Complications of the COX-2 inhibitors parecoxib and valdecoxib after cardiac surgery. N Engl J Med 2005;352(11):1081–91.

78. Farkouh ME, Kirshner H, Harrington, RA, et al. Comparison of lumiracoxib with naproxen and ibuprofen in the Therapeutic Arthritis Research and Gastrointestinal Event Trial (TARGET), cardiovascular outcomes, randomized controlled trial. Lancet 2004;364:675–84.

79. Ray WA, Stein CM, Daugherty JR, Hall K, Arbogast PG, Griffin MR. COX-2 selective nonsteroidal anti-inflammatory drugs and risk of serious coronary heart disease. Lancet 2002;360:1071–73.

80. Solomon DH, Schneeweiss S, Glynn RJ, Kiyota Y, Levin R, Mogun H, et al. Relationship between selective COX-2 inhibitors and acute myocardial infarction. Circulation 2004;109:2068–73.

81. Schneeweiss S, Glynn RJ, Tsai EH, Avorn J, Solomon DH. Adjusting for unmeasured confounders in pharmacoepidemiologic claims data using external information: The example of COX-2 inhibitors and myocardial infarction. Epidemiology 2005;16:17–24.

82. Graham DJ, Campen D, Hui R, Spence M, Cheetham C, Levy G, et al. Risk of acute myocardial infarction and sudden cardiac death in patients treated with cyclo-oxygenase 2 selective and non-selective non-steroidal anti-inflammatory drugs: Nested case-control study. Lancet 2005;365:475–81.

83. Kimmel SE, Berlin JA, Reilly M, Jaskowiak J, Kishel L, Chittams J, et al. Patients exposed to rofecoxib and celecoxib have different odds of nonfatal myocardial infarction. Ann Intern Med 2005;142:157–64.

84. Mamdani M, Rochon P, Juurlink DN, et al. Effect of selective cyclooxygenase 2 inhibitors and naproxen on short-term risk of acute myocardial infarction. Arch Intern Med 2003;163:481–86.

85. Shaya FT, Blume SW, Blanchette CM, Weir MR, Mullins CD. Selective cyclooxygenase-2 inhibition and cardiovascular effects. Arch Intern Med 2005;165:181–86.

86. Catella-Lawson F, Reilly MP, Kapoor SC, Cucchiara AJ, DeMarco S, Tournier B, et al. Cyclooxygenase inhibitors and the antiplatelet effects of aspirin. N Engl J Med 2001;345:1809–17.

87. MacDonald TM, Wei L. Effect of ibuprofen on cardioprotective effect of aspirin. Lancet 2003;361:573–74.

88. Kimmel SE, Berlin JA, Reilly M, Jaskowiak J, Kishel L, Chittams J, et al. The effects of nonselective non-aspirin non-steroidal anti-inflammatory medications on the risk of nonfatal myocardial infarction and their interaction with aspirin. J Am Coll Cardiol 2004; 43:985–90.

89. Kurth T, Glynn RJ, Walker AM, Chan KA, Buring JE, Hennekens CH, et al. Inhibition of clinical benefits of aspirin on first myocardial infarction by nonsteroidal antiinflammatory drugs. Circulation 2003;108:1191–95.

90. Curtis JP, Wang YF, Portnay EL, Masoudi FA, Havranek EP, Krumholz HM. Aspirin, ibuprofen, and mortality after myocardial infarction: Retrospective cohort study. Br Med J 2003;327:1322–23.

91. Patel TN, Goldberg KC. Use of aspirin and ibuprofen compared with aspirin alone and the risk of myocardial infarction. Arch Intern Med 2004;164:852–56.

92. Garcia Rodriguez LA, Varas-Lorenzo C, Maguire A, Gonzalez-Perez A. Nonsteroidal antiinflammatory drugs and the risk of myocardial infarction in the general population. Circulation 2004;109:3000–06.

93. Solomon DH, Goodson NJ. The cardiovascular system in rheumatic disease: The next "extra-articular" manifestation? J Rheumatol 2005;32:1415–18.

94. Swan SK, Rudy DW, Lasseter KC, Ryan CF, Buechel KL, Lambrecht LJ, et al. Effect of cyclooxygenase-2 inhibition on renal function in elderly persons receiving a low-salt diet: A randomized, controlled trial. Ann Intern Med 2000;133(1):1–9.

95. Rossat J, Maillard M, Nussberger J, Brunner HR, Burnier M. Renal effects of selective cyclooxygenase-2 inhibition in normotensive salt-depleted subjects. Clin Pharmacol Ther 1999;66:76–84.

96. Catella-Lawson F, McAdam B, Morrison BW, Kapoor S, Kujubu D, Antes L, et al. Effects of specific inhibition of cyclooxygenase-2 on sodium balance, hemodynamics, and vasoactive eicosanoids. J Pharmacol & Exp Ther 1999;289(2):735–41.

97. Griffin MR, Yared A, Ray WA. Nonsteroidal antiinflammatory drugs and acute renal failure in elderly persons. Am J Epidemiol 2000;151(5):488–96.

98. Perez Gutthann S, Garcia Rodriguez LA, Raiford DS, Duque Oliart A, Ris Romeu J. Nonsteroidal anti-inflammatory drugs and the risk of hospitalization for acute renal failure. Arch Intern Med 1996;156(21):2433–39.

99. Perneger TV, Whelton PK, Klag MJ. Risk of kidney failure associated with the use of acetaminophen, aspirin, and nonsteroidal antiinflammatory drugs. N Engl J Med 1994;331(25):1675–79.

100. Sandler DP, Burr FR, Weinberg CR. Nonsteroidal anti-inflammatory drugs and the risk for chronic renal disease. Ann Intern Med 1991;115(3):165–72.

101. Alanko K, Stubb S, Kauppinen K. Cutaneous drug reactions: Clinical types and causative agents. A five-year survey of in-patients (1981–1985). Acta Dermato-Venereologica 1989; 69(3):223–26.

102. http://www.fda.gov/cder/drug/infopage/COX2/default.htm. Accessed 29 July 2005.

103. Curhan GC, Bullock AJ, Hankinson SE, Willett WC, Speizer FE, Stampfer MJ. Frequency of use of acetaminophen, nonsteroidal anti-inflammatory drugs, and aspirin in US women. Pharmacoepidemiol Drug Safety 2002;11:687–93.

104. Solomon DH, Schneeweiss S, Glynn RJ, Levin R, Avorn J. Determinants of selective cyclooxygenase-2 inhibitor prescribing: Are patient or physician characteristics more important? Am J Med 2003;115(9):715–20.

105. Dai C, Stafford RS, Alexander GC. National trends in cyclooxygenase-2 inhibitor use since market release: Nonselective diffusion of a selectively cost-effective innovation. Arch Intern Med 2005;165(2):171–77.

106. Solomon DH, Schneeweiss S, Glynn RJ, Levin R, Avorn J. Determinants of selective cyclooxygenase-2 inhibitor prescribing: Are patient or physician characteristics more important? Am J Med 2003;115(9):715–20.

107. Patino FG, Allison J, Olivieri J, Mudano A, Juarez L, Person S, et al. The effects of physician specialty and patient comorbidities on the use and discontinuation of coxibs. Arthritis Rheum 2003;49(3):293–99.

108. Greenberg JD, Bingham CO III, Abramson SB, Reed G, Sebaldt RJ, Kremer J. Effect of cardiovascular comorbidities and concomitant aspirin use on selection of cyclooxygenase inhibitor among rheumatologists. Arthritis Rheum 2005;53(1):12–17.

109. Smalley W, Stein CM, Arbogast PG, Eisen G, Ray WA, Griffin M. Underutilization of gastroprotective measures in patients receiving nonsteroidal antiinflammatory drugs. Arthritis Rheum 2002;46(8):2195–2200.

110. Solomon DH, Schneeweiss S, Glynn RJ, Levin R, Avorn J. Determinants of selective cyclooxygenase-2 inhibitor prescribing: Are patient or physician characteristics more important? Am J Med 2003;115(9):715–20.

111. Spiegel BM, Targownik L, Dulai GS, Gralnek IM. The cost-effectiveness of cyclooxygenase-2 selective inhibitors in the management of chronic arthritis. Ann Intern Med 2003;138(10):795–806.

112. Maetzel A, Krahn M, Naglie G. The cost effectiveness of rofecoxib and celecoxib in patients with osteoarthritis or rheumatoid arthritis. Arthritis Rheum 2003;49(3):283–92.

113. Smalley W, Stein CM, Arbogast PG, Eisen G, Ray WA, Griffin M. Underutilization of gastroprotective measures in patients receiving nonsteroidal antiinflammatory drugs. Arthritis Rheum 2002;46(8):2195–2200.

114. Stein CM, Griffin MR, Taylor JA, Pichert JW, Brandt KD, Ray WA. Educational program for nursing home physicians and staff to reduce use of non-steroidal anti-inflammatory drugs among nursing home residents: A randomized controlled trial. Medical Care 2001;39(5):436–45.

# 12 Complementary and Alternative Medicine in Osteoarthritis

Amanda Tiffany and Lan X. Chen

## INTRODUCTION

Complementary and alternative medicine (CAM) represents a diverse and large group of products, therapies, and health care systems that are not considered a part of conventional medicine. During the past few decades, the interest in and popularity of CAM have been rapidly growing among adults in the United States. It has been estimated that about 60% of adults used at least one form of alternative therapy in 2002, spending billions of dollars out-of-pocket. The increase in use of CAM may be explained by market forces, the desire of patients to be proactive in their health care, access to information on the Internet, and frustration or dissatisfaction with conventional medicine.[1]

The majority of people use CAM therapies as a complement to conventional medicine. In the 2002 National Health Interview Survey conducted by the Centers for Disease Control and Prevention, respondents were more likely to use CAM if they believed such therapies combined with conventional medicine would improve their health and/or if they were simply interested in trying the alternative practices.[1] Eisenberg et al. reported that out of 831 people who saw a medical doctor and used a CAM during the past year, 79% believed the combination was superior to either practice alone.[2]

Users of complementary and alternative practices are more likely to be female than male, to be college educated, and to have chronic conditions. The most common reason for CAM use is to treat musculoskeletal conditions or other conditions associated with chronic pain.[1] Studies have estimated that one-third to two-thirds of patients followed in private and university-based rheumatology practices have used some form of alternative therapy in the past year.[3] In a cross-sectional survey of patients in an outpatient rheumatology clinic, about 42% of patients reported using CAM. Acupuncture and homeopathy were the most common alternative practices. Patients with fibromyalgia used significantly more CAM therapies per person than patients with other rheumatologic conditions. Self-perceived efficacy of alternative therapies was greatest in patients with osteoarthritis (OA) and spondyloarthropathies, whereas satisfaction was lowest in rheumatoid arthritis (RA), vasculitis, and connective tissue disorders.[4]

Because complementary and alternative therapy use is prevalent among patients with OA, it is important for health care practitioners to have some knowledge about these therapies and objective evidence of efficacy and safety. This chapter focuses on the most common and well-studied alternative practices used to treat OA, including acupuncture, herbal therapies, mind-body therapies, tai chi, and yoga.

## ACUPUNCTURE

It has been estimated that more than 15 million Americans have used acupuncture, primarily for pain relief.[5] Pain, of course, is one of the most common symptoms of our patients with OA. Throughout Asia, acupuncture is often used not only to treat diseases but to maintain health. Acupuncture is based on the theory that essential life energy (qi), the blood, and essence of body fluid are fundamental substances in the human body that help sustain normal vital activities. The qi flows through the body along channels called meridians, which connect with various tissues and organs. There are more than 300 major acupuncture points that lie along these meridians. Disorders (including physical and emotional disturbance) can unbalance the energy flow (qi) in the meridians and connected tissues and organs.

Out-of-balance qi can cause a variety of symptoms and pain. Stimulation and manipulation of specific points along the meridians are proposed to restore the flow of qi to optimize health or to relieve pain.[6] Acupuncture has evolved over several thousands of years in China. The earliest major source of acupuncture theory is the *Huang Di Nei Jing* (*Yellow Emperor's Inner Classic*), dated to the Han dynasty in the second century BC. It views the human body as a microcosmic reflection of the universe and considers acupuncture a tool for regulating and maintaining the body's harmonious balance.[7] Most Americans heard of acupuncture in 1972, when President Nixon visited China.

In a front-page article in the *New York Times*, journalist James Reston described how acupuncture needles alleviated his postoperative pain from an emergency appendectomy.[8] In 1997, a National Institutes of Health (NIH) panel published its *Consensus Development Statement on Acupuncture*.[9] They concluded that acupuncture showed efficacy in alleviating adult postoperative and chemotherapy nausea and vomiting and in alleviating postoperative dental pain. Other situations (such as addiction, stroke rehabilitation, headache, menstrual cramps, tennis elbow, fibromyalgia, myofascial pain, low back pain, carpal tunnel syndrome, asthma, and OA) were only considered possible situations in which acupuncture might be useful as an adjunct treatment, acceptable alternative, or part of a comprehensive management program. In the last few years, three large randomized controlled trials (RCTs) studying the role of acupuncture in knee OA have been published.[6,10,11]

Berman et al. examined whether acupuncture provides greater pain relief and improved function compared with sham acupuncture or education in patients with OA of the knee. This RCT enrolled 570 patients with OA of the knee (mean age [SD], 65.5; 8.4 years). Twenty-three true acupuncture sessions were given over 26 weeks. Controls received six 2-hour sessions over 12 weeks or 23 sham acupuncture sessions over 26 weeks. Primary outcomes were changes in the Western Ontario and McMaster Universities Osteoarthritis Index (WOMAC) pain and function scores at 8 and 26 weeks. Secondary outcomes were patient global assessment, 6-minute walk distance, and physical health scores of the 36-Item Short-Form Health Survey (SF-36).

Participants in the true acupuncture group experienced greater improvement in WOMAC function scores than the sham acupuncture group at 8 weeks (mean difference −2.9 [95% CI, −5.0 to −0.8]; p = 0.01) but not in WOMAC pain score (mean difference, −0.5 [CI, −1.2 to 0.2]; p = 0.18) or the patient global assessment (mean difference 0.16 [CI, −0.02 to 0.34]; p > 0.2). At 26 weeks, the true acupuncture group experienced significantly greater improvement than the sham group in the WOMAC function score (mean difference −2.5 [CI, −4.7 to −0.4]; p = 0.01), WOMAC pain score (mean difference, −0.87 [CI, −1.58 to −0.16]; p = 0.003), and patient global assessment (mean difference 0.26 [CI, 0.07 to 0.45]; p = 0.02).[10] In this study, it

seems acupuncture provided improvement in function and pain relief as an adjunctive therapy for OA of the knee when compared with sham acupuncture control and education control groups.

Vas et al. analyzed the efficacy of acupuncture as a complementary therapy to the pharmacologic treatment of OA of the knee with respect to pain relief, reduction of stiffness, and increased physical function during treatment; to modifications in the consumption of diclofenac during treatment; and to changes in the patient's quality of life. They have done a randomized, controlled, single blind trial, with blinded evaluation and statistical analysis of results. Ninety-seven outpatients with OA of the knee were recruited. Patients were randomly separated into two groups: one receiving acupuncture plus diclofenac (n = 48) and the other placebo acupuncture plus diclofenac (n = 49).

The clinical variables examined included intensity of pain as measured by a visual analogue scale; pain, stiffness, and physical function subscales of the WOMAC OA index; dosage of diclofenac taken during treatment; and the profile of quality of life in the chronically ill (PQLC) instrument, evaluated before and after the treatment. Eighty-eight patients completed the trial. In the intention-to-treat analysis, the WOMAC index had a greater reduction in the intervention group than in the control group (mean difference 23.9, 95% confidence interval 15.0 to 32.8).

The reduction was greatest in the subscale of functional activity. The same result was observed in the pain visual analogue scale, with a reduction of 26.6 (18.5 to 34.8). The PQLC results indicate that acupuncture treatment produces significant changes in physical capability (p = 0.021) and psychologic functioning (p = 0.046). Three patients reported bruising after the acupuncture sessions.[11] This RCT trial demonstrated that acupuncture plus diclofenac is more effective than placebo acupuncture plus diclofenac for the symptomatic treatment of OA of the knee. Thus, acupuncture can be a part of a comprehensive management program for patients with knee OA.

There is another recently published acupuncture study that showed that after 8 weeks of acupuncture treatment pain and joint function were improved more with acupuncture than with minimal acupuncture or no acupuncture in patients with OA of the knee. However, this benefit decreases over time. Patients with chronic OA of the knee (Kellgren grade < or = 2) were randomly assigned to acupuncture (n = 150), minimal acupuncture (superficial needling at non-acupuncture points; n = 76), or a waiting-list control (n = 74). Specialized physicians in 28 outpatient centers administered acupuncture and minimal acupuncture in 12 sessions over 8 weeks.

Patients completed standard questionnaires at baseline and after 8 weeks, 26 weeks, and 52 weeks.

The primary outcome was the WOMAC index at the end of week 8 (adjusted for baseline score). All main analyses were by intention to treat. A total of 294 patients were enrolled, with eight patients lost to follow-up after randomization but included in the final analysis. The mean baseline-adjusted WOMAC index at week 8 was 26.9 (SE 1.4) in the acupuncture group, 35.8[1.9] in the minimal acupuncture group, and 49.6[2.0] in the waiting-list group (treatment difference of acupuncture versus minimal acupuncture −8.8 [95% CI −13.5 to −4.2], p = 0.0002; acupuncture versus waiting list −22.7 [−27.5 to −17.9], p < 0.0001). However, after 52 weeks the difference between the acupuncture and minimal acupuncture groups was no longer significant (p = 0.08).[6]

In these three RCT trials, acupuncture consistently demonstrated effectiveness in function improvement and pain relief for patients with knee OA (Fig. 12.1). Acupuncture can also be used with non-steroidal anti-inflammatory drugs (NSAIDs) as an adjunctive therapy for pain relief with minimal side effects. Further studies are needed to study the effective duration of acupuncture. Optimal acupuncture protocols may still need to be established in the management of knee OA. Chen, Farrar, and the authors at the University of Pennsylvania have been conducting an NIH-sponsored sham-needle controlled acupuncture study to evaluate combining acupuncture with physical therapy in knee OA.[12] In the study, we have tested a newly developed method of sham needling in which the needle is placed in the true acupuncture point but does not penetrate the skin. The appearances of true and sham needles are indistinguishable by patients (Fig. 12.1).[13]

Hip and knee are the two common joints involved in OA. Two studies have examined the role of acupuncture in managing hip OA. Stener-Victorin et al. have done a study to evaluate the therapeutic effect of electro-acupuncture (EA) and hydrotherapy, both in combination with patient education or with patient education alone, in the treatment of OA in the hip. Forty-five patients aged 42 to 86 years with radiographic changes consistent with OA in the hip, pain related to motion, pain on load, and aching during day or night were chosen. They were randomly allocated to EA, hydrotherapy, both in combination with patient education, or patient education alone.

Outcome measures were the disability rating index (DRI), global self-rating index (GSI), and visual analogue scale (VAS). Assessments were done before the intervention and immediately after the last treatment, as well as 1, 3, and 6 months after the last treatment. It was found that pain related to motion and pain on load was for the hydrotherapy group reduced for as long as 3 months after the last treatment and for the EA group as long as 6 months. Aching during the day was significantly improved in both the EA and hydrotherapy groups—for as long as 3 months after the last treatment. Aching during the night was reduced in the hydrotherapy group for as long as 3 months after the last treatment and in the EA group for as long as 6 months.

Disability in functional activities was improved in EA and hydrotherapy groups for as long as 6 months after the last treatment. Quality of life was also improved in EA and hydrotherapy groups (as long as 3 months after the last treatment). There were no changes in the education group alone.[13] It seems that EA and hydrotherapy, both in combination with patient education, induce long-lasting effects—evidenced in reduced pain and ache and in increased functional activity and quality of life.

**Fig. 12.1** True needles (left) and sham needles (right).

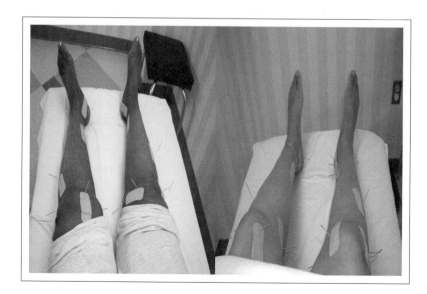

Auricular acupuncture (AA) is reported to be effective in the treatment of various pain conditions. In AA, acupuncture needles are applied to the ears at sites obviously distant from the hip. Usichenko et al. tested whether AA of specific points is superior to sham acupuncture for complementary analgesia after total hip arthroplasty in a patient/anesthesiologist/evaluator/analyst-blinded study. The patients were randomly allocated to receive true AA (lung, shenmen, thalamus, and hip points) or sham procedure (four non-acupuncture points on the auricular helix). Permanent-press AA needles were retained in situ for 3 days following surgery. Postoperative pain was treated with intravenous piritramide (opioid receptor agonist with analgesic potency of 0.7 compared with morphine) using a patient-controlled analgesia (PCA) pump.

The time to the first analgesic request, the amount of postoperative piritramide via PCA, and pain intensity on a 100-mm VAS (VAS-100) were used to evaluate postoperative analgesia. Intraoperative anesthetic requirement, incidence of analgesia-related side effects, inflammation parameters, and success of patients' blinding were also recorded. Fifty-four patients (29 AA and 25 controls) completed the study. Piritramide requirement during 36 hours following surgery in the AA group was lower than in control: 3,718 versus 5,421 mg; mean SD; p = 0.004. Pain intensity on VAS-100 and incidence of analgesia-related side effects were similar in both groups. The differences between the groups as regards patients' opinions concerning success of blinding were not significant.[14] This study demonstrates that AA could be used to reduce postoperative analgesic requirement.

Although acupuncture appears to be relatively safe, patients should be advised of certain infrequent risks (such as fainting, bruising, local pain, needle retention, and infection).[15,16] Patients should confirm that their acupuncture practitioner is certified or licensed. It would be advisable that patients keep written notes about their responses to the acupuncture and communicate such responses with their acupuncturist and physicians.

As rheumatologists, we should be willing to continuously rethink and revise therapeutic guidelines as new data become available. Hopefully in the future we will be able to advise our patients on the grounds of evidence-based medicine, in contrast to the reliance of alternative medicine tradition and belief. The NIH has established the National Center for Complementary and Alternative Medicine to encourage basic and clinical research on alternative medicine under Dr. Stephen Straus's leadership. Treatments using alternative medicine whose efficacy can be demonstrated by high-quality controlled trials will be likely to be incorporated into medical practice. As rheumatologists, we are in an era with more options for treating rheumatologic disease. We should evaluate not only the new medications guided by evidence-based medicine but the treatments of alternative medicine by the same standards.

## HERBAL THERAPIES

Plants and herbs have been used for medicinal purposes since ancient times, and have been an important part of many cultures and traditional health systems throughout the world. Thousands of herbs and plant products are believed to have healing properties and are used to treat a variety of conditions, including OA. Herbal therapies have been growing in popularity since the 1960s among the American public, with use increasing more than fivefold during the 1990s (from 2.1% in 1990 to 12.1% in 1997).[17]

According to the 2002 National Health Interview Survey (conducted by the National Center for Health Statistics at the Centers for Disease Control and Prevention), about 19% (more than 38 million) of adults in the United States used some form of natural product—including herbal medicines, food products such as garlic, and animal-based products such as glucosamine—during the 12 months surveyed. The natural products used by more than 10% of these respondents included echinacea, ginseng, ginkgo biloba, garlic supplements, glucosamine, St. John's wort, fish oils, and ginger supplements.[1] Between 1998 and 2002, use doubled in adults over the age of 65.[18]

An analysis of national survey data from 2000 showed that one-sixth of U.S. women took at least one herbal product within the past year. Factors significantly associated with use of the most commonly reported herbal therapies were being non-Hispanic white, 35 to 64 years of age, college educated, not poor, residents of southern or western states, current alcohol users, and having a functional disability or chronic disease.[19]

The most commonly cited reasons for using herbal medicines include overall health improvement and chronic conditions such as headache, memory loss, arthritis, and fatigue.[20] People typically use these therapies as an adjunct to allopathic medical therapies. The Slone national telephone survey conducted in 1998 to 1999 showed that 16% of adults taking prescription medications were using an herbal product simultaneously.[18]

Allopathic health care practitioners are frequently unaware of the concurrent use of prescription and herbal medicines by their patients. It has been estimated from a national survey that about 60 to 70% of patients do not disclose the use of a complementary and alternative therapy to their allopathic physician. The main reasons reported for not disclosing this information are that the patient thought it was not important or that the doctor did not ask.[2] People often perceive herbal therapies as safe because they are "natural" and because the person does not consider them to be drugs. In addition, some patients may be embarrassed to tell their doctor or believe that their doctor will disapprove.[21]

Many people who suffer from OA turn to herbal products for relief of symptoms. They are usually motivated by curiosity, frustration with the inability of conventional medicine to provide a cure for the condition or to fully relieve symptoms, or lack of tolerance to the side effects of conventional pharmaceutical medicines used to treat OA.[22] The herbal products are often used without knowledge of their efficacy, potential for interactions with other medicines, and side effects. Due to the rapid rise in use by patients with OA during the past two decades, the medical community has been increasingly concerned with the lack of objective evidence of efficacy and safety. As a result, many RDTs have been conducted investigating the use of herbs and nutritional supplements in the treatment of OA.

A large number of different herbal medicines have been studied. The quality and quantity of evidence vary for each. The natural products with promising and moderately strong evidence (resulting from two or more RCTs, for or against efficacy) include devil's claw, avocado/soybean unsaponifiables, ginger, and capsaicin cream. (Avocado/soybean unsaponifiables, ginger, and capsaicin are generally considered food products rather than herbs and are therefore explored in another chapter.) In addition, other studies have investigated herbal preparations containing mixtures of multiple herbs. Phytodolor is one herbal mixture for which there is moderately strong evidence from multiple trials supporting efficacy in the treatment of OA.

Devil's claw is the common name for a perennial plant, *Harpagophytum procumbens*, which is indigenous to southern and eastern areas of Africa. It received this common name because the fruit of the plant is covered with sharp curved thorns. It is also referred to as the wood spider and the grapple plant. Substances from the tuber of devil's claw are used in traditional African medical therapies in the treatment of arthritis, low back pain, headaches, neuralgias, indigestion, and fevers. The medicinal properties of the heterogeneous mixture of substances found in the tuber are attributed to compounds that belong to the iridoid glycoside family. The fraction of each constituent in herbal products made from this plant depends on the extraction process used.[21]

Evidence from controlled and uncontrolled trials suggests that devil's claw is an effective therapy for symptoms of OA. Two randomized placebo-controlled trials were cited in a systematic review of herbal therapies for OA. The interventions consisted of *Harpagophytum* extracts with 1.5 and 3% iridoid glycoside content taken three times daily for 3 weeks and 2 months, respectively. A statistically significant reduction in pain and improved mobility in patients with OA of the knee and hip was associated with the use of devil's claw extracts in both studies.[23]

Chantre et al. compared the efficacy of *Harpagophytum* powder with the weak NSAID diacerein in the treatment of OA of the knee and hip for 4 months. Although pain and function (measured by the Lequesne's index) were improved in both groups, the difference was not statistically significant. Use of the herbal product was associated with significantly fewer side effects, decreased use of NSAIDs for breakthrough pain, and improved global tolerance assessment compared to diacerein. The most common side effect in both groups was diarrhea, occurring in 8.1% and 26.7% of patients in the *Harpagophytum* and diacerein groups (respectively).[24] The results of this study suggest that the herbal product made from the tuber of devil's claw is as efficacious as a weak NSAID in the treatment of OA of the hip and knee and is superior in safety.

Mild gastrointestinal distress is the main side effect reported with the use of devil's claw extract. Contraindications for use may include patients with gastric or duodenal ulcers, gallstones, or diabetes. Currently no data exist concerning long-term toxicities and drug interactions.[21]

The mechanism by which *Harpagophytum* extract may be effective in reducing side effects of OA is thought to be anti-inflammatory in nature. A series of in vitro studies has demonstrated that the active component in the extract inhibits arachidonic acid metabolism and eicosanoid biosynthesis. Although this inhibition depends on the concentration of the active iridoid glycoside in the tuber extract, samples containing the pure component have less inhibitory activity than the extract. This suggests that different components of the extract may act synergistically.[21] More research, including in vivo studies, is needed to further clarify the therapeutic mechanism of action.

Phytodolor is an herbal product containing alcoholic extracts of *Populus tremula*, *Fraxinus excelsior*, and *Solidago virgaurea* in the ratio of 3:1:1. There are multiple proposed active ingredients, including salicin, salicyl alcohol, flavonoids, and triterpensaponines. Standard preparations of this herbal medicine contain 1 mg/ml of salicin, 0.07 mg/ml of flavonoids, and 0.14 mg/ml of isofraxidine.[23]

According to a systematic review, several RCTs of good methodologic quality have found significant reductions in pain and NSAID use and improved mobility associated with the use of Phytodolor compared to placebo. In addition, studies have shown this herbal preparation to be as effective as certain NSAIDs (such as diclofenac) in reducing pain. Adverse effects associated with Phytodolor appear to be minimal and infrequent. They may include gastrointestinal distress, diarrhea, nausea, pruritis, allergic reaction, fatigue, and vertigo.[23] The potential for interactions between this herbal product and other medications is unclear but of concern.

Different mechanisms of action of this herbal mixture have been proposed based on animal and in vitro studies. The therapeutic effect may in part be explained by the suppression of inflammatory mediators by inhibition of arachidonic acid metabolism.[25] A few studies have suggested that the individual components of Phytodolor may also have anti-oxidative properties, which may contribute to the activity of the combination.[26] Further work is needed to evaluate these proposed mechanisms.

Although certain herbal products appear to be effective in improving pain and function with minimal side effects and drug interactions in patients with OA, a major concern regarding the general safety of herbal therapy use remains to be addressed. In the United States, herbal products are currently categorized as dietary supplements. The Dietary Supplement and Health Education Act of 1994 stated that supplements can be sold without the prior approval of or regulation by the Food and Drug Association. As a result of this lack of regulation, the herbal products available to patients vary in quality, efficacy, and safety.

Hundreds of different commercial brands are available for many common herbal therapies. The quality of an herbal preparation depends on the particular plant species and part of the plant used; how the plant was grown, harvested, and stored; and how the herbal product was processed.[27] In addition, inaccurate labeling of herbal products has been reported. The herbal content or fraction of different active substances may not match the information given on the label.[28] Infrequently, certain commercial products (including those containing Ayurvedic and Traditional Chinese Medicine herbal therapies) have been reported to be contaminated with pharmaceuticals, lead, mercury, and arsenic.[29,30]

Given the varying degree of evidence for or against the efficacy of certain herbs, the potential for drug interactions and side effects, and the lack of regulation and standardization, it is important to counsel patients concerning their use. When taking a medication history, health care providers can ask patients if they are taking or planning to take any herbal products. Physicians and patients should discuss the existence of and strength of evidence supporting the use of certain herbal products in the treatment of OA. Patients should be warned about the risk of adverse events and variation in quality and purity of different commercial products. Renal and hepatic insufficiency may increase risk for side effects and require dose adjustments. Older adults who are taking several prescription medications may be at increased risk of herb/drug interactions. Use of certain herbs can be recommended or discouraged based on these factors. Physicians should monitor closely the efficacy and safety of herbal product use in each patient.

## MIND-BODY THERAPIES

Many people with the same chronic illness often experience different symptoms, degrees of pain, and levels of disability. During the past few decades, researchers and health care practitioners have been describing the influence of emotional and psychologic factors on the quantity and quality of pain and disability a person experiences.[22] The interaction between the mind and an individual's overall health is a concept that has been an integral part of Traditional Chinese Medicine, Ayurvedic medicine, and other ancient medical practices—including those of Europe prior to the Renaissance.

Interest in the use of mind-body therapies in the management of health and illness has been increasing in the United States since the early part of the twentieth century. Meditation, relaxation, biofeedback, cognitive-behavioral therapy, hypnosis, and guided imagery are practices referred to as mind-body therapies. (Yoga and tai chi, both of which combine mind-body techniques with physical activity, are often included in this group. They are discussed separately in this chapter.) According to the NIH, mind-body therapies are "interventions that focus on the interactions among the brain, mind, body, and behavior, and the powerful ways in which emotional, mental, social, spiritual, and behavioral factors can directly affect health."[31]

The therapies are based on the principal belief in the mind's ability to affect how the body functions. This approach to health emphasizes self-knowledge, self-care, and personal growth—often with the guidance of a health care professional. The techniques of mind-body therapies are used to relieve stress, to develop coping skills, to relax the mind and body, and to facilitate cognitive restructuring.[32] Table 12.1 outlines each type of mind-body therapy in greater detail.

Mind-body therapies are commonly practiced by diverse populations of adults throughout the United States. In a national phone survey conducted from 1997 to 1998, among 2,055 randomly selected participants 28.9% of respondents reported having used a mind-body therapy—with 18.9% reporting usage within the last year. The most common forms were meditation, guided imagery, and yoga. These therapies were mainly practiced as a part of individual self-care, with only 20% reporting a visit to a trained instructor.

| TABLE 12.1 ALTERNATIVE TREATMENTS | | |
|---|---|---|
| Type of Therapy | Description[22,33] | Prevalence (%) in 2002[1] |
| Meditation | Meditation originated as part of ancient religions and spiritual practices. It was developed as a means of achieving spiritual growth or a transcendental experience. Transcendental and mindfulness meditation are the two types of meditation that have been the subject of most research. In transcendental meditation, the practitioner silently repeats and focuses on a phrase, or mantra, in order to quiet mental thoughts and obtain peacefulness of the body and mind. | 7.6 |
| Relaxation | A variety of relaxation techniques are used to increase the practitioner's awareness of tension and stress and to enhance the ability to release that tension. These techniques include breathing exercises, body scan, and progressive muscle relaxation. The goal of another form of relaxation, Benson's relaxation response, is to reduce sympathetic arousal. | 11.6 (deep breathing exercises), 3.0 (progressive relaxation) |
| Hypnosis | Hypnosis is a technique of using altered consciousness to achieve relaxation and to focus attention. The main components of hypnosis include intense concentration, dissociation of external experiences from normal conscious awareness, and increased acceptance of instructions or guidance from an external source. | 0.2 |
| Guided imagery | Visualization and guided imagery are techniques that involve the generation of sensory or affective mental images with the goal of reaching a state of relaxation or achieving a specific outcome, such as decreased pain or symptoms. These techniques can be practiced individually or in groups with or without the guidance of a practitioner. | 2.1 |
| Biofeedback | Biofeedback involves the use of electronic monitors to teach an individual how to use the mind to affect body functions, such as decreasing the pain associated with migraine headaches or increasing body temperature to relieve symptoms of Raynaud's phenomenon. | 0.1 |
| Cognitive behavioral therapy | Cognitive behavioral therapy emphasizes the ability of cognitive processes to affect emotional, mental, and physical experiences. For instance, anxiety and anger are considered results of non-rational thinking. | — |

Most respondents used mind-body therapies (88.9%) as an adjunct to their allopathic medical care.

A multivariable logistic regression model showed that factors independently and positively associated with the use of mind-body therapies included being between 40 and 49 years of age, being not married, being college educated, and having used another complementary or alternative medical therapy in the last year.[33] In another study, based on data from the 1999 U.S. National Health Interview survey, level of education was the strongest independent predictor of the use of mind-body therapies. In addition, men were less likely to use these therapies than women, and respondents from western states were more likely to use mind-body therapies than people living in other parts of the United States.[1]

The 2002 National Health Interview survey (conducted by the National Center for Health Statistics) among 31,044 adults over the age of 18 estimated that one-third of the population used a form of mind-body therapy in 2002.[34] Table 12.1 shows the percentage of survey respondents who reported using each specific therapy during the past year.

Many prospective RCTs have investigated the use of mind-body therapies in the treatment of chronic pain associated with OA and other conditions. There is strong evidence from the trials suggesting that specific therapies may be effective as adjunctive treatments for recurrent headaches, chronic low back pain, cancer symptoms and treatment side effects, and pain during and following surgical and medical procedures.[32,35] In response to this evidence, the 1996 NIH consensus panel recommended and supported the use of mind-body therapies as an adjunctive treatment for chronic pain.[1]

A few studies have investigated the use of multimodal patient education therapies (including a combination of relaxation, biofeedback, cognitive therapies, and education) in the treatment of RA, OA, and fibromyalgia. Findings from a prospective study of participants in the Arthritis Self Management program conducted in the early 1980s suggested that a community-based program of education, cognitive restructuring, relaxation, and exercise may help reduce pain and disability in patients with arthritis. An analysis of 500 patients, which included 340 patients with OA, showed that pain reductions after participation in the interventional program were maintained after 4 years of follow-up. In addition, health care visits for arthritis decreased by 40%.[33]

In a meta-analysis of 19 controlled trials of patient educational interventions, which included relaxation techniques, the average effect size of pain reduction in patients with OA and RA was 0.17—with the effect being greater in RA compared to OA. Most of these patients were using NSAIDs throughout the trials. The authors also compared results of this meta-analysis to a meta-analysis of placebo-controlled trials of NSAID treatments. They report that the patient education and relaxation techniques may provide about 20 to 30% additional benefit in pain relief to that achieved from NSAIDs.[36] Currently, mind-body therapies have not been directly compared to NSAIDs or other pharmaceutical drugs in an RCT.

Few studies have evaluated adverse effects associated with the use of mind-body therapies. This may be due to the lack of a standardized or well-developed method of assessing adverse events.[35] Relaxation-induced anxiety is one reported complication of mind-body therapies involving relaxation techniques. In a study of 30 patients with chronic anxiety, 17% of the patients experienced increased anxiety during progressive relaxation techniques. This event may be associated with a fear of becoming anxious or of losing control.[37] Other negative effects associated with relaxation techniques that have been reported include intrusive thoughts, floating, dizziness, myoclonic jerks, muscle spasms, and feelings of vulnerability.

A survey of 116 psychologists, whose practice involved the use relaxation techniques, revealed that the therapists prematurely ended treatment sessions with about 4% of their patients due to serious side effects. Studies of hypnotic therapies suggest that patients may experience side effects that include headaches, drowsiness, confusion, nausea, or dizziness. Some researchers have attributed these negative effects to inappropriate use of hypnosis.[35] Given the risk of adverse effects associated with the use of mind-body therapies, it is important that these therapies be used only after careful evaluation of each patient and after tailoring the therapy to their unique individual response.[38]

The mechanisms explaining how mind-body therapies may help reduce pain in patients with OA are currently unclear. It has been suggested that the effect may be a result of modification in the cognitive and emotional components of pain perception.[1] Studies of functional brain mapping using fMRI have shown that the practice of meditation activates parts of the brain involved in attention and control of the autonomic nervous system.[39] An RCT of mindfulness meditation in healthy subjects showed that subjects practicing meditation had a statistically significant increase in activation of areas of the brain associated with positive affect and a significant improvement in immune function (measured as antibody titers to the influenza vaccine).[40]

Although there is some evidence to suggest that mind-body therapies (when used as a multimodal therapy in combination with education and behavioral counseling) are effective as adjunctive treatments for OA, that evidence is limited. Effect sizes in the studies have been small and have diminished with time. Studies differ in the type of mind-body therapy or combination of therapies used. Few studies have evaluated the use of mind-body therapies on patients with OA alone rather than combined with RA and other rheumatic conditions.

More RCTs need to be conducted to further evaluate the efficacy of mind-body therapies in the management of OA. It would be useful to compare different types or combinations of mind-body therapies directly and to compare mind-body therapies combined with standard therapies, including NSAIDs and exercise, to standard therapies alone. In addition to evaluating the relative clinical efficacy of different mind-body therapies, future research should investigate the role of patient characteristics in influencing outcomes, cost effectiveness of these therapies, and mechanisms of action.[35]

Evidence from epidemiologic studies suggests that a small percentage of patients with musculoskeletal problems, including OA, are using mind-body therapies. In a study of data from the U.S. 1999 National Health Interview survey, although respondents with musculoskeletal pain were almost twice as likely as those without to report using a mind-body therapy within the past year this represented only 9% (1 out of 10) of respondents with musculoskeletal pain.[1]

Only 14.8% of respondents with OA, from a telephone survey conducted among 2,055 American adults in 1997 to 1998, reported using mind-body therapies. Almost half the respondents with OA who used mind-body therapies found them to be helpful for these conditions.[33] The infrequent use of mind-body therapies by patients with OA suggests the existence of important barriers, which may occur at the patient, physician/provider, and/or institutional levels.[1] Further work needs to be done to improve understanding of

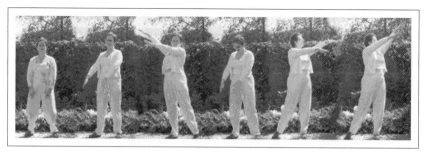

**Fig. 12.2** "Bridge over water." (Courtesy of *http://www.everyday-taichi.com*.)

these barriers and to facilitate wider application of these therapies as adjunctive treatments for OA.

## TAI CHI

Tai chi is an ancient Chinese martial art and exercise that involves slow repetitive movements, changes in the center of balance, and meditation.[41] It has been practiced in other countries for centuries as a treatment for many acute and chronic conditions. Many different styles or schools of tai chi have evolved, with the principal schools being the Sun, Chen, Hao, Hu Lei, Wu, and Yang styles.[42] The basic movements of each style include weight shifting between the right and left legs, knee flexion and extension, flexion and rotation of head and trunk, and asymmetrical arm and leg movements.

Fig. 12.2 depicts the sequences of three different sets of tai chi motions. Tai chi focuses on balance, flexibility, strength, relaxation, and body alignment. The intensity of this low-impact exercise can be varied by adjusting the heights of postures, duration of each training session, and the practice style. In addition, it does not require expensive equipment and can be performed anywhere individually or in groups. These features allow tai chi to be accessible to people of all ages, aerobic capacity, and previous exercise experience[43] (Figs. 12.2 through 12.4).

Exercise and physical therapy are important parts of a multidisciplinary approach to the management of OA. Evidence from RCTs has suggested that aerobic exercise, strength training, and flexibility can have beneficial effects for patients with OA. By strengthening muscles, providing joint stability, improving joint circulation, and assisting in weight loss, regular exercise can help reduce arthritic pain and improve functional status.[44] Current guidelines from the American College of Rheumatology recommend that aerobic exercise, range of motion, and quadriceps resistance training be integrated into standard practice for patients with OA of the knee.[45] The goal of exercise for patients with OA of the hip should be "to preserve at least 30 degrees of flexion and full extension of the hip and to strengthen the hip abductors and extensors."[46]

During the past few decades, tai chi has been gradually emerging as a popular exercise form in Western societies. According to the National Center for Health Statistics, about 1.3% of the adult population practiced tai chi in 2002.[1] Many centers for older adults offer tai chi classes.[47] It has also gained the attention of health practitioners and researchers as an exercise that may potentially benefit older adults and patients with OA. In that the principal elements of tai chi are slow movement; low weight bearing; and emphasis on posture, balance, relaxation, and stretching, it may help protect joints from injury by strengthening muscles

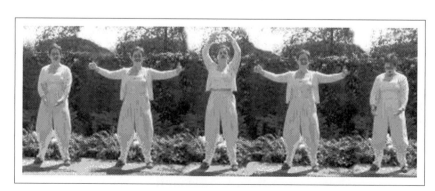

**Fig. 12.3** Rolling the arms. (Courtesy of *http://www.everyday-taichi.com*.)

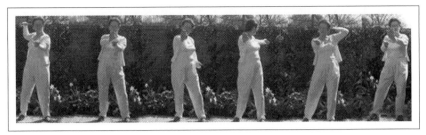

**Fig. 12.4** "Wild goose looks for food." (Courtesy of *http:// www.everyday-taichi.com*.)

and preventing falls through improvements in balance and gait.[48]

A number of controlled trials have investigated the use of tai chi in the elderly. Sattin et al. reported a statistically significant decrease in fear of falling in a group of older adults randomized to a tai chi treatment group compared to subjects in a wellness education group after 8 and 12 months of intervention.[49] A within-subject analysis involving 69 women over the age of 65 from retirement communities found a statistically significant improvement in balance, functional mobility, and fear of falling after 3 months of twice-weekly 30-minute tai chi instruction.[41] In a nonrandomized study, Choi et al. found no significant difference in incidence of falls between ambulatory adults over 60 years of age who were assigned to a 12-week tai chi treatment group compared to a nonequivalent control group.

Although the results were not statistically significant, the relative risk of falling was 0.62 in the treatment group compared to controls, and the tai chi participants had significantly greater confidence in their ability to avoid falls. The authors also report a statistically significant improvement in flexibility, mobility, and strength of knee and ankle flexors and extensors in the tai chi group.[50] The Atlanta FICSIT (Frailty and Injuries: Cooperative Studies of Intervention and Techniques) trial randomized 200 people over 70 years of age living in Atlanta to one of three groups: tai chi, computerized balance training, and education.

The interventions (conducted for 15 weeks) consisted of twice-weekly 1-hour tai chi classes, a computerized program requiring subjects to balance their center of mass while standing on a transducer platform, and an education program instructing patients to continue usual exercise levels while receiving education about other issues of interest to older adults. At the conclusion of the study, subjects in the tai chi group had reduced ambulation speed, reduction in systolic blood pressure after a 12-minute walk, and less loss in grip strength compared to the balance training and education groups. In addition, there was a statistically significant decrease in fear of falling and in rate of falls after participating in tai chi compared to the education group.[51]

The evidence suggests that tai chi is a form of exercise that can lead to improvements in balance, mobility, muscle strength, and joint flexibility and reductions in rate of fall and fear of falling in frail older adults. It should be noted that many of these studies have involved small sample sizes and have varied in subject demographics, forms of tai chi practiced, methods of evaluation, outcomes measured, and study quality. In addition, because most of the study subjects have been Caucasian women the results may not be able to be generalized to other populations of older adults. Nonetheless, the findings are important because falls among the older population in the United States constitute a major public health problem.[41]

It has been estimated that about 30% of people over 65 years of age fall each year.[50] Falls result in significant morbidity, mortality, and health care spending among the elderly. Fall-related injuries and fear of falling often inhibit further activity and lead to loss of independence and self-care capabilities.[41] In addition, patients with lower extremity OA are at risk for falling, and the injuries that result can be a serious complication.

To date only two trials have evaluated the efficacy of tai chi as a treatment for OA. An exercise program consisting of 12 tai chi movements in the Sun style has recently been developed specifically for patients with OA.[52] The movements in this program are performed at a high stance, which limits the amount of stress placed on the lower extremities. To study the effects of this tai chi program on arthritic symptoms and physical functioning, Sun et al. randomized 72 Korean women over the age of 55 with OA to a tai chi exercise group or to a non-exercise control group.

The women in the treatment group were expected to complete the specific exercises for 20 minutes per day for a minimum of three times per week. Prior to and after 12 weeks, the K-WOMAC (Korean version of the WOMAC) was used to assess self-reported symptoms and an exercise physiologist (blinded to group assignments) measured physical functioning, flexibility, balance, muscle strength, body mass index, and cardiovascular fitness. The results showed a statistically significant improvement in pain, stiffness, and physical functioning of 35%, 29%, and 29% (respectively) for these three measures in the exercise group compared to the control group. In addition, patients who performed tai chi demonstrated significantly improved balance and abdominal muscle strength after 12 weeks.

Although no significant differences between the groups were found in cardiovascular functioning, flexibility, and knee muscle strength, the authors suggest that the tai chi program may need to be carried out longer than 12 weeks in order to see an improvement in these factors. Out of 72 patients randomized, 22 and 21 subjects in the exercise and control groups (respectively) completed the study. This dropout rate of 43% reduces the ability of the study to accurately detect significant group differences and limits the generalizability of the findings.[48]

In a second study investigating the use of tai chi in the management of OA, 33 Springfield (Massachusetts) patients with lower extremity OA were randomized to either an exercise program consisting of tai chi training for 2 hours per week for 12 weeks or to a control group. Subjects in the control group were instructed to continue their usual physical activity and had the opportunity to discuss issues relating to OA as a group three times during the 12 weeks and with a health care practitioner every 2 weeks by telephone.

Outcome measures (which included arthritis-related pain and function, quality of life, and lower extremity mobility) were assessed at baseline and after 12 weeks using the Arthritis Self Efficacy Scale (ASES), Arthritis Impact Measurement Scale (AIMS), the 50-foot walking speed test, the one-leg balance test, and the "time to rise from a chair" test. After 12 weeks, the tai chi group experienced significant improvement in arthritis symptoms, tension, and satisfaction with general health status.[53] The interpretation of the results from the study is limited by the small sample size and multiple statistical comparisons. Although there was no statistically significant difference between the two groups in baseline demographic characteristics, the subjects in the tai chi group reported more baseline pain and less satisfaction with health status. This difference may weaken the statistical and clinical significance of the improvements in self-efficacy in the intervention group.

The findings from the two studies suggest that tai chi may benefit patients with OA by improving symptoms and function. However, both of these studies involved small numbers of patients and assessed patients only in the short term following a 12-week tai chi program. In order to further evaluate the efficacy of tai chi as a treatment for OA, RCTs involving larger patient populations and with short- and long-term follow-up

need to be conducted. It may be useful for future studies to focus on particular joints affected by OA. In addition, tai chi interventions should be compared to other exercise programs currently used as part of the management of this condition.

When designing a future study, certain other factors should be considered. First, the intervention may have differential benefits among subgroups of patients within the treatment group. A reanalysis of results from an RCT evaluating the health benefits of tai chi among healthy older adults showed that subjects in the tai chi group with lower levels of physical function at baseline experienced greater rate and degree of improvement in physical functioning compared to subjects within the group with higher initial functional status.[54]

This evidence suggests that tai chi programs may need to be tailored to individual levels of baseline physical functioning. Active older adults may receive greater benefit from a more vigorous tai chi intervention. When subjects in the intervention group differ in pre-intervention characteristics, the use of a group mean to estimate effect size may be misleading. Because the presence or absence of subgroup differences may influence whether a difference is detected between the intervention and control groups, a subgroup analysis based on pre-intervention characteristics of the subjects in the treatment group should be conducted.

A second factor that should be taken into consideration is the generalizability of results. Subjects in most studies are usually volunteers. In one study, involving 69 women (from three different retirement communities in Atlanta) who volunteered to participate in a 6-month tai chi intervention study, the subjects represented only 10% of the total female populations from the three community homes. In addition, the dropout rate for most exercise intervention studies ranges from 25 to 64%.[41] The motivational factors influencing whether or not a patient volunteers to participate or completes a study need to be addressed.

Third, the availability of social support may influence whether patients participate in and benefit from tai chi exercise programs. Family members, physicians, instructors, health care center staff, retirement center staff, and other sources often provide significant encouragement and support to study participants.[41] The role of these support groups on participation and outcomes in an exercise intervention study needs to be further investigated.

The exact mechanism by which tai chi may reduce symptoms and improve function in patients with OA is not clear. Current theories speculate that tai chi allows patients to exercise, increase flexibility, and strengthen their joints while simultaneously increasing awareness of posture and weight bearing during exercise.

By improving balance and gait, leading to a decrease in the risk of falls, tai chi may prevent further injury to joints. In addition, evidence from a meta-analysis suggests that this form of exercise improves aerobic capacity in both healthy subjects and patients with chronic diseases.[43] Further work needs to be done to evaluate potential mechanisms of tai chi.

## YOGA

Yoga is a philosophy and discipline originating from the ancient civilizations of India. The term *yoga* is derived from the Sanskrit root *yug*, meaning to join together or to unify. The goal of this discipline is to consciously achieve union between one's body, mind, emotions, and spirit.[55] According to the yogic philosophy, this union can be achieved by following a moral code of conduct, meditation, *asanas* (postures), and *pranayama* (controlled breathing).[56] The end result is a sense of well-being that can greatly impact health and disease. According to B.K.S. Iyengar (a world renowned teacher and master), yoga maintains good health, prevents the development of disease, and aids in the recovery from ill health.[57]

Although there are many types of yogic disciplines, Hatha yoga is well known and has been subjected to the most clinical research. It was initially developed as a means of meditating or of calming the mind. Given the focus on activity and exercise, it is currently mainly practiced for health and vitality in Western countries.[58] Multiple styles reflecting a different approach to the *asanas* have arisen within Hatha yoga. Iyengar yoga (based on the teachings of B.K.S. Iyengar) is a particular Hatha style that has become widely popular in the United States. It is unique in that it is designed to be accessible to everyone. The use of props (such as chairs, belts, blankets, and blocks) allows the practitioner to assume precise and appropriate positioning without straining the joints or muscles.[59]

During the past few decades, the physical postures (*asanas*) used in yoga have become a popular form of exercise in the Western cultures. The prevalence of the use of yoga among adults in the United States in 2002 was estimated to be about 5.1%, which increased from 3.7% in 1997.[1,60] Yoga has increasingly been commercialized as a trendy means of maintaining fitness and reducing stress, usually without regard to the intended goal of achieving wholeness and self-realization.[55] Many patients ask their health professionals about the health benefits of yoga and are often referred to yoga instructors or programs.

Multiple research studies have shown that Hatha yoga can improve muscle strength and flexibility. In addition, there has been some evidence to suggest that yoga may help control blood pressure, respiration, heart rate, and metabolic rate.[55] In that the static postures of yoga emphasize stretching and improve strength and flexibility, it has been considered an alternative form of exercise to be used in the treatment of OA.[56] Similar to that of tai chi, the role of yoga in the management of OA has received little objective evaluation. Only two prospective studies have been completed, which respectively investigated the use of Hatha yoga as a treatment for OA of the hand and knee.

Garfinkel et al. randomly assigned 17 patients with OA of the hand to either a yoga treatment program or to a control group. The subjects were greater than 50 years of age and included both men and women. The intervention consisted of supervised Iyengar Hatha yoga instruction for 1 hour once a week for 8 weeks. Subjects in the control group continued their baseline treatment regimen, which included medications received by both groups. The primary outcomes measured were hand pain, hand function as measured by the Stanford Hand Assessment Questionnaire, and range of motion, tenderness, and circumference of the finger joints.

Patients who completed the yoga program demonstrated statistically significant improvement in pain during activity, range of motion, and tenderness after 8 weeks compared to the control group. Although no significant difference was found in finger circumference and grip strength between the groups, there was a trend toward greater improvement in the intervention group.[61] The results in this study are limited by the small sample size and short study duration. Some researchers have suggested that the personal attention and social support a patient receives from participating in an intervention may provide some benefit independent of the effect from the treatment itself. Because the subjects in the control group did not receive any intervention, the influence of the supportive group format of yoga on the differences in results between the two groups should not be discounted.

Kolasinski et al. conducted an open-labeled pilot study investigating the use of Iyengar Hatha yoga as a treatment for symptoms of OA of the knee. Eligible participants were greater than 50 years of age and sedentary, with symptomatic OA in at least one knee for at least 6 months. The intervention consisted of 8 weeks of once-weekly yoga sessions lasting 1 to 1.5 hours and led by a certified Iyengar yoga teacher. Participants were required to attend five of eight sessions, and were assessed (via WOMAC, the Arthritis Impact Measurement Scale 2 (AIMS2) social and psychologic subsets, the 50-foot walk time test, and the Patient and Physician Global Assessments) prior to and after completing the intervention.[59]

Out of 11 subjects enrolled in the study, seven women participated for the duration of the study (and six of these seven patients were obese). The authors report statistically significant reductions in pain and physical function assessed by the WOMAC after 8 weeks compared to pre-intervention status. Although there was a decrease in WOMAC stiffness, the results were not statistically significant. Subjects also showed significant improvement in affect, as measured by the AIMS2, and large but non-significant changes in AIMS2 symptoms. Improvements in the Physician Global Assessment and the Patient Global Assessment were observed, but the trends did not reach statistical significance. There was no change in 50-foot walk time after 8 weeks. No adverse effects, including injuries, were reported throughout the study.[59]

This pilot study demonstrates that yoga may be a safe and feasible form of exercise for previously yoga-naive, obese, female patients over 50 years of age.[59] Although the findings suggest that yoga may reduce pain and disability in patients with OA of the knee, the results are limited by the small sample size, short study duration, and lack of a control group.

Because only two studies (both methodologically limited) have investigated the efficacy of yoga as a treatment for OA, concrete recommendations concerning the use of yoga cannot be made at this time. Larger RCTs need to be conducted to support the findings in these studies for OA of the knee and hand. The use of yoga should also be evaluated for other joints affected by OA, including the hip and shoulder. Goals for future research include larger sample sizes, use of male and female subjects, longer duration of treatment, short- and long-term follow-up, and comparison to other non-pharmacologic interventions for OA (such as education, range-of-motion and muscle-strengthening exercises, and walking). The role of yoga in the prevention of OA may also be a direction for future investigation.

Although the exact mechanisms responsible for the possible benefits of yoga for symptoms of OA are currently unknown, some hypotheses have been proposed. For instance, yogic postures that emphasize knee extension and flexion may help reduce symptoms of OA of the knee by strengthening the quadriceps. The use of certain props, such as ropes and bands, to stretch the knee joint may also play a role.[56] Other mechanisms may include improvements in cardiovascular fitness, flexibility, and awareness of body positioning at rest and during exercise.[59]

In a study involving 20 college students who were previously untrained in yoga, participation in 6 weeks of yoga resulted in significantly increased levels of serum lactate dehydrogenase (LDH).[55] This evidence suggests that yoga may also improve cardiovascular endurance in older adults and patients with OA. In addition, researchers have begun to investigate the physiologic effects of exercise. Changes in muscle cell shape that occur during exercise can alter gene regulation and expression of proteins involved in cell interaction with the extracellular matrix and other cells, ultimately affecting cell function.[56] From attaining and holding yogic postures, the stretching and conditioning of skeletal muscle cells result in increased oxidation capacity and decrease glycogen utilization.

Physicians should also be aware of potential risks or problems associated with yoga as well as the benefits. It should be noted that if the postures are done incorrectly or without prior stretching injuries to joints or muscles may occur. With the increasing availability and accessibility of personal-use yoga guides (such as video- and audiotapes, DVDs, and books), patients are trying to practice yoga in the convenience of their own homes and may be more likely to perform postures with incorrect alignment.

This problem may be avoided with supervised yoga instruction. In addition, there are a variety of approaches to and styles of yoga available that may differ in effectiveness as a treatment for OA. Before recommendation or referring a patient to a yoga instructor, it is important to be aware of the instructor's credentials and style of practice. Patients should also be advised against any form of instruction that makes extravagant or inappropriate claims.[56]

## REFERENCES

1. Barnes PM, Powell-Griner E, McFann K, Nahin RL. Complementary and alternative medicine use among adults: United States, 2002. Adv Data 2004;343:1–19.
2. Eisenberg DM, Kessler RC, Van Rompay MI, Kaptchuk TJ, Wilkey SA, Appel S, et al. Perceptions about complementary therapies relative to conventional therapies among adults who use both: Results from a national survey. Ann Intern Med 2001:135:344–51.
3. Rao JK, Kroenke K, Mihaliak KA, Grambow SC, Weinberger M. Rheumatology patients' use of complementary therapies: Results from a one-year longitudinal study. Arthritis Rheum 2003;49:619–25.
4. Breuer GS, Orbach H, Elkayam O, Berkun Y, Paran D, Mates M, et al. Perceived efficacy among patients of various methods of complementary alternative medicine for rheumatologic diseases. Clin Exp Rheumatol 2005;23:693–96.
5. Eisenberg DM, Kessler RC, Foster C, et al. Unconventional medicine in the United States: Prevalence, costs, and patterns of use. N Engl J Med 1993;328:246.
6. Witt C, Brinkhaus B, Jena S, Linde K, Streng A, Wagenpfeil S, et al. Acupuncture in patients with osteoarthritis of the knee: A randomised trial. Lancet 2005;366:100–01.
7. Helms JM. Acupuncture Energetic: A Clinical Approach for Physicians. Berkeley, California: Medical Acupuncture Publishers 1995.
8. Reston J. Now about my operation in Peking. The New York Times, 26 July 1971:1,6.

9. Ramsey DJ, Bowman MA, Greenman PE, et al. National Institutes of Health Consensus Development Statement on Acupuncture. JAMA 1997;15:1–34.

10. Berman BM, Lao L, Langenberg P, Lee WL, Gilpin AM, Hochberg MC. Effectiveness of acupuncture as adjunctive therapy in osteoarthritis of the knee: A randomized, controlled trial. Ann Intern Med 2004;141:901–10.

11. Vas J, Mendez C, Perea-Milla E, Vega E, Panadero MD, Leon JM, et al. Acupuncture as a complementary therapy to the pharmacological treatment of osteoarthritis of the knee: Randomised controlled trial. BMJ 2004;329(7476):1216.

12. Chen LX, Farrar JT. Can sham needling be successfully blinded for acupuncture research in osteoarthritis? Arthrit Rheum 2003;48:S72.

13. Stener-Victorin E, Kruse-Smidje C, Jung K. Comparison between electro-acupuncture and hydrotherapy, both in combination with patient education and patient education alone, on the symptomatic treatment of osteoarthritis of the hip. Clin J Pain 2004;20:179–85.

14. Usichenko TI, Dinse M, Hermsen M, Witstruck T, Pavlovic D, Lehmann Ch. Auricular acupuncture for pain relief after total hip arthroplasty: A randomized controlled study. Pain 2005;114:320–27.

15. Yamashita H, Tsukayama H, Hori N, et al. Incidence of adverse reactions associated with acupuncture. J Altern Complement Med 2000;6:345–50.

16. Yamashita H, Tsukayama H, Tanno Y, et al. Adverse events in acupuncture and moxibustion treatment: A six-year survey at a national clinics in Japan. J Altern Complement Med 1999;5:229–36.

17. Eisenberg DM, Davis RB, Ettner SL, Appel S, Wilkey S, Van Rompay M, et al. Trends in alternative medicine use in the United States, 1990–1997: Results of a follow-up national survey. JAMA 1998;280:1569–75.

18. Kelly JP, Kaufman DW, Kelley K, Rosenberg L, Anderson TE, Mitchell AA. Recent trends in use of herbal and other natural products. Arch Intern Med 2005;165:281–86.

19. Yu SM, Ghandour RM, Huang ZJ. Herbal supplement use among U.S. women, 2000. J Am Med Womens Assoc 2004;59:17–24.

20. Kaufman DW, Kelly JP, Rosenberg L, Anderson TE, Mitchell AA. Recent patterns of medication use in the ambulatory adult population of the United States: The Slone survey. JAMA 2002;287:337–44.

21. Setty AR, Sigal LH. Herbal medications commonly used in the practice of rheumatology: Mechanisms of action, efficacy, and side effects. Semin Arthritis Rheum 2005;34:773–84.

22. Horstman J. The Arthritis Foundation's Guide to Alternative Therapies. Atlanta: Arthritis Foundation 1999.

23. Long L, Soeken K, Ernst E. Herbal medicines for the treatment of osteoarthritis: A systematic review. Rheumatology (Oxford) 2001;40:779–93.

24. Chantre P, Cappelaere A, Leblan D, Guedon D, Vandermander J, Fournie B. Efficacy and tolerance of Harpagophytum procumbens versus diacerein in treatment of osteoarthritis. Phytomedicine 2000;7:177–83.

25. von Kruedener S, Schneider W, Elstner EF. A combination of Populus tremula, Solidago virgaurea and Fraxinus excelsior as an anti-inflammatory and antirheumatic drug: A short review. Arzneimittelforschung 1995;45:169–71.

26. Meyer B, Schneider W, Elstner EF. Antioxidative properties of alcoholic extracts from Fraxinus excelsior, Populus tremula and Solidago virgaurea. Arzneimittelforschung 1995;45:174–76.

27. Ernst E. Harmless herbs? A review of the recent literature. Am J Med 1998;104:170–78.

28. Garrard J, Harms S, Eberly LE, Matiak A. Variations in product choices of frequently purchased herbs: Caveat emptor. Arch Intern Med 2003;163:2290–95.

29. Ko RJ. A U.S. perspective on the adverse reactions from traditional Chinese medicines. J Chin Med Assoc 2004;67:109–16.

30. Saper RB, Kales SN, Paquin J, Burns MJ, Eisenberg DM, Davis RB, et al. Heavy metal content of ayurvedic herbal medicine products. JAMA 2004;292:2868–73.

31. http://nccam.nih.gov/health/backgrounds/mindbody.html.

32. Astin JA. Mind-body therapies for the management of pain. Clin J Pain 2004;20:27–32.

33. Wolsko PM, Eisenberg DM, Davis RB, Phillips RS. Use of mind-body medical therapies. J Gen Intern Med 2004;19:43–50.

34. Astin JA, Shapiro SL, Eisenberg DM, Forys KL. Mind-body medicine: state of the science, implications for practice. J Am Board Fam Pract 2003;16:131–47.

35. Tindle HA, Wolsko P, Davis RB, Eisenberg DM, Phillips RS, McCarthy EP. Factors associated with the use of mind body therapies among United States adults with musculoskeletal pain. Complement Ther Med 2005;13:155–64.

36. Superio-Cabuslay E, Ward MM, Lorig KR. Patient education interventions in osteoarthritis and RA: A meta-analytic comparison with nonsteroidal anti-inflammatory drug treatment. Arthritis Care Res 1996;9:292–301.

37. Braith JA, McCullough JP, Bush JP. Relaxation-induced anxiety in a subclinical sample of chronically anxious subjects. J Behav Ther Exp Psychiatry 1988;19:193–98.

38. Carlson CR, Nitz AJ. Negative side effects of self-regulation training: Relaxation and the role of the professional in service delivery. Biofeedback Self Regul 1991;16:191–97.

39. Lazar SW, Bush G, Gollub RL, Fricchione GL, Khalsa G, Benson H. Functional brain mapping of the relaxation response and meditation. Neuroreport 2000;11:1581–85.

40. Davidson RJ, Kabat-Zinn J, Schumacher J, Rosenkranz M, Muller D, Santorelli SF, et al. Alterations in brain and immune function produced by mindfulness meditation. Psychosom Med 2003;65:564–70.

41. Taggart HM. Effects of Tai Chi exercise on balance, functional mobility, and fear of falling among older women. Appl Nurs Res 2002;15:235–42.

42. http://www.chebucto.ns.ca/Philosophy/Taichi/styles.html.

43. Taylor-Piliae RE, Froelicher ES. Effectiveness of Tai Chi exercise in improving aerobic capacity: A meta-analysis. J Cardiovasc Nurs 2004;19:48–57.

44. Kovar PA, Allegrante JP, MacKenzie CR, Peterson MG, Gutin B, Charlson ME. Supervised fitness walking in patients with osteoarthritis of the knee: A randomized, controlled trial. Ann Intern Med 1992;116:529–34.

45. Hochberg MC, Altman RD, Brandt KD, Clark BM, Dieppe PA, Griffin MR, et al. Guidelines for the medical management of osteoarthritis. Part II. Osteoarthritis of the knee. American College of Rheumatology. Arthritis Rheum 1995;38:1541–46.

46. Hochberg MC, Altman RD, Brandt KD, Clark BM, Dieppe PA, Griffin MR, et al. Guidelines for the medical management of osteoarthritis. Part I. Osteoarthritis of the hip. American College of Rheumatology. Arthritis Rheum 1995;38:1535–40.

47. Burks K. Osteoarthritis in older adults: Current treatments. J Gerontol Nurs 2005;31:11–19.

48. Song R, Lee EO, Lam P, Bae SC. Effects of tai chi exercise on pain, balance, muscle strength, and perceived difficulties in physical functioning in older women with osteoarthritis: A randomized clinical trial. J Rheumatol 2003;30:2039–44.

49. Sattin RW, Easley KA, Wolf SL, Chen Y, Kutner MH. Reduction in fear of falling through intense tai chi exercise training in older, transitionally frail adults. J Am Geriatr Soc 2005;53:1168–78.

50. Choi JH, Moon JS, Song R. Effects of Sun-style Tai Chi exercise on physical fitness and fall prevention in fall-prone older adults. J Adv Nurs 2005;51:150–57.

51. Wolf SL, Barnhart HX, Kutner NG, McNeely E, Coogler C, Xu T. Reducing frailty and falls in older persons: An investigation of Tai Chi and computerized balance training. Atlanta FICSIT Group. Frailty and Injuries: Cooperative Studies of Intervention Techniques. J Am Geriatr Soc 1996;44:489–97.

52. Lam P. New horizons: Developing tai chi for health care. Aust Fam Physician 1998;27:100–01.

53. Hartman CA, Manos TM, Winter C, Hartman DM, Li B, Smith JC. Effects of Tai Chi training on function and quality of life indicators in older adults with osteoarthritis. J Am Geriatr Soc 2000;48:1553–59.

54. Li F, Fisher KJ, Harmer P, McAuley E. Delineating the impact of Tai Chi training on physical function among the elderly. Am J Prev Med 2002;23(2):92–7.

55. http://www.everyday-taichi.com.

56. Raub JA. Psychophysiologic effects of Hatha Yoga on musculoskeletal and cardiopulmonary function: A literature review. J Altern Complement Med 2002;8:797–812.

57. Garfinkel M, Schumacher HR Jr. Yoga. Rheum Dis Clin North Am 2000;26:125–32.

58. Iyengar BKS, Evans JJ, Abrams D. *Light on Life: The Yoga Journey to Wholeness, Inner Peace, and Ultimate Freedom*. Emmaus, PA: Rodale 2005.

59. http://www.yogaworld.org/.

60. Kolasinski SL, Garfinkel M, Tsai AG, Matz W, Dyke AV, Schumacher HR. Iyengar yoga for treating symptoms of osteoarthritis of the knees: a pilot study. J Altern Complement Med 2005;11:689–93.

61. Tindle HA, Davis RB, Phillips RS, Eisenberg DM. Trends in use of complementary and alternative medicine by US adults: 1997–2002. Altern Ther Health Med 2005;11:42–9.

62. Garfinkel MS, Schumacher HR Jr., Husain A, Levy M, Reshetar RA. Evaluation of a yoga based regimen for treatment of osteoarthritis of the hands. J Rheumatol 1994;21:2341–43.

# 13 Future Directions in Physical Therapy for Knee Osteoarthritis

Kim Bennell, Rana Hinman, and Tim Wrigley

## INTRODUCTION

As knee osteoarthritis (OA) is essentially an incurable condition, contemporary management has centered on the alleviation of symptoms and the maintenance or improvement of physical function. Due to the heterogeneity of the disease, a variety of symptoms may be associated with knee OA—including pain, muscle weakness, joint stiffness, swelling, and instability. Impairments in the local mechanical environment and neuromotor control systems (such as mal-alignment, joint laxity, and altered muscle activity patterns) also exist. The combined effect of these disease-associated symptoms and impairments is often one of declining physical function and ultimately a reduction in quality of life.

Treatment options for knee OA may be classified as nonpharmacologic, pharmacologic, or surgical. Given their relatively low toxicity and cost, nonpharmacologic strategies (such as physical therapy, including exercise) are recommended by clinical guidelines as the first-line treatment for knee OA.[1,2] Physical therapy is integral to the management of patients with knee OA, and there is abundant evidence demonstrating its beneficial clinical effects in patients (see Table 13.1). The primary goals of physical therapy are to reduce pain, decrease disability, and optimize participation in social, domestic, occupational, and recreational pursuits.[3] Physical therapy encompasses a variety of treatment modalities for knee OA, including manual joint mobilization, exercise prescription, hydrotherapy, massage, knee taping, transcutaneous electrical nerve stimulation (TENS), knee braces, and shoe insoles. Although such treatments may be applied in isolation, clinical practice generally utilizes multiple treatment strategies concurrently.

Although alleviation of symptoms is the major concern for most patients with knee OA, rising health care costs and the increasing prevalence of OA due to population aging[4] necessitate a focus on preventing disease incidence in the first place and on slowing its progression once disease is established. However, most physical therapy research to date has focused on symptomatic and functional outcomes. It is feasible that physical therapy interventions could influence structural disease, probably via reductions in knee load. Effects are likely to differ according to the type of intervention and the local mechanical environment operating within each individual.

This chapter discusses the role of knee loading in the development and progression of knee OA and the influence of local mechanical factors on knee load and intervention outcomes. Current and novel physical therapy interventions for knee OA with the potential for disease-modifying effects are also discussed. The emphasis here is on tibiofemoral rather than patellofemoral OA, in that the latter may require different rehabilitative approaches and currently there is very little research on OA in the patellofemoral compartment.

## ROLE OF KNEE LOADING IN KNEE OSTEOARTHRITIS

Knee loading plays a major role in knee OA development and progression. This is highlighted by in vivo animal experiments[5] and by the positive relationship of knee OA to obesity[6,7] and to occupations involving repetitive knee bending.[8] Because direct measurement of joint loads in vivo is not feasible in humans, 3D gait analysis providing kinetics (forces and moments) and kinematics (motions) is a valuable tool for inferring dynamic loading conditions. During the stance phase of gait, high loads are applied to the knee in both sagittal and frontal planes. For knee OA, the most relevant and widely studied load is the external knee adduction moment (AM) in the frontal plane—generated because the ground reaction force vector passes medial to the joint center.[9]

This moment forces the knee laterally into varus and is resisted by an internal abduction moment, resulting in compression of the medial joint compartment and stretching of the lateral structures (Fig. 13.1). The AM

| TABLE 13.1 SUMMARY OF EFFICACIOUS PHYSICAL THERAPY INTERVENTIONS IN KNEE OSTEOARTHRITIS | |
|---|---|
| **Intervention** | **Effects** |
| Aerobic exercise | Decreased knee pain, improved physical function, increased respiratory capacity, decreased joint tenderness |
| Strengthening exercise | Increased muscle strength, decreased knee pain, improved physical function, improved quality of life |
| Hydrotherapy | Decreased knee pain, improved physical function |
| Knee taping | Decreased knee pain, improved physical function |
| TENS | Decreased knee pain |
| Unloading knee braces | Decreased knee pain, reduced loading across the knee, improved physical function |
| Laterally wedged shoe insoles | Decreased knee pain, reduced loading across the knee |
| Combined treatments | Decreased knee pain, increased muscle strength, improved physical function, improved quality of life |

TENS = transcutaneous electrical nerve stimulation.

Source: Fransen FM, McConnell S, Bell M. Therapeutic exercise for people with osteoarthritis of the hip or knee: A systematic review. J Rheumatol 2002;29:1737; Fransen M, McConnell S, Bell M. Exercise for osteoarthritis of the hip or knee (Cochrane Review). *The Cochrane Library*. Chichester, UK: John Wiley & Sons 2003; Foley A, Halbert J, Hewitt T, et al. Does hydrotherapy improve strength and physical function in patients with osteoarthritis?: A randomised controlled trial comparing a gym based and a hydrotherapy based strengthening program. Ann Rheum Dis 2003;62:1162; Wyatt F, Milam S, Manske R, et al. The effects of aquatic and traditional exercise programs on persons with knee osteoarthritis. J Strength Conditioning Res 2001;15:337; Cushnaghan J, McCarthy C, Dieppe P. Taping the patella medially: A new treatment for osteoarthritis of the knee joint? Brit Med J 1994;308:753; Hinman R, Bennell K, Crossley K, et al. Immediate effects of adhesive tape on pain and disability in individuals with knee osteoarthritis. Rheumatol 2003;42:865; Hinman R, Crossley K, McConnell J, et al. Efficacy of knee tape in the management of knee osteoarthritis: A blinded randomised controlled trial. Brit Med J 2003;327:135; Osiri M, Welch V, Brosseau L, et al. Transcutaneous electrical nerve stimulation for knee osteoarthritis (Cochrane Review). *The Cochrane Library*. Oxford, UK: John Wiley & Sons 2005; Deyle GD, Henderson NE, Matekel RL, et al. Effectiveness of manual physical therapy and exercise in osteoarthritis of the knee: A randomized, controlled trial. Ann Int Med 2000;132:173; Fransen M, Crosbie J, Edmonds J. Physical therapy is effective for patients with osteoarthritis of the knee: A randomized controlled trial. J Rheumatol 2001;28:156; Quilty B, Tucker M, Campbell R, et al. Physiotherapy, including quadriceps exercises and patellar taping, for knee osteoarthritis with predominant patello-femoral joint involvement: randomized controlled trial. J Rheumatol 2003;30:1311.

influences the load distribution between the medial and lateral plateaus. The higher the AM the greater the load on the medial plateau relative to the lateral plateau.[9] The AM is higher in people with knee OA than in controls,[10] and it strongly predicts medial compartment knee OA severity[11] and outcome from surgical procedures.[12] Importantly, the AM during gait is one of only a few factors known to predict OA progression in humans. A 20- to 30% increase in the AM is associated with a 2.8- to 6.5-fold increase in the risk of progression.[13,14]

Impact loading occurs when the moving foot contacts the ground at the beginning of the stance phase of gait. This causes a shock wave to be transmitted up the skeleton. This impact loading may manifest itself as a heel-strike transient—a short spike of force typically seen 10 to 20 ms after heel strike on the ground reaction force trace (Fig. 13.2). There is variability in the magnitude and rate of the heel-strike transient depending on factors such as the properties of the foot (mass and velocity) and the interface (thickness, elasticity, and viscosity).[15]

About a third of the normal population demonstrates a clear heel-strike transient.[16] Although it is often suggested that these transient forces play a role in

knee OA, there is only indirect evidence for this (largely from animal studies).[17,18] One of the few human studies to lend support to this theory found that young adults with "pre-arthritic" knee pain had a 37% greater rate of loading than a group of age-matched controls[16] (which the authors suggested may predispose them to future development of knee OA). Further research is needed to clarify what effect transient forces have at the knee joint and whether they are important in the development and/or progression of knee OA.

Physical therapy interventions that reduce knee load could potentially play a role in reducing the onset, progression, and symptoms of knee OA. To date, there is little research evaluating their effect on knee load and much of our understanding remains speculative.

## LOCAL MECHANICAL FACTORS MAY INFLUENCE KNEE LOADING AND PHYSICAL THERAPY OUTCOMES

The effectiveness of physical therapy interventions in knee OA is likely to differ depending on local mechanical factors. The main local mechanical factors particularly relevant to knee OA are mal-alignment and laxity. To date, outcomes of specific physical therapy interventions

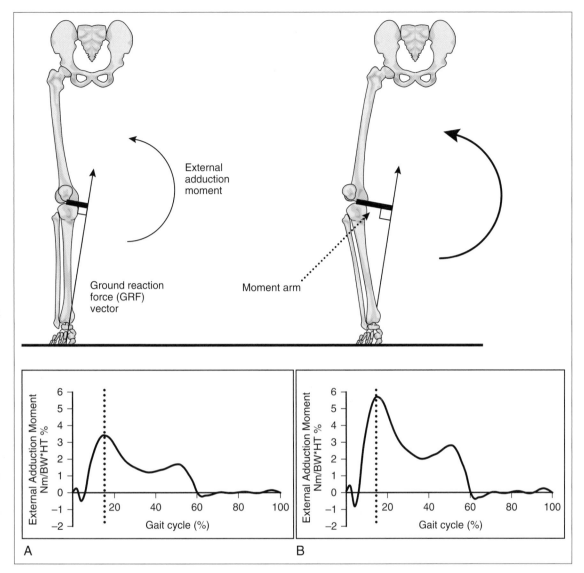

**Fig. 13.1** Ground reaction force vector and external knee adduction moment in (a) normally aligned and (b) varus mal-aligned knees. The external knee adduction moment is greater in the varus mal-aligned knee because the moment arm between the ground reaction force vector and the knee joint center is longer. (See Color Plate 6.)

have not been evaluated in subgroups characterized according to the local mechanical environment.[19]

## Mal-alignment

The mechanical alignment of the lower limb influences distribution of loads across the medial and lateral knee joint compartments. Preexisting mal-alignment may contribute to the development of OA and/or mal-alignment may arise as a consequence of the osteoarthritic process due to cartilage loss, bony attrition, and meniscal damage. In a neutrally aligned knee, the ground reaction force vector passes slightly medial to the knee joint center. In a varus mal-aligned knee, the vector is

displaced even more medially to the knee joint center and thus increases knee AM and compressive load across the medial compartment.[20] In a valgus knee, the ground reaction force vector passes initially closer to the knee joint center and then more laterally—with increasing valgus, thus increasing load across the lateral compartment (Fig. 13.1).

Varus mal-alignment is most common in people with knee OA due to the prevalence of medial tibiofemoral joint OA.[21] Several longitudinal cohort studies have found that the degree of mal-alignment at baseline predicts the subsequent risk of progression of OA disease.[22-24] For example, one study showed that

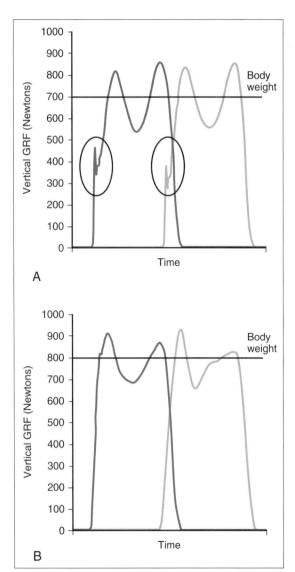

**Fig. 13.2** Vertical ground reaction forces for patients (A) with and (B) without heel-strike transients.

Dynamic stability relies on the integrity of the passive structures together with the coordinated activity of muscles around the knee joint. Proprioceptive input from the extremities is important in controlling reflex and centrally driven muscle activity, and proprioception is known to be impaired in people with knee OA.[29,30] Declines in joint stability can lead to a change in load distribution. The cartilage may then be less able to withstand applied loads and this may lead to degeneration.

In some cases, abnormal joint motion during gait may manifest itself as a varus thrust. This is observed as a bowing out of the knee laterally during the stance phase and the return to a less varus position during the swing phase of gait. It has been found that this can be reliably assessed by visual observation.[31] The frequency of a varus thrust in knee OA patients has not been well reported, but in one study cohort was shown to be 17%.[31] In this cohort, the presence of a varus thrust was associated with a higher AM and with a fourfold greater likelihood of disease progression in the medial compartment over an 18-month period.[31]

This effect was seen over and above the detrimental effect of static varus mal-alignment but only in those with 5(o) varus. This suggests that in this subgroup of patients interventions may be needed that reduce the presence of a varus thrust. However, research is needed to identify why patients exhibit this feature. Do such patients have more joint laxity but normal muscle activity unable to compensate or do altered muscle activation patterns allow a varus thrust to occur in the absence of lesser amounts of passive laxity? An understanding of the causes underlying a varus thrust will help design the most appropriate intervention to stabilize the knee and reduce this phenomenon.

Failure to dynamically control frontal plane laxity at the knee joint may also result in symptomatic knee instability (buckling, slipping, or giving way of the knee) during functional activities. This has recently been identified as a problem in a significant proportion of individuals with knee OA. In a cohort of 105 people, 44% reported instability that affected their ability to function.[32] Instability is likely to be multifactorial, resulting from factors such as passive joint laxity, structural damage, muscle weakness, pain, and altered neuromuscular control. Further research needs to examine the extent to which these factors contribute to the symptom of instability in knee OA, in that this will influence treatment strategies utilized.

## PHYSICAL THERAPY INTERVENTIONS FOR KNEE OSTEOARTHRITIS

Although there are a number of physical therapy and rehabilitative interventions available for knee OA, this

varus mal-alignment at baseline was associated with a fourfold increase in the odds of medial joint progression.[24] It also predicts deterioration in physical function.[25] Mal-alignment has been shown to be a mediator for the effects of other factors (such as obesity) on disease progression.[26,27] Because load is less well distributed in mal-aligned knees, the detrimental effect of obesity appears to be magnified.

## Laxity

Passive knee laxity generally refers to abnormal motion of the tibia with respect to the femur in the unloaded state. It is determined by ligaments, joint capsule, other soft tissues, and the joint surfaces. Varus-valgus laxity has been found to be greater in people with knee OA.[28]

chapter focuses on those that may be able to change the disease course by enhancing muscle function and neuromuscular control, by minimizing instability, or by attenuating load and improving load distribution. However, there is little direct research of such interventions—with most information currently based on theoretical and biomechanical considerations or indirect evidence.

## Strengthening Specific Muscles

### Quadriceps Muscle Strengthening

Muscle weakness (particularly of the quadriceps) is a well-recognized impairment in people with knee OA.[33] It has been associated with increased pain[34] and a greater deterioration in function over time.[25] Quadriceps strengthening has formed the cornerstone of traditional OA exercise therapy, and clinical trials of various types of quadriceps strengthening exercise have consistently found significant reductions in pain and improvements in physical function.[35] However, whether quadriceps strengthening is also beneficial for structural outcomes is unclear.

The relationship between quadriceps strength and knee load is controversial. The quadriceps act eccentrically to control the amount and rate of knee flexion immediately following heel strike.[36] It has long been proposed that strong quadriceps are necessary to absorb the transient forces that occurs at heel strike. This is supported by a study comparing sedentary and strength-trained women.[37] The sedentary group with lower quadriceps and hamstring strength had higher rates of loading and a greater frequency of heel-strike transient occurrence than the trained group. However, the timing of quadriceps activity during stance may be too late to absorb transient forces because the peak of stance phase knee flexion occurs about 150 ms after initial contact—whereas the heel-strike transient occurs during the first 20 ms of stance.[15] Thus, the relationship between quadriceps strength and the heel-strike transient requires further evaluation before appropriate interventions can be tested.

The quadriceps muscles play a large role in resisting the AM.[9] A recent experimental study by Torry et al.[38] in healthy individuals showed that quadriceps weakness induced via a knee joint effusion significantly increased the knee AM. Conversely, in a cross-sectional study of 40 people with knee OA by the authors a significant relationship between isometric quadriceps strength and the AM was not observed (unpublished data).

Results of cohort studies investigating the relationship between quadriceps strength and disease incidence or progression also conflict. Slemenda et al.[39] found that in women, but not men, stronger quadriceps muscles reduced the risk of developing radiographic

knee OA. A recent study supports these findings. Hootman et al.[40] evaluated 3,081 community-dwelling adults free of OA, joint symptoms, and injuries. Women with a moderate to high isokinetic quadriceps strength had respectively a 55 and 64% reduced risk of developing hip or knee OA.

Increased muscle mass has also been associated with greater knee cartilage volume and a reduction in the loss of both medial and lateral tibial cartilage volume.[41,42] However, co-inheritance of thicker cartilage (as well as stronger muscles rather than local muscle hypertrophy arising from exercise) may be a more likely explanation of these relationships. Thus, it remains to be seen whether implementing a quadriceps-strengthening program reduces the risk of knee OA in healthy individuals.

A possible role for quadriceps-strengthening exercise in slowing disease progression was first explored in 1999.[43] However, this longitudinal cohort study failed to find a relationship between quadriceps strength and disease progression (possibly due to limited statistical power). A more recent study showed that *higher* baseline quadriceps strength was associated with a *greater* risk of disease progression in knee OA patients with mal-alignment and laxity.[44] In neutrally aligned and stable knees, there was no relationship between strength and progression. This suggests that loads placed on the knee by strong muscles may be more detrimental to cartilage in knees that are mechanically abnormal.

An intervention study of quadriceps strengthening is needed to definitively assess the effects of increasing quadriceps strength on knee load and progression. However, this study does imply that exercise has differential effects (depending on patient presentation) and highlights the need for specificity of exercise prescription. It may be that other interventions designed to alter mal-alignment and laxity are needed in combination with quadriceps strengthening in these patient subgroups.

### Hamstring Muscle Strengthening

Weakness of the hamstring muscles has been found in patients with knee OA.[45] Control of varus-valgus laxity is largely produced by co-contraction of the quadriceps and hamstring muscles.[9,46] Thus, if the hamstring muscles are weak this could reduce the ability to resist external loads applied to the knee and increase symptoms of knee instability. Knee muscle strength imbalance has been suggested as a contributing factor to altered muscle activation patterns (see material following). In one study, an increase in hamstring strength between baseline and 18 months was associated with less deterioration in function in people with knee OA.[25] This might highlight the need to strengthen the hamstrings as well as the quadriceps in the rehabilitation of patients with knee OA.

### Hip Muscle Strengthening

It has been proposed that strengthening the hip muscles responsible for controlling pelvic position in the frontal plane may reduce knee loads and slow disease progression. During walking, the hip abductor and adductor muscles stabilize the pelvis on the hip joint. Weakness may cause a drop in the level of the pelvis, thereby shifting the center of mass and increasing the knee AM. This is supported by a recent study showing that people with less severe knee OA can use their hip abductor muscles to position their upper body over the stance leg and reduce their knee AM.[47] Importantly, a recent longitudinal cohort study found that those with a lower external hip AM (indicating less use of the hip abductor muscles) had more rapid knee OA progression.[48] Because the posterior fibers of the hip abductor muscles also act as hip external rotators, strengthening these muscles could reduce knee load by increasing toe-out during gait (see material following).

Less is known about the hip adductor muscles in relation to knee OA, but they may assist in resisting the knee AM—particularly in a varus mal-aligned knee. By virtue of their attachment to the distal medial femoral condyle, the adductors could eccentrically restrain the tendency of the femur to move into further varus (Fig. 13.3). Yamada et al.[49] found that patients with knee OA had stronger hip adductors compared with age-matched controls, and that those with more severe OA had even stronger adductors than their less severe counterparts. They hypothesized that this increased strength may be due to greater use of the hip adductors in an attempt to lower the knee AM.

Given that hip mechanics can alter knee load and potentially neuromuscular control, hip strengthening could be a novel intervention for rehabilitation of knee OA patients. This has not been formally evaluated.

## Other Strengthening Considerations

Much research and clinical emphasis has been on maximal strength of muscles. However, it is important to realize that when performing activities of daily living muscles are not generally required to act maximally. What may be more important is the degree of muscle endurance or fatiguability. This has implications for the design of specific knee-OA-patient strengthening programs that traditionally focus on maximizing strength, with little attention directed toward endurance. It is not known whether any differences exist in outcomes from muscle-strengthening versus muscle-endurance programs.

Another factor that may influence treatment is the degree to which the reduction in muscle strength is due to muscle atrophy from disuse or to an impairment in the central nervous system's (CNS's) ability to volitionally activate the muscle, often referred to as arthrogenous muscle inhibition (AMI).[33,50] AMI may be due to the presence of effusion or pain—and as such may require targeted interventions such as ice, compression bandaging, anti-inflammatory medication, and other pain-relieving modalities to remove the source of the inhibition. It is not possible to measure AMI in the clinical setting, although discrepancies between muscle bulk and muscle strength could indicate the presence of a degree of AMI. These other interventions may be reserved for cases for which traditional strengthening does not seem to provide the expected increases in muscle strength.

Other factors that may influence the choice of strengthening exercise are the coexistence of symptoms arising from the patellofemoral joint or the presence of obesity. In these cases, strengthening may need to be performed in positions that minimize the patellofemoral contact forces and knee loading (for example, in lesser degrees of knee flexion and in non weight bearing). Exercise prescription may need to emphasize lower loads and a greater number of repetitions. Hydrotherapy may also be a useful way to strengthen muscles while minimizing joint loading, particularly in the obese or in those with more advanced stages of knee OA or with greater abnormalities in the local mechanical environment.

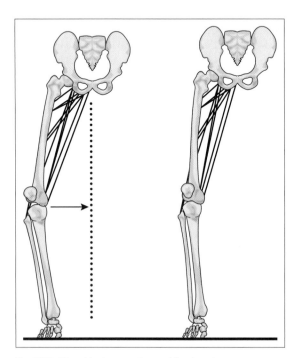

**Fig. 13.3** Hip adductor muscles could reduce knee varus by virtue of their distal attachment to the proximal femur.

## NEUROMUSCULAR RETRAINING/PERTURBATION PROGRAMS

Exercise specifically targeting neuromuscular control may have greater disease-modifying effects than strengthening alone. Data are beginning to highlight the complexity of muscle strategies adopted by the CNS to compensate for joint derangement. The paradox is that these strategies may actually increase disease progression by increasing joint compressive forces.

As described previously, the knee sustains substantial loads during functional activities such as gait—with adduction loading particularly relevant for knee OA. The CNS may adopt a number of different neural strategies to counter external loads during gait. However, two generalized strategies have been suggested.[51] The first involves selected activation of muscles with moment arms that are best able to counter the external load. For example, to counteract an AM the lateral gastrocnemius, lateral hamstrings (biceps femoris), and tensor fascia latae would be activated.[52] The second strategy is generalized co-contraction involving coactivation of hamstring and quadriceps muscles with no selectivity of specific muscular components.

This strategy would involve greater compressive loads applied through the joint. Studies have shown that both strategies are used by the CNS to stabilize the knee joint during isometric varus tasks.[46] However, it seems that the greatest muscular contribution to AM control is provided by quadricep and hamstring contraction, largely as a by-product of their activity in controlling sagittal loads.[9] Given the small cross-sectional area of lateral muscles with a larger moment arm, the contribution of these muscles to countering the AM has been considered less important.[46] However, for medial compartment OA use of these lateral muscles is preferable because they provide stability while minimizing increased medial compartment loading. Interventions designed to preferentially activate these muscles warrant investigation.

In OA, the muscular strategies employed by the CNS appear to differ from those in healthy individuals. Recently, differences in both the timing and amplitude of muscle activity in patients with knee OA compared with healthy controls have been identified in cross-sectional electromyographic studies.[53-56] Childs et al.[53] found that the lower limb muscles were activated for 1.5 times longer in OA patients compared to controls during walking and stair ascent/descent. Greater muscle coactivation between the vastus lateralis and the medial hamstrings was also evident in the OA group. Others have similarly reported increased levels of co-contraction, with greater activation of the hamstrings.[55,56]

Lewek et al.[55] reported greater co-contraction levels of muscles on the medial but not the lateral side comparing OA patients and controls. Other differences were greater medial joint space opening on X-ray under a valgus load, a higher AM, and more self-reported instability in the OA group. These authors suggest that given the greater medial joint space opening the greater medial muscle co-contraction is an attempt at stabilization. However, this strategy is likely to result in greater medial joint compressive loads and thus may hasten disease progression.

These neuromuscular alterations in knee OA most likely represent coping strategies in combating pain, muscle weakness, or local mechanical changes (including joint laxity). Although such strategies may have short-term benefits, they may have long-term negative consequences by altering the distribution and increasing the magnitude of load and potentially speeding disease progression (Fig. 13.4). This has led to the recommendation that novel exercise approaches designed to reduce levels of co-contraction should be developed to address these neuromuscular changes.[53,56] However, if co-contraction is an adaptive response removing this strategy without addressing more appropriate means of controlling joint stability may be detrimental. It is currently unknown what form of physical therapy would be most effective.

One option may be a structured agility and perturbation training program. In a case study, a program modified from that used for younger patients with anterior cruciate ligament insufficiency reduced symptoms of instability in an older woman with knee OA.[57] The program included activities such as side stepping, braiding, front and back crossover steps, shuttle walking, obstacle course, and perturbations applied by a therapist while the patient tried to balance on various surfaces. However, it is not known whether the change in instability symptoms was accompanied by altered muscle activation patterns or knee load.

Another strategy may be to train patients to activate appropriate selective muscles using real-time biofeedback and motor control relearning. In this, the movement is broken down into smaller components and the person is made aware of the muscle activity required. Repetition and feedback are key components. The patient could commence by practicing the activity of late swing to early stance phase. Another method may be to apply a varus force to the knee using a thera-band while the patient is positioned in a stride-standing or single-leg-stance position (Fig. 13.5). The patient is instructed to maintain a neutral knee alignment, thereby having to use muscle activity to resist the varus-directed force at the knee. Whether these techniques are effective has not been tested.

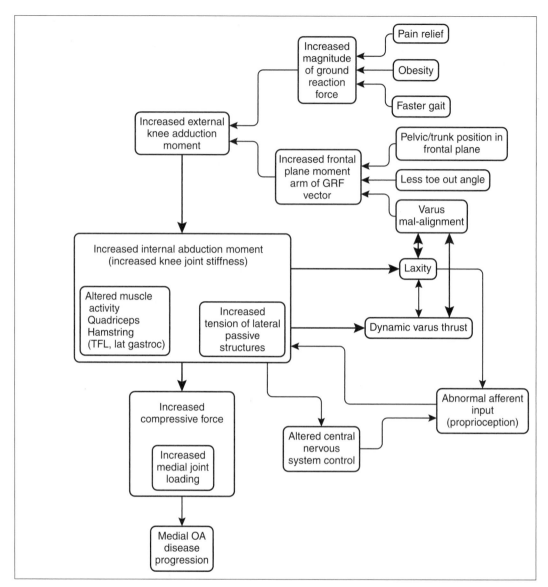

**Fig. 13.4** Interactions among local mechanical factors, neuromuscular control, knee loading, and disease progression.

## Gait Retraining

Gait patterns can influence loading at the knee joint, and thus changing them through gait retraining could slow disease progression. Parameters worthy of altering include toe-out angle, walking speed, and location of loading under the foot during stance. Although patients may be able to alter their gait pattern when instructed in the clinic, the use of novel biofeedback devices, leg/foot taping, or other strategies may be necessary to allow the pattern to become habitual.

Toe-out angle refers to the angle between the long axis of the foot and the straightforward line of progression of the body. A greater toe-out angle is associated with a lower AM in the late stance phase[20,58] because it shifts the ground reaction force vector closer to the knee joint center. However, there does not seem to be a relationship between toe-out angle and the larger peak AM in early stance. A longitudinal study showed that there was a 10% reduction in the odds of structural disease progression per additional 1 degree of toe-out angle.[59] Thus, small alterations in toe-out angle may have clinically relevant effects.

Walking speed is another factor associated with knee load, with faster walking speeds increasing all knee loads (including the knee AM). Indeed, people with knee OA often walk more slowly than the average, which is thought to be an adaptive mechanism in reducing knee loads. Recently, Mundermann et al.[60] showed that the relationship between walking speed and knee AM was greatest in those with less severe

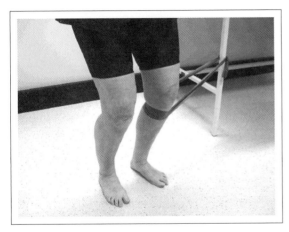

**Fig. 13.5** Use of theraband to apply a varus force to the knee joint while performing quadriceps-strengthening exercises.

knee OA compared to their more severe counterparts. This suggests that teaching the patient to walk more slowly would be more likely to benefit those with less severe knee OA. However, because walking speed is already slower in patients with knee OA compared with healthy age-matched individuals it may not be the most appropriate intervention in reducing knee loads (particularly given its likely impact on function).

## Aerobic Exercise

Aerobic exercise (including cycling, swimming, and walking) has been found to be effective for relieving symptoms in knee OA.[61] Such exercise could also have benefits for longer-term joint health by assisting with weight reduction. Obesity is a well-known risk factor for both the onset and progression of knee OA.[27,62] A recent randomized clinical trial showed that the combination of dietary weight loss and exercise (including both aerobic and resistance components) was more effective in improving function and pain in people with knee OA compared to either intervention alone.[63] There was no effect on joint space width, although this may relate to the relatively modest weight loss achieved. In the obese, non weight-bearing exercise such as cycling may allow greater exercise intensities to be achieved while minimizing joint loading.

## Knee Braces

Mechanical correction of knee mal-alignment can be achieved with the application of a knee brace designed to provide support in the frontal plane. In particular, valgus "unloader" braces (which provide an external AM about the knee) are advocated for reducing loads on the medial knee joint compartment and for relieving symptoms in patients with medial tibiofemoral joint OA. Numerous studies demonstrate that the

use of a valgus knee brace results in reduced pain, improved function, and increased quality of life in these patients.[64-66]

Although mixed biomechanical effects of valgus braces have been reported in the literature, research suggests that bracing can significantly reduce medial compartment loads at the knee. Lindenfeld et al.[65] reported a mean 10% decrease in the peak external AM with a brace in a group of middle-aged people with medial OA. Individual responses varied, with one patient demonstrating a reduction by as much as 32%. Importantly, this reduction in the AM appears to directly reduce medial compartment joint load. Pollo et al. demonstrated a mean reduction in net AM about the knee of 13% with valgus bracing, and a reduction in medial compartment load by an average of 11%.[66] It is believed that a direct alteration in mechanical alignment of the lower limb underlies the changes in AM observed with bracing. Given that a reduction in the AM of about 10% corresponds to a 3.3-fold decrease in the risk of disease progression,[13] valgus bracing offers great potential for knee OA. Long-term studies are required to evaluate the effects of bracing on joint structure.

Knee bracing may also impart sensorimotor benefits to the patient with knee OA. Birmingham et al.[67] demonstrated a significant improvement in knee joint proprioception in patients with knee OA while wearing a knee brace. However, the mean difference between the braced and unbraced conditions was only 0.7%—which renders the clinical significance of these findings questionable. It is feasible that enhanced sensory input at the knee with a brace may favorably influence muscle activation patterns. However, this has not been investigated to date in patients with OA.

## FOOTWEAR AND INSOLES

### Lateral Wedges

Wedged insoles were first proposed as a treatment for knee OA in the 1980s by Japanese researchers.[68,69] Wedged insoles exert a mechanical effect on the lower limb by altering the magnitude, temporal pattern, and plantar location of the ground reaction force acting on the foot during gait. By virtue of the lower limb's closed kinetic chain during weight-bearing activities, wedged insoles in the shoes can modify moments acting upon the knee joint. Due to the predominance of medial tibiofemoral joint disease,[21] which often results in varus mal-alignment of the knee due to medial joint space loss, lateral wedges have been subjected to the most research. Unpublished data of the authors and other biomechanical studies demonstrate that insertion of lateral wedges in the shoes results in a reduction in the AM moment of 5 to 8%[70,71] (Fig. 13.6).

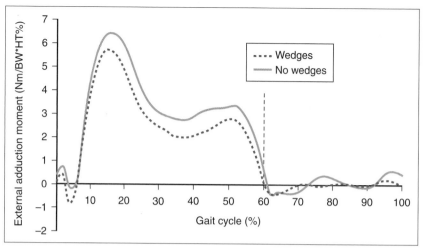

**Fig. 13.6** Change in peak external knee adduction moment with the insertion of lateral wedges in the shoes.

This corresponds to a 3.2% reduction in peak medial knee load, primarily due to the reduction in the AM.[70]

The exact mechanism underpinning the change in the AM with wedges is unclear at present. Some studies suggest that lateral wedges increase the external subtalar joint valgus moment via a lateral shift in the center of pressure,[72-75] thereby reducing the moment arm of the knee AM arm in the frontal plane (Fig. 13.7). Studies demonstrating an increase in the valgus angulation of the subtalar joint and calcaneum with lateral wedges lend support to this hypothesis.[69,76] Combining a laterally wedged insole with strapping to restrict talar motion

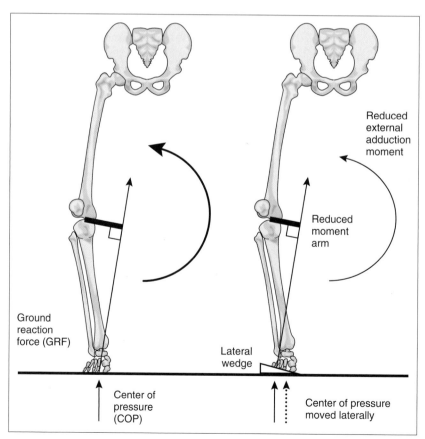

**Fig. 13.7** Proposed mechanism of biomechanical effects at the knee joint with lateral wedge.

leads to a more valgus alignment in the frontal plane at the knee,[69,76,77] an effect that does not occur with insertion of a wedge alone.[69,78]

This suggests that (via strapping) restriction of talar motion forces the calcaneum laterally, thereby altering the static mechanical axis of the lower limb and leading to a more valgus knee alignment—which may also contribute to the lower knee AM observed with laterally wedged insoles. A similar effect may be observed in patients who are already at end-range subtalar joint pronation, although this has not been studied directly. Unpublished data of the authors, demonstrating a correlation between heel angle and symptomatic response to lateral wedges after 3 months, support this hypothesis.

Non- and quasi-experimental clinical studies demonstrate pain-relieving effects of lateral wedges in many, but not all, patients with knee OA.[68,79-81] These findings conflict with those of a randomized controlled trial that failed to demonstrate a change in pain with wedged insoles for medial compartment OA.[82,83] However, the decrease in NSAID consumption combined with better compliance in the treatment group favors a beneficial effect of the wedges. Given the individual variation in response evident in most biomechanical studies, it is probable that not all patients with medial knee OA will benefit clinically from laterally wedged insoles and that certain subgroups of patients (such as those with a more valgus heel angle) are most likely to benefit. Further research is needed to identify which patient factors best predict clinical outcome with lateral wedges. In contrast to current clinical practice, customized prescription of lateral wedges with regard to the degree of inclination will most likely optimize outcome.

Given their effectiveness at reducing the knee AM, lateral wedges have great potential for slowing OA progression when used over the long term. Structural effects of wedges have been evaluated in a 2-year randomized controlled trial. However, no effect on joint space narrowing rate (as measured by X-ray) was observed.[83] This may in part be due to the relative insensitivity of the measurement technique (compared to magnetic resonance imaging) or due to the heterogeneous patient sample selected. Further studies are warranted to better evaluate the long-term structural effects of lateral wedges.

Despite the beneficial effects of lateral wedges in patients with medial knee OA, this intervention remains underutilized in clinical practice. In light of their biomechanical effects, lateral wedges may serve their greatest benefit when combined with other interventions that have a symptomatic effect only, such as aerobic exercise. Such a combination may allow both symptoms and risk of disease progression to be addressed concurrently, thus optimizing patient management.

## Shock-absorbing Insoles

In patients with knee OA, where reducing loads applied across the lower limb is vital, modifications to footwear or the use of shock-absorbing insoles may offer great potential in rehabilitation. Viscoelastic materials used in footwear or in insoles augment body tissues (particularly the heel pad) in reducing the magnitude of the heel-strike transient.[15] With age, heel pad structure alters and results in a loss of shock-absorbing capacity.[84] Viscoelastic insoles can attenuate transient forces incurred during walking, running, stair climbing, and jumping activities.[85,86] Their success appears to depend on the viscosity and thickness of the material utilized.

Although the efficacy of viscoelastic materials in reducing the symptoms of knee OA has not been studied, evidence of their symptomatic effectiveness is available from other patient populations. A study in military recruits revealed that training in modified basketball shoes with viscoelastic soles resulted in a lower incidence of metatarsal stress fractures and foot overuse injuries compared with standard infantry boots.[87] In patients with low back pain, use of viscoelastic shoe inserts and light flexible shoes resulted in improvements in pain and mobility in approximately 80% of patients.[88]

Similar inserts worn daily for 18 months in various patient groups with clinical symptoms of osteoarthritic joint disease (including knee OA) have shown similar results, with 78% reporting disappearance of clinical symptoms. In the patients with knee pain, 63% reported no pain after 18 months, 26% reported periodic pain of moderate intensity, and only 11% reported no improvement.[89] It is unclear what effect shock-absorbing insoles may have on the incidence or progression of knee OA. However, a potential benefit certainly exists.

## Textured Insoles

As discussed previously, neuromotor control is important at the knee for dynamic absorption of loads during gait. Timely and accurate muscle activity depends on accurate and coordinated tactile, visual, and proprioceptive information. Mechano-receptors in the skin of the foot respond to pressure, skin deformation, and vibration, and provide sensory input to the CNS. This information is then used by the brain to modulate muscular activity throughout the lower limb. Any intervention that enhances sensory input from the periphery may improve neuromuscular control of knee stability. Shoe insoles in intimate contact with the foot's plantar surface represent a potentially simple means of activating mechano-receptors. Textured insoles may provide greater stimulation than that arising from smooth-surfaced insoles.

Waddington et al.[90,91] evaluated the effects of textured finger profile rubber insoles (with four nodules/cm[2]) on ankle movement discrimination in sports people. They found that the addition of textured insoles to the shoes restored movement discrimination ability back to barefoot levels. Although no research has been conducted on the effects of textured insoles in elderly patients or those with knee OA, vibrating insoles have been shown to reduce postural sway in younger and elderly subjects—with the elderly gaining more in motor control performance than the younger participants.[92] It is possible that textured insoles may lead to changes in lower limb muscle activity patterns as a result of enhanced afferent input, offering additional benefits to knee OA patients—although this too has not been investigated to date.

## Footwear Modifications

In clinical practice, the insertion of insoles into the shoes may be problematic because many shoes worn by patients with knee OA are not spacious enough to accommodate the insole.[71] Foot discomfort or blistering may arise, or the clinician may be forced to prescribe an insole of insufficient wedging or thickness to achieve a clinical benefit. For patients with knee OA, it may be easier to provide wedging or shock absorption through the heel of the actual shoe rather than by inserting an insole. This area has not been the subject of much research in knee OA.

## Type of Footwear

The type of footwear worn by patients with knee OA can potentially increase the risk of disease progression. Thus, shoe choice is an easily modifiable risk factor and health professionals should advise patients with knee OA regarding the most appropriate footwear for their condition. Kerrigan et al.[93] have demonstrated that healthy women wearing stiletto high-heeled shoes increased the normal varus torque at the knee by an average of 23% during the stance phase of level walking, thus increasing the load across the medial knee compartment. A prolonged knee flexor torque was also observed, suggesting increased work of the quadriceps, prolonged strain through the patellar tendon, and prolonged pressure across the patello-femoral joint—all of which may contribute to the development of osteoarthritic change within this compartment.

A subsequent study[94] demonstrated similar effects with wide-based high-heeled shoes (Fig. 13.8). In contrast, shoe styles typically worn by men (firm-soled dress shoes and rubber-soled sneakers) have minimal effect on knee joint torques compared to barefoot walking once the slightly faster walking speed with shoes is accounted for.[95] Studies suggest that shock absorption at heel strike can be enhanced by containing the heel pad within a firm heel counter of a shoe.[96,97] Although this has not been studied in knee OA, the potential of such shoes in reducing the magnitude of the heel-strike transient (and possibly symptoms) warrants consideration. Appropriate choice of footwear can offer additional benefits in knee OA.

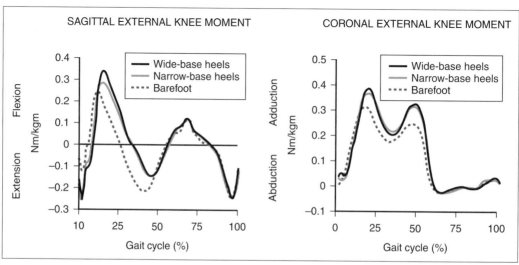

**Fig. 13.8** Effect of high-heeled shoes on sagittal and coronal knee torques in healthy women. (Modified and reprinted with permission from Elsevier, *The Lancet* 2001;357:1097–98.)

Individuals with knee OA demonstrate poorer balance and an increased risk of falls compared to their non-osteoarthritic counterparts.[33,98-100] Wearing shoes with low heels and large contact areas may help patients with knee OA reduce the risk of a fall in everyday activities.[101] A laboratory study in healthy elderly men has shown that shoes with thin hard soles result in better balance than those with thick, soft midsoles,[102] which may partially be related to the fact that these types of soles enhance foot position awareness.[103] However, laboratory studies may not necessarily emulate real-life situations, as an examination of footwear between elderly fallers and non-fallers demonstrated that athletic shoes and sneakers were the style of footwear associated with the lowest risk of a fall.[104] These findings are encouraging, given that this type of footwear with its viscoelastic soles is probably most beneficial in terms of shock absorption for the patient with knee OA.

## SUMMARY

In that knee joint loading plays a major role in the onset and progression of knee OA, physical therapy strategies that aim to reduce knee load may be beneficial. Because the knee functions as part of a closed kinetic chain during weight-bearing functional activities, these strategies may not only be directed specifically at the knee joint but also at foot/ankle complex and the hip, trunk, and pelvis. Although there is currently little direct evidence, novel physical therapy interventions have the potential to influence knee loading or disease course. Future research needs to be directed at evaluating these interventions.

## REFERENCES

1. Jordan K, Arden N, Doherty M, et al. EULAR recommendations 2003: An evidence-based approach to the management of knee osteoarthritis, report of a task force of the Standing Committee for International Clinical Studies Including Therapeutic Trials (ESCISIT). Ann Rheum Dis 2003;62:1145.
2. American College of Rheumatology Subcommittee on Osteoarthritis. Recommendations for the medical management of osteoarthritis of the hip and knee, 2000 update. Arthritis Rheum 2000;43:1905.
3. Vogels E, Hendriks H, van Baar M, et al. Clinical practice guidelines for physical therapy in patients with osteoarthritis of the hip or knee. Royal Dutch Society for Physical Therapy, 2003, www.fysionet.nl/index.html?dossier_id=81&dossiers=1.
4. Hamerman D. Clinical implications of osteoarthritis and aging. Ann Rheum Dis 1995;54:82.
5. Radin E, Paul I. Response of joints to impact loading. I. In vitro wear. Arthritis Rheum 1971;14:356.
6. Ledingham J, Regan M, Jones A, et al. Factors affecting radiographic progression of knee osteoarthritis. Ann Rheum Dis 1995;54:53.
7. Schouten J, van den Ouweland F, Valkenburg H. A 12-year follow up study in the general population on prognostic factors of cartilage loss in osteoarthritis of the knee. Ann Rheum Dis 1992;51:932.
8. Felson D, Hannan M, Naimark A, et al. Occupational physical demands, knee bending, and knee osteoarthritis: Results from the Framingham Study. J Rheumatol 1991;18:1587.
9. Schipplein OD, Andriacchi TP. Interaction between active and passive knee stabilizers during level walking. J Orthop Res 1991;9:113.
10. Bailunas A, Hurwitz D, Ryals A, et al. Increased knee joint loads during walking are present in subjects with knee osteoarthritis. Osteoarthritis Cartilage 2002;10:573.
11. Sharma L, Hurwitz DE, Thonar E, et al. Knee adduction moment, serum hyaluronan level, and disease severity in medial tibiofemoral osteoarthritis. Arthritis Rheum 1998;41:1233.
12. Prodomos CC, Andriacchi TP, Galante JO. A relationship between gait and clinical changes following high tibial osteotomy. JBJS 1985;67A:1188.
13. Miyazaki T, Wada M, Kawahara H, et al. Dynamic load at baseline can predict radiographic disease progression in medial compartment knee osteoarthritis. Ann Rheum Dis 2002;61:617.
14. Sharma L, Dunlop D, Andriacchi T, et al. The adduction moment and knee osteoarthritis (OA): A longitudinal study. 67th ACR/ARHP Annual Scientific Meeting, 23–28 October 2003, Orlando, Florida.
15. Whittle M. Generation and attenuation of transient impulsive forces beneath the foot: A review. Gait Posture 1999;10:264.
16. Radin EL, Yang KH, Riegger C, et al. Relationship between lower limb dynamics and knee joint pain. J Orthop Res 1991;9:398.
17. Simon SR, Radin EL, Paul IL, et al. The response of joints to impact loading II: In vivo behaviour of subchondral bone. J Biomech 1972;5:267.
18. Radin EL, Orr RB, Kelman JL, et al. Effect of prolonged walking on concrete on the knees of sheep. J Biomech 1982;15:487.
19. Sharma L. Local factors in osteoarthritis. Curr Opinion Rheumatol 2001;13:441.
20. Hurwitz D, Ryals A, Case J, et al. The knee adduction moment during gait in subjects with knee osteoarthritis is more closely correlated with static alignment than radiographic disease severity, toe out angle and pain. J Orthop Res 2002;20:101.
21. Ledingham J, Regan M, Jones A, et al. Radiographic patterns and associations of osteoarthritis of the knee in patients referred to hospital. Ann Rheum Dis 1993;52:520.
22. Cerejo R, Dunlop D, Cahue S, et al. The influence of alignment on risk of knee osteoarthritis progression according to baseline stage of disease. Arthritis Rheum 2002;46:2632.
23. Cicuttini F, Wluka A, Hankin J, et al. Longitudinal study of the relationship between knee angle and tibiofemoral cartilage volume in subjects with knee osteoarthritis. Rheumatol 2004;43:321.
24. Sharma L, Song J, Felson D, et al. The role of knee alignment in disease progression and functional decline in knee osteoarthritis. JAMA 2001;286:188.
25. Sharma L, Cahue S, Song J, et al. Physical functioning over three years in knee osteoarthritis: Role of psychosocial, local mechanical, and neuromuscular factors. Arthritis Rheum 2003;48:3359.
26. Sharma L, Lou C, Cahue S, et al. The mechanism of the effect of obesity in knee osteoarthritis: The mediating role of malalignment. Arthritis Rheum 2000;43:568.
27. Felson D, Goggins J, Niu J, et al. The effect of body weight on progression of knee osteoarthritis is dependent on alignment. Arthritis Rheum 2004;50:390.
28. Sharma L, Lou C, Felson D, et al. Laxity in healthy and osteoarthritic knees. Arthritis Rheum 1999;42:861.
29. Pai Y-C, Rymer WZ, Chang RW, et al. Effect of age and osteoarthritis on knee proprioception. Arthritis Rheum 1997;40:2260.
30. Sharma L. Proprioceptive impairment in knee osteoarthritis. Rheum Dis Clinics North Am 199;25:299.
31. Chang A, Hayes K, Dunlop D, et al. Thrust during ambulation and the progression of knee osteoarthritis. Arthritis Rheum 2004;50:3897.

32. Fitzgerald G, Piva S, Irrgang J. Reports of joint instability in knee osteoarthritis: Its prevalence and relationship to physical function. Arthritis Rheum (Arthritis Care Res) 2004;51:941.

33. Hassan B, Mockett S, Doherty M. Static postural sway, proprioception, and maximal voluntary quadriceps contraction in patients with knee osteoarthritis and normal control subjects. Ann Rheum Dis 2001;60:612.

34. O'Reilly SC, Jones A, Muir KR, et al. Quadriceps weakness in knee osteoarthritis: The effect on pain and disability. Ann Rheum Dis 1998;57:588.

35. Pelland L, Brosseau L, Wells G, et al. Efficacy of strengthening exercises for osteoarthritis (Part I): A meta-analysis. Physical Ther Rev 2004;9:77.

36. Jefferson RJ, Collins JJ, Whittle MW, et al. The role of the quadriceps in controlling impulsive forces around heelstrike. Proc Inst Mech Eng 1990;204:21.

37. Mikesky AE, Meyer A, Thompson KL. Relationship between quadriceps strength and rate of loading during gait in women. J Orthop Res 2000;18:171.

38. Torry M, Pflum M, Shelburne K, et al. The effects of quadriceps weakness on the knee adductor moment during gait. Med Sci Sports Ex 2004;36:S46.

39. Slemenda C, Heilman D, Brandt K, et al. Reduced quadriceps strength relative to body weight: A risk factor for knee osteoarthritis in women? Arthritis Rheum 1998;41:1951.

40. Hootman J, Fitzgerald S, Macera C, et al. Lower extremity muscle strength and risk of self-reported hip or knee osteoarthritis. J Phys Activity Health 2004;1:321.

41. Cicuttini F, Teichtahl A, Wluka A, et al. The relationship between body composition and knee cartilage volume in healthy, middle-aged subjects. Arthritis Rheum 2005;52:461.

42. Hudelmaier M, Glaser C, Englmeier K, et al. Correlation of knee-joint cartilage morphology with muscle cross-sectional areas vs anthropometric variables. Anat Rec 2003;270:175.

43. Brandt KD, Heilman DK, Slemenda C, et al. Quadriceps strength in women with radiographically progressive osteoarthritis of the knee and those with stable radiographic changes. J Rheumatol 1999;26:2431.

44. Sharma L, Dunlop D, Cahue S, et al. Quadriceps strength and osteoarthritis progression in malaligned and lax knees. Ann Int Med 2003;138:613.

45. Fransen M, Crosbie J, Edmonds J. Isometric muscle force measurement for clinicians treating patients with osteoarthritis of the knee. Arthritis Rheum (Arthritis Care Res) 2003;49:29.

46. Lloyd D, Buchanan T. Strategies of muscular support of varus and valgus isometric loads at the human knee. J Biomech 2001;34:1257.

47. Mundermann A, Dyrby CO, Andriacchi T. Gait compensation in patients with medial compartmental knee osteoarthritis: Increased load at the ankle, knee and hip during walking. 51st Meeting of the Orthopaedic Research Society Washington DC. 2005;1406.

48. Chang A, Hayes K, Cahue S, et al. The hip abduction moment and progression of knee osteoarthritis (OA). Osteoarthritis Cartilage 2004;12:S24.

49. Yamada H, Koshino T, Sakai N, et al. Hip adductor muscle strength in patients with varus deformed knee. Clin Orthop 2001;386:179.

50. Pap G, Machner A, Awiszus F. Strength and voluntary activation of the quadriceps femoris muscle at different severities of osteoarthritic knee joint damage. J Orthop Res 2004;22:96.

51. Besier TF, Lloyd DG, Ackland T. Muscle activation strategies at the knee during running and cutting maneuvers. Med Sci Sports Ex 2003;35:119.

52. Zhang L-Q, Wang G. Dynamic and static control of the human knee joint in abduction-adduction. J Biomech 2001;34:1101.

53. Childs J, Sparto P, Fitzgerald G, et al. Alterations in lower extremity movement and muscle activation patterns in individuals with knee osteoarthritis. Clin Biomech 2004;19:44.

54. Hinman RS, Bennell KL, Metcalf BR, et al. Delayed onset of quadriceps activity and altered knee joint kinematics during stair stepping in individuals with knee osteoarthritis. Arch Phys Med Rehabil 2002;83:1080.

55. Lewek M, Rudolph K, Snyder-Mackler L. Control of frontal plane laxity during gait in patients with medial compartment knee osteoarthritis. Osteoarthritis Cartilage 2004;12:745.

56. Hortobagyi T, Westerkamp L, Beam S, et al. Altered hamstring-quadriceps muscle balance in patients with knee osteoarthritis. Clin Biomech 2005;20:97.

57. Fitzgerald G, Childs J, Ridge T, et al. Agility and perturbation training for a physically active individual with knee osteoarthritis. Phys Ther 2002;82:372.

58. Andrews M, Noyes F, Hewett T, et al. Lower limb alignment and foot angle are related to stance phase knee adduction in normal subjects: A critical analysis of the reliability of gait analysis data. J Orthop Res 1996;14:289.

59. Chang A, Hurwitz D, Hayes K, et al. Toe-out angle during gait and protection against progression of medial tibiofemoral knee osteoarthritis. Arthritis Rheum 2004;50:S252.

60. Mundermann A, Dyrby CO, Hurwitz D, et al. Potential strategies to reduce medial compartment loading in patients with knee OA of varying severity: Reduced walking speed. Arthritis Rheum 2004;50:1172.

61. Brosseau L, Pelland L, Wells G, et al. Efficacy of aerobic exercises for osteoarthritis (Part II): A meta-analysis. Phys Ther Rev 2004;9:125.

62. Felson D, Anderson J, Naimark A, et al. Obesity and knee osteoarthritis: The Framingham study. Ann Intern Med 1988;109:18.

63. Messier S, Loeser R, Miller G, et al. Exercise and dietary weight loss in overweight and obese older adults with knee osteoarthritis. Arthritis Rheum 2004;50:1501.

64. Kirkley A, Webster-Bogaert S, Litchfield R, et al. The effect of bracing on varus gonarthrosis. JBJS (Am) 1999;4:539.

65. Lindenfeld T, Hewett T, Andriacchi T. Joint loading with valgus bracing in patients with varus gonarthrosis. Clin Orthop 1997;344:290.

66. Pollo F, Otis J, Backus S, et al. Reduction of medial compartment loads with valgus bracing of the osteoarthritic knee. Am J Sports Med 2002;30:414.

67. Birmingham T, Kramer J, Kirkley A, et al. Knee bracing for medial compartment osteoarthritis: Effects on proprioception and postural control. Rheumatol 2001;40:285.

68. Sasaki T, Yasuda K. Clinical evaluation of the treatment of osteoarthritic knees using a newly designed wedged insole. Clin Orthop 1987;221:181.

69. Yasuda K, Sasaki T. The mechanics of treatment of the osteoarthritic knee with a wedged insole. Clin Orthop 1987;215:162.

70. Crenshaw S, Pollo F, Calton E. Effects of lateral-wedged insoles on kinetics at the knee. Clin Orthop 2000;375:185.

71. Kerrigan D, Lelas J, Goggins J, et al. Effectiveness of a lateral-wedge insole on knee varus torque in patients with knee osteoarthritis. Arch Phys Med Rehabil 2002;83:889.

72. Kakihana W, Akai M, Yamasaki N, et al. Changes of joint moments in the gait of normal subjects wearing laterally wedged insoles. Am J Phys Med Rehabil 2004;83:273.

73. Nester C, van der Linden M, Bowker P. Effect of foot orthoses on the kinematics and kinetics of normal walking gait. Gait Posture 2003;17:180.

74. Van Gheluwe B, Dananberg H. Changes in plantar foot pressure with in-shoe varus or valgus wedging. J Am Pod Med Assoc 2004;94:1.

75. Nigg B, Stergiou P, Cole G, et al. Effect of shoe inserts on kinematics, center of pressure, and leg joint moments during running. Med Sci Sports Exerc 2003;35:314.

76. Toda Y, Segal N, Kato A, et al. Effect of a novel insole on the subtalar joint of patients with medial compartment osteoarthritis of the knee. J Rheumatol 2001;28:2705.

77. Toda Y, Tsukimura N. A six-month followup of a randomized trial comparing the efficacy of a lateral-wedge insole with subtalar strapping and an in-shoe lateral-wedge insole in patients with varus deformity osteoarthritis of the knee. Arthritis Rheum 2004;50:3129.

78. Maly M, Culham E, Costigan P. Static and dynamic biomechanics of foot orthoses in people with medial compartment knee osteoarthritis. Clin Biomech 2002;17:603.

79. Keating E, Faris P, Ritter M, et al. Use of lateral heel and sole wedges in the treatment of medial osteoarthritis of the knee. Orthop Rev 1993;22:921.

80. Ogata K, Yasunaga M, Nomiyama H. The effect of wedged insoles on the thrust of osteoarthritic knees. Int Orthop 1997;21:308.

81. Tohyama H, Yasuda K, Kaneda K. Treatment of osteoarthritis of the knee with heel wedges. Int Orthop 1991;15:31.

82. Maillefert J, Hudry C, Baron G, et al. Laterally elevated wedged insoles in the treatment of medial knee osteoarthritis: A prospective randomised controlled study. Osteoarthritis Cartilage 2001;9:738.

83. Pham T, Maillefert J, Hudry C, et al. Laterally elevated wedged insoles in the treatment of medial knee osteoarthritis: A two-year prospective randomized controlled study. Osteoarthritis Cartilage 2003;12:46.

84. Jorgensen U, Bojsen-Moller F. Shock absorbency of factors in the shoe/heel interaction, with special focus on role of the heel pad. Foot Ankle 1989;9:294.

85. Johnson G. The effectiveness of shock-absorbing insoles during normal walking. Prosthet Orthot Int 1988;12:91.

86. Windle C, Gregory S, Dixon S. The shock attenuation characteristics of four different insoles when worn in a military boot during running and marching. Gait Posture 1999;9:31.

87. Milgrom C, Finestone A, Shlamkovitch N, et al. Prevention of overuse injuries of the foot by improved shoe shock attenuation: A randomized prospective study. Clin Orthop 1992;281:189.

88. Wosk J, Voloshin A. Low back pain: Conservative treatment with artificial shock absorbers. Arch Phys Med Rehabil 1985;66:145.

89. Volshin A, Wosk J. Influence of artificial shock absorbers on human gait. Clin Orthop 1981;160:52.

90. Waddington G, Adams R. Textured insole effects on ankle movement discrimination while wearing athletic socks. Phys Ther Sport 2000;1:119.

91. Waddington G, Adams R. Football boot insoles and sensitivity to extent of ankle inversion movement. Br J Sports Med 2003;37:170.

92. Priplata A, Niemi J, Harry J, et al. Vibrating insoles and balance control in elderly people. Lancet 2003;362:1123.

93. Kerrigan DC, Todd MK, Riley PO. Knee osteoarthritis and high-heeled shoes. Lancet 1998;351:1399.

94. Kerrigan D, Lelas J, Karvosky M. Women's shoes and knee osteoarthritis. Lancet 2001;357:1097.

95. Kerrigan D, Karvosky M, Lelas J, et al. Men's shoes and knee joint torques relevant to the development and progression of knee osteoarthritis. J Rheumatol 2003;30:529.

96. Jorgensen U. Body load in heel-strike running: The effect of a firm heel counter. Am J Sports Med 1990;18:177.

97. Jorgensen U, Ekstrand J. Significance of heel pad confinement for the shock absorption at heel strike. Int J Sports Med 1988;9:468.

98. Hinman R, Bennell K, Metcalf B, et al. Balance impairments in individuals with symptomatic knee osteoarthritis: A comparison with matched controls using clinical tests. Rheumatol 2002;41:1388.

99. Wegener L, Kisner C, Nichols D. Static and dynamic balance responses in persons with bilateral knee osteoarthritis. J Orthop Sports Phys Ther 1997;25:13.

100. Pandya N, Draganich L, Mauer A, et al. Osteoarthritis of the knees increases the propensity to trip on an obstacle. Clin Orthop 2005;431:150.

101. Tencer A, Koepsell T, Wolf M, et al. Biomechanical properties of shoes and risk of falls in older adults. J Am Ger Soc 2004;52:1840.

102. Robbins S, Gouw G, McClaran J. Shoe sole thickness and hardness influence balance in older men. J Am Ger Soc 1992;40:1089.

103. Robbins S, Waked E, Allard P, et al. Foot position awareness in younger and older men: The influence of footwear sole properties. J Am Ger Soc 1997;45:61.

104. Koepsell T, Wolf M, Buchner D, et al. Footwear style and risk of falls in older adults. J Am Ger Soc 2004;52:1495.

# 14 Management of Limb Osteoarthritis

Maxime Dougados

## INTRODUCTION

Osteoarthritis (OA) is a heterogeneous condition with varied patterns of expression. These attributes explain in part the variety of treatment modalities for OA. It has been proposed that management begins only when OA has been definitively diagnosed (curative approach). In fact, management might also be viewed as concerning the person at risk for developing OA (preventive approach). With such an approach in mind, at present the greatest impact in management of knee OA might be derived from adequate prevention and/or treatment of obesity and injury. This chapter deals with the curative approach of OA. A discussion of OA management is centered on two key areas.

- *Assessment of OA patient:* Which data should be collected to help in the therapeutic decision? How should such data be collected?
- *The treatment:* What are the available therapeutic modalities? What are their optimal indications?

This chapter reviews both of these areas crucial to the management of OA.

## ASSESSMENT OF OSTEOARTHRITIS

### Points to Consider in Optimal Management

The data to be collected at each visit should facilitate therapeutic decisions. Such therapeutic decisions should be made with regard to the present subjective symptoms and in relation to the following questions (see Table 14.1).

- What is the localization of the OA?
- Is the OA active?
- How severe is the OA and what is the extent of joint damage that has already occurred?
- What is the potential for severe progressive OA?
- Is the OA refractory?
- What co-morbidities are present and what is their severity?

### Localization of Osteoarthritis

In daily practice, the management of OA is aided by awareness of the major symptomatic joints and whether the patient has more generalized OA. Although at present treatment to relieve symptoms is not greatly influenced by these issues, it is clear that risk factors for disease progression (and very likely symptoms) differ by joint site and OA subset. Local non-pharmacologic treatment options and prognostic education differ by joint site.

In theory, emerging systemic therapies may be ultimately more appropriate in those with generalized OA.[1] Concerning the target joint, prognosis and treatment modalities might differ according to site of OA disease. For example, specific exercise recommendations are different for patellofemoral than tibiofemoral OA and physicians more often elect to treat hand OA that involves the proximal interphalangeals (PIPs) or metacarpophalangeals (MCPs) than the commonly less severe distal interphalangeal (DIP) disease. At the hip, prognosis is worse for superolateral than superomedial migration of the femoral head.

### Activity of the Disease

The concept of "activity" alludes to inflammatory phases of OA disease. Awareness of level of inflammatory activity can inform the therapeutic decision regarding whether to emphasize pain management of more mechanical cause versus more inflammatory cause. Intra-articular steroid injection may be more beneficial in the presence of symptoms of inflammation.

### Severity of the Disease

The concept of severity refers to structural damage. There is much research interest at present in how severity influences therapeutic decisions such as for total joint replacement. Disease severity impacts the choice of medication (anti-inflammatory, analgesic, narcotic), how to combine medication, and the likelihood of response to medications (often declines at more advanced stages of OA disease).

| TABLE 14.1  POINTS FOR OPTIMAL MANAGEMENT OF OSTEOARTHRITIS PATIENTS |
|---|
| Which localization? |
| • Generalized OA versus localized OA |
| • Specific localization within a single joint (e.g., medial, lateral tibiofemoral, patellofemoral at the knee level) |
| Is the disease "active" (inflammatory phase)? |
| • Night pain |
| • Morning stiffness |
| • Hydarthrodial effusion |
|   • Synovitis detected by ultrasonography, MRI |
|   • Subchondral bone edema detected by MRI and the like |
| Is the disease "severe" (cartilage breakdown)? |
| • Abnormal attitudes (flexion, instability, and so on) |
| • Peri-articular amyotrophy |
| • Radiological joint space narrowing |
| Is the disease "potentially severe"? |
| • Presence of inflammation |
| • Interest of biomarkers? |
| • Is the disease refractory? |

## Potentially Severe Disease

This concept has been recognized more extensively in the field of rheumatoid arthritis than in OA. However, there is an increasing body of evidence that the presence of synovial inflammation, subchondral bone marrow abnormality, and mal-alignment may contribute to both the presence of symptoms and the risk of disease progression.[2-5] Ultimately, such parameters may serve to identify persons for emerging disease-modifying treatment.

Most physicians restrict their investigation to the clinical interview and physical examination. Whether or not investigations beyond knee radiography (such as ultrasonography, MRI, and full-limb radiography) are useful in OA management will require further study.

## Refractory Severe Disease

In the management of OA, the concept of refractory severe disease is particularly important in two clinical situations.

- In the decision to perform total joint replacement (well recognized).
- In the decision to use a specific medication or non-pharmacologic intervention with the objective of a sparing effect on the current treatment. This less recognized approach is especially important in situations in which the current treatment has the potential for adverse effects.

## Disease Versus Patient

Therapeutic decisions in OA are also influenced by the patient's condition apart from OA, including both the presence and severity of co-morbidities. For example, the history or the concomitant presence of cardiovascular diseases might eliminate use of non-steroidal anti-inflammatory drugs (NSAIDs) or at least prevent their daily intake.

## Assessment of Osteoarthritis Patients

### Concept

OA assessment should be focused on the main domains of interest (e.g., pain, function, inflammation, range of motion, structural damage, and concomitant therapies). A specific tool has to be chosen for each domain, and for each tool a threshold has to be chosen above or below which a therapeutic decision has to be made.[6] This process typically occurs in the mind of the physician on an individual basis. Specific thresholds are not established for most aspects of OA management. To assess pain, a visual analogue scale was recommended and is widely used in clinical studies.[7] It has previously been recommended that a therapeutic decision should be considered with a value above 40 mm.

### Domains Versus Osteoarthritis Characteristics

Unfortunately, the domains of assessment in the clinic are not well suited to address the key points for OA management summarized previously (i.e., activity, severity, potential severity, and refractory). For example, the level of pain and/or functional impairment can be related to both an "active" (inflammatory) and a "severe" (advanced with structural damage) disease.

In clinical trials, it is clear that the domains "pain" and "functional impairment" have to be precisely (using specific tools) evaluated. In daily practice, interest in the use of such tools is not common. Two areas that receive particular emphasis in the clinic are evidence of inflammation and evidence of severe advanced disease (e.g., periarticular muscle atrophy and loss of range of motion).

### Tools

#### Pain

In clinical trials, there is a large body of evidence for the use of specific tools (see Table 14.2).

#### Functional Impairment

This domain can be evaluated at three levels.

- By a generic tool (e.g., whatever the disease, a tool used to evaluate functional disability—such as the Health Assessment Questionnaire, HAQ)[8]
- By a regional tool such as a hand disability index
- By a specific OA tool

| **TABLE 14.2 ASSESSMENT OF OSTEOARTHRITIS PATIENTS** | |
|---|---|
| Domain | Tool |
| Pain | Visual Analogue Scale, Lequesne's index (hip, knee), WOMAC pain sub-scale (hip, knee) |
| Function | WOMAC function subscale (hip); Neer (shoulder); AUSCAN, Cochin, Dreizer (hand) |
| Inflammation | Night pain, morning stiffness, hydarthrodial effusion |
| Range of motion | Joint specific |
| Abnormal attitudes | Joint specific |
| Concomitant therapies | Dose of NSAIDs, number of intra-articular injections of steroids |
| Co-morbidities | Disease specific (e.g., renal failure) |

To our knowledge, an OA functional impairment tool that can be used whatever the localization of the disease is not available. At variance, there are several tools (e.g., WOMAC[9]) that evaluate specific regional OA such as hip or knee Lequesne.[10] In daily practice, the use of such tools (pain, function) might facilitate exchanges between health professionals, and there is evidence that their use improves patient satisfaction with care.[11]

History and physical examination are important tools in the evaluation of inflammation in OA. Symptoms and exam findings of OA were associated with synovitis by ultrasound.[12,13] The remaining question is whether investigations (e.g., ultrasonography, MRI, and the like) have to be performed in order to adequately assess this domain both in clinical studies and daily practice.

## Range of Motion

This domain is frequently evaluated by the orthopedic surgeon and/or the physiotherapist and less frequently by the rheumatologist and/or the general practitioner.

## Abnormal Attitudes

As previously discussed, the presence of abnormal attitudes are important factors to consider in daily practice in order to evaluate the severity of the disease and therefore to facilitate the therapeutic decision (e.g., indication of surgery, physiotherapy, and so on).

## Concomitant Therapies

The amount of symptomatic treatment required by the patient in order to obtain an acceptable symptom state is also important to consider because such doses could be considered unacceptable with regard to the risk of toxicity and therefore rule out the tool as a

benefit in therapeutic decision making (e.g., indication to a specific anti-OA drug, or indication to surgery). This concept is usually applied in the context of two commonly used symptomatic therapies.

- Intra-articular injection of steroids
- NSAIDs

The remaining question concerns the threshold above which one could consider such treatment unacceptable.

## Composite Indices

Finally, if everybody agrees that the optimal way to monitor a patient is to obtain information related to different domains (pain, function, and so on), the use of composite index combining the information from different domains might be considered attractive. To our knowledge, two types of composite indices have been developed.

- For evaluating the response to therapy
- For considering time to surgery

A third category is missing: an OA Disease Activity Score such as that used in rheumatoid arthritis.

- *Alpha OMERACT-OARSI responder criteria:* This composite index includes information from the domains "pain," "function," and "patient global assessment."[14] This composite index is used to conduct and report clinical trials but is not used in daily practice (Table 14.3).
- *Beta sets of criteria for considering total articular replacement:* To the author's knowledge, five sets of criteria for total articular replacement have been proposed:[15-21] National Institutes of Health,[15] Western Ontario and McMaster Universities osteoarthritis

| **TABLE 14.3 OMERACT-OARSI RESPONDER CRITERIA FOR HIP/KNEE OSTEOARTHRITIS[14]** | |
|---|---|
| High improvement in pain or in function ≥50% and absolute change ≥20 | |
| ↗ | ↘ |
| Yes | No |
| ⇩ | ⇩ |
| Response | Improvement in at least two of the following: |
| | • Pain ≥20% and absolute change ≥10 |
| | • Function ≥20% and absolute change ≥10 |
| | • Patient's global assessment ≥20% and absolute change ≥10 |
| ↗ | ↘ |
| Yes | No |
| ⇩ | ⇩ |
| Response | No response |

index,[16] New Zealand criteria,[17] Lequesne index,[10,18,19] and the Hôpital Cochin composite index.[20,21]

The number of proposed sets of criteria indicates clearly that no consensus presently exists with respect to the optimal time for a patient to undergo total articular replacement. They require validation in future studies conducted in various cohorts of patients and in different countries.

## TREATMENT MODALITIES

### Objectives

Treatment aims at educating the patient about OA, lowering pain, improving or at least maintaining function, and preventing or retarding progression of damage to joint tissues (cartilage, bone, ligament, muscle). Current treatments include a wide range of non-pharmacologic, pharmacologic, and surgical modalities. Based on a combined evidence-based medicine and expert-opinion approach, a European League Against Rheumatism (EULAR) task force proposed recommendations for management of OA.

These recommendations include all modality categories. Because there are specific issues related to site of OA involvement, the recommendations are joint specific. To date, EULAR recommendations are available for the hip and knee (Tables 14.4 and 14.5).[22,23] EULAR hand OA treatment guidelines are under development. Concomitantly, the American College of Rheumatology has also prepared recommendations for management of hip and knee OA (Table 14.6).[24]

### Non-pharmacologic Therapies

#### Education

This treatment modality is well recognized[25] and is included in the EULAR recommendations. Two areas need to be elucidated.

- The best content of such treatment
- The route of administration

Content should include information concerning OA pathophysiology, clinical presentations, how the disease is assessed, its natural course, and the indications and expected results of various treatment modalities. A major objective of education is to improve patient

| N° | Proposition |
|---|---|
| | **TABLE 14.4  EULAR RECOMMENDATIONS FOR MANAGEMENT OF KNEE OSTEOARTHRITIS[22]** |
| 1 | The optimal management of knee OA requires a combination of non-pharmacologic and pharmacologic treatment modalities. |
| 2 | The treatment of knee OA should be tailored according to: |
| | (a)  Knee risk factors (obesity, adverse mechanical factors, physical activity) |
| | (b)  General risk factors (age, co-morbidity, poly-pharmacy) |
| | (c)  Level of pain intensity and disability |
| | (d)  Sign of inflammation (e.g., effusion) |
| | (e)  Location and degree of structural damage |
| 3 | Non-pharmacologic treatment of knee OA should include regular education, exercise, appliances (stick, insoles, knee bracing), and weight reduction. |
| 4 | Paracetamol is the oral analgesic to try first, and if successful is the preferred long-term oral analgesic. |
| 5 | Topical applications (NSAID, capsaicin) have clinical efficacy and are safe. |
| 6 | NSAIDs should be considered in patients unresponsive to paracetamol. In patients with an increased gastrointestinal risk, nonselective NSAIDs and effective gastro-protective agents or selective COX-2 inhibitors should be used. |
| 7 | Opioid analgesics, with or without paracetamol, are useful alternatives in patients in whom NSAIDs (including COX-2-selective inhibitors) are contraindicated, ineffective, and/or poorly tolerated. |
| 8 | SYSADOA (glucosamine sulfate, chondroitin sulfate, ASU, diacerein, hyaluronic acid) have symptomatic effects and may modify structure. |
| 9 | Intra-articular injection of long-acting corticosteroid is indicated for flare of knee pain, especially if accompanied by effusion. |
| 10 | Joint replacement has to be considered in patients with radiographic evidence of knee OA who have refractory pain and disability. |

OA, osteoarthritis; NSAIDs, nonsteroidal anti-inflammatory drugs; SYSADOA, symptomatic slow-acting drugs for osteoarthritis.

## TABLE 14.5 EULAR RECOMMENDATIONS FOR MANAGEMENT OF HIP OSTEOARTHRITIS[23]

| N° | Proposition |
|----|-------------|
| 1 | The optimal management of hip OA requires a combination of non-pharmacologic and pharmacologic treatment modalities. |
| 2 | The treatment of hip OA should be tailored according to: |
| | (a) Hip risk factors (obesity, adverse mechanical factors, physical activity, dysplasia) |
| | (b) General risk factors (age, gender, co-morbidity, co-medications) |
| | (c) Level of pain intensity, disability, and handicap |
| | (d) Location and degree of structural damage |
| | (e) Wishes and expectations of the patient |
| 3 | Non-pharmacologic therapy of hip OA should include regular education, exercise, appliances (stick, insoles), and weight reduction if obese or overweight. |
| 4 | Because of its efficacy and safety, paracetamol (up to 4 g/day) is the oral analgesic of first choice for mild to moderate pain, and if successful is the preferred long-term oral analgesic. |
| 5 | NSAID, at the lowest effective dose, should be added or substituted in patients who respond inadequately to paracetamol. In patients with increased gastrointestinal risk, nonselective NSAIDs plus a gastro-protective agent or a selective COX-2 inhibitor (coxib) should be used. |
| 6 | Opioid analgesics, with or without paracetamol, are useful alternatives in patients in whom NSAIDs—including COX-2-selective inhibitors (coxibs)—are contraindicated, ineffective, and/or poorly tolerated. |
| 7 | SYSADOA (glucosamine sulfate, chondroitin sulfate, diacerein, avocado soybean unsaponifiable, and hyaluronic acid) have symptomatic effect and low toxicity, but effect sizes are small, suitable patients are not well defined, and clinically relevant structure modification and pharmaco-economic aspects are not well established. |
| 8 | Intra-articular steroid injections (guided by ultrasound or X-ray) may be considered in patients with a flare that is unresponsive to analgesic and NSAID. |
| 9 | Osteotomy and joint-preserving surgical procedures should be considered in young adults with symptomatic hip OA, especially in the presence of dysplasia or varus/valgus deformity. |
| 10 | Joint replacement has to be considered in patients with radiographic evidence of hip OA who have refractory pain and disability. |

OA, osteoarthritis; NSAIDs, nonsteroidal anti-inflammatory drugs; SYSADOA, symptomatic slow-acting drugs for osteoarthritis.

knowledge in order to integrate him or her into the decision-making team. Moreover, such education should improve treatment compliance. Obviously, the route of administration is not well established and could include one-on-one discussions with health professionals, didactic sessions, group discussion, or self-reviewed materials (e.g., booklets, web sites).

### Exercise

The ultimate goal of exercise in OA is to prevent or delay disability. An exercise program[26] should incorporate elements to lessen pain during activity and to increase or at least maintain joint range of motion, periarticular muscle strength, joint stability, and aerobic capacity or level of conditioning.[27] A systematic review of 11 randomized controlled trials of different exercise therapy programs in patients suffering from hip or (more frequently) knee OA[28] revealed adequate methodologic quality in 6 of the 11 studies. This review concludes that exercise decreases pain and improves function in the short term. Improvements over the control group in these studies ranged from 15 to 25% after 3 to 6 months of therapy.[29]

The evidence appeared less convincing for hip than for knee OA, but the paucity of hip OA exercise trials makes it difficult to make a definitive statement.[30] Exercise in OA should be adapted according to the presence and severity of pain. In painful episodes, isometric exercise or exercise in a non weight-bearing (e.g., biking, rowing with adapted tools) or in a partial weight-bearing position (e.g., aquatic exercises) should be recommended. In painless (or at least less painful) periods, the exercise program may include progressive muscle performance exercises.

The best route of administration is at present not clear. Key issues in determining the best route for an individual patient include the best route to ensure correct exercise performance and what is the best route to

| TABLE 14.6 ACR RECOMMENDATIONS FOR MANAGEMENT OF OSTEOARTHRITIS OF THE HIP AND KNEE[25] |
| --- |
| **Nonpharmacologic therapy for patients with osteoarthritis:** |
| • Patient education |
| • Self-management programs (e.g., Arthritis Foundation Self-Management program) |
| • Personalized social support through telephone contact |
| • Weight loss (if overweight) |
| • Aerobic exercise programs |
| • Physical therapy |
| • Range-of-motion exercises |
| • Assistive devices for ambulation |
| • Patellar taping |
| • Lateral-wedged insoles (for genu varum) |
| • Bracing |
| • Occupational therapy |
| • Joint protection and energy conservation |
| • Assistive devices for activities of daily living |
| **Pharmacologic therapy for patients with osteoarthritis:** |
| • Oral |
|   • Acetaminophen |
|   • COX-2-specific inhibitor |
|   • Nonselective NSAID plus misoprostol or a proton pump inhibitor |
| • Nonacetylated salicylate |
| • Other pure analgesics |
|   • Tramadol |
|   • Opioids |
| • Intraarticular |
|   • Glucocorticoids |
|   • Hyaluronan |
| • Topical |
|   • Capsaicin |
|   • Methylsalicylate |

maximize long-term compliance. Published reports suggest some benefit with a variety of approaches, including when therapy was initiated in the hospitalized and monitored at the patient's home by a visiting nurse,[25] a supervised home-based program,[31] and even an unsupervised home-based program.[11]

Whatever the mode of administration, it appears that the exercise should be performed at least three times per week and perhaps even as frequently as seven times per week. The optimal frequency is not known and may differ according to patient characteristics. Efficacy is better in compliant patients. Motivation and compliance should be addressed regularly, possibly through a combination of in-person visits and phone calls.

### Weight Loss
This treatment modality has only been evaluated in knee OA. The impact of weight loss on OA at other sites is not known. At the knee, being overweight and obesity seem to be important factors in the occurrence of OA, and (especially in varus mal-aligned knees) in the progression of medial tibiofemoral disease.[32-34] Weight loss and exercise have been associated with improvement in pain and physical function in knee OA. In a recent study, a sustained weight loss of 8% in one year resulted in a 19% improvement in WOMAC score.[35]

Exercise therapy is recommended in knee OA in order to both improve symptoms and reduce body weight in those who are overweight or obese.[36] A mean weight reduction of 6, 10, and 14 kg has been observed in patients performing an exercise therapy program of less than 150 minutes/week, between 150 and 200 minutes, and more than 200 minutes per week, respectively.[37] Despite the demonstration of its efficacy, such treatment is not initiated often enough. Only 34% of 1,000 obese individuals who had visited a doctor in the previous year were advised to perform exercise.[38]

### Orthotics and Bracing
The main objective of orthotics is to improve symptoms, but orthotics may also be used to prevent articular deformity. Intermittent bracing may also be applied during a flare of symptoms. In trapezio-metacarpal joint OA, a splint maintaining the thumb in abduction can improve symptoms and may help to prevent a common deformity (i.e., thumb adductus).[39] In distal interphalangeal joint OA, a splint maintaining the joint in extension may be indicated in the case of a painful and/or inflammatory episode (in order to prevent a lateralizing deformity). In hip OA, one uncontrolled study suggested that a heel lift may reduce symptoms.[40]

There are more reports dealing with orthotics in knee OA. Modalities under study include insoles and braces. Studies have demonstrated that wearing lateral wedged insoles led to a reduction in knee pain and/or in NSAID requirement in persons with medial compartment knee OA.[41-44] Knee braces have been evaluated as well (i.e., valgus bracing of patients with medial compartment OA). There is still insufficient data from rigorous randomized controlled trials on which to base recommendations regarding braces. Medial taping of the patella of patients with patellofemoral OA may be beneficial.[45]

### Use of a Cane and/or Crutches

A cane, along with education about its correct use, might be helpful in those with knee or hip OA who are experiencing symptom flares. Although usually a cane is proposed for short periods (2 to 4 weeks),[46] longer-term use may be beneficial in persons with chronic mechanical pain due to severe hip OA.[47]

### Modifications of Activities of Daily Living and Sports Activities

Based on clinical experience, a diminution in activity is advisable during inflammatory phases of the disease. In contrast, at all other times maintaining physical activity (if it is adequate) or increasing it should be recommended. There are enormous benefits to physical activity in OA—on well-being, psychological status, cardiovascular fitness, pain reduction, and potentially disability prevention.

Some specific advice is advisable in terms of athletic activity. OA may begin at a relatively early age in adult life, in certain sports (soccer, rugby, racket sports, and other track-and-field sports) and under certain conditions (in highly competitive settings). In healthy joints, recreational athletic activity does not appear to increase the risk of OA development. There is very little in the published literature dealing with sports activity in the setting of established OA.[48]

Occupational therapy and related assistive devices will improve performance of activities of daily living. These may include an elevated toilet seat or shower bench in someone with lower extremity OA, or appliances designed to help with the opening of jars in a patient with hand OA.

## PHARMACOLOGIC TREATMENT MODALITIES

### Topical Agents

The two most widely used types are preparations containing capsaicin and those containing NSAIDs. Capsaicin preparations[49,50] and topical NSAIDs (particularly diclofenac and eltenac[51-53]) have been tested in double-blind placebo-controlled trials of OA of the hand and knee. Topical agents should be considered, especially in patients intolerant, at risk of intolerance, or unwilling to take oral analgesics and/or oral NSAIDs.

### Analgesics

#### Acetaminophen (Paracetamol)

Acetaminophen (known as paracetamol outside the United States) as a treatment for symptoms of OA is recommended as a first-line treatment by EULAR,[22,23] ACR,[24] and North of England.[54] Of the three issues

efficacy, safety, and cost, efficacy and safety were reexamined recently. Placebo-controlled studies evaluating acetaminophen in OA are limited and often shortlived. Recommendations for the use of acetaminophen as an efficient symptom-modifying drug were based until recent years on two placebo-controlled trials: one using a crossover design and the other a parallel group design.[55,56]

These studies demonstrated the superiority of oral acetaminophen 3 to 4 g/day. However, another placebo-controlled trial using a parallel group design failed to demonstrate any superiority of acetaminophen for treating symptomatic OA of the knee.[57] Pincus et al. in two different placebo-controlled trials using a crossover design reported superiority of acetaminophen versus placebo in a single trial.[58]

A large (779 patients) 6-week placebo-controlled trial in painful knee OA patients evaluating a 4-g/day dose of paracetamol failed to reveal a statistically significant difference between acetaminophen and placebo.[59] However, a post hoc analysis suggested that the treatment effect was significant in a subset with chronic mechanical knee pain without inflammatory symptoms.

In terms of safety, hepatic toxicity was reported in patients taking high doses (≥4 grams) concomitantly with alcohol consumption. Results of an epidemiologic study also suggest that high (≥4 grams) doses of acetaminophen may convey the same risk for upper gastrointestinal complications as traditional NSAIDs.[60] The mechanism of high-dose acetaminophen's apparent upper gastrointestinal toxicity may be related to its ability to function as a weak inhibitor of cyclooxygenase-1.[61]

Another concern is the potential for a patient's concomitant use of over-the-counter products containing acetaminophen. Despite these data, because of the relatively higher risk of toxicity of NSAIDs and narcotic analgesics acetaminophen remains the recommended first-line therapy.

### Narcotic Analgesics

Codeine and propoxyphene have been used effectively in patients with OA, especially in combination with acetaminophen.[62] Tramadol is also available alone or in combination with acetaminophen.[63] Pure opioids are rarely indicated in OA. However, in patients with very severe OA who are unable to take other symptom-modifying agents this treatment modality can be considered with close monitoring. All of these agents (codeine, propoxyphene, tramadol, pure opioids) have potential side effects, including nausea, dizziness, somnolence, and constipation—each of which might be clinically relevant, particularly in elderly patients.

## Non-steroidal Anti-inflammatory Agents

NSAIDs are used widely for the management of OA. A detailed description of mechanisms of action and the potential gastrointestinal and cardiovascular toxicity observed in both nonselective NSAIDs and COX-2 selective inhibitors can be found elsewhere in this book. All clinical trials evaluating NSAIDs in OA clearly demonstrate some short-term symptomatic effect. However, several questions remain—some of which are currently being reexamined.

- Is their therapeutic effect better than that observed with analgesics?[57,58,64-68]
- Is their therapeutic effect maintained when using COX-2-specific inhibitors?
- Is their therapeutic effect modified positively or negatively by a structure-modifying effect?[69-75]
- Is a systematic daily intake of better benefit than an "at request" (on demand, PRN) intake?

## Specific Anti-osteoarthritic Drugs

### Treatment Specificities

Drugs (e.g., glucosamine sulfate, doxycycline, diacerein, and so on) other than pure analgesics and NSAIDs have been proposed or are being developed for the management of OA patients. These compounds have also been called SYSADOA (symptomatic slow-acting disease osteoarthritis) compounds. The main differences between these compounds and NSAIDs are as follows.

- A probably lower effect on symptoms effect. For example, whereas NSAIDs result in a 15- to 20-mm decrease in visual analogue scale (VAS) pain beyond that seen with placebo,[66,67] avocado/soybean unsaponifiables and diacerein were only associated with a change of 7 to 8 mm over the magnitude of placebo change.[76,77]
- A delayed onset of action. In an 8-week trial comparing placebo, tenoxicam, and diacerein, the treatment effect of tenoxicam (i.e., the effect observed in the tenoxicam group over that observed in the placebo group) was stable at 17 to 18% during the 8 weeks of the study. By contrast, the diacerein effect was 0, 5, 11, and 12% (respectively) at weeks 2, 4, 6, and 8.[76]
- A carryover effect (i.e., effect on symptoms after the drug has been discontinued). In the study evaluating diacerein and diclofenac, the relief of pain obtained with diclofenac was no longer observed 4 weeks after discontinuation of the drug. On the other hand, the relief of pain obtained at month 4 in the diacerein group (i.e., the end of the treatment period) was maintained until the end of the follow-up (i.e., at months 5 and 6).[78]
- It is believed that these drugs may lessen NSAID requirement, although this has not been formally examined.
- A potential beneficial structural effect.

### Diacerein

Diacerein is a rhein derivative developed empirically for the treatment of OA. Based on a number of clinical trials, diacerein is approved to treat symptoms of OA in several countries.[79] Several studies (both in vitro and in animal models) suggest that diacerein may inhibit interleukin-1 (IL-1) production[80,81] and reduce cartilage breakdown[82] and the development of cartilage lesions.[83,84] In vitro studies of rabbit chondrocytes have shown that diacerein inhibits collagenase production and modulates IL-1 inhibition of proteoglycan (PG) synthesis.[85] Diacerein has also been implicated in the regulation of transforming growth factor (TGF) β1 and β2 in articular chondrocytes.[86] In several reports, diacerein was superior to placebo in the treatment of OA symptoms. The magnitude of the diacerein effect was typically small, however.[76,87]

The potential structural effect was investigated in a 3-year placebo-controlled trial in 507 patients suffering from painful hip OA.[88] Adiographic progression (i.e., using a life-table approach in which the time to progression, 0.5-mm loss of joint space width, was determined) was significantly less frequent and occurred later in the diacerein group compared to the placebo group.

### Glucosamine

The American College of Rheumatology and the European League Against Rheumatism consider it premature to make specific recommendations because of methodologic limitations of reported studies.[89,90] Glucosamine is commercially derived from chitin, the specially processed exoskeleton of shrimps, lobsters, and crabs. There are no dietary sources of glucosamine, and it is available commercially as a nutritional supplement in three forms: glucosamine hydrochloride, glucosamine sulfate, and N-acetyl-glucosamine.

For several years, the counter anion of the glucosamine salt (i.e., chloride or sulfate) was not considered likely to play a role in the action or pharmacokinetics of glucosamine. However, there is some evidence that a component of the activity of glucosamine sulfate is related to sulfate residues.[91,92] It has been suggested that glucosamine may delay or prevent cartilage degradation and even possibly stimulate production of new cartilage, but basic biologic and biochemical studies on possible mechanisms of action of glucosamine in cartilage remain incomplete.

Clinical trials evaluating not only the symptomatic but structural effect have been conducted using a placebo-controlled randomized design. Concerning the short-term (≤6 months) symptomatic efficacy of glucosamine, both a Cochrane review and a recent meta-analysis are available.[93-95]

The conclusion of the Cochrane review was that there is good evidence that glucosamine is effective and safe in treating symptoms of OA. However, the long-term effectiveness and toxicity of glucosamine remain unclear. In addition, whether different glucosamine preparations proposed by different manufacturers are equally effective is not known.[94] In addition, only one of the 15 evaluated placebo-controlled trials was independent from manufacturer support, and it has been demonstrated that commercially funded studies can induce biased interpretation of results.[96] More recently, a study failing to demonstrate a symptomatic effect of glucosamine has been reported.[97]

Concerning the structural effect, two placebo-controlled randomized trials have been conducted in painful knee OA.[98,99] Both showed a statistically significant reduction in radiologic joint space narrowing with glucosamine when compared to placebo (+0.06 versus –0.31 mm in one trial[98] and +0.04 versus –0.19 mm in the other[99] trial).

Because of these findings (i.e., the possibilities of a symptomatic effect and a structure effect versus potential biases of the reported studies) and because of the importance of the consequences for management of patients in daily practice, the National Institutes of Health is sponsoring a large (3,238 patients) multicenter U.S. study of glucosamine in painful knee OA (the GAIT trial).[100] This study was a priori designed to have two parts: an evaluation of the symptomatic effect in the first 6 months and evaluations of both symptomatic and structural effects over 24 months. The five treatment arms of the study are placebo, celecoxib 200 mg daily, glucosamine HIC 500 mg three times per day, sodium chondroitin sulfate 400 mg three times per day, and glucosamine plus chondroitin sulfate.

In an early report (as yet unpublished) at the 2005 ACR meeting,[100] compared to placebo there was a significant difference in the primary variable (i.e., response defined by an improvement of at least 20% in pain) in favor of celecoxib (70.4 versus 60.1% responder rate) and a non-significant trend in favor of glucosamine, chondroitin sulfate, or the combination (percentage responders: 64.0, 65.4, 66.6%, respectively). However, subanalyses performed in those with more severe pain at entry revealed a significant difference of the combination (glucosamine plus chondroitin sulfate) versus placebo (percentage responders 79.2 versus 54.3%, respectively). Until these results have been formally reported, it will be difficult to know how to apply them to clinical practice. The results of the second phase are not yet available.

## Chondroitin Sulfate

Chondroitin sulfate is a macromolecule that contributes to (like hyaluronic acid) a framework for collagen formation. The rationale for use and the discussion concerning the available data for symptomatic efficacy are very similar to those discussed previously for glucosamine, except that the number of well-conducted placebo-controlled trials is much smaller with chondroitin sulfate.[90]

A recent double-blind placebo-controlled 2-year trial focused on the evaluation of both the symptomatic and structural effect of 800 mg chondroitin sulfate.[101] This study failed to show a significant difference in terms of symptoms but did reveal a significant difference in terms of radiologic joint space progression (0.00 ± 0.53 versus 0.14 ± 0.61 mm in the chondroitin versus placebo group, respectively). As with glucosamine, chondroitin sulfate seems to be very safe.

## Avocado/Soybean Unsaponifiables

Avocado/soybean unsaponifiables (ASU) can be considered either a diet supplement or a drug. Despite the fact that ASU is commonly used in OA, the evidence of its efficacy is quite poor. Concerning the symptomatic efficacy, a 6-month placebo-controlled trial revealed a significant (albeit weak) difference in the changes in symptoms (e.g., pain by VAS and function by Lequesne index) and concomitant NSAID consumption (48 versus 63% in the ASU versus the placebo group).[77]

A structural effect of ASU was not found in a 2-year placebo-controlled trial in painful hip OA. However, in a post hoc analysis ASU was shown to reduce the progression of joint space narrowing in the subgroup of patients with advanced joint space narrowing.[102] These results prompted an ongoing placebo-controlled trial in hip OA with stratification based on a baseline structural parameter (radiographic joint space width).

## Glycosaminoglycan Polysulfuric Acid

Glycosaminoglycan polysulfuric acid (GAGPS), known as the trade names Arteparon and Adequan, is a highly sulfated glycosaminoglycan. Human studies suggested a potential short-term symptomatic effect.[103,104] However, potentially serious allergic and heparin-like effects were observed. GAGPS is not available for human use.

## Glycosaminoglycan-peptide Complex

Glycosaminoglycan-peptide complex (GP-C), known as the trade name Rumalon, is a highly sulfated polysaccharide derived from bovine tracheal cartilage and bone marrow.[105] Despite some previous data indicating a potential beneficial symptomatic effect, a well-conducted placebo-controlled trial failed to confirm such an effect and also failed to show any structural effect[106] in the entire group of patients. However, in the subanalysis focused on the group of hip OA patients there was a trend in favor of a structural effect of Rumalon. Because of the extraction of the compound (bovine cartilage) and the associated potential risk of serious infection, this compound is no longer available in many countries.

## Pentosan Polysulfate (Cartrofen)

Cartrofen is a purified extract of beech hemicellular. Data concerning both its symptomatic and structural efficacy are lacking and/or only presented in abstract form.[107]

## Risedronate

Risedronate is a potent bisphosphonate with a well-established anti-osteoclastic activity effect. The rationale to evaluate this compound in OA is based on the potential role of subchondral bone in both the occurrence and progression of OA and on data derived from animal models of OA. For example, in a study using the guinea pig OA model the pyridinyl bisphosphonate risedronate was shown to slow disease progression (as measured by the size and severity of cartilage lesions and the size of osteophytes) by up to 40%.[108,109] Based on these pre-clinical studies, risedronate was evaluated in two placebo-controlled trials in painful knee OA. The first one (the British study of risedronate in structure and symptoms of knee OA [BRISK] trial), conducted in 284 patients, was 1 year in duration and showed a trend toward less joint space narrowing in the group receiving 15 mg risedronate.[110]

These first results prompted the conduct of a larger trial. Results of this trial (not yet published) include a lack of effect on either structure (radiographic) or symptoms, but did include a significant difference between persons receiving risedronate versus placebo in biomarkers reflecting cartilage breakdown such as CTX-II. Elucidation of risedronate's effect will require additional studies.

## Doxycycline

Doxycycline is a tetracycline antibiotic. The rationale of evaluation of doxycycline as a potential disease-modifying OA drug was based on results of in vitro studies showing that doxycycline inhibited the degradation of type XI collagen (one of the minor collagens of articular cartilage)[111] and that doxycycline inhibited messenger RNA for inducible nitric oxide synthase, an enzyme present in large quantities in OA cartilage—the activity of which results in secretion of matrix metalloproteinases by the chondrocytes.[112,113]

In vivo studies have been conducted in a canine nitrate-deficiency model of OA. These studies showed that doxycycline markedly reduced the evidence and progression of joint pathology.[114] Such findings were in accordance with those obtained in the guinea pig spontaneous OA model.[115] Based on these findings, the National Institutes of Health sponsored a 30-month placebo-controlled trial in obese women with unilateral radiographic knee OA comparing 100 mg doxycycline to placebo.[116] The predefined primary efficacy criterion was the incidence of radiologic contralateral knee OA.

In terms of this criterion, the study failed to demonstrate a therapeutic effect. However, subanalyses showed less radiographic progression in the affected knee in participants receiving doxycycline than those receiving placebo (0.30 ± 0.60 versus 0.45 ± 0.70 mm, respectively). During the study, there was no significant difference between the two groups in pain or in functional limitation. However, the frequency of follow-up visits at which the subjects reported a ≥25% increase in pain in the baseline affected knee relative to the previous visit was reduced among those receiving doxycycline.[116] It is not as yet clear how these results should be applied in practice. Treatments targeting metalloproteinases should be further developed and examined in clinical trials.

### Ongoing Studies with Potential Candidates

With advances in knowledge of mechanisms of cartilage breakdown has come a shift in investigation away from compounds such as cartilage extracts and toward drugs with a specific mechanism of action; namely, targeted therapies. Such targeted therapies include inhibition of specific enzymes such as metalloproteinases, but also growth factor and cytokine manipulation.[117,118] Gene therapy has been attempted as well, but to our knowledge not in humans. Concerning chondrocyte and stem cell transplants, it has to be noted that such therapeutic procedures are indicated only in the case of small and well-demarcated cartilage defects (usually post-traumatic in young people) but not (at least at present) in patients with primary OA.[119]

## Intra-articular Injections

### Steroids

Intra-articular steroids are recommended in several guidelines for the management of patients with peripheral joint OA.[22,24] They are widely used. A survey of rheumatologists in the United States suggested that more than 95% use them at least sometimes, and 53% frequently.[120] Evidence of the efficacy of intra-articular injections of steroids in OA is based on somewhat contradictory data and results are difficult to interpret, in particular because of a powerful response to placebo.[121-125] Data on joints other than the knee are very limited. Onset of efficacy tends to be rapid (i.e., within 24 to 48 hours). Maximal efficacy is reached in less than 1 week but lasts only from 1 to 4 weeks.[126,127]

There is limited evidence that the presence of joint effusion predicts a better response to the intra-articular injection of steroids.[122,128,129] Knee effusion may reflect the presence of inflammatory synovitis, which would explain a good response to intra-articular steroid. At the hip, it has been suggested that patients with an atrophic pattern respond less well than those with a hypertrophic or mixed-type pattern.[130]

The commonly raised question from the patient is the potential deleterious (local and/or systemic) effect of repeated intra-articular injections of steroids. Despite the fact that intra-articular injection of steroids has been commonly used for several decades there is insufficient data in the literature on which to base an answer to this question. In a recent placebo-controlled trial of repeated intra-articular steroid injections every three months for up to 2 years no greater risk of side effects with the steroid injections was detected.[125]

The structural effect of intra-articular injection of steroids has been studied in a number of animal models, with conflicting results. The previously mentioned 2-year placebo-controlled trial failed to demonstrate any significant difference between groups—at least in terms of radiologic joint space narrowing.[125]

### Hyaluronic Acid

Visco-supplementation refers to the intra-articular injection of hyaluronic acid (HA), a high-molecular-weight polysaccharide that is a major component of synovial fluid and cartilage, in order to relieve pain and improve function. Several HA preparations are currently available, in two categories: low molecular weight (0.5 to 2 MDa) and high molecular weight (cross-linked HA, 6 to 7 MDa). Published reports include three systematic reviews and one additional randomized controlled trial comparing hyaluronan preparations with placebo.[127,131,132] Most studies in humans have been carried out in patients with knee OA. The main conclusion is that a course (three to five injections at weekly intervals) has a significant but weak symptomatic effect.

In a systematic review comparing Hyalgan with various steroids, Ayral found five placebo-controlled trials reporting similar benefits of hyaluronic acid and steroids at 1 month—but with modest superiority of Hyalgan after a few months.[132] Studies suggest that the benefit obtained with hyaluronan was similar to that of NSAIDs for pain, and with fewer gastrointestinal adverse effects. Most studies agree that onset of efficacy is delayed by 2 to 5 weeks, the plateau of efficacy is reached in 1 to 2 months, and efficacy is maintained for 4 to 12 months. The absence of joint effusion[132] or of advanced disease[133] may predict a better short-term response. Clinical predictive factors of hyaluronan efficacy have not been specifically evaluated in prospective clinical trials.

Potential structure-modifying effects of hyaluronic acid in OA have been suggested in animal models, but results conflict.[134] Limited studies in humans have been performed. Listrat et al. reported in a pilot-controlled randomized study of 36 patients with medial knee OA that those who received three series of three Hyalgan injections at 3-month intervals showed less progression of the disease 1 year later, as judged by arthroscopy, than controls who received conventional treatment but not hyaluronan injections.[135] Recently, 408 patients assigned randomly to receive three courses of three intra-articular injections of Hyalgan or placebo had radiographic evaluations again after 1 year.[136] Analysis showed no difference in medial femorotibial joint space narrowing between the two groups in the full sample. However, post hoc analyses suggest that the intervention may have had an effect in knees with greater joint space width at baseline.

### Other Intra-articular Drug Injections
#### Alpha Synoviorthesis

Radioactive injections (isotope synoviorthesis) and osmic acid (chemical synoviorthesis) have been used for many years in inflammatory diseases.[137] Their place is probably limited in OA, and there are no placebo-controlled trials evaluating them in this indication.

#### Beta Experimental Treatments

Several compounds usually administered either intravenously or intra-muscularly have been investigated in open uncontrolled studies (e.g., methotrexate, rifampicin).[138] Intra-articular injection of interleukin-1 inhibitor has been reported to be of potential benefit.[139] However, a recent placebo-controlled trial evaluating a single injection of either 50 or 150 mg of IL1-receptor failed to demonstrate a short-term (12 weeks) symptomatic effect.[140] However, the short half-life of this treatment might limit benefits of a single injection. Further studies are required in this field.

## SURGICAL INTERVENTIONS

Surgical interventions in OA can be categorized in three groups based on the rationale and/or the main objective of the treatment.

- The first aimed at improving current symptoms (e.g., lavage and joint debridement).
- The second aimed at preventing the risk of structural progression (e.g., osteotomy).
- The third aimed at improving the symptoms related to an advanced disease (e.g., joint replacement).

### Lavage and Joint Debridement

In theory, lavage of the joint (through a large needle or by arthroscopy) removes debris such as microscopic or macroscopic fragments of cartilage or calcium phosphate crystals that may induce synovitis, a likely source of pain. Tidal irrigation is a similar process, but uses only one entry site.

Arthroscopic debridement consists of smoothing rough fibrillated articular and meniscal surfaces, shaving tibial-spine osteophytes that interfere with the motion of the joint, and removing inflamed synovium.

Despite the availability of some randomized controlled trials,[124,141-144] the evidence of symptomatic efficacy of these treatment modalities is weak. Onset of efficacy is rapid (less than 1 week). In those trials showing a positive symptomatic effect of lavage or arthroscopy, efficacy is maintained for up to 6 months.[124] The predisposing factors of response to such therapies are not well established. For most patients with knee OA, lavage and debridement are probably not as efficient a treatment as once was hoped. The exact place of lavage in knee OA remains to be established.

## Osteotomy

Mal-alignment has been recognized as an important predisposing factor for further structural progression. Therefore, the correction of an abnormality was tempting.[145,146] Observational open studies suggest that osteotomy should be considered in patients with the following characteristics.

- Painful condition
- Moderate cartilage loss
- Specific localization of OA

A specific indication might be the constitutional genu varum observed in patients with mild to moderate medial tibiofemoral OA or moderate superolateral hip

OA occurring in a patient with evident hip dysplasia.[147] However, the lack of evaluation of a safety/efficacy profile of this treatment modality makes impossible any formal recommendation—explaining the huge inter-country variability of the use of such treatment.

## Articular Replacement

Articular replacement is highly effective in providing pain relief and improving function in many patients with OA. Hip and knee joint replacement are the most common. A major remaining question relates to the optimal time for surgery. As noted previously, there are several sets of criteria that have been proposed in this field for different purposes (prioritization of patients who are on a waiting list, epidemiologic studies evaluating the over- or underuse of such therapy,[148] and the endpoint for clinical trials evaluating potential disease-modifying drugs). In daily practice at the individual level, the decision should at least be based on the following.

- Level of symptomatic severity and disability
- Level of structural severity
- Level of required symptomatic therapies
- Co-morbidity
- Patient's willingness

## REFERENCES

1. Dougados M, Nakache JP, Gueguen A. Criteria for generalized and focal osteoarthritis. Rev Rhum Engl Ed 1996;63:569–75.
2. Felson DT, McLaughlin S, Goggins J, et al. Bone marrow edema and its relation to progression of knee osteoarthritis. Ann Intern Med 2003;139:330–36.
3. Dieppe P, Cushnagan J, Young P, Kirwan J. Prediction of the progression of joint space narrowing of the knee by bone scintigraphy. Ann Rheum Dis 1993;52:557–63.
4. Ayral X, Pickering EH, Woodworth TG, et al. Synovitis: A potential predictive factor of structural progression of medial tibio-femoral knee osteoarthritis, results of a 1-year longitudinal arthroscopic study in 422 patients. Osteoarthritis Cartilage 2005; 13:361–67.
5. Dougados M. Structural progression is also driven by clinical symptoms in patients with osteoarthritis. Arthritis Rheum 2004;50:1360–65.
6. Dougados M. Monitoring osteoarthritis progression and therapy. Osteoarthritis Cartilage 2004;12(A):S55–60.
7. GREES. Osteoarthritis section: Recommendations for the registration of drugs used in the treatment of osteoarthritis. Ann Rheum Dis 1996;55:552–57.
8. Fries JF, Spitz P, Kraines RG, et al. Measurement of patient outcome in arthritis. Arthritis Rheum 1980;23:137–45.
9. Bellamy N, Buchanan WW, Goldsmith CH, et al. Validation of WOMAC: A health status instrument for measuring clinically important patient relevant outcomes to anti-rheumatic drug therapy in patients with osteoarthritis of the hip or knee. J Rheumatol 1995;15:1833–40.
10. Lequesne M. Arthrose de la hanche et du genou, critères de diagnostic: Indices de mesure de la douleur, de la fonction et du résultat thérapeutique. In JG Peyron (ed.), L'arthrose: Problèmes Cliniques et Fondamentaux Actuels. Paris: Ciba-Geigy 1985.
11. Ravaud P, Giraudeau B, Logeart I, et al. Management of osteoarthritis (OA) with an unsupervised home based exercise program and/or patient administered assessment tools: A cluster randomized controlled trial with a 2×2 factorial design. Ann Rheum Dis 2004;63:703–08.
12. d'Agostino MA, Conaghan P, Le Bars M, et al. EULAR report on the use of ultrasonography in painful knee osteoarthritis, part 1: Prevalence of inflammation in osteoarthritis. Ann Rheum Dis 2005;64(12):1703–09.
13. Conaghan P, d'Agostino MA, Ravaud P, et al. EULAR report on the use of ultrasonography in painful knee osteoarthritis, part 2: Exploring decision rules for clinical utility. Ann Rheum Dis 2005;64(12):1710–14.
14. Pham T, van der Heijde D, Altman RD, et al. OMERACT-OARSI initiative: Osteoarthritis Research Society International set of responder criteria for osteoarthritis clinical trials revisited. Osteoarthritis Cartilage 2004;12:389–99.
15. NIH consensus development panel on total hip replacement. JAMA 1995;273:1950–56.
16. Hawker GA, Wright JG, Coyre PC, et al. Differences between men and women in the rate of use of hip and knee arthroplasty. N Engl J Med 2000;342:1016–22.
17. Hadorn HC, Holmes AC. Education and debate: The New Zealand priority criteria project. Part 1: overview. Br Med J 1997;314:131–34.
18. Lequesne M. The algofunctional indices for hip and knee osteoarthritis. J Rheumatol 1997;24:779–81.
19. Lequesne M, Taccoen A. Clinical and radiographic status of patients in the ECHODIAH study who underwent THA: Pertinence of the pain-function index for operative decision making. Presse Med 2002;31:4518–19.
20. Maillefert JF, Gueguen A, Nguyen M, et al. A composite index for total hip arthroplasty in patients with hip osteoarthritis. J Rheumatol 2002;29:347–52.
21. Maillefert JF, Dougados M. Is time to joint replacement a valid outcome measure in clinical trials of drugs for osteoarthritis? Rheum Dis Clin North Am 2003;29:831–45.
22. Jordan K, Arden NK, Doherty M, et al. EULAR recommendations 2003: An evidence-based approach to the management of knee

osteoarthritis. Report of a Task Force of the Standing Committee for International Clinical Studies Including Therapeutic Trials (ESCISIT). Ann Rheum Dis 2003;62:1145–55.

23. Zhang, Doherty M, Arden N, et al. EULAR evidence-based recommendations for the management of hip osteoarthritis: Report of a task force of the EULAR Standing Committee for International Clinical Studies Including Therapeutics (ESCISIT). Ann Rheum Dis 2005;64:669–81.

24. ACR. ACR subcommittee on osteoarthritis guidelines: Recommendations for the medical management of osteoarthritis of the hip and knee. Arthritis Rheum 2000;43:1905–15.

25. Mazzuca SA, Brandt KD, Katz BP, et al. effects of self-care education on the health status of inner-city patients with osteoarthritis of the knee (see comments). Arthritis Rheum 1997;40:1466–74.

26. Dougados M, Ravaud P. Exercise therapy in patients with osteoarthritis of the hip or knee. Curr Rheumatol Rep 2001;3:353–54.

27. Minor MA. Exercise in the treatment of osteoarthritis. Rheum Dis Clin North Am 1999;25:397–415.

28. van Baar ME, Assendelft WJJ, Dekker J, et al. Effectiveness of exercise therapy in patients with osteoarthritis of the hip or knee: A systematic review of randomized clinical trials. Arthritis Rheum 1999;42:1361–69.

29. Ettinger W, Burns R, Messier S, et al. A randomized trial comparing aerobic exercise and resistance exercise with a health education program in older adults with knee osteoarthritis: The Fitness Arthritis and Senior trial (FAST). JAMA 1997;277:25–31.

30. van Baar ME, Dekker J, Oostendorp RAB, et al. The effectiveness of exercise therapy in patients with osteoarthritis of the hip or knee: A randomized clinical trial. J Rheumatol 1998;25:2432–39.

31. Deyle CD, Hendersony NE, Matekel RL, et al. Effectiveness of manual physical therapy and exercise in osteoarthritis of the knee. Ann Intern Med 2000;132:173–81.

32. Felson DT, Zhang Y, Anthony JM, et al. Weight loss reduces the risk for symptomatic knee osteoarthritis in women. Ann Intern Med 1992;116:535–39.

33. Sharma L, Lou C, Cahue S, Dunlop DD. The mechanism of the effect of obesity in knee osteoarthritis: The mediating role of mal-alignment. Arthritis Rheum 2000;43:568–75.

34. Cooper C, Snow S, McAlindon TE, et al. Risk factors for the incidence and progression of radiographic knee osteoarthritis. Arthritis Rheum 2000;43:995–1000.

35. Christensen R, Astrup A, Bliddal H, et al. Sustained weight loss as treatment of knee osteoarthritis in obese patients: Long-term results from a randomized trial. Ann Rheum Dis 2005;64(III):66.

36. Toda Y, Toda T, Takemura S, et al. Change in body fat, but not body weight or metabolic correlates of obesity, is related to symptomatic relief of obese patients with knee osteoarthritis after a weight control program. J Rheumatol 1998;25:2181–86.

37. Jakicic JM, Winters C, Lang W, Wing R. Effects of intermittent exercise and use of home exercise equipment on adherence, weight loss, and fitness in overweight women: A randomized trial. JAMA 1999;282:1554–60.

38. Fontanarosa P. Patients, physicians, and weight control. JAMA 1999;282:1581–82.

39. Berggren M, Joost-Davidsson A, Lindstrand J, et al. Reduction in the need for operation after conservative treatment of osteoarthritis of the first carpometacarpal joint: A seven year prospective study. Scand J Plast Reconstr Surg Hand Surg 2001;35:415–17.

40. Ohsawa S, Ueno R. Heel lifting as a conservative therapy for osteoarthritis of the hip: Based on the rationale of Pauwels' intertrochanteric osteotomy. Prosthet Orthot Int 1997;21:153–58.

41. Sasaki T, Yasuda K. Clinical evaluation of the treatment of osteoarthritis knees using a newly designed wedged insole. Clin Orthop 1987;221:181–87.

42. Maillefert JF, Hudry C, Baron G, et al. Laterally elevated wedged insoles in the treatment of medial knee osteoarthritis: A prospective randomized controlled study. Osteoarthritis Cartilage 2001;9:738–45.

43. Pham T, Maillefert JF, Hudry C, et al. Laterally elevated wedged insoles in the treatment of medial knee osteoarthritis: A two-year prospective randomized controlled study. Osteoarthritis Cartilage 2004;12:46–55.

44. Pollo FE, Otis JC, Backus SI, et al. Reduction of medial compartment loads with valgus bracing of the osteoarthritic knee. Am J Sports Meid 2002;30:414–21.

45. Hinman RS, Crossley KM, McConnell J, Bennell KL. Efficacy of knee tape in the management of osteoarthritis of the knee: Blinded randomised controlled trial. BMJ 2003;327:35.

46. Amor B. Congestive outbreak of osteoarthritis: Chondrolysis and cartilage repair. Rev Prat 1993;43:601–03.

47. Brandt RA, Crowninshield RD. The effect of cane use on hip contact force. Clin Orthop 1980;147:181–84.

48. Lequesne MG, Dang N, Lane NE. Sport practice and osteoarthritis of the limbs. Osteoarthritis Cartilage 1997;5:75–6.

49. McCarty GM, McCarthy DJ. Effect of topical capsaicin in the therapy of painful osteoarthritis of the hands. J Rheumatol 1992;19:604–07.

50. Deal CL, Schnitzer TJ, Lipstein E, et al. Treatment of arthritis with topical capsaicin: A double-blind trial. Clin Ther 1991;13:383–95.

51. Grace D, Rogers J, Skeith K, Anderson K. Topical diclofenac versus placebo: A double blind, randomized clinical trial in patients with osteoarthritis of the knee. J Rheumatol 1999;26:2659–63.

52. Sandelin J, Harilainen A, Crone H, et al. Local NSAID gel (eltenac) in the treatment of osteoarthritis of the knee: A double blind study comparing eltenac with oral diclofenac and placebo gel. Scand J Rheumatol 1997;26:287–92.

53. Tugwell PS, Wells GA, Shainhouse JZ. Equivalence of a topical diclofenac solution (pennsaid) compared with oral diclofenac in symptomatic treatment of osteoarthritis of the knee: A randomized controlled trial. J Rheumatol 2004;31:2002–12.

54. Eccles M, Freemantle N, Mason J, for the North of England NSAIDs drug guideline development group. North of England evidence based guideline development project summary guideline for NSAIDs versus basic analgesic in treating the pain of degenerative arthritis. Br Med J 1998;317:526–30.

55. Zoppi M, Peretti G, Boccard E. Placebo-controlled study of the analgesic efficacy of an effervescent formulation of 500 mg acetaminophen in arthritis of the knee or the hip. Eur J Pain 1996;16:42–8.

56. Amadio P, Cummings DM. Evaluation of acetaminophen in the management of osteoarthritis of the knee. Curr Ther Res 1983;34:59–66.

57. Case JP, Baliunas AJ, Block JA. Lack of efficacy of acetaminophen in treating symptomatic knee osteoarthritis: A randomized, double-blind, placebo-controlled comparison trial with diclofenac sodium. Arch Int Med 2003;163:169–78.

58. Pincus T, Koch G, Lei H, et al. Patient preference for placebo, acetaminophen (paracetamol) or celecoxib efficacy studies (PACES): Two randomized, double-blind, placebo controlled, crossover clinical trials in patients with knee or hip osteoarthritis. Ann Rheum Dis 2004;63:931–39.

59. Miceli-Richard C, Le Bars M, Schmideley N, Dougados M. Paracetamol in osteoarthritis of the knee. Ann Rheum Dis 2004;63:923–30.

60. Garcia Rodriguez LA, Hernandez Diaz S. The relative risk of upper gastrointestinal complications among users of acetaminophen and non-steroidal anti-inflammatory drugs. Epidemiology 2001;12:570–76.

61. Warner TD, Guilliao F, Vojnovic I, et al. Non-steroid drug selectivities for cyclo-oxygenase 1 rather than cyclo-ocygenase 2 are associated with human gastrointestinal toxicity: A full in vitro analysis. Proc Natl Acad Sci USA 1999;96:7563–68.

62. Mullican WS, Lacy J. TRAMAP-ANAG-006 Study Group Tramadol/acetaminophen combination tablets and codeine/acetaminophen combination capsules for the management of chronic pain: A comparative trial. Clin Ther 2001;23:1429–45.

63. Silvenfield JC, Kamin M, WU SC, et al. Tramadol/acetaminophen combination tablets for the treatment of osteoarthritis flare pain: A multicenter, outpatient, randomized, double-blind placebo-controlled, parallel-group, add-on study. Clin Ther 2002;24:282–97.

64. Wolfe F, Zhao S, Lane N. Preference for non-steroidal anti-inflammatory drugs over acetaminophen by rheumatic disease patients. Arthritis Rheum 2000;43:378–85.

65. Pincus T, Swearingen C, Cummins P, Callahan LF. Preference for non-steroidal anti-inflammatory drugs versus acetaminophen

and concomitant use of both types of drugs in patients with osteoarthritis. J Rheumatol 2000;27:1020–27.

66. Geba GP, Weaver AL, Polis AB, et al. Efficacy of rofecoxib, celecoxib and acetaminophen in osteoarthritis of the knee: A randomized trial. JAMA 2002;287:64–71.

67. Ehrich EW, Schnitzer TJ, McIlwain H, et al., for the rofecoxib osteoarthritis pilot study group. Effect of specific Cox-2 inhibition in osteoarthritis of the knee: A 6-week double-blind, placebo controlled pilot study of rofecoxib. J Rheumatol 1999;26:2438–47.

68. Bensen WG, Fiechtner JJ, McMillen JI, et al. Treatment of osteoarthritis with celecoxib, a cyclooxygenase-2 inhibitor: A randomized controlled trial. Mayo Clin Proc 1999;74: 1095–105.

69. Pelletier JP, Martel-Pelletier J. Effects of nimesulide and naproxen on the degradation and metalloprotease synthesis of human osteoarthritic cartilage. Drugs 1993;46:34–9.

70. Pelletier JP, Mineau F, Fernades J, et al. Two NSAIDs, nimesulide and naproxen, can reduce the synthesis of urokinase and IL-6 while increasing PAI-1 in human OA synovial fibroblasts. Clin Exp Rheumatol 1997;15:393–98.

71. Huskisson EC, Berry H, Gihsen P, et al., on behalf of the LINK Study Group. Effects of anti-inflammatory drugs on the progression of osteoarthritis of the knee. J Rheumatol 1995;22:1941–46.

72. Rashad S, Revell P, Hemingway A, et al. Effect of non-steroidal anti-inflammatory drugs on the course of osteoarthritis. Lancet 1989;I:519–22.

73. Williams HJ, Ward JR, Egger MJ, et al. Comparison of naproxen and acetaminophen in a two-year study of treatment of osteoarthritis of the knee. Arthritis Rheum 1993;36:1196–1206.

74. Dieppe P, Cushnighan J, Jasani MK, et al. A two-year, placebo-controlled trial of non-steroidal anti-inflammatory therapy in osteoarthritis of the knee joint. Br J Rheumatol 1993;32:595–600.

75. Buckland-Wright JC, McFarlane DG, Lynch JA, et al. Quantitative microfocal radiography detects changes in osteoarthritis knee joint space width in patients in placebo controlled trial of NSAID therapy. J Rheumatol 1995;22:934–43.

76. Nguyen M, Dougados M, Berdah L, et al. Diacerein in the treatment of osteoarthritis of the hip. Arthritis Rheum 1994;37:529–36.

77. Maheu E, Mazieres B, Valat JP, et al. Symptomatic efficacy of avocado/soybean unsaponifiables in the treatment of osteoarthritis of the knee and hip: A prospective, randomized, double-blind, placebo-controlled, multicenter clinical trial with a six-month treatment period and a two-month follow-up demonstrating a persistent effect. Arthritis Rheum 1998;41:81–91.

78. Lequesne M, Berdah L, Gerentes I. Efficacy and tolerance of diacerein in the treatment of gonarthrosis and coxarthrosis. Rev Prat 1998;48:31–5.

79. Falgarone G, Dougados M. Diacerein as a disease-modulating agent in osteoarthritis. Curr Rheumatol Rep 2001;3:479–83.

80. Martel-Pelletier J, Mineau F, Jolicoeur FC, et al. In vitro effects of diacerein and rhein on interleukin 1 and tumor necrosis factor-alpha systems in human osteo-arthritic synovium and chondrocytes. J Rheumatol 1998;25:753–62.

81. Yaron M, Shieazi I, Yaron I. Anti-interleukin-1 effects of diacerein and rhein in human osteoarthritic synovial tissue and cartilage cultures. Osteoarthritis Cartilage 1999;7:272–80.

82. Moore AR, Greenslade KJ, Alam CA, Willoughby DA. Effects of diacerein on granuloma induced cartilage breakdown in the mouse. Osteoarthritis Cartilage 1998;6:19–23.

83. Smith GN Jr., Myers SL, Brandt KD, et al. Diacerein treatment reduces the severity of osteoarthritis in the canine cruciate-deficiency model of osteoarthritis. Arthritis Rheum 1999;42:545–54.

84. Mazieres B, Berdah L, Thiechart M, Viguier G. Diacetylrhein on a post-contusion model of experimental osteoarthritis in the rabbit. Rev Rhum Ed Fr 1993;60:77S–81S.

85. Boittin M, Redini F, Loyau G, Pujol JP. Effect of diacerein (ART 50) on the matrix synthesis and collagenase secretion by cultured joint chondrocytes in rabbits. Rev Rhum Ed Fr 1993;60:68S–76S.

86. Felisaz N, Boumediene K, Ghayor C, et al. Stimulating effect of diacerein on TGF-beta 1 and beta 2 expression in articular chondrocytes cultured with and without interleukin-1. Osteoarthritis Cartilage 1999;7:255–64.

87. Pelletier JP, Yaron M, Haraoui B, et al. Efficacy and safety of diacerein in osteoarthritis of the knee. Arthritis Rheum 2000;43:2339–48.

88. Dougados M, Nguyen M, Berdah L, et al., for the ECHODIAH investigators study group. Evaluation of the structure-modifying effects of diacerein in hip osteoarthritis: ECHODIAH, a 3-year placebo-controlled trial. Arthritis Rheum 2001;44: 2539–47.

89. Zerkak D, Dougados M. The use of glucosamine therapy in osteoarthritis. Curr Rheumatol Rep 2004;6:41–5.

90. McAlindon TE, Biggee BA. Nutritional factors and osteoarthritis: recent developments. Curr Opin Rheumatol 2005;17:647–52.

91. van der Kraan PM, de Vries BJ, Vitters EL, et al. Inhibition of glycosaminoglycan synthesis in anatomically intact rat patellar cartilage by paracetamol-induced serum sulfate depletion. Biochem Pharmacol 1988;37:3683–90.

92. van der Kraan PM, de Vries BJ, Vitters EL, van der Berg WB. High susceptibility of human articular cartilage glycosaminoglycan synthesis to changes in inorganic sulfate availability. J Orthop Res 1990;8:656–71.

93. Towheed TE, Anastassiades TP, Shea B, et al. Glucosamine therapy for treating osteoarthritis. Cochrane Database Syst Rev 2001;1:CD002946.

94. Houpt JB, McMillan R, Wein C, Paget-Dellio SD. Effect of glucosamine hydrochloride in the treatment of pain osteoarthritis of the knee. J Rheumatol 1999;26:2294–97.

95. McAlindon TE, LaValley MP, Gulin JP, Felson DT. Glucosamine and chondroitin for treatment of osteoarthritis: A systematic quality assessment and meta-analysis. JAMA 2000;283: 1469–75.

96. Chard JA, Tallon D, Dieppe PA. Epidemiology of research into intervention for the treatment of osteoarthritis of the knee joint. Ann Rheum Dis 2000;59:414–18.

97. Hughes R, Catt A. A randomized, double-blind, placebo-controlled trial of glucosamine sulfate as an analgesic in osteoarthritis of the knee. Rheumatology 2002;241:279–84.

98. Reginster JY, Deroisy R, Rovati LC, et al. Long-term effects of glucosamine sulfate on osteoarthritis progression: A randomized, placebo-controlled clinical trial. Lancet 2000;357:251–56.

99. Pavelka K, Gatterova J, Olejarova M, et al. Glucosamine sulfate use and delay of progression of knee osteoarthritis: A 3-year, randomized, placebo-controlled, double-blind study. Arch Intern Med 2002;162:2113–23.

100. Clegg DO, Reda DJ, Harris CL, Klein MA for the GAIT Investigators. The efficacy of glucosamine and chondroitin sulfate in patients with painful knee osteoarthritis (OA): The Glucosamine/chondroitin Arthritis Intervention Trial (GAIT). Arthritis Rheum 2005;52:S256 (abstr. 622).

101. Michel BA, Stucki G, Frey D, et al. Chondroitins 4 and 6 sulfate in osteoarthritis of the knee: A randomized, controlled trial. Arthritis Rheum 2005;52:779–86.

102. Lequesne M, Maheu E, Cadet C, et al. Structural effect of avocado/soybean unsaponifiables on joint space loss in osteoarthritis of the hip. Arthritis Rheum 2002;47:508.

103. Rejholec V. Long-term studies on anti-osteoarthritic drugs: An assessment. Semin Arthritis Rheum 1987;17(1):35–53.

104. Pavelka K Jr., Sedlackova M, Gatterova J, et al. Glycosaminoglycan polysulfuric acid (GAGPS) in osteoarthritis of the knee. Osteoarthritis Cartilage 1995;3:15–23.

105. Moskowitz RW, Reese JH, Young RG, et al. The effects of Rumalon, a glycosaminoglycan peptide complex, in a partial meniscectomy model of osteoarthritis in rabbits. J Rheumatol 1991;18:205–09.

106. Pavelka K, Gatterova J, Gollerova V, et al. A 5-year randomized controlled, double-blind study of glycosaminoglycan polysulphuric acid complex (Rumalon) as a structure modifying therapy in osteoarthritis of the hip and knee. Osteoarthritis Cartilage 2000;8:335–42.

107. Gosh P, Edelman J, March L, et al. Pentosan polysulfate, a rational therapy for the treatment of osteoarthritis: Results of a double blind placebo controlled clinical trial. Ann Rheum Dis 2005;64(III):487 (abstr. SAT0246).

108. Meyer JM, Dansereau SM, Farmer RW, et al. Bisphosphonates structurally similar to Risedronate (actonel) slow disease progression in the guinea pig model of primary osteoarthritis. Arthritis Rheum 2001;44:S307(abstr.1527).

109. Meyer J, Farmer R, Prenger MC. Risedronate but not alendronate slow disease progression model of primary osteoarthritis. J Bone Miner Res 2001;S305 (abstr. SA47).

110. Spector TD, Conaghan PG, Buckland-Wright JC, et al. Effect of risedronate on joint structure and symptoms of of knee osteoarthritis: results of the BRISK randomized, controlled trial [ISRCTN01928173]. Arthritis Res Ther 2005;7:R625–33.

111. Yu LP, Smith GN, Hasty KA, Brandt KD. Doxycycline inhibits type XI collagenolytic activity of extracts from human osteoarthritic cartilage and gelatinase. J Rheumatol 1991;18:1450–52.

112. Amin AR, Attur MG, Thakker GD, et al. A novel mechanism of action of tetracyclines: Effects on nitric oxide synthases. Proc Natl Acad Sci USA 1996;93:14014–19.

113. Lotz M. The role of nitric oxide in articular cartilage damage. Rheum Dis Clin North Am 1999;25:269–82.

114. Yu LP Jr., Smith GN Jr., Brandt KD, et al. Reduction of the severity of canine osteoarthritis by prophylactic treatment with oral doxycycline. Arthritis Rheum 19992;35:1150–59.

115. Greenwald RA. Treatment of destructive arthritis disorders with MMP inhibitors. Ann NY Acad Sci 1994;731:181–98.

116. Brandt KD, Mazzuca SA, Katz BP, et al. Effects of doxycycline on progression of osteoarthritis: Results of a randomized, placebo-controlled, double-blind trial. Arthritis Rheum 2005;52:2015–25.

117. Caron JP, Fernandes JC, Martel-Pelletier J, et al. Chondroprotective effects of intra-articular injections of interleukin-1 receptor antagonist in experimental osteoarthritis: Suppression of collagenase-1 expression. Arthritis Rheum 1996;39:1535–44.

118. Hernandes J, Tardif G, Martel-Pelletier J, et al. In vivo transfer of interleukin-1 receptor antagonist gene in osteoarthritic rabbit knee joints: Prevention of osteoarthritis progression. Am J Pathol 1999;154:1159–69.

119. Doherty PJ, Zhang H, Tremblay L, et al. Resurfacing of articular cartilage explants with genetically-modified human chondrocytes in vitro. Osteoarthritis Cartilage 1998;6:153–59.

120. Hochberg MC, Perlmutter DL, Hudson JI, Altman RD. Preferences in the management of osteoarthritis of the hip and knee: Results of a survey of community based rheumatologists in the United States. Arthritis Care Res 1996;9:170–76.

121. Wright V, Chandler GN, Morison RA, Harfall SJ. Intra-articular therapy in osteoarthritis: Comparison of hydrocortisone acetate and hydrocortisone tertiary butylacetate. Ann Rheum Dis 1960;19:257–61.

122. Friedman DM, Moore ME. The efficacy of intra-articular steroids in osteoarthritis: A double blind study. J Rheumatol 1980;7:850–56.

123. Valtonen E. Clinical comparison of triamcinolone hexacetonide and bethamethasone in the treatment of osteoarthritis of the knee joint. Scand J Rheumatol 1981;41:1–7.

124. Ravaud P, Moulinier L, Giraudeau B, et al. Effects of joint lavage and steroid injection in patients with osteoarthritis of the knee: Results of a multicenter, randomized, controlled trial. Arthritis Rheum 1999;42:475–82.

125. Raynauld JP, Buckland-Wright C, Ward R, et al. Safety and efficacy of long-term intra-articular steroid injections in osteoarthritis of the knee: A randomized, double-blind, placebo-controlled trial. Arthritis Rheum 2003;48:370–77.

126. Gossec L, Dougados M. Intra-articular treatments in osteoarthritis: From the symptomatic to the structure modifying. Ann Rheum Dis 2004;63:478–82.

127. Kirwan JR, Jankin E. Intra-articular therapy in osteoarthritis. Baillieres Clin Rheumatol 1997;11:769–94.

128. Gaffney K, Ledingham J, Perry JD. Intra-articular triamcinolone hexacetonide in knee osteoarthritis: Factors influencing the clinical response. Ann Rheum Dis 1995;54:379–81.

129. Jones A, Doherty M. Intra-articular corticosteroids are effective in osteoarthritis but there are no clinical predictors of response. Ann Rheum Dis 1996;55:829–32.

130. Plant MJ, Borg AA, Dziedzik K, et al. Radiographic patterns and response to corticosteroid hip injection. Ann Rheum Dis 1997;56:476–80.

131. Maheu E, Ayral X, Dougados M. A hyaluronan preparation (500-730 kDa) in the treatment of osteoarthritis: A review of clinical trials with Hyalgan. Int J Clin Pract 2002;56:804–13.

132. Xayral X. Injections in the treatment of osteoarthritis. Best Pract Res Clin Rheumatol 2001;15:609–26.

133. Lussier A, Cividino AA, McFarlane CA, et al. Viscosupplementation with hylan for the treatment of osteoarthritis: Findings from clinical practice in Canada. J Rheumatol 1996;23:1579–85.

134. Brandt KD, Smith GN, Simon LS. Intra-articular injection of hyaluronan on treatment for knee osteoarthritis: What is the evidence? Arthritis Rheum 2000;43:1192–1203.

135. Listrat V, Ayral X, Paternello F, et al. Arthroscopic evaluation of potential structure modifying activity of hyaluronan: Hyalgan in osteoarthritis of the knee. Osteoarthritis Cartilage 1997;5:153–60.

136. Jubb RW, Piva S, Beinat L, et al. A one-year, randomized, placebo (saline) controlled clinical trial of 500-730 kDa sodium hyaluronate (Hyalgan) on the radiological change in osteoarthritis of the knee. Int J Clin Pract 2003;57:467–74.

137. Hilliquin P, Le Devic P, Menkes CJ. Comparaison de l'efficacitédes synoviorthèses et du lavage articulaire dans la gonarthrose avec épanchement. Rev Rhum Ed Fr 1996;63:99–108.

138. Blyth T, Stirling A, Coote J, et al. Injection of the rheumatoid knee: does intra-articular methotrexate or rifampicin add to the benefits of triamcinolone hexacetonide? Br J Rheumatol 1998;37:770–72.

139. Chevalier X, Giraudeau B, Conrozier T, et al. Safety study of intra-articular injection of interleukin 1 receptor antagonist in patients with painful knee osteoarthritis: A multicenter study. J Rheumatol 2005;32:1317–23.

140. Chevalier X, Goupille P, Beaulieu AD, et al. MRI evaluation placebo controlled, multicenter trial of a single-intra-articular injection of Anakinra (Kineret) in patients with osteoarthritis of the knee. Arthritis Rheum 2005;52(9):S507 (abstr.1339).

141. Chang RW, Falconer J, Stulberg SD, et al. A randomized controlled trial of arthroscopic surgery versus closed-needle joint lavage of patients with osteoarthritis of the knee. Arthritis Rheum 1993;36:289–96.

142. Ike RW, Arnold WJ, Rotschild EW, Shaw HL. Tidal irrigation versus conservative medical management in patients with osteoarthritis of the knee: A prospective randomized study. Tidal Irrigation Cooperating Group. J Rheumatol 1992;19:772–79.

143. Kalunian KC, Moreland LW, Klashman DJ, et al. Visually-guided irrigation in patients with early knee osteoarthritis: A multicenter randomized, controlled trial. Osteoarthritis Cartilage 2000;8:412–18.

144. Bradley JD, Heilman DK, Katz BP, et al. Total irrigation as treatment for knee osteoarthritis: A sham-controlled, randomized, double-blinded evaluation. Arthritis Rheum 2002;46:100–08.

145. Amendola A, Panarella L. High tibial osteotomy for the treatment of unicompartmental arthritis of the knee. Orthop Clin North Am 2005;36:497–504.

146. Wright JM, Crockett HC, Slawski DP, et al. High tibial osteotomy. J Am Acad Orthop Surg 2005;13:279–89.

147. Ito H, Matsuno T, Minami A. Chiari pelvic osteotomy for advanced osteoarthritis in patients with hip dysplasia. J Bone Surg Am 2005;87(2):213–25.

148. Hawker GA, Wright JG, Badley EM, Coyte PC. Perceptions of, and willingness to consider, total joint arthroplasty in a population-based cohort of individuals with disabling hip and knee arthritis. Arthritis Rheum 2004;15:635–41.

# 15 Nutritional and Nutritional Supplement Interventions for Osteoarthritis

Timothy E. McAlindon and Grace H. Lo

## INTRODUCTION

The relationship between diet and arthritis is of great public interest. Patients frequently ask their physicians questions about the influence of nutritional supplements on osteoarthritis (OA). Speculative lay publications on this subject abound, and health food stores offer a plethora of nutritional supplements represented as therapies for arthritis.[1] The over-the-counter consumption of such nutritional remedies is substantial, with glucosamine and chondroitin together ranking third among all top-selling nutritional products in the United States—with annual sales amounting to $369 million.[2] Surveys suggest that 5 to 8% of adults in the United States have used at least one of these products at some time.[3]

There are numerous mechanisms by which micronutrients might influence OA processes. However, unlike the situation in another widespread age-related skeletal disorder (osteoporosis)—for which numerous studies have demonstrated associations with dietary factors—it is surprising to find that there has been relatively little focus in traditional scientific studies on the relationship between OA and nutritional factors (other than obesity).

## WEIGHT LOSS

Epidemiologic studies have shown that overweight people are at considerably increased risk for the development of OA in their knees, and may be more susceptible to OA in both hip and hand joints.[4] Because overweight individuals do not necessarily have increased load across their hand joints, investigators have wondered whether systemic factors (such as dietary factors or other metabolic consequences of obesity) may mediate some of this association. Indeed, early laboratory studies using strains of mice and rats suggested that there is an interaction among body weight, genetic factors, and diet—although attempts to demonstrate a direct effect of dietary fat intake have proven inconclusive.[5,6]

The fact that adipocytes share a common stem cell precursor with connective tissue cells such as osteoblasts and chondrocytes has prompted investigation into the possibility that the metabolic milieu might influence their phenotypic differentiation.[7] In fact, fat and fatty acids have been associated with osteoarthritic changes in joints and can influence prostaglandin and collagen synthesis in vitro.[7,8] Preliminary evidence also suggests that leptin, an adipose-tissue-derived hormone, may have anabolic effects in osteoarthritic cartilage.[9]

Based on these observations, weight loss is considered a priority in the management of overweight individuals with OA. However, there have been relatively few rigorous studies testing weight loss as a therapeutic intervention to reduce symptoms, prevent disability, or delay disease progression. The recent Arthritis, Diet, and Activity Promotion Trial (ADAPT) is thus significant in examining whether long-term exercise and dietary weight loss are effective interventions for functional impairment, pain, and mobility in older overweight individuals with knee OA.[10] The results suggest that diet-induced weight loss alone is effective but that the combination of the two is additive and more effective than either alone. Exercise alone was not more effective than the placebo arm. Only the combination treatment consistently showed a significant effect by all outcome measures in the treatment of knee OA in this trial.

In this study, investigators recruited 316 adults with knee OA and a body mass index (BMI) of at least 28 kg/m,[2] and randomized them to one of four interventions: healthy lifestyle (i.e., participants met monthly for 1 hour for 3 months to listen to a lecturer or to watch a videotape on topics concerning OA, obesity, and exercise), diet only, exercise only, and diet plus exercise. The primary outcome was the Western Ontario and McMaster Universities Osteoarthritis Index (WOMAC) physical function score at 18 months of follow-up.

Secondary outcomes included weight loss, 6-minute walk distance, stair-climb time, and WOMAC pain and stiffness scores. Eighty percent of the participants completed the 18-month study. Adherence ranged from 60 (exercise only) to 73% (healthy lifestyle). The main finding of the trial was that the diet intervention led to significant benefits at 18 months of follow-up, with the effect being larger with the addition of exercise (see Table 15.1). (A decrease in WOMAC physical function is consistent with improved function.)

The reduction in WOMAC physical function at 18 months' follow-up in the combination group and the diet-only group were both significantly different (p < 0.05) compared with healthy lifestyle. The diet and exercise group lost more weight than the diet-only group (5.7 versus 4.9% of their body weight), whereas the exercise-only group lost 3.7% and the healthy lifestyle group lost 1.2%—suggesting that the improvement in symptoms is likely related to the amount of weight that is lost, irrespective of the means by which this is achieved.

A more recent study by Christensen et al.[11] contrasts with the ADAPT trial both in design and conclusions. On the basis that weight loss might relieve knee OA symptoms both through biomechanical effects and influences on body fat,[12] they set out to test the effectiveness of a rapid diet-induced weight loss intervention on overweight individuals with knee OA.

They enrolled 96 people (mostly women) with knee OA into a comparison of a low-energy diet (LED) intervention (i.e., participants were only allowed a dietary intake of 3.4 MJ/day; approximately 800 kcal/day) with a control or "hypoenergetic" diet (i.e., 5 MJ/day; approximately 1,200 kcal/day). The LED diet consisted of a nutrition powder taken as six daily meals that met the recommendations for a daily intake of high-quality protein such that 37% of the energy provided from the powder was from soy protein.

The hypoenergetic diet consisted of a traditional low-calorie high-protein diet taken in the form of ordinary foods individually chosen by participants based on recommendations from a 2-hour nutritional advice session. The LED group also had weekly dietary sessions, whereas the control group was given a booklet describing weight loss practices. The primary outcome was self-reported pain and physical function limitation measured by the WOMAC index at 8 weeks of follow-up. They also examined changes in body weight and body composition as independent predictors of changes in knee OA symptoms.

In total, there were 80 participants enrolled in this trial with only nine dropouts, mainly due to noncompliance. The dropouts appeared to be nondifferential, and thus the investigators performed an analysis based on completers. The LED group lost considerably more weight than the controls (11.1 versus 4.3%), with a mean difference of 6.8% (95%; CI 5.5 to 8.1%). The LED group also loss 2.2% more body fat (95%; CI 1.5 to 3.0%).

A substantially greater fall in WOMAC scores was observed in the LED group. The mean between-group difference for the total WOMAC index was 219.3 mm (p = 0.005). Oddly, this was not reflected in the Lequesne index assessment, which detected no between-group difference. In subsidiary analyses, they estimated that the "number needed to treat" to obtain an improvement in WOMAC score of 50% or greater in at least one patient was 3.4. They also found that the changes in WOMAC score were best predicted by reduction of body fat, with a 9.4% improvement in WOMAC score for each percent of body fat reduced (p = 0.0005).

These results suggest that rapid and substantial weight loss may by itself translate into reduced pain and improved function in overweight patients with knee OA. However, some caution needs to be exerted in interpreting these results. The long-term effectiveness of this short-term intervention is uncertain. Their participants were very heavy mean BMI 36 kg/(m²), and the results may not be generalizable to a less overweight population. Although the authors assert that the groups were balanced at the end of the study, it is unclear whether censoring the participants who discontinued the intervention preserved the equal distribution of participants afforded by randomization.

The higher WOMAC scores at baseline in the LED group compared to the hypoenergetic group provides evidence that the groups were not balanced at baseline. This difference makes it difficult to attribute the differences seen in the two arms at follow-up to the effect of either intervention. The greater effect of LED as measured by a greater change in WOMAC may have resulted from a stronger tendency for regression to the mean in the LED group. Support for this assertion is that both groups had comparable mean Lequesne indices at baseline, a measure that was not different in the two groups at 8 weeks of follow-up.

| TABLE 15.1 WOMAC PHYSICAL FUNCTION | | |
|---|---|---|
| | Mean Change at 18 Months | 95% CI |
| Healthy lifestyle | −3.40 | −0.48 to −6.32 |
| Exercise only | −3.07 | −1.91 to −6.13 |
| Diet only | −4.23 | −1.27 to −7.19 |
| Diet and exercise | −5.73 | −2.63 to −8.83 |

Another issue regarding this study is that the LED group preferentially received more attention with weekly sessions for 8 weeks, with a dietician likely encouraging a high degree of compliance—whereas the hypoenergetic group only met with the dietician for once at the beginning of the study. This is a difference that was not controlled for in their analyses. Finally, the study was also essentially unblinded—which may also have led to between-group biases.

Nevertheless, these data are of considerable interest and underscore a need for further research into potential benefits from more extreme weight reduction interventions. Preliminary results from a study of musculoskeletal complaints among morbidly obese patients undertaking gastric bypass surgery showed a 52% reduction in the number of symptomatic sites, and an approximately 50% reduction in WOMAC score 6 to 12 months following the procedure.[13] Full details of this study will likely provide additional insight regarding this issue.

## ANTIOXIDANTS

Reactive oxygen species are chemicals with unpaired electrons. These are formed continuously in tissues via endogenous and some exogenous mechanisms.[14] It has been estimated that 1 to 2% of electrons leak from the mitochondrial respiratory chain, forming superoxide anions ($O_2[\bullet-]$).[15] Other endogenous sources include release by phagocytes during the oxidative burst (generated by mixed-function oxidase enzymes) and in hypoxia-reperfusion events.[16] Reactive oxygen species are capable of causing damage to many macromolecules (including cell membranes, lipoproteins, proteins, and DNA[17]) and are implicated in the development of many common human diseases associated with aging,[14,18-20] including OA.[21]

Laboratory studies have shown that chondrocytes are potent sources of reactive oxygen species and that oxidative damage to cartilage is physiologically important.[22-25] Superoxide anions can damage collagen structure, depolymerize synovial fluid hyaluronate, and damage mitochondria.[21,22,24,26,27] Mitochondrial damage probably also contributes to the age-related loss of chondrocyte function.[21] Evidence of oxidative damage due to overproduction of nitric oxide and other reactive oxygen species has been demonstrated in aging and osteoarthritic cartilage[28] and has been correlated with the extent of cartilage damage.[29] Patients with chondral or meniscal lesions also have increased levels of reactive oxygen species in their synovial fluid.[30]

In fact, the human body has extensive and multilayered antioxidant defense systems.[14] Intracellular defense is provided primarily by antioxidant enzymes, including superoxide dismutase, catalase, and peroxidases.

In joints, hyaluronic acid may also have an antioxidant function.[31] In addition, a number of small molecule antioxidants may have an important role in the extracellular space (where antioxidant enzymes are sparse).[32]

These include vitamins A, C, and E. The concentrations of these antioxidants in the blood are primarily determined by dietary intake. Micronutrient antioxidants might provide further defense against tissue injury when intracellular enzymes are overwhelmed. Therefore, it would be reasonable to anticipate that high dietary intake of these micronutrients may protect against age-related disorders. Because higher intake of dietary antioxidants appears beneficial with respect to outcomes such as cataract extraction and coronary artery disease,[18-20,33] it is plausible that they may confer similar benefits for OA.

### Vitamin C

Vitamin C (ascorbic acid, ascorbate) is a water-soluble vitamin found naturally in many foods—such as citrus fruits, strawberries, brussels sprouts, broccoli, cabbage, peppers, potatoes, and parsley (Fig. 15.1). In addition to being an antioxidant, vitamin C plays several functions in the biosynthesis of cartilage molecules. First, through the vitamin-C-dependent enzyme lysyl hydroxylase vitamin C is required for the post-translational hydroxylation of specific prolyl and lysyl residues in procollagen, a modification essential for stabilization of the mature collagen fibril.[18-20,33-35] Vitamin C also appears to stimulate collagen biosynthesis by pathways independent of hydroxylation, perhaps through lipid peroxidation.[36] In addition, by acting as a carrier of sulfate groups vitamin C participates in glycosaminoglycan synthesis.[37] Thus, relative deficiency of vitamin C may impair not only the production of cartilage but its biomechanical quality.

Recent work on the impact of oxidative stress on cartilage has added insight into the biologic mechanisms of OA progression. Yudoh et al. studied this from the viewpoint of genomic instability and replicative senescence in human chondrocytes.[29] They isolated chondrocytes from articular cartilage from patients with knee OA, looking to measure oxidative damage histologically by immunohistochemistry for

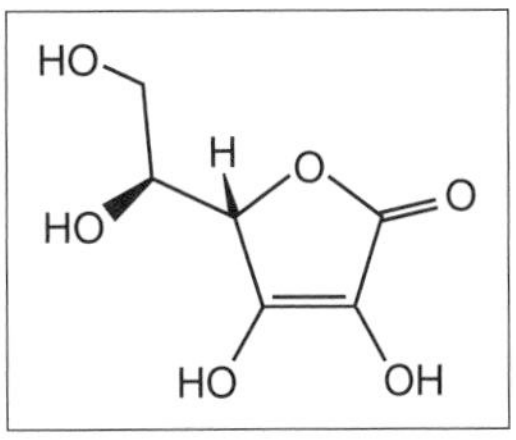

Fig. 15.1 Chemical structure of vitamin C.

nitrotyrosine (a marker of oxidative damage). They then assessed cellular replicative potential, telomere instability, and glycosaminoglycan production both under conditions of oxidative stress and in the presence of an antioxidant (ascorbic acid). Similarly, in the tissue cultures of the articular cartilage explants they measured the presence of oxidative damage, chondrocyte telomere length, and loss of glycosaminoglycans in the presence or absence of reactive oxygen species or in the presence or absence of ascorbic acid.

They found lower antioxidative capacity and stronger staining of nitrotyrosine in osteoarthritic regions compared with normal regions within the same cartilage explants. Oxidative damage correlated with the severity of histologic damage. During continuous culture of the chondrocytes, the telomere length, replicative capacity, and glycosaminoglycan production were all decreased in the presence of oxidative stress.

In contrast, treatment of cultured chondrocytes with ascorbic acid resulted in greater telomere length and replicative life span of the cells. Similarly, in the tissue cultures of the cartilage explants chondrocyte telomere length and glycosaminoglycan production in the cartilage tissue subjected to oxidative stress were lower than in the control groups—whereas those treated with ascorbic acid exhibited a tendency to maintain the chondrocyte telomere length and glycosaminoglycan production. These results suggest that oxidative stress induces chondrocyte telomere instability and catabolic changes in cartilage matrix structure and composition. This process may contribute to the development and/or progression of OA.

Further animal in vitro and in vivo studies support this hypothesis. In guinea pigs deprived of vitamin C, Peterkovsky et al. observed decreased synthesis of cartilage collagen and proteoglycan molecules. Furthermore, addition of ascorbate to tissue cultures of adult bovine chondrocytes resulted in decreased levels of degradative enzymes and increased synthesis of type II collagen and proteoglycans.[37,38] Schwartz et al. and Meacock et al. found that vitamin C supplementation in a guinea pig model of surgically induced OA reduced the extent of joint damage on a macroscopic level.[39,40]

Epidemiologic data from the Framingham OA cohort also suggests that higher intake of vitamin C may reduce progression of OA.[41] In that study, participants had knee X-rays taken at a baseline and at follow-up approximately 8 years later. Knee OA was classified using the Kellgren–Lawrence grading system.[42] Nutrient intake, including supplement use, was calculated from dietary habits reported at the midpoint of the study using a food frequency questionnaire. In the analyses, micronutrient intakes were ranked into sex-specific tertiles and tested to see if higher intakes of vitamin C, vitamin E, and beta-carotene (compared with a panel of non-antioxidant "control" micronutrients) were associated with reduced incidence and reduced progression of knee OA.

All analyses presented (unless otherwise stated) were adjusted for age, sex, BMI, physical activity, and total energy intake. Six-hundred forty participants (mean age 70.3 years) had complete assessments. There were no significant associations with vitamin C and *incident* radiographic knee OA (e.g., adjusted OR for highest versus lowest tertile of vitamin C intake = 1.1, 95% CI 0.6 to 2.2). However, with respect to *progression* of radiographic knee OA there was a threefold reduction in risk for those in the middle and highest tertiles compared to those in the lowest tertile of vitamin C intake (adjusted OR 0.3, 95% CI 0.1 to 0.6).

Those in the highest tertile for vitamin C intake also had reduced risk of developing knee pain (OR 0.3, 95% CI 0.1 to 0.9). Reduction in risk of *progression* was also seen for beta-carotene (vitamin A) (OR 0.4, 95% CI 0.2 to 0.9) and vitamin E (OR 0.7, 95% CI 0.3 to 1.6), but these findings were less compelling in that the beta-carotene association diminished substantially after adjustment for vitamin C and the vitamin E effect was seen only in men (OR 0.07, 95% CI 0.01 to 0.6).

Vitamin C is a water-soluble compound with a broad spectrum of antioxidant activity due to its ability to react with numerous aqueous free radicals and reactive oxygen species.[14] The extracellular nature of reactive oxygen-species-mediated damage in joints and the aqueous intra-articular environment may favor a role for a water-soluble agent such as vitamin C, rather than fat-soluble molecules such as beta-carotene or vitamin E. In addition, it has been suggested that vitamin C may regenerate vitamin E at the water/lipid interface by reducing alpha-tocopherol radical back to alpha-tocopherol. Whether this occurs in vivo, however, is controversial. An alternative explanation is that the protective effects of vitamin C relate to its biochemical participation in the biosynthesis of cartilage collagen fibrils and proteoglycan molecules, rather than its antioxidant properties. No significant associations were observed for any of the micronutrients among purported non-antioxidants.

Other than potentially being a structure modifier in OA, there is suggestion that vitamin C may be effective in the treatment of OA symptoms. Recently, Baker et al. investigated the relationship of vitamin C intake (evaluated using a food frequency questionnaire) and knee pain over a 30-month period among 324 (mostly men) participants in the Boston Osteoarthritis of the Knee study—a natural history study of knee OA.[43] Pain score was computed as an average of WOMAC pain scores reported at all visits, and vitamin C status was based on the average vitamin C level from all visits in this cross-sectional analysis. They found that individuals with the lowest tertile of vitamin C intake had more knee pain after adjusting for age, BMI, and energy intake compared to those in the middle and highest tertiles of vitamin C intake—with the relation being stronger in men than in women.

There are numerous reasons to expect that vitamin C might have beneficial effects in OA, and therefore the results of a recent study of the effects of ascorbic acid supplementation on the expression of spontaneous OA in the Hartley guinea pig are surprising.[44] This rigorous investigation tested the effects of three doses of ascorbic acid on the in vivo development of histologic knee OA. The low dose represented the minimum amount needed to prevent scurvy. The medium dose was the amount present in standard laboratory guinea pig chow and resulted in plasma levels comparable with those achieved in a person consuming five fruits and vegetables daily. The high dose was the amount shown in a previous study of the guinea pig to slow the progression of surgically induced OA.[40]

They found a positive association between ascorbic acid supplementation and the severity of spontaneous OA, with a higher dose of vitamin C being associated with greater severity of arthritis. In fact, there was a dose-dependent increase in all elements of the knee joint histologic scores across the three arms of the study. Furthermore, there was a significant correlation of histologic severity score with plasma ascorbate concentration ($r = 0.38$, $p = 0.01$). Of interest, there was evidence of active TGF-$\beta$ in the guinea pigs in this study, predominantly expressed in marginal osteophytes (whereas little was seen in the extracellular matrix of the articular cartilage, remote from osteophytes).[44] TGF-$\beta$ has been implicated in the pathophysiology of OA,[45-47] and ascorbate may function on an activator of this cytokine.[48] The presence of TGF-$\beta$ in osteophytes supports a role of this cytokine in vitamin C's effects on histologic severity.

Although these findings are thought-provoking, it remains uncertain to what extent they can be generalized to the human situation. It is also possible that the model of spontaneous OA used in this study may not reflect the same pathology as OA in humans. Further, it is problematic to assume that the concentrations of vitamin C considered pathologic in guinea pigs are also pathologic in humans. Nonetheless, these findings are paradoxical to the apparently beneficial effect of dietary vitamin C found in the Framingham cohort study[41] and in the Boston Osteoarthritis of the Knee study.[43] Thus, the situation predicates a need for further studies of vitamin C in humans.

One multicenter randomized double-blind placebo-controlled case-crossover study of 133 patients with radiographically verified hip and/or knee OA has been reported that evaluated the effectiveness of 1 gm of oral calcium ascorbate.[49] Each participant received vitamin C for 14 days and placebo for 14 days, separated by a 7-day wash-out period. The participants were randomized to the sequence of administration of vitamin C and placebo (e.g., placebo and vitamin C versus vitamin C and placebo). The primary outcome was pain on visual analogue scale (VAS) in a preselected joint. Using intent-to-treat statistical methods, treatment with vitamin C resulted in a greater improvement in pain compared with placebo—with a mean difference of 4.6 mm ($p = 0.0078$).

These results are exciting and support the possibility that vitamin C is effective in improving symptoms related to knee and/or hip OA. That being said, there are several limitations to this study. First, the dosage of vitamin C used in this trial was more than 10 times that of the recommended dietary allowance. Although it has been reported that oral doses up to 3 gm daily are unlikely to cause adverse reactions, longer-term studies are needed to comprehensively quantitate adverse effects related to this treatment. In addition, this trial was relatively small and included participants with knee and/or hip OA (likely a heterogeneous population).

Finally, it is unclear whether a mean difference of 4.6 mm on VAS is a meaningful difference, although vitamin C's duration of action is unclear and treatments with a prolonged duration of action apparently will have diluted effects in studies with a case-crossover design—biasing the results toward the null. Thus, the presence of even a small effect of vitamin C may still be very meaningful. A larger randomized clinical trial in humans is needed to fully evaluate the potential role of vitamin C in the treatment of both symptoms and structural progression in OA.

## Vitamin E

Vitamin E is a collection of eight fat-soluble compounds, tocopherols (derivatives of tocol), and tocotrienols. Some sources of vitamin E include vegetable and nut oils, nuts, safflower, sunflower seeds, and whole grains. The most common and biologically active form is alpha-tocopherol (5,7,8 trimethyltocol) (Fig. 15.2).

In addition to being an antioxidant, vitamin E has diverse influences on the metabolism of arachidonic acid—a pro-inflammatory fatty acid found in all cell membranes. Vitamin E blocks formation of arachidonic acid from phospholipids and inhibits lipoxygenase activity, without having much effect on cyclo-oxygenase.[50] It is therefore possible that vitamin E reduces the modest synovial inflammation that may accompany OA.

**Fig. 15.2** Chemical structure of alpha-tocopherol.

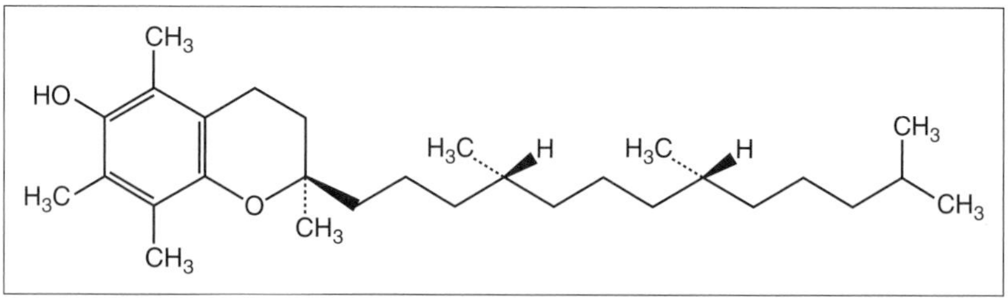

Benefit from vitamin E therapy has been suggested by several small human studies of OA,[51-54] of which the most rigorous was a company-sponsored 6-week double-blind placebo-controlled trial of 400 mg alpha-tocopherol (vitamin E) in 56 OA patients in Germany.[55] Vitamin-E-treated patients experienced greater improvement in every efficacy measure, including pain at rest (69% better in vitamin E versus 34% better in placebo, $p < 0.05$), pain on movement (62% better on vitamin E versus 27% on placebo, $p < 0.01$), and use of analgesics (52% less on vitamin E and 24% less on placebo, $p < 0.01$). The rapid response in symptoms observed in this study suggests that vitamin E does not exert a structural effect in this disorder. Instead, perhaps the beneficial effect results from some metabolic action such as inhibition of arachidonic acid metabolism.

In vitro and in vivo studies suggest that vitamin E may enhance chondrocyte growth via protection against reactive oxygen species and ultimately modulate the development of OA.[25,56] Further, in the study by McAlindon et al. in the Framingham OA cohort there was suggestion that men with higher vitamin E levels were less likely to have knee OA progression compared with those with lower levels.[41]

Although there was rationale to expect a chondroprotective effect of vitamin E, results from a 2-year double-blind placebo-controlled trial among 136 patients with knee OA do not support this role of vitamin E. Wluka et al. tested whether vitamin E (500 IU) affects cartilage volume loss in patients with knee OA.[57] The primary outcome was change in tibial cartilage volume from baseline to 2 years of follow-up measured by magnetic resonance imaging (MRI). Secondary outcomes included pain, stiffness, function, and total WOMAC scores—as well as the SF-36. One hundred seventeen subjects completed the study for a loss to follow-up rate of 14%.

Loss of medial and lateral tibial cartilage was similar in subjects treated with vitamin E and placebo (e.g., mean loss in the medial compartment 157 versus 187 $\mu m^3$, $p = 0.5$). The investigators also report that there were no significant differences between the vitamin-E- and placebo-treated groups in improvement of symptoms from baseline. There even appeared to be a slightly greater improvement in the placebo arm compared to the treatment arm, although the difference was not statistically significant. They concluded that vitamin E does not appear to benefit cartilage volume loss in people with OA.

Although the investigators of this study made efforts to evaluate this treatment in a rigorous randomized controlled study, there are limitations that should be considered in the interpretation of these results. First, although this study was a trial of 136 participants it was powered to detect a 50% reduction in the rate of cartilage loss in the treatment arm. This effect size was likely an overestimation of any effect that could have been expected from vitamin E over a 2-year follow-up period. Second, the structural outcome measure evaluated in this study was cartilage volume assessed on MRI. This is problematic because it has been shown that cartilage volume uncorrected for surface area lacks construct validity.[58]

Further, cartilage volume has not been tested for sensitivity to change as it is unclear whether a real change in cartilage volume within a given individual can be distinguished from measurement error. Cartilage volume needs to be comprehensively validated and evaluated for reliability before it replaces joint space narrowing on plain radiograph as the structural outcome measure recommended in OA clinical trials.[59] In this study, cartilage volume was the only structural outcome measured.

Although symptomatic treatment was not the primary outcome in this study, it was measured in this study. As this study is larger than the other previously mentioned smaller studies, it is more likely to reflect the true effect of vitamin E in the treatment of symptoms. The lack of effect observed in this study suggests the presence of publication bias in the publication of studies evaluating vitamin E in the treatment of OA.

## Vitamin D

Vitamin D (calciferol) is a broad category inclusive of a collection of steroid-like substances such as vitamin D2 (ergocalciferol) and vitamin D3 (cholecalciferol). Vitamin D is only found in animal sources and can be manufactured by the body with exposure to ultraviolet

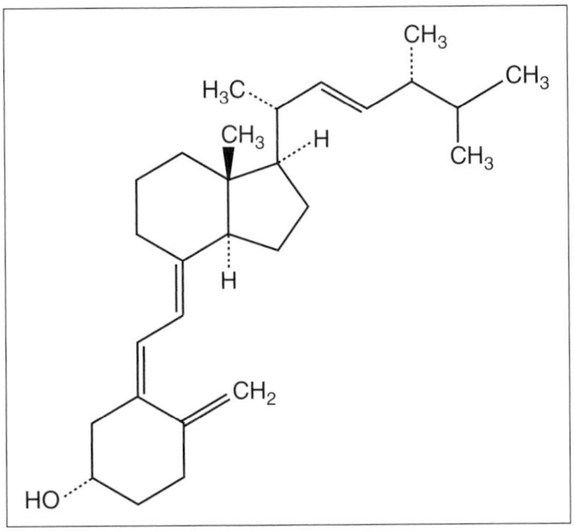

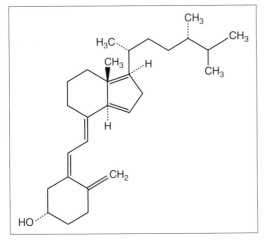

**Fig. 15.3** Chemical structure of $D_2$.

radiation (Figs. 15.3 and 15.4). Normal bone metabolism is contingent on the presence of vitamin D. Suboptimal vitamin D levels may have adverse effects on calcium metabolism, osteoblast activity, matrix ossification, and bone density.[60,61] Low tissue levels of vitamin D may therefore impair the ability of bone to respond optimally to pathophysiologic processes in OA, and predispose to disease progression.

Reactive changes in the bone underlying and adjacent to damaged cartilage are an integral part of the osteoarthritic process.[62-68] Sclerosis of the underlying bone, trabecular microfracturing, attrition, and cyst formation are all likely to accelerate the degenerative process as a result of adverse biomechanical changes.[69,70] Other phenomena, such as osteophyte (bony spur) formation, may be attempts to repair or stabilize the process.[71,72] It has also been suggested that bone mineral density may influence the skeletal

expression of the disease, with a more erosive form occurring in individuals with "softer" bone.[73]

Although some cross-sectional studies have suggested a modest inverse relationship between presence of OA and osteoporosis, recent prospective studies have suggested that individuals with lower bone mineral density are at increased risk for OA progression.[74] The idea that the nature of bony response in OA may determine outcome has been further advanced by the demonstration that patients with bone scan abnormalities adjacent to an osteoarthritic knee have a higher rate of progression than those without such changes.[75]

Animal studies suggest that vitamin D might also have direct effects on chondrocytes in osteoarthritic cartilage. They suggest that vitamin D might exert an effect on the development or progression of OA through cartilage as well as bone. Although these findings emanate from animal studies, they serve as preliminary data that these relationships may also exist in humans. During bone growth, vitamin D regulates the transition in the growth plate from cartilage to bone.

It had been assumed that chondrocytes in developing bone lose their vitamin D receptors with the attainment of skeletal maturity. Corvol et al., however, found that chondrocytes isolated from mature rabbit growth plate cartilage were able to transform 25(OH) D3 to 24,25(OH)$_2$ D3.[76,77] They also observed that 24,25(OH)$_2$ D3 could stimulate proteoglycan synthesis by mature chondrocytes, and that it increased DNA polymerase activity in chondrocytes during cell division. They also demonstrated the presence of nuclear receptors for 24,25(OH)$_2$ D3 in chondrocytes.[76]

Tetlow and Woolley were able to demonstrate a regional association of vitamin D receptor expression with matrix metalloproteinase (MMP) expression in osteoarthritic human chondrocytes, a phenomenon virtually absent in normal cartilage.[78] In further analyses using chondrocyte culture systems, they found that 1,25(OH)$_2$ D3 could up-regulate expression of matrix MMP-3 yet suppress PMA-induced production of MMP-9 and prostaglandin E2. Thus, in vitro vitamin D has both enhancing and suppressive roles in the regulation of chondrocyte products. Because these could have differential effects on cartilage, and the net overall effect is unknown, Tetlow et al. (broadly) concluded that the disparate modulatory effects of 1,25(OH)$_2$ D3 may be of relevance to the chondrolytic processes that occur in OA and that further research is needed.

McAlindon et al. also tested the association of vitamin D status on the *incidence* and *progression* of knee OA among the Framingham OA Cohort Study participants.[79] This study included both a dietary assessment and a serum assay of 25(OH) D3. Dietary intake of vitamin D and serum 25(OH) D3 levels were

**Fig. 15.4** Chemical structure of $D_3$.

unrelated to OA *incidence*. Risk of *progression* over 8 years in those with evidence of OA at baseline, however, was three- to fourfold higher for participants in the middle and lower tertiles of both vitamin D intake (OR for lowest versus highest tertile 4.0, 95% CI 1.4 to 11.6) and serum level (OR 2.9, 95% CI 1.0 to 8.2). Low serum vitamin D level also predicted cartilage loss, assessed by loss of joint space (OR 2.3, 95% CI 0.9 to 5.5) and osteophyte growth (OR 3.1, 95% CI 1.3 to 7.5).

Lane et al. tested the relationship of serum 25(OH) D3 and 1,25(OH)$_2$ D3 with the development of radiographic hip OA.[80] They studied a population of Caucasian women aged over 65 years participating in the Study of Osteoporotic Fractures. Serum vitamin D levels were measured in 237 subjects randomly selected from 6,051 women who had pelvic radiographs taken at both the baseline examination and after 8 years of follow-up.

There was an association observed between vitamin D levels and incident hip OA defined dichotomously in two ways: (1) the occurrence of joint space narrowing and (2) the development of osteophytes during the study period. They found a significantly increased risk for development of joint space narrowing among those in the lowest and middle tertile for 25(OH) D3 compared to those in the highest tertile (OR 3.3, 95% CI 1.1 to 9.9) and (OR 3.2, 95% CI 1.1 to 9.7), respectively. No increased risk of osteophyte incidence was observed and there was no association between 1,25(OH)$_2$ D3 and either incident joint space narrowing or osteophyte formation.

McLaughlin et al. examined the effects of serum 25(OH) D3 and parathyroid hormone on risk of progression among a cohort of 312 participants with symptomatic knee OA conducted at a VA hospital. This study has been reported in abstract form only at this time.[81] In contrast to the prior studies, they found no striking influence of these variables on OA progression in their analyses. Further reports are forthcoming from this preliminary analysis.

However, there are some features of this study that might account for the discordance with the Framingham data. These relate to the characteristics of the VA-hospital-based sample and the focus on joint space narrowing as the primary outcome measure. In addition, the levels of 25(OH) D3 were lower in the VA study such that the cut point between the middle and upper tertile (25 ng/ml) corresponded to the cutoff point between the lower and middle tertile for the Framingham cohort. Thus, the VA sample may not have had sufficiently high levels of vitamin D to exert a detectable effect.

These factors predicated a recent study by Carbone et al. of the relationship of antiresorptive drug use to structural findings and symptoms of knee OA.[82] This examined the cross-sectional association between use of medications that have a bone anti-resorptive effect with structural features and symptoms of knee OA among participants in the Women in the Health, Aging and Body Composition Study. The investigators found associations of use of alendronate and/or estrogen with decreased structural lesions and lower pain scores.[82] However, as pointed out by DeMarco[83] the original report did not account for potential influence of vitamin D on these associations.

Carbone et al. therefore reanalyzed their results to adjust for a possible effect of vitamin D supplement use (as they did not have serum 25[OH]D levels).[84] Sixteen percent of participants in this study used vitamin D supplements at any dosage. This variable was not associated with structural changes of OA or pain severity, nor did its inclusion as a covariate in the statistical models change the formerly observed associations.

Of note, this study was not originally designed to study the effects of vitamin D in OA. Therefore, caution should be used in the interpretation of these results. First, the lack of influence of including vitamin D supplement use into the multivariate model evaluating the effect of anti-resorptive agents on structural features and symptoms of knee OA suggests that this measurement is not a confounder in the relation between anti-resorptive agents and knee OA. However, vitamin D could still potentially exert an independent effect on knee OA.

Second, only a small portion of the participants used vitamin D supplements and likely at widely varying dosages. Finally, as this was an observational study the lack of effect seen with the use of vitamin D supplementation could potentially be secondary to confounding by indication (i.e., those who have been identified to be deficient in vitamin D would have been more likely to have been started on these supplements), not because vitamin D supplementation does not truly exert an effect on OA symptoms and structural progression.

If low vitamin D levels are indeed associated with OA progression, vitamin D supplementation could potentially act as a disease-modifying OA drug (DMOAD). Despite a fairly compelling biologic rationale, results from observational studies about the role of vitamin D in OA progression are conflicting. To rigorously address this issue, a randomized placebo-controlled clinical trial of a vitamin D intervention for knee OA was begun in the fall of 2005, evaluating both OA symptoms and structural progression longitudinally over 2 years.

## VITAMIN K

The primary form of vitamin K, a fat-soluble vitamin, in the diet is phylloquinone (vitamin K$_1$)—which is concentrated in dark green leafy vegetables and vegetable oils (Fig. 15.5). Although there is some endogenous production of vitamin K, a subclinical deficiency can be created by limiting dietary intake of phylloquinone. Further, low dietary intake of vitamin K is common, and studies evaluating biochemical measures of vitamin K status suggest that inadequate intake of vitamin K is widespread among U.S. and UK adults.[85,86]

Vitamin K has bone and cartilage effects that may be relevant to OA. Post-translational γ-carboxylation of glutamic acid residues to form γ-carboxyglutamic acid (Gla) residues confers functionality to these Gla proteins.[87] Vitamin K is an essential cofactor for this process.[87] Multiple coagulation, bone, and cartilage proteins are dependent on vitamin K because the Gla residues are required for these proteins to function appropriately. Bone and cartilage Gla proteins include growth-arrest-specific protein 6 (Gas-6) and the skeletally expressed extracellular matrix proteins osteocalcin and matrix Gla protein (MGP).[87-90]

The vitamin-K-dependent γ-carboxylation of these bone and cartilage proteins is important to their normal functioning. Gas-6, through its interactions with the axl tyrosine kinase receptor, prevents chondrocyte apoptosis and is involved in chondrocyte growth and development.[88] Low levels of vitamin K could lead to inadequate levels of functional Gas-6, contributing to increased chondrocyte apoptosis and attendant mineralization. Another Gla protein is osteocalcin, the most abundant noncollagenous protein in bone and a potent inhibitor of hydroxyapatite mineralization.

MGP, a protein that plays a role in chondrocyte development and maturation, is associated with mineralization in hypertrophic chondrocytes and endochondral ossification—the same process through which osteophytes form.[91,92] In addition, MGP may inhibit mineralization via its interaction with bone morphogenetic protein-2 (BMP-2). BMP-2 is a known inducer of chondrocyte and osteoblast differentiation that signals through Smad1, together enhancing bone formation. Interference by MGP leads to diminished bone-forming capacity.[93] Conversely, under-carboxylated MGP could lead to increased bone-forming capacity.

Beyond being a necessary cofactor for γ-carboxylation, vitamin K compounds also exhibit anti-inflammatory properties—reducing prostaglandin E2 and interleukin-6 production and inhibiting interleukin-1 and prostaglandin E2 mediated bone resorption.[94,95] The effects of inadequately functioning vitamin-K-dependent proteins has been seen in warfarin (vitamin K antagonist) embryopathy, Keutel syndrome (a genetic disorder in which MGP is deficient), and an MGP knockout mouse model—all of which exhibit growth plate cartilage abnormalities.[96-98]

These abnormalities may reflect a process similar to osteophyte formation in that both cartilage plate abnormalities and osteophyte formation involve endochondral ossification. Thus, vitamin K (an important regulator of bone and cartilage mineralization and function) may play a role in OA. Neogi et al. has investigated the potential association between vitamin K and OA in the Framingham osteoarthritis cohort. In their first assessment, they examined the relationship between dietary vitamin K intake (evaluated using a food frequency questionnaire) and radiographic evidence of osteophytes.[99]

They demonstrated an association between higher vitamin K intake and lower osteophyte prevalence, but the association was not significant with prevalence ratios of osteophytes from lowest to highest vitamin K intake quartiles of 1.0 (reference), 1.1, 0.8, and 0.9 (p for trend = 0.2). As a follow-up study, Neogi et al. subsequently measured vitamin K levels using plasma vitamin levels because they are more reliable than levels estimated from dietary questionnaires.[100]

In this study, they showed an association between plasma phylloquinone and severity of radiographic OA (particularly of osteophytes) in the hand and knee (after adjusting for age, sex, BMI, femoral neck bone mineral density, total energy intake, and plasma vitamin D). The prevalence of hand and knee osteophytes in those in the highest plasma phylloquinone quartile was 40% lower than in those in the lowest quartile. No significant associations were noted for control nutrients (vitamins B1 and B2), suggesting that a healthy lifestyle does not account for these results.

Based on these two observational studies, it is unclear whether there is an association between vitamin K and OA. However, it would be reasonable

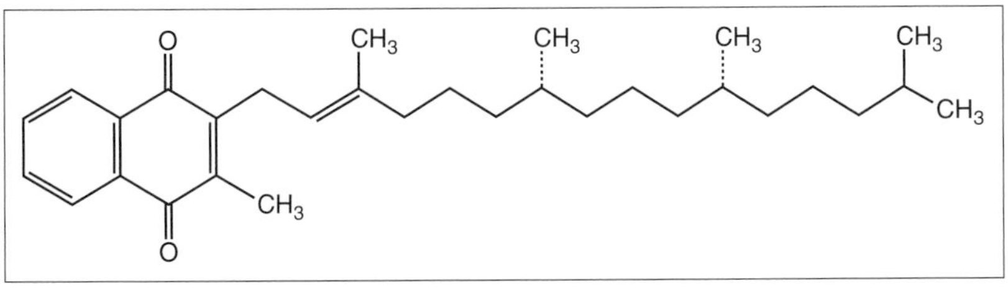

**Fig. 15.5** Chemical structure of phylloquinone (vitamin K$_1$).

to expect that plasma levels of micronutrients are a more accurate measure compared with dietary intake measures, lending more credibility to the latter study supporting the presence of a relationship between vitamin K and osteophytes.

As mentioned, to date no pharmacologic agent has been identified as an ever-elusive (DMOAD). However, with data suggestive that vitamin K deficiency is associated with features of OA and OA severity vitamin K *supplementation* has the potential of being classified as a DMOAD. To address this possibility, Neogi and others are involved in conducting a randomized double-blind placebo-controlled trial evaluating longitudinal structural and symptom effects of vitamin K supplementation on OA.

## SELENIUM AND IODINE: STUDIES OF KASHIN-BECK DISEASE

Selenium is an integral component of iodothyronine deiodinase as well as glutathione peroxidase. Kashin-Beck disease is an osteoarthropathy of children and adolescents that occurs in geographic areas of China in which deficiencies of both selenium and iodine are endemic. Strong epidemiologic evidence exists supporting the environmental nature of this disease.[101] Although the clinical and radiologic characteristics of Kashin-Beck disease differ from OA, its existence raises the possibility that environmental factors also play a role in the occurrence of this disorder.

Selenium deficiency together with pro-oxidative products of organic matter in drinking water (mainly fulvic acid) and contamination of grain by fungi have been proposed as environmental causes for Kashin-Beck disease. The efficacy of selenium supplementation in preventing the disorder, however, is controversial. Moreno-Reyes et al. studied iodine and selenium metabolism in 11 villages in Tibet in which Kashin-Beck disease was endemic and one village in which it was not.[102] They found iodine deficiency to be the main determinant of Kashin-Beck disease in these villages.

It should be noted, however, in the three groups, people with disease in villages with Kashin-Beck disease, people without disease in villages with Kashin-Beck disease, and people in a control village without Kashin-Beck disease, all had selenium levels that were very low (and those in the latter group had the lowest levels). In an accompanying editorial, Utiger inferred that Kashin-Beck disease probably results from a combination of deficiencies of both of these elements, and speculated that growth plate cartilage is both dependent on locally produced triiodothyronine and sensitive to oxidative damage.[101] It should be noted that there is little evidence, if any, to suggest that Kashin-Beck disease has any similarities with adult-onset spontaneous OA.

Recently reported in abstract form at the Annual Scientific Meeting of the American College of Rheumatology, Jordan et al. evaluated the relationship between selenium and knee OA in a cross-sectional observational study of a community-based population (the Johnston County Osteoarthritis Project).[103] Nine hundred forty participants submitted toenail clippings for a selenium assessment by instrumental neutron activation analysis. Radiographic knee OA was scored using a definition of Kellgren–Lawrence grade >2. Mean selenium levels were 0.76 parts per million (ppm)$^+$.[102] Compared with those in the lowest tertile of selenium, those in the highest tertile had an OR of 0.62 (95% CI 0.37 to 1.02) for having prevalent knee OA and an OR of 0.56 (95% CI 0.31 to 0.97) for having bilateral knee OA. Based on these findings, low selenium levels appear to be associated with prevalent knee OA (particularly bilateral disease).

Although results from this study are thought-provoking, there are several limitations to this study. First, although the measurement of selenium via toenail clippings has been used in the past, the duration of exposure to different selenium levels cannot be ascertained using this measurement.

Second, given that Kashin-Beck disease was the model from which selenium deficiency was hypothesized to be associated with OA information on iodine status would have been of interest in this study—although admittedly with the supplementation of iodine in salt within the United States, it is less likely to find people severely deficient in iodine. However, if iodine status were predictive of OA in participants with low selenium levels (as has been seen in Kashin-Beck disease) it would be important in enhancing our understanding of the role of selenium in OA pathophysiology. Finally, it is possible that selenium levels could be a surrogate for some unmeasured micronutrient. A randomized controlled trial of selenium supplementation (perhaps in factorial design with iodine supplementation) is needed to evaluate whether it would be effective as a DMOAD.

Little research exists evaluating the efficacy of selenium in treating OA symptoms. There is one small published clinical trial of supplemental selenium in which Hill and Bird conducted a 6-month double-blind placebo-controlled study of selenium-ACE—a proprietary nutritional supplement in the UK—among 30 patients with either primary or secondary hip or knee OA.[104] The "active" treatment contained on average 144 µg of selenium as well as 450 µg, 90 mg, and 30 mg of vitamins A, C, and E (respectively). In fact, the "placebo" also contained 2.9 µg of selenium. Pain and stiffness scores remained similar for the two groups at both 3 and 6 months of follow-up. The authors concluded that their data did not support efficacy for selenium-ACE in relieving OA symptoms.

It is unlikely that the aforementioned clinical trial will provide any insight regarding the efficacy of selenium in the treatment of symptoms in OA. With just 30 participants in the trial, it is underpowered to detect even a moderate effect of selenium. Even if investigators would have found an effect of the active treatment, it would have been impossible to attribute the effects to selenium because the active treatment also contained moderate to high doses of vitamins A, C, and E. A larger randomized placebo-controlled clinical trial evaluating selenium supplementation should be conducted to evaluate its efficacy in the treatment of symptoms related to OA.

## GLUCOSAMINE AND CHONDROITIN SULFATE

Glucosamine (an amino monosaccharide found in chitin, glycoproteins, and glycosaminoglycans) is also known as 2-amino-2-deoxyglucose or 2-amino-2-deoxy-beta-D-glucopyranose. As a nutritional supplement, it is available commercially in three forms: glucosamine hydrochloride, glucosamine sulfate, and N-acetyl-glucosamine (Fig. 15.6).

Chondroitin sulfate is a glycosaminoglycan consisting of linear repeating units containing D-galactosamine and D-glucuronic acid. This compound is found in humans in cartilage, bone, cornea, skin, and the arterial wall. Chondroitin sulfate comes in three forms: A, B, and C. The two most common found in chondroitin sulfate nutritional supplements are types A (chondroitin 4-sulfate) and C (chondroitin 6-sulfate). Chondroitin sulfate is found primarily in fish and shark cartilage, as well as in cartilaginous rings of bovine trachea and pork ears and snouts (Fig. 15.7).

Glucosamine and chondroitin sulfate are cartilage extracellular matrix components that have been widely promulgated as a remedy for OA on the basis that they might provide a substrate for matrix synthesis and repair. However, the mechanisms by which they might do this remain something of a conundrum. According to our understanding of the metabolic pathways

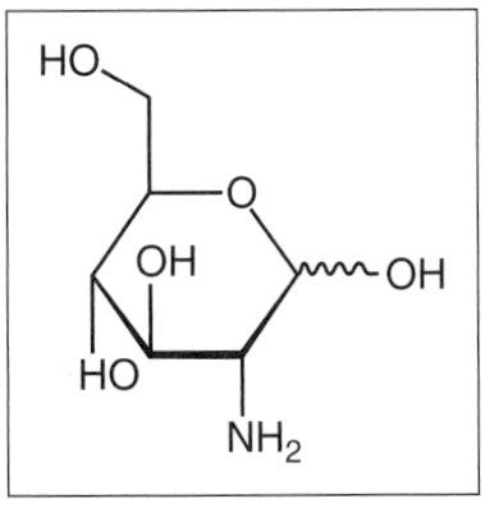

Fig. 15.6 Chemical structure of glucosamine.

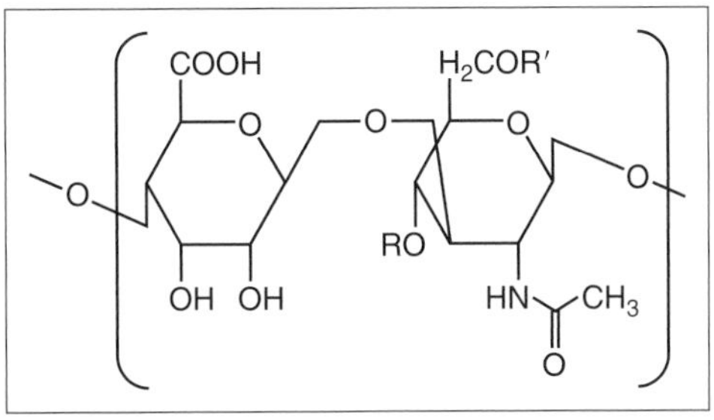

Fig. 15.7 Chondroitin sulfate A R = SO3H R1 = H chondroitin sulfate C R = H R1 = SO3H.

involved, glucosamine (as an amino sugar) should be rapidly degraded by the liver during first-pass metabolism. Early pharmacodynamic studies assessed absorption of the compounds only indirectly.[105,106]

A recent pharmacokinetic study in dogs, using a refined high-performance liquid chromatographic (HPLC) assay, demonstrated that glucosamine (hydrochloride) is absorbed with a bioavailability of approximately 10 to 12% from single or multiple doses.[107] Furthermore, laboratory work in rats has suggested that glucosamine is substantially degraded in the lumen of the GI tract.[108] To evaluate the absorption of glucosamine sulfate in humans, Bigee et al. performed a small study evaluating 10 participants with OA, measuring serum levels of glucosamine every 15 to 30 minutes over 3 hours after ingestion of the recommended 1,500 mg of oral glucosamine sulfate.[109]

Nine out of ten subjects had detectable serum glucosamine beginning to rise at 30 to 45 minutes and peaking at 90 to 180 minutes, with the mean maximal serum level being 12 μmols/L. This would provide <2% of ingested glucosamine to blood and interstitial fluid combined. Based on the very small serum levels seen in this study, Bigee et al. concluded that ingestion of standard glucosamine sulfate is unlikely to stimulate cartilage chondroitin synthesis. Persiani et al. also evaluated both serum and synovial fluid levels of glucosamine in five people with knee OA both before and after administration of 2 weeks of daily oral glucosamine and found similar increase in levels of serum glucosamine of 7.9 μmols/L and a similar increase in synovial fluid, 7.2 μmols/L.[110]

In addition to the fact that serum levels of glucosamine are very low, the notion that exogenous glucosamine might be incorporated into the structure of hyaluronan or cartilage proteoglycans is also problematic because although glucosamine can enter the glycosaminoglycan biosynthetic pathway after its conversion to UDP-N-galactosamine glucose is a much more abundant substrate. That being said, recent in vitro and in vivo studies in animals have shown increases in proteoglycan synthesis by chondrocytes after addition of glucosamine to the culture medium—suggesting that instead of providing substrate for hyaluronan or cartilage proteoglycans glucosamine sulfate's mechanism of action may be an anti-inflammatory effect.[105,106]

The biologic fate of orally administered chondroitin sulfate is less clear, but some evidence exists to suggest that the compound may be absorbed following oral administration—possibly as a result of pinocytosis.[111] Chondroitin sulfate is able to cause an increase in RNA synthesis by chondrocytes,[112] which appears to correlate with an increase in the production of proteoglycans and collagens.[113-116] In addition, there is evidence that chondroitin sulfate partially inhibits leukocyte elastase and may therefore reduce the degradation of cartilage collagen and proteoglycans prominent in the osteoarthritic process.[117-120]

A potential adverse effect of glucosamine was recently highlighted in a report from the Institute of Medicine.[121] Glucosamine may lead to an increase in insulin dysregulation among individuals predisposed to such problems. These concerns are based on the known ability of glucosamine to bypass the glutamine/fructose-6-phosphate aminotransferase step of hexosamine biosynthesis and desensitize glucose transport.[122] Insulin dysregulation is of particular interest to individuals with OA because high BMI is a risk factor for both OA and insulin resistance (and/or diabetes mellitus).

Whereas the effects of glucosamine have been well documented in animal models, less is known about its effects on glucose metabolism in humans. Although preliminary studies have been reassuring, their interpretation has been limited by the considerable variability in measures and small numbers of participants.[123,124] In a study by Bigee et al., three individuals with evidence of radiographic OA with normal screening serum glucose levels and without a preexisting history of diabetes mellitus all had abnormal glucose tolerance tests. These three individuals all had worsening of their glucose tolerance tests after glucosamine administration.[125]

## Sulfate

Cartilage proteoglycans are highly sulfated. The amount of sulfate made available to cells is an important factor in the degree of proteoglycan sulfation.[126,127] Some in vitro experiments on cultured cells suggest that increases in serum sulfate concentration enhance glycosaminoglycan synthesis.[128] It has also been found that the rate of sulfated glycosaminoglycan synthesis in human articular cartilage is sensitive to small deviations from physiologic sulfate concentrations.[129] In addition, sulfate pools in humans are among the smallest of all species,[130] making them especially susceptible to physiologically relevant small changes. Interestingly, sulfate balance in humans is poorly understood and may vary based on dietary factors or on dietary supplements.

One study measured human urinary sulfate excretion after ingestion of methionine or chondroitin sulfate supplements in the setting of high- or low-protein diets. They found that more sulfate was excreted in the urine in those with a background of high-protein diets compared to those with low-protein diets. This suggests that the body increased sulfate retention from supplements in the low-protein state.[131] These observations raise the possibility that sulfate supplementation may have a beneficial role in cartilage health.

## Efficacy for Osteoarthritis Symptoms

Glucosamine and chondroitin sulfate have been the subject of numerous clinical trials in Europe and Asia, all of which (until recently) demonstrated favorable effects.[132-146] In 2000, McAlindon et al. performed a meta-analysis and quality assessment of 15 eligible double-blind placebo-controlled clinical trials of glucosamine and chondroitin compounds (six of glucosamine and nine of chondroitin).[147] Most of these trials were sponsored by a manufacturer of the product, all reporting positive results. Not surprisingly, there was evidence of publication bias with an asymmetric funnel plot ($p < 0.01$).

There were also numerous methodologic quality issues in the 15 trials included in the meta-analysis, with only one study describing adequate allocation concealment and just two reporting intent-to-treat analyses. In this study, there was heterogeneity among the chondroitin trials ($p < 0.001$), but when one outlier trial was removed heterogeneity was no longer significant. In this review, the aggregated effect sizes (standardized mean differences, SMDs) were 0.44 (95% CI 0.24 to 0.64) and 0.78 (95% CI 0.60 to 0.95) for glucosamine and chondroitin (respectively). When evaluating, the author identified primary outcome of each trial (excluding the one outlier trial), results were similar when including only pain as an outcome. As a reference, 0.2 is considered a small effect, 0.5 a moderate effect, and 0.8 a large effect.[148]

At the same time, Towheed et al. performed a structured literature search and systematic review of randomized controlled trials comparing glucosamine against placebo or non-steroidal anti-inflammatory drugs (NSAIDs).[149] They identified 16 eligible randomized controlled trials (13 placebo-controlled and 3 with an NSAID comparator). Their report emphasized considerable heterogeneity among the trials in terms of mode of glucosamine administration, classification of OA, joint sites evaluated, and outcomes measured. They also pointed out that

15 trials tested glucosamine sulfate but only one tested glucosamine hydrochloride.

Most of the trials were noted to have some form of affiliation with Rotta, an Italian manufacturer of glucosamine sulfate. Comparing glucosamine to placebo, the authors derived a pooled SMD for pain reduction (using a random effects model) of 1.40 (95% CI 0.65 to 2.14)—a clinically significant treatment benefit as effective as or more effective than a total joint replacement (which does not seem reasonable).[150,151] The SMD using a fixed effects model was 0.84 (95% CI 0.71 to 0.97).

Results for function, measured by the Lequesne index, were positive but just missed the $\alpha = 0.05$ level of significance—with an SMD of 0.63 (95% CI −0.04 to 1.29). When comparing glucosamine to NSAID, the pooled SMD for pain reduction from three randomized controlled trials was 0.86 (95% CI 0.58 to 1.14)—suggesting that glucosamine sulfate is also superior to NSAIDs. Finally, the safety profile of glucosamine was considered excellent in that of approximately 1,000 participants randomized to glucosamine only 14 withdrew because of toxicity.

A second meta-analysis of chondroitin sulfate trials was also performed. Leeb et al. included seven double-blind randomized controlled studies in their review evaluating a total of 703 patients in those trials.[152] The pooled Glass scores (i.e., [pain at study termination$_{treatment arm}$ minus pain at study termination$_{placebo arm}$]/[standard deviation of placebo arm]) for pain was 0.9 (95% CI [estimated from a figure] ~ 0.8 to 1.0) and for function was 0.74 (95% CI [estimated from a figure] ~ 0.65 to 0.85). Study termination dates varied from as short as 56 days to as long as 1,095 days, with the majority of studies lasting from 90 to 180 days.

Leeb et al. concluded that pooled data from eligible trials suggested that the product may be useful in OA. However, they acknowledged several major problems in interpreting the data—including small numbers of participants in the eligible trials and no study was evaluated using intent-to-treat analysis. Further, there was evidence of publication bias in this review (although details of these evaluation methods were not provided)—suggesting that it led to a relative error of 30%. The presence of publication bias likely led to an overestimation of the effect sizes.[152]

Disagreement in the conclusions drawn from the meta-analyses of glucosamine by McAlindon and Towheed may have resulted from the more restrictive inclusion criteria for higher-quality trials imposed by McAlindon et al. In addition, in the Towheed review the presence of discordant SMDs when evaluating pain using fixed versus random effects models suggests that there is excessive heterogeneity[153] in the population of trials aggregated. Further, there were only three trials

that compared glucosamine to NSAIDs (each being relatively small, with n < 100)—which may be too few to pool in a meta-analysis.

The results from the two meta-analyses of chondroitin corroborated each other, suggesting that chondroitin has a moderate to large effect. That being said, the effect of chondroitin estimated at being close to or exceeding that of a total knee replacement does not seem reasonable. Further, the presence of publication bias observed in both reviews further supports that the effect sizes are likely an overestimate of the effect of chondroitin. The one chondroitin sulfate intervention trial that has been published since these meta-analyses showed no effect of chondroitin sulfate in the improvement of OA symptoms supporting this conclusion drawn by both meta-analyses.[154]

Since the publication of the two glucosamine meta-analyses, the body of evidence concerning this treatment's efficacy has been altered by the publication of four independently funded clinical trials—three of which had completely null results.[155-158] The first of these enrolled 114 knee OA patients from a VA medical center and randomized them into a 2-month placebo-controlled trial of glucosamine sulfate of 500 mg tid.[158] The participants were required to have radiographic OA with a Kellgren–Lawrence grade > 1 and naïve to both glucosamine and chondroitin prior to enrollment into the study. Sixteen participants were lost to follow-up or withdrew. No difference was seen in pain outcomes between the treatment and placebo groups after either 30 days or 60 days of treatment.

Hughes and Carr performed a double-blind placebo-controlled randomized controlled trial of glucosamine sulfate (1.5 g per day) in patients recruited from a rheumatology clinic.[157] Participants had relatively severe knee OA from both a symptomatic and radiographic perspective. Twenty-three percent had a Kellgren–Lawrence grade of 4, the mean WOMAC score was 9.2 (SD 3.5), and many were frequently using NSAIDs (46%) or other analgesics (23%).

No significant between-group differences were found in the primary endpoint (VAS overall assessment of pain in the affected knee) or any of the secondary pain assessments in this study at 6, 12, and 24 weeks of follow-up. The two treatment groups were also similar in the measures of range of motion, except for range of knee flexion—which showed a mean increase of 4 degrees in the glucosamine group and a decrease of 9 degrees in the placebo arm (p for the difference = 0.02). The authors were skeptical about the credibility of this finding because the magnitude of the difference is less than the minimal detection limit of a goniometer.

Cibere et al. performed a glucosamine withdrawal trial in 137 people with knee OA who were already using the product and reported at least moderate benefit.[155] The design was a four-center 6-month randomized double-blind placebo-controlled glucosamine discontinuation trial in which enrollees were randomly assigned to placebo or to the treatment, where participants continued taking glucosamine sulfate.

The primary outcome was the proportion of disease flares among the groups analyzed using an intent-to-treat analysis. Secondary outcomes included time to flare, analgesic use, the severity of flare, and change in pain, stiffness, function, and quality of life. Ultimately, disease flares occurred in 28 (42%) of the placebo arm and 32 (45%) of the glucosamine arm (difference −3%, 95% CI −19 to 14). In the Cox regression analysis, after adjustment for sex, study site, and OA radiographic severity time to disease flare was not significantly different between the glucosamine and the placebo group (hazard ratio of flare = 0.8; $p = 0.4$). At final study visit, acetaminophen was used in 27 and 21% of placebo and glucosamine patients, respectively ($p = 0.4$), non-steroidal anti-inflammatory drugs in 29% and 30% ($p = 0.9$), and both in 20 and 21% ($p = 0.8$).

No differences were found in severity of disease flare or other secondary outcomes between placebo and glucosamine patients. Thus, in patients with knee OA and at least moderate subjective improvement with prior glucosamine use there was no symptomatic benefit from continued use of glucosamine sulfate. Cibere et al. also analyzed samples for type II collagen degradation biomarkers as a proxy for OA progression.[159] They found no statistically significant effect of glucosamine sulfate on type II collagen fragment levels, with the primary outcome being the ratio of $C_1,C_2$ epitope to C2C epitope in the urine and serum at baseline and at 4, 12, and 24 weeks of follow-up.

This study represents an interesting and innovative approach to testing such products. It selects for a group of people who potentially are the most likely to respond to a treatment, a population in which the treatment is the most likely to show an effect. However, as a new study design it is subject to a new set of potential flaws and limitations. For example, if the duration of effectiveness of glucosamine is prolonged the period of follow-up in the previously cited study may have been insufficient. In addition, the heterogeneity of glucosamine products on the market could have biased any differences to the null.

Motivated in part by the heterogeneity of glucosamine trial results and by interest in including the previously cited non industry-sponsored clinical trials, Towheed et al. recently updated the Cochrane review of available data with an additional intent of investigating the differences in the trials in an effort to explain the heterogeneity observed.[160] This review included 20 trials

in total, with a statistically significant SMD for pain and function of 0.61 (95% CI 0.28 to 0.95)—consistent with a moderate effect of glucosamine. However, when the analysis was restricted to the eight studies of higher quality that reported adequate allocation concealment no benefit of glucosamine for pain and WOMAC function was seen with an SMD of 0.19 (95% CI −0.11 to 0.50).

In the subset of trials that tested the Rotta preparation of glucosamine (n = 10), glucosamine was superior for pain and function with SMDs of 1.31 (95% CI 0.64 to 1.99) and 0.51 (95% CI 0.05 to 0.96), respectively. Pooled results for pain in those trials in which a non-Rotta preparation of glucosamine was compared to placebo did not reach statistical significance, with an SMD of 0.15 (95% CI −0.05 to 0.35). The authors concluded that studies that tested a non-Rotta preparation or used inadequate allocation concealment procedures failed to show benefit in pain and WOMAC function—whereas those evaluating the Rotta preparation show benefit in the treatment of symptomatic OA.[160]

It should be noted that in the subgroup analysis limited to the trials evaluating a Rotta preparation the SMD for pain[1,3] was as large as the effect of a total joint replacement. This magnitude of effect does not seem reasonable, particularly because there is no biologic reason to expect why the Rotta preparation would have such a disparate effect compared with the other glucosamine preparations. Although not explicitly evaluated in this study, perhaps most of the trials of the Rotta preparation were industry sponsored and many of the non-Rotta formulation studies were not industry sponsored. If true, this would provide further support for the presence of publication bias.

As an attempt to settle the question of glucosamine's and chondroitin's efficacy in symptomatic improvement in OA, the National Institutes of Health has sponsored the largest multi-center randomized controlled trial of this treatment.[161] The results of this study have been printed in abstract form at the time of this publication. A total of 1,583 participants were randomized, and 1,258 (80%) completed the study. Participants were randomized to one of five arms (placebo, celecoxib, glucosamine 500 mg tid only, and chondroitin sulfate 400 mg tid only) or the combination of glucosamine HCl and chondroitin sulfate.

The primary outcome in this study was a 20% improvement in WOMAC pain at 24 weeks of follow-up from baseline. The respective response rates were 60.1, 70.1, 64.0, 65.4, and 66.6%. The difference between combination treatment and placebo was reported as near statistically significant ($p = 0.09$). In a subgroup analysis of participants with a higher WOMAC score at baseline, the response rates were 54.3, 69.4, 65.7, 61.4, and 79.2%. In this analysis, the combination treatment was significantly different from placebo (p = 0.002). The authors concluded that the combination therapy is effective in treating moderate to severe knee pain due to OA.

These findings were presented at the 2005 Annual Scientific Meeting of the American College of Rheumatology. At that time, the conclusions were tempered by the representation of the combination treatment effect as null. Further, it was pointed out that the placebo response rates were unusually high in this study. In addition, although not explicitly stated the subgroup analysis looking at those with higher baseline pain scores appeared to be a post hoc analysis in which the placebo response rate was slightly lower and the combination treatment response rate was slightly higher. Given the controversy existing around the interpretation of results from this large well-designed clinical trial, there appears to be little hope that the question of glucosamine and chondroitin's efficacy will be settled anytime soon.

## Efficacy as Disease-modifying Agents

Rotta Pharmaceuticals sponsored two large multi-center randomized controlled trials to examine the possibility that glucosamine might reduce rate of loss of articular cartilage.[162,163] These enrolled about 200 outpatients with primary knee OA into 3-year randomized controlled trials comparing once-daily 1.5 g of Rotta glucosamine sulfate with placebo. The primary outcome in each trial was based on joint space measurements obtained from conventional extended-view standing anteroposterior knee radiographs (a recommended radiographic approach at that time). Both trials showed quantitatively similar benefits in the glucosamine treatment arms with respect to the rate of loss of joint space width and symptoms.

Unfortunately, the approach that was used to estimate joint space width in these randomized controlled trials has proved to be problematic, even though it was the recommended technique at the inception of the trials.[164] Precise measurement of this variable is contingent on highly reproducible radio-anatomic positioning of the joint, and may be biased by the presence of pain. If those in the glucosamine group had less pain at their follow-up X-ray, they may have stood with the knee more fully extended (a non-physiologic position that may be associated with the femur riding up on the tibial edge)—giving the appearance of a better preserved joint space. What appeared to have been a slower rate of joint space loss may have reflected between-group differences in the degree of knee extension at the follow-up X-ray.

Michel et al. recently reported the results of a 2-year randomized double-blind controlled trial of 800 mg chondroitin sulfate or placebo once daily among 300 patients with knee OA.[154] The primary outcome was joint space loss over 2 years as assessed by a posteroanterior radiograph of the knee in mild flexion (a better-validated technique).[165] Secondary outcomes included pain and function. The participants in the placebo arm exhibited significant joint space loss, with a mean cumulative joint space loss of 0.14 mm$^{+0}$(61) at two years of follow-up compared to no change in the chondroitin arm (0.00 mm$^{+0}$[53]). In the intent-to-treat analysis, the between-group difference in mean joint space loss was 0.14 + 0.57 mm (p = 0.04).

In contrast, the differences in the symptom outcomes between the groups were trivial and non-significant. However, chondroitin was well tolerated, with no significant differences in rates of adverse events between the two groups. Although the authors focused on the results providing evidence of structure damage modification by chondroitin, vexing questions remain about the internal validity of joint space width as a measure of cartilage loss and its relevance to the clinical state of the patient with knee OA—especially in the absence of any overt impact on symptomatic outcomes.

## OTHER NUTRITIONAL PRODUCTS

There appears to be an increasing number of nutritional remedies being promulgated for purported benefits in arthritis. A number of these have now been tested in controlled clinical trials. Four trials of avocado/soybean unsaponifiables, for example, were pooled in a meta-analysis that had guardedly positive results.[166] Trials of S-adenosylmethionine have also had apparently positive results, albeit somewhat limited by adverse effects and high dropout rates.[167-172] A ginger-derived product has also been tested in a trial that had moderately positive results.[173]

## CONCLUSIONS AND RECOMMENDATIONS

Studies evaluating diet and exercise interventions suggest that treatment with the combination is more effective than either intervention alone in the improvement of symptoms related to OA. Epidemiologic data and animal studies strongly suggest that vitamin C may be effective in the treatment of both OA symptoms and structural progression. One moderate-sized randomized controlled trial suggests that vitamin C supplementation may be effective in treating OA symptoms.

Good rationale also supports the expectation that vitamin E would be effective in treatment of symptoms and structural progression. Several small industry-sponsored randomized controlled trials do support effectiveness of vitamin E in OA symptoms. However, one moderate-sized study reported a lack of symptomatic effect of vitamin E. No chondroprotective effects of vitamin E were seen in this study, although the presence of serious limitations to this study suggests that further investigation is warranted.

Vitamin D is important in bone health and may have direct chondroprotective effects. Epidemiologic data are conflicting regarding the effect of vitamin D on OA progression in the knee and hip. A randomized controlled trial with 2 years of follow-up evaluating the effects of vitamin D supplementation on both symptoms and structural progression is currently under way.

Similarly, there are data that vitamin K has both bone and cartilage effects. Epidemiologic data for vitamin K as a disease-modifying micronutrient in OA are conflicting. A randomized controlled trial with 2 years of follow-up is currently under way to address the efficacy of vitamin K in both the treatment of symptoms and structural progression in OA.

With rationale to expect that selenium could prevent structural progression, recent epidemiologic data suggest that higher selenium levels may be protective of prevalent OA radiographic features in one large population-based cohort. One small poorly designed randomized clinical trial did not support efficacy of selenium supplementation in the treatment of OA symptoms. Further evaluation of selenium supplementation in the treatment of OA symptoms and structural progression is warranted.

Of all of the supplements of interest, glucosamine and chondroitin have been the most frequently studied. The mechanism of action of these two treatments as providing substrate for matrix synthesis and repair has not been substantiated. Multiple randomized controlled trials have been conducted evaluating the efficacy of these treatments. Meta-analyses of both treatments have been conducted in an attempt to assimilate the data from existing clinical trials. That being said, the question of efficacy of these treatments with respect to symptomatic improvement and structural progression still lingers. Hopefully, detailed results from a large multi-center non industry-sponsored clinical trial evaluating the efficacy of both glucosamine and chondroitin will bring us closer to clarifying the efficacy of these treatments in OA.

## REFERENCES

1. Theodosakis J, Adderly B, Fox B. *The Arthritis Cure*. New York: St. Martin's Press 1997.
2. Marra J. The state of dietary supplements: Even slight increases in growth are better than no growth at all. Nutraceuticals World 2002;5:32–40.
3. U.S. nutrition industry: Top 70 supplements 1997–2001. Nutrition Business Journal 2001 (chart 14).
4. Felson DT. Weight and osteoarthritis. J Rheumatol 1995;22(43):7–9.
5. Sokoloff L, Mickelsen O. Dietary fat supplements, body weight and osteoarthritis in DBA/2JN mice. J Nutr 1965;85:117–21.
6. Sokoloff L, et al. Experimental obesity and osteoarthritis. Am J Physiol 1960;198:765–70.
7. Aspden RM, Scheven BA, Hutchison JD. Osteoarthritis as a systemic disorder including stromal cell differentiation and lipid metabolism. Lancet 2001;357:1118–20.
8. Lippiello L, Walsh T, Fienhold M. The association of lipid abnormalities with tissue pathology in human osteoarthritic articular cartilage. Metabolism 1991;40:571–76.
9. Dumond H, et al. Evidence for a key role in leptin in ostoearthritis. Arthritis Rheum 2003;48:S282.
10. Messier SP, et al. Exercise and dietary weight loss in overweight and obese older adults with knee osteoarthritis: The Arthritis, Diet, and Activity Promotion Trial. Arthritis Rheum 2004;50:1501–10.
11. Christensen R, Astrup A, Bliddal H. Weight loss: The treatment of choice for knee osteoarthritis? A randomized trial. Osteoarthritis Cartilage 2005;13:20–7.
12. Toda Y, et al. Change in body fat, but not body weight or metabolic correlates of obesity, is related to symptomatic relief of obese patients with knee osteoarthritis after a weight control program. J Rheumatol 1998;25:2181–86.
13. Hooper MM, et al. Musculoskeletal findings in morbidly obese subjects before and after weight loss due to gastric bypass surgery. Arthritis Rheum 2004;50(9):S699.
14. Frei B. Reactive oxygen species and antioxidant vitamins: Mechanisms of action. Am J Med 1994;97(3A):5S–13S.
15. Boveris A, Oshino N, Chance B. The cellular production of hydrogen peroxide. Biochem J 1972;128:617–30.
16. Blake DR, et al. Hypoxic-reperfusion injury in the inflamed human. Lancet 1989;11:290–93.
17. Ames BN, Shigenaga MK, Hagen TM. Oxidants, antioxidants and the degenerative diseases of aging. Proc Natl Acad Sci USA 1993;90:7915–22.
18. Jacques PF, Chylack LT, Taylor A. Relationships between natural antioxidants and cataract formation. In B Frei (ed.), *Natural Antioxidants in Human Health and Disease*. San Diego: Academic Press 1994:515–33.
19. Gaziano JM. Antioxidant vitamins and coronary artery disease risk. Am J Med 1994;97(3A):18S–21S.
20. Hennekens CH. Antioxidant vitamins and cancer. Am J Med 1994;97(3A):2S–4S.
21. Martin JA, Buckwalter JA. Aging, articular cartilage chondrocyte senescence and osteoarthritis. Biogerontology 2002;3:257–64.
22. Henrotin Y, et al. Production of active oxygen species by isolated human chondrocytes. Br J Rheumatol 1993;32:562–67.
23. Henrotin Y, et al. Active oxygen species, articular inflammation, and cartilage damage. EXS 1992;62:308–22.
24. Rathakrishnan C, et al. Release of oxygen radicals by articular chondrocytes: A study of luminol-dependent chemoluminescence and hydrogen peroxide secretion. J Bone Miner Res 1992;7:1139–48.
25. Tiku ML, et al. Malondialdehyde oxidation of cartilage collagen by chondrocytes. Osteoarthritis Cartilage 2003;11:159–66.
26. Greenwald RA, Moy WW. Inhibition of collagen gelation by action of the superoxide radical. Arthritis Rheum 1979;22:251–59.
27. McCord JM. Free radicals and inflammation: Protection of synovial fluid by superoxide dismutase. Science 1974;185:529–30.
28. Loeser RF, et al. Detection of nitrotyrosine in aging and osteoarthritic cartilage: Correlation of oxidative damage with the presence of interleukin-1beta and with chondrocyte resistance to insulin-like growth factor 1. Arthritis Rheum 2002;46:2349–57.
29. Yudoh K, et al. Potential involvement of oxidative stress in cartilage senescence and development of osteoarthritis: Oxidative stress induces chondrocyte telomere instability and downregulation of chondrocyte function. Arthritis Res Ther 2005;7:R380–91.
30. Haklar U, et al. Oxygen radicals and nitric oxide levels in chondral or meniscal lesions or both. Clin Orthop 2002;403:135–42.

31. Sato H, et al. Antioxidant activity of synovial fluid, hyaluronic acid, and two subcomponents of hyaluronic acid: Synovial fluid scavenging effect is enhanced in rheumatoid arthritis patients. Arthritis Rheum 1988;31:63–71.

32. Briviba K, Seis H. Non-enzymatic antioxidant defense systems. In B Frei (ed.), *Natural Antioxidants in Human Health and Disease*. San Diego: Academic Press 1994:107–128.

33. Hankinson SE, et al. Nutrient intake and cataract extraction in women: A prospective study. BMJ 1992;305:335–39.

34. Peterkofsky B. Ascorbate requirement for hydroxylation and secretion of procollagen: Relationship to inhibition of collagen synthesis in scurvy. AM J Clin Nutr 1991;54: 1135S–40S.

35. Spanheimer RG, Bird TA, Peterkofsky B. Regulation of collagen synthesis and mRNA levels in articular cartilage of scorbutic guinea pigs. Arch Biochem Biophys 1986;246:33–41.

36. Houglum KP, Brenner DA, Chijkier M. Ascorbic acid stimulation of collagen biosynthesis independent of hydroxylation. Am J Clin Nutr 1991;54:1141S–43S.

37. Schwartz ER, Adamy L. Effect of ascorbic acid on arylsulfatase activities and sulfated proteoglycan metabolism in chondrocyte cultures. J Clin Invest 1977;60:96–106.

38. Sandell LJ, Daniel LC. Effects of ascorbic acid on collagen mRNA levels in short-term chondrocyte cultures. Connect Tiss Res 1988;17:11–22.

39. Meacock SCR, Bodmer JL, Billingham MEJ. Experimental OA in guinea pigs. J Exp Path 1990;71:279–93.

40. Schwartz ER, Oh WH, Leveille CR. Experimentally induced osteoarthritis in guinea pigs: Metabolic responses in articular cartilage to developing pathology. Arthritis Rheum 1981;24: 1345–55.

41. McAlindon TE, Jacques P, Zhang Y, Hannan MT, Aliabadi P, Weissman B, et al. Do antioxidant micronutrients protect against the development and progression of knee osteoarthritis? Arthritis Rheum 1996;39:648–56.

42. Kellgren J, Lawrence JS. *The Epidemiology of Chronic Rheumatism: Atlas of Standard Radiographs. Volume 2*. Oxford: Blackwell Scientific 1963.

43. Baker K, et al. The effects of vitamin C intake on pain in knee osteoarthritis (OA). Arthritis Rheum 2003;48:S422.

44. Kraus VB, et al. Ascorbic acid increases the severity of spontaneous knee osteoarthritis in a guinea pig model. Arthritis Rheum 2004;50:1822–31.

45. Bakker AC, et al. Overexpression of active TGF-beta-1 in the murine knee joint: Evidence for synovial-layer-dependent chondro-osteophyte formation. Osteoarthritis Cartilage 2001;9:128–36.

46. Scharstuhl A, et al. Inhibition of endogenous TGF-beta during experimental osteoarthritis prevents osteophyte formation and impairs cartilage repair. J Immunol 2002;169:507–14.

47. van Beuningen HM, et al. Osteoarthritis-like changes in the murine knee joint resulting from intra-articular transforming growth factor-beta injections. Osteoarthritis Cartilage 2000;8:25–33.

48. Barcellos-Hoff MH, Dix TA. Redox-mediated activation of latent transforming growth factor-beta 1. Mol Endocrinol 1996;10: 1077–83.

49. Jensen NH. Reduced pain from osteoarthritis in hip joint or knee joint during treatment with calcium ascorbate: A randomized, placebo-controlled cross-over trial in general practice. Ugeskr Laeger 2003;165:2563–66.

50. Panganamala RV, Cornwell DG. The effects of vitamin E on arachidonic acid metabolism. Ann NY Acad Sci 1982;393: 376–91.

51. Hirohata K, et al. Treatment of osteoarthritis of the knee joint at the state of hydroarthrosis. Kobe Med Sci 1965;11:65–66.

52. Doumerg C. Etude clinique experimentale de l'alpha-tocopheryle-quinone en rheumatologie et en reeducation. Therapeutique 1969;45:676–78.

53. Machetey I, Quaknine L. Tocopherol in osteoarthritis: A controlled pilot study. J Am Ger Soc 1978;26:328–30.

54. Scherak O, et al. Hochdosierte vitamin-E-therapie bei patienten mit aktivierter arthrose. Z Rheumatol 1990;49:369–73.

55. Blankenhorn G. Clinical efficacy of spondyvit (vitamin E) in activated arthroses. A multicenter, placebo-controlled, double-blind study. Z Orthop 1986;124:340–43.

56. Kaiki G, Tsuji H, Yonezawa T, Sekido H, Takano T, Yamashita S, et al. Osteoarthrosis induced by intra-articular hydrogen peroxide injection and running load. J Orthop Res 1990;8:731–40.

57. Wluka AE, et al. Supplementary vitamin E does not affect the loss of cartilage volume in knee osteoarthritis: A 2 year double blind randomized placebo controlled study. J Rheumatol 2002;29:2585–91.

58. Hunter DJ, et al. Cartilage volume must be normalized to bone surface area in order to provide satisfactory construct validity: The Framingham study. Osteoarthritis Cartilage 2004;12(B):M4.

59. Altman R, et al. Design and conduct of clinical trials in patients with osteoarthritis: Recommendations from a task force of the Osteoarthritis Research Society. Results from a workshop. Osteoarthritis Cartilage 1996;4:217–43.

60. Kiel DP. Vitamin D, calcium and bone: Descriptive epidemiology. In IH Rosenberg (ed.), *Nutritional Assessment of Elderly Populations: Measurement and Function*. 1995, New York: Raven Press. 1995:277–90.

61. Parfitt AM, et al. Vitamin D and bone health in the elderly. AM J Clin Nutr 1982;36:1014–31.

62. Radin EL, Paul IL, Tolkoff MJ. Subchondral changes in patients with early degenerative joint disease. Arthritis Rheum 1970;13:400–05.

63. Layton MW, et al. Examination of subchondral bone architecture in experimental osteoarthritis by microscopic computed axial tomography. Arthritis Rheum 1988;31:1400–05.

64. Milgram JW. Morphological alterations of the subchondral bone in advanced degenerative arthritis. Clin Orthop Rel Res 1983;173:293–312.

65. Kellgren JH, Lawrence JS. *The Epidemiology of Chronic Rheumatism: Atlas of Standard Radiographs. Volume 2*. Oxford, UK: Blackwell Scientific 1963.

66. Cartilage and bone in osteoarthrosis. Brit Med J 1976;2:4–5.

67. DequeckerJ, Mokassa L, Aerssens J. Bone density and osteoarthritis. J Rheumatol 1995;22(43):98–100.

68. Dedrick DK, et al. A longitudinal study of subchondral plate and trabecular bone in cruciate-deficient dogs with osteoarthritis followed up for 54 months. Arthritis Rheum 1993;36:1460–67.

69. Ledingham J, et al. Radiographic progression of hospital-referred osteoarthritis of the hip. Ann Rheum Dis 1993; 52:263–67.

70. Radin EL, Rose RM. Role of subchondral bone in the initiation and progression of cartilage damage. Clin Orthop Rel Res 1986;213:34–40.

71. Pottenger LA, Phillips FM, Draganich LF. The effect of marginal osteophytes on reduction of varus-valgus instability in osteoarthritic knees. Arthritis Rheum 1990;33:853–58.

72. Perry GH, Smith MJG, Whiteside CG. Spontaneous recovery of the joint space in degenerative hip disease. Ann Rheum Dis 1972;31:440–48.

73. Smythe SA. Osteoarthritis, insulin and bone density. J Rheumatol 1987;14:91–3.

74. Zhang Y, et al. Bone mineral density and risk of incident and progressive radiographic knee osteoarthritis in women: The Framingham Study. J Rheumatol 2000;27:1032–37.

75. Dieppe P, et al. Prediction of the progression of joint space narrowing in osteoarthritis of the knee by bone scintigraphy. Ann Rheum Dis 1993;52:557–63.

76. Corvol MT. Hormonal control of cartilage metabolism. Bull Schweiz Akad Med Wiss 1981;37:205–09.

77. Corvol MT, et al. Cartilage and vitamin D in vitro. Ann Endocrinol (Paris) 1981;42:482–87.

78. Tetlow LC, Woolley DE. Expression of vitamin D receptors and matrix metalloproteinases in osteoarthritic cartilage and human articular chondrocytes in vitro. Osteoarthritis Cartilage 2001;9:423–31.

79. McAlindon TE, et al. Relation of dietary intake and serum levels of vitamin D to progression of osteoarthritis of the knee among participants in the Framingham Study. Ann Intern Med 1996;125:353–59.

80. Lane NE, et al. Serum vitamin D levels and incident changes of radiographic hip osteoarthritis: A longitudinal study. Study of Osteoporotic Fractures Research Group. Arthritis Rheum 1999;42:854–60.

81. McLaughlin S, et al. Effect of 25-hydroxyvitamin D and parathyroid hormone on progression of radiographic knee osteoarthritis. Arthritis Rheum 2002;46(9):S299.

82. Carbone LD, et al. The relationship of antiresorptive drug use to structural findings and symptoms of knee osteoarthritis. Arthritis Rheum 2004;50:3516–25.

83. Demarco PJ, Constantinescu F. Does vitamin D supplementation contribute to the modulation of osteoarthritis by bisphosphonates? Arthritis Rheum 2005;52:1622–23.

84. Carbone LD, Barrow KD, Nevitt MC. Reply. Arthritis Rheum 2005;52:1623.

85. Thane CW, et al. Intake and sources of phylloquinone (vitamin K1): Variation with socio-demographic and lifestyle factors in a national sample of British elderly people. Br J Nutr 2002;87: 605–13.

86. Booth SL, Suttie JW. Dietary intake and adequacy of vitamin K. J Nutr 1998;128:785–88.

87. Furie B, Bouchard BA, Furie BC. Vitamin K-dependent biosynthesis of gamma-carboxyglutamic acid. Blood 1999;93: 1798–1808.

88. Loeser RF, et al. Human chondrocyte expression of growth-arrest-specific gene 6 and the tyrosine kinase receptor axl: Potential role in autocrine signaling in cartilage. Arthritis Rheum 1997;40:1455–65.

89. Hale JE, Fraser JD, Price PA. The identification of matrix Gla protein in cartilage. J Biol Chem 1988;263:5820–24.

90. Price PA. Gla-containing proteins of bone. Connect Tissue Res 1989;21:51–7; discussion 57–60.

91. Newman B, et al. Coordinated expression of matrix Gla protein is required during endochondral ossification for chondrocyte survival. J Cell Biol 2001;154:659–66.

92. Yagami K, et al. Matrix GLA protein is a developmental regulator of chondrocyte mineralization and, when constitutively expressed, blocks endochondral and intramembranous ossification in the limb. J Cell Biol 1999;147:1097–1108.

93. Zebboudj AF, Imura M, Bostrom K. Matrix GLA protein, a regulatory protein for bone morphogenetic protein-2. J Biol Chem 2002;277:4388–94.

94. Hara K, et al. Menatetrenone inhibits bone resorption partly through inhibition of PGE2 synthesis in vitro. J Bone Miner Res 1993;8:535–42.

95. Reddi K, et al. Interleukin 6 production by lipopolysaccharide-stimulated human fibroblasts is potently inhibited by naphthoquinone (vitamin K) compounds. Cytokine 1995;7:287–90.

96. Neuropathic joints: Degenerative joint disease. Arthritis Rheum 1970;13:571–78.

97. Hall JG, Pauli RM, Wilson KM. Maternal and fetal sequelae of anticoagulation during pregnancy. Am J Med 1980;68:122–40.

98. Luo G, et al. Spontaneous calcification of arteries and cartilage in mice lacking matrix GLA protein. Nature 1997;386:78–81.

99. Neogi T, et al. Is there an association between osteophytes and vitamin K intake? Arthritis Rheum 2004;50:S305.

100. Neogi T, et al. Low vitamin K is associated with osteoarthritis. Arthritis Rheum 2005;52:S455.

101. Utiger RD, Kashin-Beck disease: Expanding the spectrum of iodine-deficiency disorders. N Engl J Med 1998;339:1156–58.

102. Moreno-Reyes R, et al. Kashin-Beck osteoarthropathy in rural Tibet in relation to selenium and iodine status. N Engl J Med 1998;339:1112–20.

103. Jordan JM, et al. Low selenium levels are associated with increased risk for osteoarthritis of the knee. Arthritis Rheum 2005;52(9):1189.

104. Hill J, Bird HA. Failure of selenium-ace to improve osteoarthritis. Br J Rheumatol 1990;29:211–13.

105. Setnikar I, et al. Pharmacokinetics of glucosamine in man. Drug Res 1993;43:1109–13.

106. Setnikar I, Giachetti C, Zanolo G. Absorption, distribution and excretion of radio-activity after a single I.V. or oral administration of [14C]glucosamine to the rat. Pharmatherapeutica 1984;3:358.

107. Adebowale A, et al. The bioavailability and pharmacokinetics of glucosamine hydrochloride and low molecular weight chondroitin sulfate after single and multiple doses to beagle dogs. Biopharm Drug Dispos 2002;23:217–25.

108. Aghazadeh-Habashi A, et al. Single dose pharmacokinetics and bioavailability of glucosamine in the rat. J Pharm Sci 2002; 5:181–84.

109. Biggee BA, et al. Human serum glucosamine and sulfate levels after ingestion of glucosamine sulfate. Arthritis Rheum 2004;50(9):S657.

110. Persiani S, et al. Oral bioavailability and dose-proportionality of crystalline glucosamine sulfate in man. Arthritis Rheum 2004;50(9):S146.

111. Theodore G. Untrsuchung von 35 arhrosefallen, behandelt mit chondroitin schwefelsaure. Schweiz Rundschaue Med Praxis 1977;66.

112. Vach J, et al. Efect of glycosaminoglycan polysulfate on the metabolism of cartilage RNA. Arzneim Forsch/Drur Res 1984;34:607–09.

113. Ali SY. The degrdation of cartilage matrix by an intracellular protease. Biochem J 1964;93:611.

114. Hamerman D, et al. Glycosaminoglycans produced by human synovial cell cultures collagen. Rel Res 1982;2:313.

115. Lilja S, Barrach HJ. Normally sulfated and highly sulfated glycosaminoglycans affecting fibrillogenesis on type I and type II collagen in vitro. Exp Pathol 1983;23:173–81.

116. Knanfelt A. Synthesis of articular cartilage proteoglycans by isolated bovine chondrocytes. Agents Actions 1984;14:58–62.

117. Baici A, et al. Inhibition of human elastase from polymorphonuclear leucocytes by gold sodium thiomalate and pentosan polysulfate (SP-54). Biochem Pharmacol 1981;30:703–08.

118. Baici A. Interactions between human leucocytes elastase and chondroitin sulfate. Chem Biol Interactions 1984;51:11.

119. Marossy K. Interaction of the antitrypsin and elastase-like enzyme of the human granulocyte with glycosaminoglycans. Biochim Biophys Acta 1981;659:351–61.

120. De Gennaro F, et al. Effet du traitement par le sulfate de galactosaminoglucuronoglycane sur l'estase granulocytaire synovial de patients atteints d'osteoarthrose. Litera Rhumatologica 1992;14:53–60.

121. Committee on the Framework for Evaluating the Safety of the Dietary Supplements, National Research Council. Glucosamine: Prototype monograph summary. In Gail Spears (ed.), Dietary Supplements: A Framework for Evaluating Safety. Washington D.C.: National Academies Press 2005:363–64.

122. Marshall S, Yamasaki K, Okuyama R. Glucosamine induces rapid desensitization of glucose transport in isolated adipocytes by increasing GlcN-6-P levels. Biochem Biophys Res Commun 2005;329:1155–61.

123. Tannis AJ, Barban J, Conquer JA. Effect of glucosamine supplementation on fasting and non-fasting plasma glucose and serum insulin concentrations in healthy individuals. Osteoarthritis Cartilage 2004;12:506–11.

124. Yu JG, Boies SM, Olefsky JM. The effect of oral glucosamine sulfate on insulin sensitivity in human subjects. Diabetes Care 2003;26:1941–42.

125. Biggee BA, et al. The effect of oral glucosamine sulfate on oral glucose tolerance test in subjects with osteoarthritis. Arthritis Rheum 2005;52:1343.

126. Humphries DE, Silbert CK, Silbert JE. Glycosaminoglycan production by bovine aortic endothelial cells cultured in sulfate-depleted medium. J Biol Chem 1986;261:9122–27.

127. Silbert CK, et al. Effects of sulfate deprivation on the production of chondroitin/dermatan sulfate by cultures of skin fibroblasts from normal and diabetic individuals. Arch Biochem Biophys 1991;285:137–41.

128. Silbert JE, Sugumaran G, Cogburn JN. Sulphation of proteochondroitin and 4-methylumbelliferyl beta-D-xyloside-chondroitin formed by mouse mastocytoma cells cultured in sulphate-deficient medium. Biochem J 1993;296(1):119–26.

129. van der Kraan PM, et al. High susceptibility of human articular cartilage glycosaminoglycan synthesis to changes in inorganic sulfate availability. J Orthop Res 1990;8:565–71.

130. Morris ME, Levy G. Serum concentration and renal excretion by normal adults of inorganic sulfate after acetaminophen, ascorbic acid, or sodium sulfate. Clin Pharmacol Ther 1983;33:529–36.

131. Cordoba F, Nimni ME. Chondroitin sulfate and other sulfate containing chondroprotective agents may exhibit their effects by overcoming a deficiency of sulfur amino acids. Osteoarthritis Cartilage 2003;11:228–30.

132. D'Ambrosio E, et al. Glucosamine sulphate: a controlled clinical investigation in arthrosis. Pharmatherapeutica 1981;2: 504–08.

133. Crolle G, D'Este E. Glucosamine sulphate for the management of arthrosis: A controlled clinical investigation. Curr Med Res Opin 1980;7:104–09.

134. Drovanti A, Bignamini AA, Rovati AL. Therapeutic activity of oral glucosamine sulfate in osteoarthrosis: A placebo-controlled double-blind investigation. Clin Ther 1980;3:260–72.

135. Noack W, et al. Glucosamine sulfate in osteoarthitis of the knee. Osteoarthritis Cart 1994;2:51–9.

136. Pujalte JM, Llavore EP, Ylescupidez FR. Double-blind clinical evaluation of oral glucosamine sulphate in the basic treatment of osteoarthrosis. Curr Med Res Opin 1980;7:110–14.

137. Reichelt A, et al. Efficacy and safety of intramuscular glucosamine sulfate in osteoarthritis of the knee: A randomized, placebo-controlled, double-blind study. Drug Res 1994;44: 75–80.

138. Vaz AL. Double-blind clinical evaluation of the relative efficacy of ibuprofen and glucosamine sulphate in the management of osteoarthrosis of the knee in out-patients. Curr Med Res Opin 1982;8:145–49.

139. Vajaradul Y. Double-blind clinical evaluation of intra-articular glucosamine in outpatients with gonarthrosis. Clin Ther 1981;3:336–43.

140. Tapadinhas MJ, Rivera IC, Bignamini AA. Oral glucosamine sulphate in the management of arthrosis: Report on a multi-centre open investigation in Portugal. Pharmatherapeutica 1982;3: 157–68.

141. Vetter VG. Glukosamine in der therapie des degenerativen rheumatismus. Duet Med J 1965;16:446–49.

142. L'Hirondel JL. Klinische doppelblind-studie mit oral verabreichtem chondroitinsulfat gegen placebo bei der tibiofemoralen gonarthrose (125 patienten). Litera Rhumatologica 1992;14:77–84.

143. Kerzberg EM, et al. Combination of glycosaminoglycans and acetylsalicylic acid in knee osteoarthrosis. Scand J Rheumatol 1987;16:377–80.

144. Mazieres B, et al. Chondroitin sulfate in the treatment of gonarthrosis and coxarthrosis: 5-month results of a multicenter double-blind controlled prospective study using placebo. Rev Rhum Mal Osteoartic 1992;59:466–72.

145. Rovetta G. Galactosaminoglycuronoglycan sulfate (matrix) in therapy of tibiofibular osteoarthritis of the knee. Drugs Exptl Clin Res 1991;17:53–7.

146. Muller-Fassbender H, et al. Glucosamine sulfate compared to ibuprofen in osteoarthritis of the knee. Osteoarthritis and Cartilage 1994;2:61–9.

147. McAlindon TE, et al. Glucosamine and chondroitin for treatment of osteoarthritis: A systematic quality assessment and meta-analysis. JAMA 2000;283:1469–75.

148. Cohen J. Statistical Power Analysis for the Behavioral Sciences, Second Edition. Hillsdale, New Jersey: Lawrence Erlbaum Associates 1988.

149. Towheed TE, et al. Glucosamine therapy for treating osteoarthritis (Cochrane Review). Cochrane Database Syst Rev 2001;1-29.

150. Liang MH, et al. Comparative measurement efficiency and sensitivity of five health status instruments for arthritis research. Arthritis Rheum 1985;28:542–47.

151. Roos EM, Nilsdotter AK, Toksvig-Larsen S. Patient expectations suggest additional outcomes in total knee replacement. ACR Abstracts 2002;46:450.

152. Leeb BF, et al. A metaanalysis of chondroitin sulfate in the treatment of osteoarthritis. J Rheumatol 2000;27:205–11.

153. Poole C, Greenland S. Random-effects meta-analyses are not always conservative. Am J Epidemiol 1999;150:469–75.

154. Michel BA, et al. Chondroitins 4 and 6 sulfate in osteoarthritis of the knee: A randomized, controlled trial. Arthritis Rheum 2005;52:779–86.

155. Cibere J, et al. Randomized, double-blind, placebo-controlled glucosamine discontinuation trial in knee osteoarthritis. Arthritis Rheum 2004;51:738–45.

156. McAlindon T, et al. Conducting clinical trials over the internet: Feasibility study. BMJ 2003;327:484–87.

157. Hughes R, Carr A. A randomized, double-blind, placebo-controlled trial of glucosamine sulphate as an analgesic in osteoarthritis of the knee. Rheumatology (Oxford) 2002;41:279–84.

158. Rindone JP, et al. Randomized, controlled trial of glucosamine for treating osteoarthritis of the knee. West J Med 2000;172:91–4.

159. Cibere J, et al. Glucosamine sulfate and cartilage type II collagen degradation in patients with knee osteoarthritis: Randomized discontinuation trial results employing biomarkers. J Rheumatol 2005;32:896–902.

160. Towheed T, et al. Glucosamine therapy for treating osteoarthritis. Cochrane Database Syst Rev 2005;2:CD002946.

161. Clegg DO, et al. The efficacy of glucosamine and chondroitin sulfate in patients with painful knee osteoarthritis (OA): The Glucosamine/chondroitin Arthritis Invervention Trial (GAIT). Arthritis Rheum 2005;52(9):622.

162. Reginster JY, et al. Long-term effects of glucosamine sulphate on osteoarthritis progression: A randomised, placebo-controlled clinical trial. Lancet 2001;357:251–56.

163. Pavelka K, et al. Glucosamine sulfate use and delay of progression of knee osteoarthritis: A 3-year, randomized, placebo-controlled, double-blind study. Arch Intern Med 2002;162: 2113–23.

164. Altman R, et al. Design and conduct of clinical trials in patients with osteoarthritis: Recomendations from a task force of the Osteoarthritis Research Society. Osteoarthritis and Cartilage 1996;4:217–43.

165. Vignon E. Radiographic issues in imaging the progression of hip and knee osteoarthritis. J Rheumatol Suppl 2004;70:36–44.

166. Ernst E. Avocado-soybean unsaponifiables (ASU) for osteoarthritis: A systematic review. Clin Rheumatol 2003;22: 285–88.

167. Muller-Fassbender H. Double-blind clinical trial of S-adenosyl-methionine versus ibuprofen in the treatment of osteoarthritis. Am J Med 1987;83(5A):81–3.

168. Konig B. A long-term (two years) clinical trial with S-adenosyl-methionine for the treatment of osteoarthritis. Am J Med 1987;83(5A):89–94.

169. Vetter G. Double-blind comparative clinical trial with S-adeno-sylmethionine and indomethacin in the treatment of osteoarthritis. Am J Med 1987;83(5A):78–80.

170. Maccagno A, et al. Double-blind controlled clinical trial of oral S-adenosylmethionine versus piroxicam in knee osteoarthritis. Am J Med 1987;83(5A):72–7.

171. Glorioso S, et al. Double-blind multicentre study of the activity of S-adenosylmethionine in hip and knee osteoarthritis. Int J Clin Pharmacol Res 1985;5:39–49.

172. Najm WI, et al. S-adenosyl methionine (SAMe) versus celecoxib for the treatment of osteoarthritis symptoms: A double-blind cross-over trial. BMC Musculoskelet Disord 2004;5:6.

173. Altman RD, Marcussen KC. Effects of a ginger extract on knee pain in patients with osteoarthritis. Arthritis Rheum 2001;44:2531–38.

# Index

Note: Page numbers followed by f indicate figures; those followed by t indicate tables.

## A

Acetabular dysplasia, 6
Acetaminophen, 238
  dosage of, 238
  efficacy of, 238
  as first-line therapy, 188
  toxicity of, 238
  usage recommendations for, 185, 185t
  vs. NSAIDs, 183, 184t
Actin cytoskeleton, 41
Activities of daily living, modification of, 238
ADAMTS-4, 120
  mouse model for, 110
Adenosine monophosphate, in chondrocyte mechano-
    transduction, 42
Adipocytes
  precursor cells for, 86
  signaling in, 88, 89–90, 95–96
  size of, 85
Adipokines, 85–98. *See also* Adiponectin; Leptin; Resistin
  age-related changes in, 79–80
  in articular tissue, 94, 94t, 96–98
  bone effects on, 95
  cartilage effects of, 94, 96–98
  cytokines and, 95–96
  definition of, 86
  discovery of, 86–87
  functions of, 86, 86f, 87f
  growth factors and, 96–97
  in inflammation, 95–96
  in OA, 92–98
  osteophytes and, 96–97
  overview of, 85
  in pathophysiology, 87
  in synovial fluid, 93
  synthesis of, 88, 94, 94t, 95
  types of, 86, 91–92
Adiponectin, 87, 87f, 91. *See also* Adipokines
  anti-inflammatory effects of, 96
  cartilage effects of, 98
  in synovial fluid, 93
  synthesis of, 94, 94t
Adipose tissue. *See also* Weight
  cell size in, 85
  components of, 85
  as endocrine organ, 85–86
  functions of, 85–86
  metabolic activity of, 85–86
  in MRI, 151
  as secretory organ, 85–86
Adipsin, 86. *See also* Adipokines
Adult articular chondrocytes, 60
  turnover of, 80–81

Advanced glycation end products (AGEs), 63, 80, 81–82, 120
Aerobic exercise, 218t, 225
Age/aging
  advanced glycation end products and, 63, 80, 81–82, 120
  aggrecan and, 79
  cartilage alterations with, 79–83, 82t
    matrix, 79–80
    microstructural, 79, 82t
  chondrocytes and, 80–83, 82t
  collagen and, 79
  oxidative stress and, 82–83
  posttraumatic OA and, 77–78
  prevalence and, 2, 77, 78f
  as risk factor, 2, 77–79
    genetic factors and, 78–79
  signaling and, 81
Aggrecan, 24, 25, 115–116, 115f
  age-related changes in, 79
  animal models of, 107, 110
  biochemical markers for, 117–118, 118t
  biomechanical properties of, 36, 37
  degradation of, 117
  in enchondral ossification, 59, 59t, 60
  structure of, 115–116, 115f
  synthesis of, 117–118
Aggrecanases, 115, 115f, 1187
Agility training, 223
Agouti-related peptide, leptin and, 90
Albumin, in synovial fluid, 116
Alendronate
  mechanism of action of, 26
  therapeutic effects of, 26
Alignment. *See* Mal-alignment
Alkaline phosphatase, bone-specific, 117, 118t
Alpha synoviorthesis, 242
Alternative therapies. *See* Complementary and alternative
    medicine
Ambulatory aids, 238
Amino-terminal propeptides, in collagen turnover,
    117, 118, 118t
AN9P1 epitope, in aggrecan turnover, 115f, 117, 118t
Anabolic activity, in cartilage metabolism, 62
  age-related changes in, 81–82
  leptin and, 94–95
Analgesia, 238–239. *See also* Drug therapy
  acetaminophen in, 185, 185t, 188, 238
  complementary and alternative medicine in, 202–214
  NSAIDs in, 178–198, 238
  opioids in, 183–185, 184t, 238
  topical agents in, 183–185, 184t, 238
Angiogenesis, 25–26
  in enchondral ossification, 57, 58, 58t
  leptin in, 90

267

Animal models, 104–111
  of defective chondrogenesis, 58–60, 58t–59t
  of experimentally induced OA, 106–111
  gender differences in, 110
  mouse, 58–60, 58t–59t, 107, 110f
  muscle weakness in, 110
  Pond-Nuki dog, 107–110
  of spontaneous OA, 107
  in therapeutic studies, 107–110
  transgenic, 110
Ank, in enchondral ossification, 59, 60t
Anterior cruciate ligament tears, 7, 34. *See also* Joint
    instability/laxity
Anticatabolic bone agents, therapeutic monitoring
    for, 127–128
Anti-osteoarthritic drugs, 27–28, 239–241
  therapeutic monitoring for, 126–128, 127f
Antioxidants, 249–254
  vitamin C, 249–251, 249f
  vitamin D, 252–254, 253f
  vitamin E, 251–252, 252f
Anti-resorptive agents
  mechanism of action of, 27–28
  therapeutic effects of, 27
Apoptosis, 80
Appetite, leptin and, 90
Arachidonic acid, age-related increase in, 80
Arthritis
  degenerative. *See* Osteoarthritis
  rheumatoid
    biochemical markers in, 128
Arthritis Foundation, Quality Indicators Project of, 185, 186t
Arthrogenous muscle inhibition, 222
Arthroplasty, total joint, 243
Articular bone plate, 17
  thickness of, 17, 18f–19f, 19
  vascularization of, 25–26. *See also* Angiogenesis
Articular cartilage. *See* Cartilage
Articular chondrocyte cell lines, 65
Articular replacement, 243
Ascorbic acid, supplemental, 249–251, 249f
Aspirin. *See also* Nonsteroidal anti-inflammatory drugs
  antithrombotic effects of, ibuprofen interference
      with, 195, 196t–197t
  development of, 178
  nonselective NSAIDs and, 193–195, 196t–197t
Assessment
  for abnormal attitudes, 233
  composite indices for, 233–234
  for concomitant therapies, 233
  disease activity scores in, 234–235
  domains of interest in, 232
  for functional impairment, 232–233
  for pain, 232
  for range of motion, 233
  in treatment planning, 232–235
Assistive devices, 238
ATF-2, in enchondral ossification, 58, 58t
Athletic activity. *See also* Exercise
  in established OA, 238
  as risk factor, 6–7, 34–35
Auricular acupuncture, 204–205
Autoantibodies, as biochemical markers, 123
Autocrine signaling. *See also* Signaling
  in chondrocyte mechano-transduction, 43–45
Autologous chondrocyte transplantation, 65, 241
Avocado/soybean unsaponifiables, 240

**B**

Basic fibroblast growth factor
  age-related changes in, 81
  in chondrocyte mechano-transduction, 45

Behavioral strategies, 247–249, 248t
Biochemical markers, 113–128
  for aggrecan, 117–118, 118t
  autoantibodies as, 123
  in bone, 117, 118t
  in cartilage, 117–121, 118t
  clearance of, 124
  clinical uses of, 124–128
  combination assays for, 122–123
  confounding factors of, 123–124
  in diagnosis, 124–125, 124f
  identification of, new methods for, 122–123
  metabolomic analysis for, 123
  in progression prediction, 125–126, 125t
  proteomic analysis for, 122–123
  in rheumatoid arthritis, 128
  sources of variability in, 124
  synovial, 118t, 121–122
  of systemic inflammation, 121
  in treatment monitoring, 126–128, 127f
  for type II collagen, 115f, 118–120, 118t, 119f
  in urine, 123–124, 123f
Biofeedback, 207–209, 208t, 223
Biomechanics. *See* Mechanical stress
Bisphosphonates, 241
  therapeutic effects of, 26
  treatment monitoring for, 127–128
Body fat. *See* Adipose tissue
Body mass index. *See also* Obesity; Weight
  as risk factor, 8, 33–34
Bone
  biochemical markers for, 117, 118t. *See also*
      Biochemical markers
  biology and biochemistry of, 113–114
  biomechanical properties of, 35–36, 35t.
      *See also* Mechanical stress
  cortical (compact), 16
  cross-talk with cartilage, 22–26
  density of
    in pathophysiology, 18–19, 21, 35–36
    as risk factor, 10
  extracellular matrix of, 16, 17–18, 113–114
  flat, 16
  formation of, 16–17. *See also* Bone remodeling/turnover
    in normal bone, 16–17
    in OA, 19–22
  functions of, 16
  lamellar, 18
  leptin effects on, 95
  long, 16
  pathologic findings in, 104, 107t
  as primary pathogenetic organ, 16, 85
  structure of, 16, 18, 18f
  subchondral. *See* Subchondral bone
  trabecular (cancellous), 16
    density of, 18–19, 21, 35–36
    MRI of, 36
Bone alkaline phosphatase, 117, 118t
Bone marrow, 16
  edema of, 26
    MRI of, 158
  lesions of, as risk factor, 9–10
  subchondral. *See also* Subchondral bone
    MRI of, 157–158
Bone matrix, 16, 17–18, 113–114
Bone mineral density
  in pathophysiology, 18–19, 21, 35–36
  as risk factor, 10
Bone morphogenetic protein, 17
  anabolic activity of, 62
    age-related changes in, 81
  for cartilage defects, 65

Bone morphogenetic protein *(Continued)*
  in chondrocyte differentiation and proliferation, 55
  in enchondral ossification, 57
  in limb development, 54, 55, 55f
  in OA, 61
Bone remodeling/turnover, 19–21
  biochemical markers for, 117, 118t
  in normal bone, 16–17
  in OA, 19–21
  osteoblasts in, 21–22
Bone resorption, 19–21
  biochemical markers for, 117, 118t
  osteoprotegerin in, 27
  RANKL in, 27
Bone sialoprotein, 104, 113–114, 118t
Bone-specific alkaline phosphatase, 117, 118t
Braces, knee, 218t, 225, 237
Bronchoconstriction, prostaglandin-induced, 181

**C**

Calciferol, 252–254, 253f
Calcification, of cartilage, age-related increase in, 79
Calcitonin, therapeutic effects of, 26
Calcium stretch-activated ion channels, 41, 41f, 45
cAMP, in chondrocyte mechano-transduction, 42
Camptodactyl-arthropathy–coxa vara–pericarditis
    syndrome, 117
Cancellous (trabecular) bone, 16. *See also* Bone;
    Subchondral bone
  density of, 18–19, 21, 35–36
  MRI of, 36
Canes, 238
Capsaicin, 238
Carboxymethyl lysine, 80
Cardiovascular system
  NSAID toxicity in, 189–195, 191t–192t, 194t
  prostaglandin effects on, 181
Cartilage. *See also* Chondrocyte(s)
  adipokines and, 94, 96–98
  age-related changes in, 79–83, 82t
  angiogenesis in, 25–26
  biochemical markers for, 117–121, 118t. *See also*
      Biochemical markers
  biochemical/metabolic changes in, 24–26
  biology and biochemistry of, 114–116
  biomechanical properties of, 36–37
  calcification of, age-related increase in, 79
  components of, 23–24
  cross-talk with bone, 22–26
  development of
    chondrocyte differentiation in, 55–57
    chondrocyte proliferation in, 55–57, 55f, 56f
    chondrogenesis in, 53–55, 55f
    steps in, 55f
  epiphyseal, 16
  exercise effects on, 37–38
  extracellular matrix of, 24, 36–37
    age-related changes in, 24, 36–37
  immobilization effects on, 37–38
  leptin in, 94
  lipids in, age-related increase in, 79–80
  loading effects on, 37–38. *See also* Mechanical stress
  micro-cracks in, 25
  normal, 23–24
  nutrition of, 22–23
  pathologic changes in, 24–25, 104, 107t
  post-traumatic changes in, 25–26, 34–35
  remodeling/turnover of, 24–25
    age-related decrease in, 79
  structure of, 23–24
  Young's modulus of, 37
Cartilage explant culture system, 64

Cartilage matrix proteins, post-translational modification of,
    119–120
Cartilage morphometry, 159–162
  MRI in, 159–162
Cartilage oligomeric matrix protein (COMP), 104, 106, 120–121
  in progression prediction, 125
Cartilage T2 mapping, 165–167, 166f
Cartilage volume
  disease progression and, 161–162
  gender differences in, 161
  height and, 161
  MRI measurement of, 160–162
Cartilage-derived morphogenetic proteins, anabolic activity of, 62
Cartrofen, 241
Catabolic activity, in cartilage metabolism, 62
  age-related changes in, 81–82
Catenin, in chondrogenesis, 58
Cathepsins, 115, 117, 118t
Celecoxib. *See also* Coxibs
  cardiovascular toxicity of, 189–190, 191t, 194t
  dosage of, 182, 182t
  pharmacokinetics of, 182, 182t
  structure of, 181, 182f
  vs. acetaminophen, 184t
Cell lines, chondrocyte, 65
Chemical-shift artifacts, in MRI, 151–152
Chemical-shift fat suppression, in MRI, 151
Chemokines, 63
Chitinase-like proteins, 118t, 121
Chondrocalcinosis, age-related increase in, 79
Chondrocyte(s), 23–25. *See also* Cartilage
  adult articular, 60
    turnover of, 80–81
  age-related changes in, 80–83, 82t
  anabolic activity in, 61–62, 81–82
  apoptosis of, 80
  catabolic activity in, 62, 81–82
  chemokines and, 63
  differentiation of, 53, 55–57
    hypertrophic, 57, 58
  in enchondral ossification, 57
  glucose transport in, 60
  hypertrophic, 57
    culture models of, 64
  hypoxia and, 60–61
  leptin and, 94–95, 97–98
  matrix remodeling in, 61
  mechanical stress on, 36–38
    response to, 38–45. *See also* Mechano-transduction
  mechano-coupling and, 38
  metabolism in, 60–61
  in normal cartilage, 23–24
  in OA, 24–25
  origin of, 53–55, 54f
  overview of, 53
  phenotypic destabilization in, 25
  phenotypic modulation in, 61
  precursor cells for, 53–55, 54f
  proliferation of, 55–57, 55f, 56f
    age and, 80–81
  replicative senescence in, 81
  signaling in, 62–63. *See also* Signaling
  therapeutic targeting of, 65–66
  transplantation of, 65, 241
  turnover of, 80–81
Chondrocyte clones, 80–81
Chondrocyte culture models, 63–66
  articular chondrocyte, 64
  cell lines for, 65
  hypertrophic chondrocyte, 64
  therapeutic applications of, 65–66
Chondrocyte reaction patterns, 111f

Chondrodysplasia *(cho/cho)* mouse, 59–60

Chondrogenesis, 53–55
  defective, mouse models of, 58–60, 58t–59t
  novel mediators of, 57–58

Chondrogenic cell lines, 65

Chondroitin sulfate, pharmacologic, 240, 257–261, 257f

Chondroitin sulfate epitopes, in aggrecan synthesis, 117–118, 118t

Chondrons, 37

Chondroprogenitor cells, 53–54, 54f

Chondrosarcoma cell lines, 65

Cigarette smoking, as risk factor, 9

Client education, 235–236

Clones, chondrocyte, 80–81

c-Maf, in enchondral ossification, 58, 58t

Codeine, 238
  vs. NSAIDs, 184–185, 184t

Cognitive behavioral therapy, 207–209, 208t

Col genes, in enchondral ossification, 57, 58, 59, 59t, 60

Colitis, NSAID-related, 189

Coll 2-1 assay, 119–120

Collagen
  age-related changes in, 79
  in bone, 17, 18, 21
  in cartilage, 24, 25, 114–115, 114f
    biomechanical properties of, 36–37
  loading-induced deformation of, MRI of, 167–168
  in OA, 61
  recapitulation of embryonic development in, 61
  in synovium, 116
  type I, 17, 18, 116
    components of, 21
    in normal bone, 17, 18
    in OA, 21, 25
  type II, 24, 114–115
    biochemical markers for, 115f, 117, 118–119, 118t, 119f
    biomechanical properties of, 36–37
    degradation of, 114–115, 118t, 119
    post-translational modification of, 119–120, 120f
    structure of, 114, 114f
    synthesis of, 114, 114f, 118, 118t
  type IIA, 61
  type III, 116
  type V, 116
  type VI, 24, 36, 37, 114, 116
  type IX, 24, 36, 37, 114
  type X, 25
  type XI, 24, 36, 114

Collagenase, 115. *See also* Matrix metalloproteinase(s)

Collagenase neoepitopes, in collagen degradation, 117, 118t, 119, 119f, 120f

Collagenase-3, 25, 26

Collagen-sensitive magnetic resonance imaging, 165–167

Compact (cortical) bone, 16
  biomechanical properties of, 35–36, 35t

Complementary and alternative medicine, 202–214. *See also* Nutritional interventions
  acupuncture in, 202–205, 204f
  herbal remedies in, 205–207
  hydrotherapy in, 204
  mind-body therapies in, 207–209, 208t
  overview of, 202
  tai chi in, 209–213, 210f, 211f
  yoga in, 213–214

Congenital joint disorders, as risk factor, 6

Congestive heart failure, NSAID-related, 190

Contrast media, in magnetic resonance imaging, 149–150

Core binding factor, 57

Cortical bone, 16. *See also* Bone
  biomechanical properties of, 35–36, 35t

Cortical end plate. *See* Subchondral bone, end plate zone of

Corticosteroids, intra-articular, 241–242

Coxibs. *See also* Nonsteroidal anti-inflammatory drugs
  adverse effects of
    cardiovascular, 189–195, 191t–192t, 194t
    central nervous system, 195, 198t
    cutaneous, 195, 198t
    gastrointestinal, 185–189, 187t, 189f
    renal, 195, 198t
  dosage of, 182, 182t
  efficacy of, 183–185
  pharmacokinetics of, 182, 182t
  structure of, 181, 183f
  usage recommendations for, 185, 185t
  utilization patterns for, 195
  vs. acetaminophen, 184t

C-propeptide, in collagen synthesis, 117, 118, 118t

C-reactive protein, 104
  as biomarker, 113
  in systemic inflammation, 121

Crutches, 238

C-telopeptide (CTX-I/II), 117, 118t
  bone marrow lesions and, 10
  in collagen degradation, 117, 118t, 119, 119f, 120f, 123f
  in progression prediction, 125, 125f, 125t, 126, 126f
  in treatment monitoring, 127–128, 127f

Culture, chondrocyte, 63–66. *See also* Chondrocyte culture models

Cutaneous drug reactions, NSAID-related, 98t, 195l

Cyclic AMP, in chondrocyte mechano-transduction, 42

Cyclooxygenase inhibitors. *See* Coxibs

Cytokines, 22, 25, 62
  in adipose tissue. *See* Adipokines
  catabolic, 62
  leptin and, 95–96
  in mechano-transduction, 43–45, 44f, 63

**D**

Debridement, 242–243

Decorin, 37

Delayed gadolinium-enhanced magnetic resonance imaging, 164–165

Dell mouse model, 110

Deoxypyridinoline, 114, 117, 118t

Developmental disorders, as risk factors, 6

Devil's claw, 206

Dexamethasone, leptin and, 88, 89t

dGERMIC magnetic resonance imaging, 164

Diacerein, 239
  vs. devil's claw, 206

Diagnostic criteria, 1–2, 3t

Diclofenac. *See also* Nonsteroidal anti-inflammatory drugs
  adverse effects of, 185–189
  dosage of, 182, 182t
  hepatotoxicity of, 188
  pharmacokinetics of, 182, 182t
  structure of, 181, 182f
  topical, 185, 238
  vs. acetaminophen, 184t
  vs. acupuncture, 203
  vs. celecoxib, 191t

Diet. *See* Nutritional interventions

Disease activity scores, 234–235

Disease progression
  cartilage volume and, 161–162
  radiographic measurement of
    in hip, 136–137, 136t
    in knee, 137–140, 138t, 139f, 139t
  risk factors for, 33

Disease-modifying osteoarthritic drugs, 27–28, 239–241
  therapeutic monitoring for, 126–128, 127f

Dislocation, congenital hip, 6

Dog models, 107–110. *See also* Animal models
Doxycycline, 241
Drug reactions, cutaneous, NSAID-related, 98t, 195l
Drug therapy
  acetaminophen in, 185, 185t, 188, 238
  in animal models, 107–110
  antibiotics in, 241
  bisphosphonates in, 26, 127–128, 241
  disease-modifying drugs in, 27–28, 126–128, 127f, 239–241
    therapeutic monitoring for, 126–128, 127f
  intra-articular steroids in, 241–242
  NSAIDs in, 178–198, 238, 239. *See also* Nonsteroidal
    anti-inflammatory drugs
  opioids in, 183–185, 184t, 238
  SYSADOA agents in, 239
  topical agents in, 183–185, 184t

**E**

Eating, leptin and, 90
Edema, bone marrow, 26
  MRI of, 158
Education, patient, 235–236
846 epitope, in aggrecan synthesis, 117–118, 118t
Elbow osteoarthritis, in throwing athletes, 7
Electro-acupuncture, 204
Eltenac, 238
Enchondral ossification, 57–58
  chondrocyte hypertrophy and, 57
  novel mediators of, 57–58
Epidemiology, 1–10
  incidence and, of symptomatic OA, 4, 4f
  key outcomes of, 5
  prevalence and
    of pathologic OA, 2
    of radiographic OA, 2–4
    of symptomatic OA, 4–5
Epiphysis, 16
Epitopes, in aggrecan turnover, 115, 115f, 117, 118t
ERK/MAPK pathway, in chondrocyte mechano-
  transduction, 43, 45
Erythema multiforme, NSAID-related, 195
Estrogen. *See also* Gender differences
  protective effects of, 9
Etoricoxib. *See also* Coxibs
  dosage of, 182, 182t
  pharmacokinetics of, 182, 182t
  structure of, 181, 182f
European League Against Rheumatism (EULAR)
  guidelines, 235, 235t
Exercise
  aerobic, 225, 236–237
  cartilage response to, 37–38
  in established OA, 238
  in pathogenesis, 6–7, 34–35
  in treatment, 218t, 225, 236–237
Exercises
  range of motion, 236–237
  strengthening, 218t, 221–222, 222f, 236–237
    hamstring, 221–222
    in motor control relearning, 223, 225f
    quadriceps, 221
    with theraband, 223, 225f
Extracellular matrix
  of bone, 16, 17–18, 113–114
  of cartilage, 24, 36–37
    age-related changes in, 24, 36–37

**F**

Fairbank's sign, 159
Falls, prevention of, 229
Fast-spin magnetic resonance imaging, 146–147, 147f, 153

Fat, body. *See* Adipose tissue
Fat suppression, in MRI, 151
Femoral head, gross pathology of, 108f
Fertility, leptin and, 90–91
Fibroblast growth factor
  anabolic activity of, 62
  in chondrocyte differentiation and proliferation, 55–56
  in limb development, 54, 55f
Fibromodulin, in enchondral ossification, 59, 59t
5D4 epitope, in aggrecan turnover, 115f, 117, 118t
Fixed flexion view, of knee, 135, 138–140, 138t, 139t
Flat bones, 16
Focal adhesions, 41
Footwear
  modified, 228
  orthotics for, 218t, 225–229, 226f, 237
  selection of, 228–229, 228f
Force attenuation, in joint components, 35, 35t
Fra2, in enchondral ossification, 58, 58t
Free radicals, oxidative stress and, 82–83, 119
Functional magnetic resonance imaging, 167–168

**G**

G proteins, in chondrocyte mechano-transduction, 42
Gadd45ß, in enchondral ossification, 57, 58, 58t, 59
Gadolinium, as MRI contrast agent, 150
Gadolinium stretch-activated ion channels, 41, 41f, 45
Gait analysis, 217–218
  varus thrust in, 220
Gait retraining, 224–225
Gastrointestinal toxicity, of NSAIDs, 185–189, 187t, 189f
Gastroprotection, for NSAIDs, 187–188, 189f
Gelatinases, 115. *See also* Matrix metalloproteinase(s)
Gender differences
  in adipokines in synovial fluid, 93
  in animal models, 110
  in cartilage volume, 161
  in incidence, 4, 4f
Gene knockout models, 110
Genetic factors
  in OA, 5–6, 22
    in chondrocyte differentiation, 55, 55f
    in free leptin levels, 97
    mechanical stress and, 46
    in mouse models, 57–60, 58t–59t
  protective, 78–79
Glc-Gal-PYD, 121–122, 122f
Glucosamine, 239–240, 257–261, 257f
Glucose transporters (GLUTs), in chondrocytes, 60
Glucosyl-galactosyl-pyridinoline, 121–122, 122f
Glycoproteins, in extracellular matrix, 17
Glycosaminoglycan(s), 24
  in aggrecan, 115–116
  exercise effects on, 37–38
  immobilization effects on, 37–38
  measurement of, dGERMIC MRI in, 164–165
  subsynovial, 117
Glycosaminoglycan polysulfuric acid, 240
Glycosaminoglycan-peptide complex, 240
Glycosaminoglycan-sensitive magnetic resonance
  imaging, 163
Gradient echo magnetic resonance imaging, 147–148, 148f
  in cartilage morphometry, 159
Grading, Kellgren-Lawrence system for, 1, 2t, 131–132
Gross pathology, 105, 109f
  early-stage, 105–106, 109f
Growth factors
  adipokines and, 96–97
  age-related changes in, 81
  in chondrocyte mechano-transduction, 43–45
  in limb development, 54, 55f

Growth plate, 16
  formation of, 55, 55f
Guided imagery, 207–209, 208t
Gyromagnetic ratio, 144

**H**

Hamstring exercises, 221–222
Hand osteoarthritis
  diagnostic criteria for, 3t
  prevalence of, 2–5, 4f
  risk factors for, 5–10, 35
*Harpagophytum procumbens* (devil's claw), 206
Heart failure, NSAID-related, 190
Helix II, in collagen degradation, 118t, 119–120, 119f, 120f
Hemangiopoietin, 116–117
Hematopoiesis, leptin in, 90
Hepatocyte growth factor, 26
Hepatotoxicity, of NSAIDs, 188–189, 238
Herbal remedies, 205–207. *See also* Complementary and
    alternative medicine
Hereditary factors, 6
High-heeled shoes, knee loading with, 229–230, 229f
Hip
  radiography of. *See also* Radiography
    in joint space measurement, 133, 134f
    in progression measurement, 136–137, 136t
  strengthening exercises for, 222, 222f
Hip dysplasia, 6
Hip osteoarthritis
  acupuncture for, 204
  diagnostic criteria for, 3t
  postoperative, 34
  prevalence of, 2–5, 4f
  risk factors for, 5–10, 34–35
Hip replacement, 243
Homeobox (Hox) genes
  in enchondral ossification, 57–58
  in limb development, 54, 55f
Hormone replacement therapy, protective effects of, 9
Human cartilage glycoprotein 39, 121
  anabolic activity of, 62
Human chondrosarcoma cell lines, 65
Hyaluronan, 116, 118t, 121
  in progression prediction, 126
Hyaluronic acid, intra-articular, 242
Hydrotherapy, 204, 218t, 222
Hydroxyapatite crystals, in extracellular matrix, 17
Hypertension, NSAID-related, 190
Hypertrophic chondrocytes, 57
  culture models of, 64
Hypnosis, 207–209, 208t
Hypoxia-inducible factor 1α, 58, 60–61

**I**

Ibuprofen. *See also* Nonsteroidal anti-inflammatory drugs
  adverse effects of, 185–189
  aspirin and, 195
  dosage of, 182, 182t
  pharmacokinetics of, 182, 182t
  structure of, 181, 182f
  vs. acetaminophen, 184t
  vs. celecoxib, 191t
  vs. lumiracoxib, 192t
Ihh (Indian hedgehog), in chondrocyte
    proliferation, 56–57
Imaging studies, 1–2. *See also* Magnetic resonance imaging;
    Radiography
Immobilization, cartilage response to, 37–38
Incidence, of symptomatic OA, 4, 4f
Indian hedgehog (Ihh), in chondrocyte proliferation, 56–57
Infertility, leptin in, 90–91

Inflammation
  adipokines in, 95–96
  biochemical markers of, 118t, 121
  cytokines in. *See* Cytokines
  prostaglandins in, 179
Insoles, 218t, 225–227, 237
  shock-absorbing, 226
  textured, 226–227
  wedged, 225–227, 226f
Instability
  animal models of, 107
  knee loading and, 220
  as risk factor, 7, 34, 107, 220
Insulin, leptin and, 88, 89t, 91
Insulin resistance, 87
  in metabolic syndrome, 92–93
Insulin-like growth factor, 21, 22
  adipokines and, 96–97
  anabolic activity of, 62
    age-related changes in, 81
  in chondrocyte mechano-transduction, 43
Insulin-like growth factor binding protein, anabolic
    activity of, 62
  age-related changes in, 81
Integrins
  age-related changes in, 81
  as chondrocyte mechano-receptors, 39–41, 40f, 43–44
  in enchondral ossification, 57, 59, 59t
  focal adhesions for, 41
Interleukin(s), 22, 25
  catabolic activity of, 62
  in chondrocyte mechano-transduction, 43–45, 44f
  leptin and, 95
  in osteophyte formation, 20
Interleukin-2 inhibitor, intra-articular, 242
Intervertebral disk disease, urinary CTX-II in, 123–124, 123f
Intra-articular injections, 241–242
  of bone morphogenetic protein, 66
  of hyaluronic acid, 242
  of interleukin-2 inhibitor, 242
  of steroids, 241–242
  of transforming growth factor-β, 66
Iodine, supplemental, 256–257
Ion channels, as chondrocyte mechano-receptors, 41, 41f, 45
Isoproterenol, leptin and, 88, 89t

**J**

JAK-STAT pathway
  in chondrocyte mechano-transduction, 43
  leptin and, 89–90
Jogging, knee OA and, 6–7, 34
Joint, normal, structure and function of, 104, 105f
Joint injuries, as risk factor, 7–8, 34–35
Joint instability/laxity
  animal models of, 107
  knee loading and, 220
  as risk factor, 7, 34, 107, 220
Joint lavage and debridement, 242–243
Joint laxity. *See* Joint instability/laxity
Joint loading
  deficient/excessive, 106f
  in knee. *See* Knee loading
  physiology of, 104, 106f
Joint replacement surgery, 243
Joint space narrowing
  as diagnostic criterion, 1
  radiographic measurement of, 131–132, 133f. *See also*
      Radiography
    in hip, 133, 134f, 136–137, 136t
    in knee, 133–135, 137–140, 138f, 139f, 139t
    in progression assessment, 136–140, 136t, 138f, 139f, 139t

**K**

Kashin-Beck disease, 256–257
Kellgren-Lawrence grading system, 1, 2t, 131–132
Keratane sulfate, in aggrecan degradation,
    115, 115f, 117, 118t
Kidney
    NSAID-related injury of, 195, 198t
    prostaglandin effects on, 181
Knee braces, 218t, 225, 237
Knee instability/laxity
    animal models of, 107
    mechanical stress and, 220
    as risk factor, 7, 34, 107, 220
Knee loading, 217–220
    analysis of, 217–218
    bracing and, 225
    contributory factors in, 224f
    deficient/excessive, 106f
    local mechanical factors in, 218–219
    mal-alignment and, 219–220, 219f, 220f
    muscle co-contraction and, 223
    neuromuscular compensatory mechanisms
        for, 223, 224f
    physiology of, 104, 106f
    shoe type and, 229–230
    toe-out angle and, 224
    walking speed and, 224–225
Knee osteoarthritis
    acupuncture for, 203–204
    diagnostic criteria for, 3t
    gait analysis in, 217–218
    mechanical stress and, 217–220
    physical therapy for, 217–229
    postoperative, 7, 8, 34
    prevalence of, 2–5, 4f
    radiography in, 133–135, 133f. See also Radiography
        in progression measurement, 137–140, 138t, 139f, 139t
    risk factors for, 5–10, 34–35
Knee replacement, 243
Knee taping, 218t
Knockout models, 110

**L**

Lamellar bone, 18. See also Bone
Larmor frequency, 144, 149
Lateral wedges, for shoes, 225–227, 226f
Lavage and debridement, 242–243
Legg-Calvé-Perthes disease, 6
Leptin, 4, 21–22, 86, 88–91. See also Adipokines
    anabolic effects of, 94–95
    in angiogenesis, 90
    in articular tissue, 94, 96–98
    biological activities of, 90
    bone effects of, 95
    cartilage effects of, 96–98
    central effects of, 90
    chondrocytes and, 94–95, 97–98
    discovery of, 86–87, 88
    in fertility and pregnancy, 90–91
    functions of, 87, 87f
    growth factors and, 96–97
    in hematopoiesis, 90
    in inflammation, 95–96
    insulin and, 91
    interleukin-2 and, 95
    matrix metalloproteinases and, 97
    in metabolic syndrome, 92–93
    ob gene and, 88, 89, 89f, 93, 97
    osteophytes and, 96–97
    peripheral effects of, 90–91
    receptors for, 89, 89f

Leptin (Continued)
    regulation of, 88, 88t
    secretion of, 89t
    in signaling, 88, 89–90, 95–96
    in synovial fluid, 93, 97
    synthesis of, 88, 94, 94t, 95
Lesquesnes' hip profile, 133, 134f
Leukotriene, 21, 26
Lifestyle interventions, 247–249, 248t
Limb alignment. See Mal-alignment
Limb development, 54–55, 55f
Lipids
    in cartilage, age-related increase in, 79–80
    metabolism of, 21–22
Lipoprotein lipase, 86. See also Adipokines
Liver disease, NSAID-related, 188–189, 238
Long bones, 16. See also Bone
Lubricin, 116
Lumiracoxib, 181–182. See also Coxibs
    cardiovascular toxicity of, 189–190, 191t, 194
    dosage of, 182, 182t
    pharmacokinetics of, 182, 182t
    structure of, 182, 183f
Lymphocytes, leptin and, 95–96
Lyon-schuss view, of knee, 135, 138–140, 138t, 139f, 139t

**M**

c-Maf, in enchondral ossification, 58, 58t
Magic angle, in MRI, 151
Magnetic resonance imaging, 1–2, 143–168
    advantages of, 143
    of articular cartilage
        focal lesions in, 153, 154t
        grade I lesions in, 155–156, 156f
        grade II lesions in, 156–157, 156f
        grade III lesions in, 157, 157f
        grade IV lesions in, 157, 157f
        normal findings in, 153–155, 154f, 154t, 155f
        parameters for, 162, 163t
        technical considerations in, 153
    artifacts in, 151–152
        chemical shift, 151–152
        magnetic susceptibility, 152
        motion, 151
        truncation, 152
    in cartilage T2 mapping, 165–167, 166f
    clinical applications of, 152–159
    collagen-sensitive, 165–167
    contrast media in, 149–150
    cost of, 142–143
    delayed gadolinium-enhanced (dGERMIC), 164–165
    diamagnetic tissues in, 151
    Fairbank's sign in, 159
    fat suppression in, 151
    ferromagnetic tissues in, 151
    functional, 167–168
    glycosaminoglycan-sensitive, 163
    gradient echo, 147–148, 148f
        in cartilage morphometry, 159
    image contrast in, 148–151
        magnetization transfer and, 150–151
        proton density and, 149
        T1 relaxation time and, 149–150
        T2 relaxation time and, 149, 150
        tissue anisotropy and, 151
    image generation in, 146
    of knee, normal findings on, 105f
    limitations of, 152–153
    magic angle in, 151
    magnetization transfer techniques in, 165
    of meniscal tears, 158–159

Magnetic resonance imaging *(Continued)*
  metallic implants in, 152
  of osteophytes, 158
  Outerbridge classification for, 153–157, 154t
  overview of, 143–144
  paramagnetic tissues in, 151
  in parametric mapping, 162–167
  physics of, 144–152
  proteoglycan-sensitive, 162–165, 163t
  pulse sequences in, 146–148
  in quantitative cartilage morphometry, 159–162
  RARE, 147, 147f
  research applications of, 143, 159–167
  scoring systems for, 153
  sensitivity of, 152–153
  signal in, 144–146
  sodium, 162, 163t
  spin echo, 145–146, 145f
    conventional, 146–147, 147f
    fast-spin, 146–147, 147f, 153
  STIR technique in, 151
  of subchondral marrow abnormalities, 157–158
  T1rho, 163
  T1-weighted images in, 149–150
  T2-weighted images in, 149, 150
  3D, 153
  tissue sensitivity of, 152–153
  of total joint involvement, 152–153
  of trabecular bone, 36
  2D, 153
  vs. radiography, 1–2
Magnetic susceptibility artifacts, in MRI, 152
Magnetization transfer, in MRI, 150, 165
Mal-alignment
  bone marrow edema and, 26
  bracing for, 225
  knee loading and, 219–220, 219f, 220f
  obesity and, 33–34
  osteotomy for, 243
  as risk factor, 4, 8, 9
Management. *See* Treatment
Mapping, MRI
  cartilage T2, 165–166
  parametric, 162–167
Marrow. *See* Bone marrow
Matrilin, in enchondral ossification, 59, 60t
Matrix metalloproteinase(s), 58–59, 58t
  in aggrecan degradation, 115f, 117, 118t
  in bone, 21
  in cartilage, 25, 26, 62
    age-related changes in, 81
  in collagen degradation, 115
  COMP and, 120
  in enchondral ossification, 57
  leptin and, 97
  in OA, 62, 121
  in synovial fluid, 121
Matrix metalloproteinase inhibitors, 120
Matrix-degrading proteinases, 62–63
Mechanical stress, 33–46, 34f
  alignment and, 33–34
  animal studies of, 37–38, 46
  bone effects of, 35–36
  cartilage effects of, 36–38
  force attenuation in joints and, 35, 35t
  gait analysis and, 217–218
  genetic factors in, 46
  on knee, 217–220, 223, 224f. *See also* Knee loading
  knee laxity and, 220
  MRI imaging studies of, 167–168
  muscle co-contraction and, 223

Mechanical stress *(Continued)*
  normal joint loading and, 104, 106f
  obesity and, 33–34
  occupational sources of, 34–35
  proteoglycan synthesis and, 38
  short- vs. long-term responses to, 38–39
  signaling pathways and, 38–45. *See also*
      Mechano-transduction
  in traumatic injuries, 34–35
  in vitro studies of, 38
  in vivo studies of, 38
  Young's modulus and, 38–39
Mechano-coupling, 38–39
Mechano-receptors, 39–41
  integrins as, 39–41, 40f, 43–44
  stretch-activated ion channels as, 41, 41f, 45
Mechano-transduction, 38–42, 38–45, 62–63.
      *See also* Signaling
  activation of, 42–45
  autocrine-paracrine signaling in, 43–45
  chondrocyte mechano-receptors in, 39–41, 40f, 41f, 43–44
  cyclic AMP in, 42
  cytokines in, 43–45, 44f, 63
  disease-related factors in, 45
  ERK/MAPK pathway for, 43, 45
  G proteins in, 42
  growth factors in, 43–45
  integrins in, 39–41, 40f, 43–44
  involved joint and, 45
  JAK-STAT pathway in, 43–45
  mechano-coupling and, 38–39
  mechano-receptors in, 39–41, 40f, 41f, 43–44
  NF-kappa B pathway for, 43
  NMDA receptors as, 39–41, 40f
  in normal vs. OA chondrocytes, 45
  phospholipase C in, 42
  protein kinases in, 42, 43, 44–45
  receptors in, 39–41, 40f, 45
  signaling pathway activation in, 42–45.
      *See also* Signaling
  stretch-activated ion channels in, 41, 41f, 45
  transduction pathways in, 42–45
Meditation, 207–209, 208t
Megakaryocyte-stimulating growth factor, 116–117
α-Melanocyte-stimulating hormone, leptin and, 90
Meniscal tears, MRI of, 158
Meniscectomy, as risk factor, 8, 34
Menopause, increased incidence after, 9
Mesenchymal stem cells
  differentiation of, 53–54, 54f
  therapeutic applications of, 66
Metabolic syndrome, 92–93
Metabolics, 123
Metallic implants, MRI artifacts from, 152
Metalloproteinases. *See* Matrix metalloproteinase(s)
Metatarsophalangeal view, of knee, 135, 138–140, 138t
Microfractures, in subchondral bone, 35
Mind-body therapies, 207–209, 208t
Misoprostol, with NSAIDs, 187–188
Mitogen-activated protein kinases (MAKPs), in chondrocyte
      mechano-transduction, 43
Morphometry, quantitative cartilage, 159–162
Motion artifacts, in MRI, 151
Motor control relearning, 223, 225f
Mouse models, 107, 110f. *See also* Animal models
  ADAMTS-4, 110
  of defective chondrogenesis, 58–60, 58t–59t
  Dell, 110
  STR, 107, 110f
  transgenic, 110
Muscle co-contraction, 223

Muscle strengthening exercises, 218t, 221–222, 222f, 236–237
  hamstring, 221–222
  in motor control relearning, 223, 225f
  quadriceps, 221
  with theraband, 223, 225f
Muscle weakness
  in animal models, 110
  as risk factor, 9, 110
  strengthening exercises for, 218t, 221–222, 222f
Myocardial infarction, NSAID-related, 193

**N**

Naproxen. *See also* Nonsteroidal anti-inflammatory drugs
  adverse effects of, 185–189
  dosage of, 182, 182t
  pharmacokinetics of, 182, 182t
  structure of, 181, 182f
  vs. lumiracoxib, 191t
  vs. NSAIDs, 184–185, 184t
  vs. rofecoxib, 191t
Narcotic analgesics, 183–185, 184t, 238
Nε-(carboxymethyl)lysine (CML), 80
Nephrotoxicity, of NSAIDs, 195, 198t
Neuromuscular retraining/perturbation programs, 223, 225f
Neuropeptide Y, leptin and, 90
Neurotoxicity, of NSAIDs, 195, 198t
NF-kappa B, in chondrocyte mechano-transduction, 43
Nifedipine stretch-activated ion channels, 45
Nitric oxide, 82–83, 119
NMDA receptors, as chondrocyte mechano-receptors, 41
Nonsteroidal anti-inflammatory
    drugs, 178–198, 239
  with acetaminophen, 188
  acupuncture with, 204
  adverse effects of
    central nervous system, 195, 198t
    cutaneous, 195, 198t
    gastrointestinal, 185–189, 187t, 189f
    hepatic, 188–189
    renal, 195, 198t
  classification of, 178
  costs of, 195–198
  development of, 178
  dosage of, 182, 182t
  efficacy of, 183–185, 184t
    vs. acetaminophen, 183, 184t
    vs. opioids, 183–185, 184t
  gastroprotection for, 187–188, 189f
  inhibitory concentration of, 182
  interactions of, 193–195, 196t–197t
  mechanism of action of, 178–181
  misoprostol with, 187–188
  nonselective, 178
    aspirin and, 193–195, 196t–197t
  pharmacokinetics of, 182, 182t
  prostaglandins and, 178–181, 180f
  proton pump inhibitors with, 187–188
  quality indicators for, 185, 186t
  respiratory effects of, 181
  selective, 178
  structure of, 181, 182f
  therapeutic effects of, 27
  topical, 185, 238
    efficacy of, 185
  usage recommendations for, 185, 185t
  utilization patterns for, 195
  utilization promotion for, 198
  vs. glucosamine, 258–259
  vs. herbal remedies, 206

N-terminal propeptide, in collagen synthesis, 117, 118, 118t
N-terminal telopeptide
  in collagen degradation, 117, 118t
  in progression prediction, 125
Nucleotide pyrophosphatase phosphodiesterase-1, in enchondral ossification, 59, 60t
Nutritional interventions, 247–262. *See also* Complementary and alternative medicine
  antioxidants in, 249–254
  avocado/soybean unsaponifiables in, 240
  chondroitin sulfate in, 240, 257–258, 257–261, 257f
  glucosamine in, 239–240, 257–258, 257–261, 257f
  glycosaminoglycan polysulfuric acid in, 240
  glycosaminoglycan-peptide complex in, 240
  iodine in, 256–257
  selenium in, 256–257
  vitamin C in, 249–251, 249f
  vitamin D in, 252–254, 253f
  vitamin K in, 254–256, 255f
  weight loss in, 237, 247–249, 248t

**O**

Ob gene, leptin and, 88, 89, 89f, 93, 97
Obesity
  adipokines and, 92–93
  complications of, 86
  fat cell size in, 85
  fat distribution in, 86
  leptin and, 90
  mal-alignment and, 33–34
  as risk factor, 8, 33–34
  weight loss interventions for, 237, 247–249, 248t
Occupational risk factors, 6, 35
Occupational therapy, 238
Omeprazole, with NSAIDs, 188
Omeract-OARSI responder criteria, 234, 234t
Opioids, 183–185, 184t, 238
Orthopedic surgery, OA after, 7, 8, 34–35
Orthotics, 218t, 225–229, 226f, 237
Ossification, enchondral, 57–58
  chondrocyte hypertrophy and, 57
  novel mediators of, 57–58
Osteoarthritis
  as bone vs. cartilage disease, 16, 85
  definitions of
    anatomic/etiologic, 1, 2t, 3t
    radiographic/functional, 1–2, 2t, 3t
  as metabolic disease, 85
  primary, 1, 2t
  secondary, 1, 2t
Osteoblasts
  leptin and, 95
  in normal bone, 16–17
  in OA, 21–22
Osteocalcin, 21, 117, 118t
Osteogenesis
  biochemical markers for, 117, 118t
  in normal bone, 16–17
  in OA, 19–22
Osteogenic protein-1, anabolic activity of, 62
  age-related changes in, 81
Osteophytes
  in athletes, 34
  formation of, 20, 24
    leptin in, 96–97
  MRI of, 158
Osteopontin, 21
Osteoprotegerin, in bone resorption, 27
Outcome measures, 5
Outerbridge classification, 153–157, 154t

Oxidative stress, 82–83, 119
 age-related, 82–83
 biochemical markers of, 119
 in pathogenesis, 82–83
Oxycodone, vs. NSAIDs, 184–185, 184t

**P**

PINP
 in collagen synthesis, 117, 118t
 in synovial synthesis, 118t
PIIANP
 in collagen synthesis, 117, 118t
 in progression prediction, 126, 126f
PIIBNP, in collagen synthesis, 117, 118t
PIICP
 in collagen synthesis, 117, 118t
 in progression prediction, 126
PIIINP, in synovial synthesis, 118t
Pain management. *See also* Drug therapy; Treatment
 acetaminophen in, 185, 185t, 188, 238
 complementary and alternative medicine in, 202–214
 NSAIDs in, 178–198, 238
 opioids in, 183–185, 184t, 238
 topical agents in, 183–185, 184t, 238
Paracetamol. *See* Acetaminophen
Paracrine signaling, in chondrocyte
  mechano-transduction, 43–45
Parathyroid hormone
 in chondrocyte differentiation and proliferation, 56–57
 osteoblast resistance to, 21
Parathyroid-related protein, in chondrocyte mechano-
  transduction, 44–45
Parecoxib/valdecoxib, cardiovascular toxicity of, 190–193, 192t
Patellar cartilage, age-related changes in, 79
Patellar subluxation, as risk factor, 107
Pathogenesis/pathophysiology
 adipokines in, 87, 92–98
 autoimmune factors in, 123
 biomechanical factors in, 35–36
 cartilage degeneration in, vs. bone changes, 16, 85
 mechanical stress in, 33–46, 34f
 oxidative stress in, 82–83, 119
 subchondral bone and, 15–30. *See also* Subchondral bone
  cross-talk with cartilage, 22–30
 two-hit hypothesis for, 77, 80
Pathologic findings
 in bone, 104, 107t
 in cartilage, 104, 107t
 early-stage, 105–106, 109f
 gross, 105, 109f
 microscopic, 109f, 110f
 in synovium, 104, 107t
 vs. symptomatic disease, 2–5
Patient education, 235–236
Pellet culture system, 64
Pentosan polysulfate, 241
Pentosidine, 80, 120. *See also* Advanced glycation end products
  (AGEs)
Peroxynitite, 119
Perturbation training, 223, 225f
Pharmacologic therapy. *See* Drug therapy
Phosphoinositide 3 kinase, in chondrocyte mechano-
  transduction, 42
Phospholipase C, in chondrocyte mechano-transduction, 42
Physical therapy, 217, 218t, 220–229, 237–238
 aerobic exercise in, 225, 228t
 gait retraining in, 224–225
 knee bracing in, 225, 228t, 237
 motor control relearning in, 223, 225f
 neuromuscular retraining/perturbation programs in, 223, 225f
 strengthening exercises in, 218t, 221–222, 222f, 236–237.
  *See also* Strengthening exercises

Phytodolor, 206–207
Pond-Nuki dog model, 107–110
Postoperative osteoarthritis, 7, 8, 34–35
Preadipocytes, 86
Pregnancy, leptin in, 90–91
Prevalence
 age and, 2, 77, 78f
 of pathologic vs. radiographic OA, 2–4, 77
*PRG4*, 116–117
Primary osteoarthritis, 1, 2t
Procollagen, type II, 114, 114f
Progression. *See* Disease progression
Progressive relaxation, 207–209, 208t
Propeptides
 in collagen synthesis, 117, 118, 118t
 in progression prediction, 126, 126f
Propoxyphene, 238
 vs. NSAIDs, 184–185, 184t
Proprioception, bracing and, 225
Prostaglandin(s), 21, 22, 26
 in arthritis, 179
 cardiovascular effects of, 180, 180f
 central nervous system effects of, 180f, 181
 functions of, 179
 gastroprotective effects of, 179–180
 genitourinary effects of, 180f, 181
 in inflammation, 179
 metabolism of, 178–179, 180f
 NSAIDs and, 178–181, 180f
 renal effects of, 180, 180f
 in signaling, 63
 in synovial fluid, 179
 synthesis of, 178–179, 181f
Prostaglandin E$_2$, 21, 22, 26
 in signaling, 63
Prostanoids, 178
Protective factors, vs. risk factors, 78–79
Protein(s), matrix. *See also* Matrix metalloproteinase(s)
 in bone, 17
 in cartilage, 24
Protein kinases, in chondrocyte mechano-transduction,
  42, 43, 63
Protein-tyrosine phosphatase, leptin and, 90
Proteoglycans
 exercise effects on, 37–38
 in extracellular matrix
  of bone, 17
  of cartilage, 24
 immobilization effects on, 37–38
 small non-aggregating, 24
Proteoglycan-sensitive magnetic resonance imaging,
  162–165, 163t
Proteomic analysis, for biochemical markers, 122–123
Proton pump inhibitors, with NSAIDs, 187–188
PTB-1B, leptin and, 90
Pyridinoline, 114, 117, 118t, 122f

**Q**

Qi, in acupuncture, 202–203
Quadriceps exercises, 221–222. *See also*
  Strengthening exercises
Quadriceps weakness
 in animal models, 110
 as risk factor, 9, 110
Quality indicators, 185, 186t
Quantitative cartilage morphometry, 159–162

**R**

Radiography, 131–140
 accuracy of, 132–135
 in grading, 1–2, 2t
 of hip, 133, 134f

Radiography *(Continued)*
   in progression measurement, 136–137, 136t
   interpretation of, 131–132
   of knee, 133–135, 133f
      in progression measurement, 137–140,
         138t, 139f, 139t
   limitations of, 131
   overview of, 131
   in progression measurement, 135–140
      in hip, 136–137, 136t
      in knee, 137–140, 138t, 139f, 139t
      scoring systems for, 131–132
      symptom correlation with, 9–10
      vs. MRI, 1–2
RAGE receptor, 63, 81–82
Range of motion
   assessment of, 234
   exercises for, 236–237
Ranitidine, with NSAIDs, 188
RANKL, in bone resorption, 27
RANTES receptors, 63
RARE magnetic resonance imaging, 147, 147f
Reactive oxygen species, 82–83, 119
Refractory severe disease, 233
Relaxation techniques, 207–209, 208t
Renal effects, of prostaglandin, 181
Renal toxicity, of NSAIDs, 195, 198t
Repetitive motion, as risk factor, 6, 35
Replicative senescence, in chondrocytes, 81
Resistin, 87, 87f, 89t, 92, 92t. *See also* Adipokines
   cartilage effects of, 98
   cytokines and, 96
   in synovial fluid, 93
   synthesis of, 94
Rheumatoid arthritis, biochemical markers in, 128
Risedronate, 241
   treatment monitoring for, biochemical
      markers in, 127–128
Risk factors, 5–10
   activity-related, 6–8
   age as, 2, 77–79. *See also* Age/aging
   animal models of, 106–111
   behavioral, 9
   bone marrow lesions as, 9–10
   bone mineral density as, 10, 18–19, 35–36
   congenital and developmental, 6
   constitutional, 5–6
   estrogen as, 9
   genetic, 5–6, 22, 46, 110
   hereditary, 5–6
   hormonal, 9
   for incident OA, 33
   joint instability as, 7, 34, 107
      animal models of, 107
   local
      mechanical, 8–9
      osseous, 9–10
      vs. systemic, 33
   mal-alignment as, 4, 9
   mechanical stress as, 33–46
   muscle weakness as, 8–9, 110
   obesity as, 8, 33–34
   occupational, 6, 35
   for progression, 33
   repetitive activity as, 6
   smoking as, 9
   sports and recreational activity as, 6–7
   surgical, 7, 8, 34–35
   for susceptibility, 33
   trauma as, 6–8, 25–26, 34–35
      age and, 77–78
   vs. protective factors, 78–79

Rofecoxib. *See also* Coxibs
   cardiovascular toxicity of, 189–190, 191t, 194t
   dosage of, 182, 182t
   pharmacokinetics of, 182, 182t
   structure of, 181, 182f, 183f
   vs. acetaminophen, 184t
Running, knee OA and, 6–7, 34
Runx2, 57, 58, 58t

**S**

Secondary osteoarthritis, 1, 2t
Selenium, supplemental, 256–257
Semiflexed views, of knee, 135, 138–140, 138t, 139t
7D4 epitope, in aggrecan synthesis, 117, 118t
Severity of disease, 232–233
Shh (Sonic hedgehog), in limb development, 54, 55f
Shock-absorbing insoles, 226
Shoes
   insoles for, 218t, 225–228, 226f, 237
   modified, 228
   selection of, 228–229, 228f
Shoulder osteoarthritis, in throwing athletes, 7
Signaling, 62–63
   age-related changes in, 81
   in chondrocyte differentiation and
      proliferation, 55–57, 55f
   cytokines in, 43–45, 44f, 63
   JAK-STAT pathway in, 43–45, 89–90
   leptin in, 88, 89–90, 95–96
   in limb development, 54–55, 55f
   mechanical, 38–45. *See also* Mechano-transduction
Slipped capital epiphysis, 6
Smad3, in enchondral ossification, 57, 58, 58t
Small non-aggregating proteoglycans, 24
Smoking, as risk factor, 9
SOCS proteins, leptin and, 90
Sodium magnetic resonance imaging, 162, 163t
Sodium stretch-activated ion channels, 41, 41f, 45
Sonic hedgehog (Shh), in limb development, 54, 55f
Spin echo magnetic resonance imaging, 145–146, 145f.
      *See also* Magnetic resonance imaging
   conventional, 146–147, 147f
   fast-spin, 147, 147f
Sports participation. *See also* Exercise
   in established OA, 238
   as risk factor, 6–7, 34–35
Stainless steel implants, MRI artifacts in, 152
STAT transcription factors, leptin and, 89–90, 94
Stem cell(s), mesenchymal
   differentiation of, 53–54, 54f
   therapeutic applications of, 66, 241
Stem cell transplantation, 66, 241
Steroids, intra-articular, 241–242
Stevens-Johnson syndrome, 195
STIR technique, in MRI, 151
STR mouse models, 107, 110f
Strengthening exercises, 218t, 221–222, 222f, 236–237
   hamstring, 221–222
   in motor control relearning, 223, 225f
   quadriceps, 221
   with theraband, 223, 225f
Stress. *See* Mechanical stress
Stretch-activated ion channels, as chondrocyte mechano-
      receptors, 41, 41f, 45
Stromelysins, 115. *See also* Matrix metalloproteinase(s)
   in progression prediction, 125
   in synovial fluid, 121
Subchondral bone, 15–30. *See also* Bone
   biomechanical properties of, 35–36, 35t
   cross-talk with cartilage, 22–26
   density of, 18–19, 21
   end plate zone of, 17

Subchondral bone *(Continued)*
thickness of, 17, 18f–19f, 19
vascularization of, 25–26. *See also* Angiogenesis
formation of
normal, 17–18
in OA, 19–22
marrow abnormalities in, MRI of, 157–158
microfractures in, 35
osteoblasts in. *See* Osteoblasts
pathologic changes in, 18–27
as cause vs. result, 15–16
major pathways in, 23f
symptoms and, 26
therapeutic implications of, 26–28
perfusion of, 17
protective functions of, 17
remodeling of
normal, 17–18
in OA, 19–22
sclerosis of, 18, 22
structure of, 17–18, 18f
trabeculae of, 18–19, 18f–19f. *See also* Trabecular bone
Subluxation, patellar, as risk factor, 107
Subsynovium, structure of, 117
Sulfate supplements, 258
Superficial zone protein, 116–117
Surgery, OA after, 7, 8, 34–35
Symptomatic disease
vs. pathologic findings, 2–5
vs. radiographic findings, 9–10
Synovial fluid, 116–117
adipokines in, 93, 97
characteristics of, 93
functions of, 93
prostaglandins in, 179
Synovial lining, components of, 116
Synoviorthesis, 242
Synovium
biochemical markers for, 118t, 121–122. *See also* Biochemical markers
biology and biochemistry of, 116–117
pathologic findings in, 104, 107t
SYSADOA agents, 239

**T**

T cells, leptin and, 95
T1 relaxation time, 149–150
T1rho magnetic resonance imaging, 163
T2 mapping, of cartilage, 165–167, 166f
T2 relaxation time, 149–150
Tai chi, 209–213, 210f, 211f
Taping, of knee, 218t
Tartrate-resistant acid phosphatase, 118t
Telopeptides, 117, 118t
TENS, 218t
Textured insoles, 226–227
Theraband exercises, 223, 225f
Thiazolinediones, leptin and, 88, 89t
3-B-3 epitope, in aggrecan synthesis, 117, 118t
Thrombosis, NSAID-related, 190
Tobacco use, as risk factor, 9
Tocopherol, 251–252, 252f
Toe-out angle, knee loading and, 224
Total joint replacement, 243
Toxic epidermal necrolysis, 195
Trabecular bone, 16. *See also* Bone; Subchondral bone
density of, 18–19, 21, 35–36
MRI of, 36
Tramadol, 238
vs. NSAIDs, 184–185, 184t
Transcription factors, in enchondral ossification, 57, 58, 58t

Transcutaneous electrical nerve stimulation, 218t
Transforming growth factor-β
adipokines and, 96–97
age-related changes in, 81
anabolic activity of, 62
age-related changes in, 81
for cartilage defects, 65
catabolic activity of, 62
in chondrocyte mechano-transduction, 43, 44–45
in enchondral ossification, 58, 59, 59t, 60
in normal bone, 17
in OA
in bone, 20, 21, 22
in cartilage, 26
in osteophyte formation, 20
Transgenic models, 110
Transplantation
chondrocyte, 65, 241
mesenchymal stem cell, 66, 241
Trauma, as risk factor, 7–8, 25–26, 34–35
age and, 77–78
Treatment, 232–243
articular replacement in, 243
assessment data for, 232–235. *See also* Assessment
bracing in, 218t, 225, 237
canes and crutches in, 238
chondrocyte transplantation in, 65, 241
co-morbidities and, 233
disease activity and, 232, 233t
disease severity and, 232–233, 233t
EULAR recommendations for, 235, 235t
exercise in, 218t, 225, 236–237
experimental, 242
guidelines for, 235, 235t, 236t
intra-articular agents in, 241–242
involved joints and, 232, 233t
lavage and debridement in, 242–243
lifestyle interventions in, 247–249, 248t
nonpharmacologic, 235–238. *See also* Complementary and alternative medicine; Physical therapy
nutritional interventions in, 247–262. *See also* Nutritional interventions
objectives of, 235
occupational therapy in, 238
orthotics in, 225–229, 237
osteotomy in, 243
patient education in, 235–236
pharmacologic, 238–242. *See also* Drug therapy
physical therapy in, 217, 220–229, 237–238. *See also* Physical therapy
stem cell transplantation in, 66, 241
strengthening exercises in, 218t, 221–222, 222f, 223, 225f, 236–237
surgical, 242–243
synoviorthesis in, 242
weight loss in, 237, 247–249
Triosephosphate isomerase (TPI), 123
Triple helix fragment (Helix II), in collagen degradation, 118t, 119–120, 119f, 120f
Truncation artifacts, in MRI, 152
Tumor necrosis factor-α, adipokines and, 96
Two-hit hypothesis, 77, 80

**U**

Ulcers, NSAID-related, 185–189, 198t
prevention of, 187–188, 189f
Unloader knee braces, 225

**V**

Valdecoxib. *See also* Coxibs
cardiovascular toxicity of, 189–194, 190–193, 191t, 192t
dosage of, 182, 182t

Valdecoxib (*Continued*)
  pharmacokinetics of, 182, 182t
  structure of, 181, 183f
Valgus knee braces, 225, 237
Varus thrust, 220
Varus/valgus alignment. *See* Mal-alignment
Vascular endothelial growth factor, 26
  in chondrocyte mechano-transduction, 44–45
  in enchondral ossification, 57, 58, 58t
Vascularization. *See* Angiogenesis
Visco-supplementation, 242
Visfatin, 87, 87f. *See also* Adipokines
Vitamin C supplements, 249–251, 249f
Vitamin D supplements, 252–254, 253f
Vitamin K supplements, 254–256, 255f

**W**

Walking speed, knee loading and, 224–225
Weakness
  animal models of, 110
  as risk factor, 9, 110
  strengthening exercises for, 218t, 221–222, 222f, 236–237

Wedged insoles, 225–227, 226f
Weight
  leptin and, 90
  as risk factor, 8
Weight loss, benefits of, 237, 247–249, 248t
Weight training, 218t
Whole Organ Magnetic Resonance Imaging Score, 153
Wnt
  in chondrogenesis, 58
  in limb development, 54, 55f
Women. *See also* Gender differences
  postmenopausal OA in, 9

**Y**

YKL-39, 118t, 121
YKL-40, 118t, 121
Yoga, 213–214
Young's modulus, of cartilage, 37